Harper's Practical Genetic Counselling
Eighth Edition

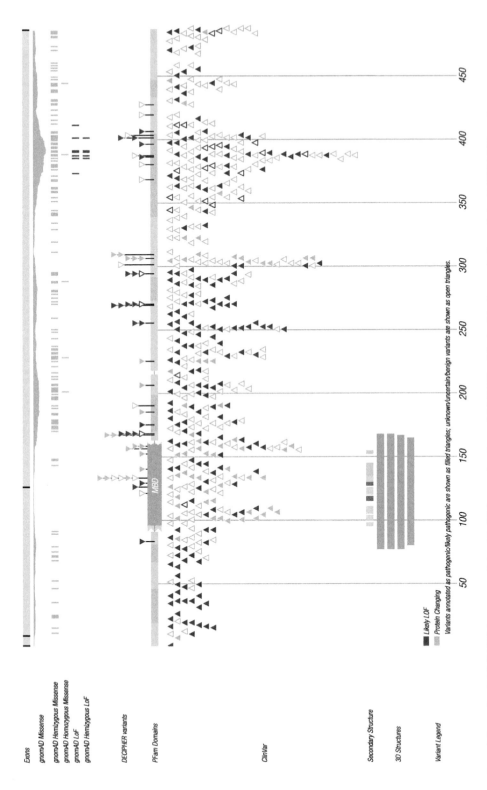

Detail from the DECIPHER browser of the MeCP2 protein view of MECP2, with the kind permission of the DECIPHER project.

Harper's Practical Genetic Counselling

Eighth Edition

Angus Clarke
Clinical Professor, Division of Cancer and Genetics
School of Medicine, University of Cardiff
Honorary Consultant, All Wales Medical Genetics Service, UK

with contributions from
Dr Alex Murray and Professor Julian Sampson

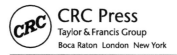

CRC Press
Taylor & Francis Group
Boca Raton London New York

CRC Press is an imprint of the
Taylor & Francis Group, an **informa** business

CRC Press
Taylor & Francis Group
6000 Broken Sound Parkway NW, Suite 300
Boca Raton, FL 33487-2742

© 2020 by Taylor & Francis Group, LLC
CRC Press is an imprint of Taylor & Francis Group, an Informa business

No claim to original U.S. Government works

Printed on acid-free paper

International Standard Book Number-13: 978-0-367-37190-6 (Hardback)
978-1-4441-8374-0 (Paperback)

Library of Congress Cataloging-in-Publication Data

Names: Clarke, Angus, 1954-author. | Harper, Peter S. Practical genetic counselling.
Title: Harper's practical genetic counselling / Angus Clarke.
Other titles: Practical genetic counselling
Description: Eighth edition | Boca Raton : CRC Press, [2020] | Preceded by Practical genetic counselling / Peter S. Harper. 7th ed. 2010. | Includes bibliographical references and index. | Summary: 'Easy to use, and useful when kept close at hand in the room where you work. The book is a pleasure to read: the style elegant and authoritative' Lancet. '...this book is a wonderful reference to enable primary physicians to be informed about their patients' Annals of Internal Medicine. Universally used across the world by genetic counsellors, medical geneticists and clinicians alike, Harper's Practical Genetic Counselling has established itself as the essential guide to counselling those at risk from inherited disorders. Increasingly, common disorders are known to have a genetic component and this book provides invaluable and up to date guidance through the profusion of new information in this area and the associated psychosocial and ethical considerations and concerns. Within its established, tried and trusted framework, the book contains new chapters on: laboratory methods, new genetic sequencing techniques and the applications of genome-wide SNP association studies, genetic susceptibility, cross-cultural aspects and the genetic counselling process. It has expanded chapters on genetic screening and screening of newborns, treatment techniques and rational approaches to treatment, non-Mendelian inheritance, free fetal DNA in prenatal screening and diagnosis. Key features: - Fully updated to provide the very latest information when in a busy consulting room or clinic - Clear and authoritative advice applicable to everyday clinical practice - Reflects the rapid development of knowledge in this area, including the implications of the human genome project and related technology. The eighth edition of this popular, best-selling text continues to be an essential source of reference for trainee and practitioner genetic counsellors, medical geneticists and clinicians. Also it provides valuable background for specialist nurses, counsellors, social scientists, ethicists as well as genetics laboratory staff.-- Provided by the publisher.
Identifiers: LCCN 2019025219 | ISBN 9781444183740 (paperback ; alk. paper) | ISBN 9780367371906 (hardback ; alk. paper) | ISBN 9780367371944 (eBook)
Subjects: MESH: Genetic Counseling--methods | Genetic Techniques | Genetic Diseases, Inborn--genetics
Classification: LCC RB155.7 | NLM QZ 52 | DDC 362.196/042--dc23
LC record available at https://lccn.loc.gov/2019025219

Visit the Taylor & Francis Web site at
http://www.taylorandfrancis.com

and the CRC Press Web site at
http://www.crcpress.com

Contents

Preface to Eighth Edition

This book, the creation of Peter Harper, has filled a valuable role over four decades in Britain and around the world. I very much hope that this revised edition will continue this into the era of genomic approaches to genetic diagnostics.

When revising *Harper's Practical Genetic Counselling*, I had three target audiences in mind:

1. Healthcare practitioners, working across the full spread of medicine, who may wish to appreciate what a referral to a medical genetics service entails and to understand the place of genetic investigations when such a diagnosis is suspected. I hope this volume may support the interested practitioner in that crucial first step of discussing cases and questions with the clinical geneticists and genetic counsellors in their local genetics service. If so, this volume will then have succeeded in promoting the appropriate mainstreaming of genetics into the rest of medicine.
2. Healthcare professionals training to work as specialists within a medical genetics service, as clinical geneticists or genetic counsellors. This book aspires to provide an initial orientation to the field and help students to gain familiarity both with the 'medical facts' of a condition and, to some extent, with the emotions that arise in this context.
3. Medical and nursing practitioners who wish to understand enough about clinical aspects of genetics to provide a basic level of genetic information and appropriate support to their patients and their patients' families. This is especially important for those working in settings where a referral to a genetics specialist is not readily available.

Let us hope that this eighth edition of this book will enable it to meet the needs of these three groups of practitioners and students as we approach the third decade of the third millennium!

Angus Clarke

Acknowledgements

I would like to thank Peter Harper for giving me the opportunity to undertake this revision of his book. However, I must also apologise to him for having taken so long to complete this task! In addition, I must thank my colleagues Dr Alex Murray and Professor Julian Sampson for their revision of the material on the genetics of cancer, which has grown from a single chapter, and to Professor Gareth Evans (of Manchester University) for his most helpful advice on Table 31.1. I am also most grateful to my colleague Dr Vinod Varghese for reading through and making helpful comments on a draft of Chapter 9, for the comments of Sian Morgan on Chapter 4 and the comments of Dr Mark Rogers on the section on 'Facioscapulohumeral Dystrophy' in Chapter 13.

I would also like to thank those who have assisted with diagrams and figures. This is especially: Jan Sharp, Medical Illustrator in Cardiff, for the new diagrams; the Wales Genomics Laboratory for permission to reproduce the array CGH results demonstrating a deletion of chromosome 15q provided by Sian Corrin; the team at DECIPHER (especially Dr Helen Firth and Julia Foreman) for their permission to represent the DECIPHER browser both in a figure and on the cover of the book; and Dr Andrew Fry for his assistance in making this interesting visually.

Of course, I am to blame for all errors that remain but I thank my colleagues heartily for their support. I am also grateful to Jane, my wife, for her understanding and forbearance.

PART 1

General aspects of genetics and genetic counselling

1

Genetics and genetic counselling: An introduction

PRELIMINARY: GENETICS IN HEALTHCARE TODAY

Scope of genetics in medicine

The context of healthcare is changing rapidly, with genetic aspects of medicine receiving progressively more prominence. Much disease is caused by a complex interaction between a person's genes and their environment over time. This may be thought of as an interaction between the person's genes, their environment and their experience, from conception onwards. This perspective broadens the scope of genetics within medicine from disease that is primarily genetic in origin to include much else as well.

A question for this volume is how far the recent development of genetics as a biomedical science plays out in the practice of genetic counselling and clinical genetics. It is apparent that the new high-throughput, genome-wide technologies of microarray and 'massively parallel' sequencing have enormously increased the information we can generate about genetic variation across the genome, but the information it yields is still applied one gene at a time. The approach in this edition – which will have to be reassessed for future editions – is that the new technologies provide a much more rapid way of identifying the genetic variant underlying a Mendelian or chromosomal disorder. However, an integrative, whole genome analysis of a patient is not yet available in the clinic. The search for specific genetic variants can be relevant to the selection of appropriate therapies for some patients, but this, again, is usually worked through one variant at a time and not in an integrated, whole genome approach because the working out of gene-gene and gene-environment interactions remains enormously challenging. Research based on this additional, genome-level information is proving enormously fruitful but has not yet reached simple clinical application: its immediate clinical utility is limited.

This book aims to set out a clinical approach to genetic disease that addresses the whole person in their family context. This has long been the aim of clinical genetics services, both clinical genetics and genetic counselling, and it is important that we do not lose sight of this in the flurry and excitement of data generated by the new genome-wide technologies. We need to use the new technologies to answer the old questions more thoroughly and more rapidly but should not be distracted by results with no clear interpretation.

While the new tools generate more and more information, our task remains to help patients and family members make sense of what their genetic analysis means for each as an individual. In addition to the 'traditional' patients in the genetic counselling clinic, with clearly inherited disease, genetics services are now also seeing patients who have had genomic investigations yielding additional or unanticipated findings and results of uncertain significance. We must all grow accustomed to investigations generating results that are potentially important despite being unconnected with the problem that triggered the investigation. Clinical genetics services then help patients to understand their results, both what they mean for the patient and what they mean for their relatives. Where there is no certainty, they may need both an explanation of, and support to deal with, the lingering uncertainties.

Far from clinical genetics services becoming outdated as genome-wide testing moves into the medical mainstream, they are becoming appreciated as a powerful resource that enables and supports the *appropriate* application of the new technologies.

WHAT DO WE MEAN BY 'GENETIC COUNSELLING'?

Although many people working in the field of medicine are familiar with the term 'genetic counselling' and have some idea what it means, many other professionals and even more patients and families are confused by the term. Closer enquiry among patients and colleagues shows a wide variation in people's concepts of what the process of genetic counselling actually entails. Some envisage an essentially supportive – even psychotherapeutic – role, akin to that of counselling processes in the social field; others see genetic counselling as primarily concerned with special diagnostic tests in inherited disease; yet others regard it as a complex mathematical process involving the estimation of risk.

All these views of genetic counselling contain a considerable element of truth, but none fully identifies what the overall process of genetic counselling actually involves. Even within the group of professionals for whom genetic counselling is a major activity, there are varied opinions as to its proper role and scope, but in essence it is a composite – hybrid – activity, made up of a series of key elements that individually are very different, but which together constitute a process that is highly distinctive in its character and its ethos.

Previous editions of this book have given various definitions of genetic counselling, but none of them is entirely satisfactory. Two approaches will be used to clarify this: we describe the activities that constitute 'genetic counselling' and then refer to a recent and widely cited definition of genetic counselling.

The elements of genetic counselling as practised are as follows:

1. Initially listening to the questions and concerns of the patient or family and establishing a relationship with appropriate empathy.
2. Addressing the diagnostic and clinical aspects, including the gathering of information from the patient and family and the checking and documentation of important clinical

---

> **BOX 1.1: Genetic counselling: The main elements**
>
> Listening to concerns and building a relationship
> Building an empathic relationship with the patient and family
> Considering diagnostic and clinical aspects (including documentation of family structure and information)
> Recognising inheritance patterns and risk estimation
> Communicating information to those being seen in the consultation and attempting to answer their questions
> Providing support to aid understanding and adjustment
> Providing practical information about medical aspects and reproduction
> Providing support for making decisions and for implementing decisions already made

information about the patient, and also about family members. This may occur in the process of a single consultation or it may become a process that takes many months.

3. Recognising the inheritance pattern and estimating risks (when relevant).
4. Communicating with those being seen and counselled, attempting to answer their questions in light of the facts.
5. Providing support for the patient and family to understand their situation and adjust to it.
6. Providing information on available options and further measures, for pursuing the diagnosis (if that remains unclear), for managing the medical aspects of the condition and for questions of reproduction.
7. Providing support for making decisions and for implementing decisions already made.

This chapter outlines these main elements, which are then dealt with in more detail in subsequent chapters of the book. It is the satisfactory synthesis of these various aspects that makes up genetic counselling as a specific process. These elements are listed in Box 1.1. A discussion of the traditional process of genetic counselling is given in more detail in Clarke (1994) and Clarke (1997) (see 'Further Reading'). We refer to current developments later, throughout this volume.

Perhaps the most authoritative recent definition of the aims of genetic counselling – what it sets out to achieve – is that of the National Society of Genetic Counsellors (Resta et al., 2006).

Genetic counselling is the 'process of helping people understand and adapt to the medical, psychological, and familial implications of genetic contributions to disease. This process integrates the following:

- Interpretation of family and medical histories to assess the chance of disease occurrence or recurrence
- Education about inheritance, testing, management, prevention, resources, and research
- Counseling to promote informed choices and adaptation to the risk or condition

This definition of the aims of genetic counselling meshes well with the description given previously of what doing genetic counselling entails in practice.

HISTORY AND DEVELOPMENT OF GENETIC COUNSELLING

The origins of genetic counselling need to be seen within the context of the overall history of human genetics, a topic until recently neglected, but which was first addressed by Reed (1955 and 1974) and has been discussed more recently in McKusick and Harper's introductory chapter for Rimoin, Pyeritz and Korf's textbook (6th edition, 2012) and in Harper's *A Short History of Medical Genetics* (2008) (see 'Further Reading').

Although human genetics research had begun to develop strongly in the first half of the twentieth century, its application at that time was confused and, to an extent, discredited by the abuses of eugenics. It was not until the World War II that the first genetic counselling clinics were opened in the United States, in Michigan in 1940 and in Minnesota in 1941. In the United Kingdom, the Hospital for Sick Children on Great Ormond Street, London, developed the first such clinic in 1946. By 1955, there were over a dozen centres in North America, and there has been a steady development since that time. As with many pioneering developments, the early centres were often the work of far-sighted eccentrics. Sheldon Reed, in his book *Counselling in Medical Genetics*, first published in 1955, gives a delightful description of Edward Dight, responsible for endowing the Dight Clinic in Minneapolis, Minnesota, who lived in a house built in a tree and who failed to file income tax returns.

Reed's book gives a vivid picture of the main areas covered in the early years of genetic counselling, and it was Reed himself who first introduced this term. Many of the problems are unchanged today, and his examples of individual cases show that the fears and concerns of families have altered little. In other respects, there have been profound changes in the more than 60 years since the book was written. Carrier detection was rarely possible and prenatal diagnosis entirely non-existent, as was oral contraception, so the options open to patients at risk were limited; either they took the risk of an(other) affected child or they did not. An even more important change has been that of the general climate of opinion among the public and the medical profession, at least in Europe and North America, in particular a greater openness in relation to inherited and familial disorders.

Reed's case histories illustrate the background of ignorance and prejudice with which his patients had to cope, and it is no wonder that he found them grateful, even when he could only give them unwelcome information or pessimistic advice. He comes across as a caring and sensitive person, upholding the concept of non-directiveness and turning his back completely on eugenics.

It is of interest that the most common cause of referral to the Dight Clinic was regarding skin colour and whether a child for adoption would 'pass for white'. Several other problems among the 20 most common causes for referral listed by Reed are today encountered only infrequently, including eye colour, twinning and Rhesus haemolytic disease. The last of these provides a real example of advance in treatment and prevention; the others reflect changes in social attitudes and the availability of better methods of paternity testing. Many others of Reed's most common problems remain equally important today, including mental handicap, schizophrenia, facial clefting, neural tube defects and Huntington's disease.

Most of the early genetic counselling clinics were run by non-medical scientists (like Reed himself) or by those who were not experienced clinicians. With the growth in knowledge of genetic disorders and the emergence of medical genetics as a distinct specialty from the 1960s, genetic counselling progressively became medicalized, representing one of the key components of clinical genetics. It was not, though, until later that the importance of a firm psychological basis was recognised and became an essential part of genetic counselling. The writings of Seymour Kessler made a particular contribution to this.

From around 1970, beginning in the United States, non-medical genetic counsellors with specific training in the field have become increasingly prominent, the graduate course based at Sarah Lawrence College, New York, becoming the model for other centres in the United States, Britain and many other countries. As the demand for genetic counselling has grown, it has become clear that not all consultations require the clinical expertise of the medical geneticist, though careful coordination and mutual respect of the two groups are essential for an optimal genetic counselling service.

At the time of the first edition of this book, almost 40 years ago, the intended readership was largely the general hospital clinician or family doctor, who were also expected to be the main provider of genetic counselling, at least for relatively straightforward situations. It has been interesting that, at least in the United Kingdom and the United States, only a few general clinicians have developed such a role; this is perhaps in part because of the lack of time, the most precious commodity for good genetic counselling. It may also reflect the fact that many clinicians wish to spend most of their time seeing and managing sick patients, whereas much of genetic counselling involves the problems and concerns of entirely healthy relatives.

As genetics progressively broadens out in its applications to clinical management beyond specialist genetics centres and genetics units, into more 'mainstream' medicine, there will be a growing need for clinicians in different fields to engage actively with the genetic counselling needs of those whom they see and also to link more closely with their local medical genetics and genetic counselling centre. Both specialists and generalists will need to communicate effectively during this process of transition, as the application of genetics enters the full range of medical practice.

It is important to recognise that the healthcare context differs greatly between countries. In some countries, there is no profession of 'genetic counsellor' as distinct from clinical (medical) geneticist, and in some countries there is still little or no recognition for the role of clinical geneticist either. Elsewhere, the role of genetic counsellor is well established. In such countries, it is most important for the genetic counsellor and clinical geneticist to work closely together. There should not be a hard and fast line between their activities and responsibilities because these depend upon the training and experience – that is, the competence – of the particular individuals working together in a team. This book does not attempt to allocate or distribute the work of 'genetic counselling' between these professional roles as that would, unhelpfully, limit the book's application to one moment of time in one healthcare system.

CONSTRUCTING A FAMILY TREE

Collecting genetic information is one of the essential early steps in genetic counselling and is best achieved by drawing up a family tree or pedigree. The use of clear and consistent symbols allows genetic information to be set out much more clearly than does a long list of relatives. Note that the whole process will often take time. Allowance must be made for this, and it should also be acknowledged that the time spent on gathering information to prepare a family history brings benefits in addition to the diagram that is constructed. One learns much about how the disorder affects various family members and about the character of particular individuals. One also learns about the relationships between affected and unaffected individuals in the family and their patterns of communication. These insights can be important when establishing relationships with a family that may persist for some years or even decades. Delegating the collection of family history information to a junior, often transient member of the team may be necessary when time is limited, but it sends unfortunate signals to the family and to one's colleagues. If the person who takes the family history is not present in the principal consultation with the family, then much of the additional value of the process beyond the diagram itself will, sadly, be lost.

Drawing a satisfactory pedigree is not difficult, although it is remarkable how rarely those clinicians without an interest in genetics will attempt the process. A clearly drawn pedigree has a certain aesthetic appeal, but its chief value is to provide an unambiguous and permanent record of the genetic information in a particular family. Although computer programs are essential

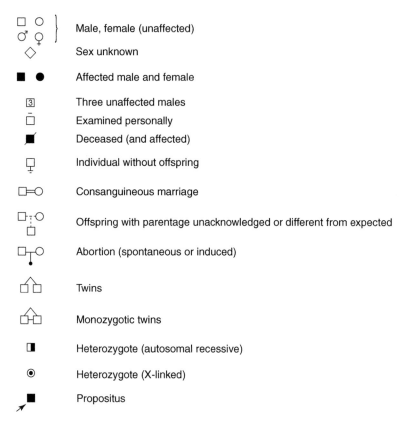

Figure 1.1 Symbols used in drawing a pedigree.

for some risk calculations and for the effective coordination of care for extended families, they are no substitute for a clearly drawn pedigree constructed by hand at the time of the interview.

Figure 1.1 shows the main symbols used in constructing pedigrees. The symbols shown for the sexes (□, ○) are preferred to the alternatives (♂, ♀), which tend to be confused at a distance. Heterozygous carriers can be denoted by half-shaded symbols or, in the case of an X-linked disorder, by a central dot. Although the sign for an early abortion (spontaneous or induced) can also be used for a stillbirth, it is preferable to denote the sex of the latter with an appropriate symbol and indicate beneath the symbol that it was a stillbirth. The previous use of a broken line for an offspring from an outside marriage is no longer appropriate, as 'illegitimacy' is no longer a meaningful concept in most Western societies. However, employing a broken line in a pedigree is still useful to represent the situation where parentage is unknown or unacknowledged or a relationship has broken down.

The proband – also called the propositus (male) or proposita (female) – should be clearly indicated with an arrow. The proband is the individual through whom the family is ascertained. Large families will commonly have several probands. The proband is generally an affected individual, but the person primarily seeking advice may well not be affected. The term 'consultand' is conveniently used for this individual.

Multiple marriages and complex consanguinity can cause problems in constructing a pedigree diagram, and artistry will have to be sacrificed for accuracy in such cases. It is usually wise to start near the middle of the pedigree sheet and to leave more room than one thinks will be needed, so that particularly prolific family branches do not become crowded out. Figure 1.2 shows examples of the 'working pedigree', one simple and one more complex.

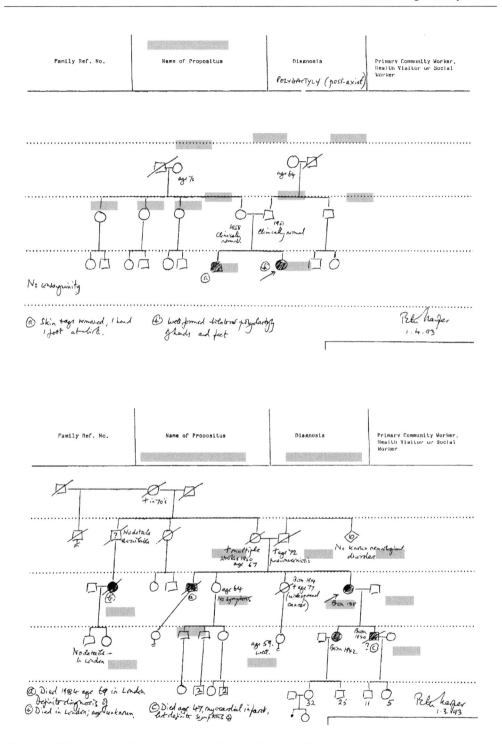

Figure 1.2 Two examples of the 'working pedigree'. These two pedigrees – one simple, the other more extensive – show how family data can be easily and clearly recorded at the time of the interview. A simple lined sheet is used; more detailed information on individuals can be recorded at the foot of the pedigree or on the back. Identifying details have been deleted.

The following practical points deserve emphasis:

- Enquire specifically about infant deaths, stillbirths and abortions. These may be highly relevant, especially if structural abnormalities of the chromosomes prove to have been present; the fact that the information had not been volunteered may be significant. Thus, two children 'lost at birth' by the mother of a woman seen for counselling proved to have both had spina bifida, a fact that considerably altered the risks.
- Consanguinity should be directly asked about and may be the clue that suggests autosomal recessive inheritance (see Chapter 10). Equally, though, the background level for consanguinity in the population concerned must be taken into account before attributing the problem to consanguinity. When most marriages in a community are consanguineous, most cases of dominant, sex-linked and chromosomal disorders will also occur within a consanguineous family unit.
- Mistaken or unacknowledged paternity must be borne in mind, especially in a puzzling situation. A family doctor or nurse, particularly in a small community, may well be able to clarify this possibility, but increasingly families are more open about it, recognising its importance in the context of genetic risk. Definitive tests of paternity based on DNA (see Chapter 10) can help to resolve these problems more easily, but DNA-based diagnostic tests may equally produce new difficulties by the detection of unsuspected non-paternity.
- Always take at least basic details about both sides of the family, even in a dominantly inherited disorder clearly originating from one side. Unexpected findings may emerge. The family that insists that there is 'nothing on our side' should be regarded with suspicion until this is verified. Taking details about both sides may also help to avoid, or at least mitigate, feelings of guilt or blame resting exclusively on one member of a couple. Guilt is always an important factor but is particularly important in some cultural and social situations.
- Record dates of birth where possible rather than ages and the date when the pedigree was drawn up.
- Record maiden names of women. This is especially significant for X-linked disorders, where the surname of affected members is likely to change with each generation.
- Note the addresses of key relevant members, though this is best done on a separate sheet. This may prove invaluable in obtaining hospital records or in later contact with relatives.

Most of these points are obvious, yet it is surprising how often vital information is not obtained unless a systematic approach is used.

In constructing a pedigree, it is not generally necessary to trace a person's ancestry back more than three or four generations; medical details often become inaccurate at this early period. Sometimes, though, it may be important to link kindreds or to establish a common ancestor, in which case genealogical records will be useful. These are surprisingly abundant in many European countries, especially Scandinavia. Online resources are now widely available and often very useful. Even in mobile populations such as in the United States, the growth of interest in family history has considerably increased people's knowledge of their ancestors.

DIAGNOSTIC INFORMATION

It has already been emphasised that a clear diagnosis is the essential basis for accurate genetic counselling. Unfortunately, this basis is all too often a shaky one, and one of the principal tasks of anyone involved in genetic counselling is to ensure that it is made as firm as possible before risk estimates are given to those seeking advice. One should not simply assume that the diagnosis reported in another family member, perhaps someone who has died, is correct. If confirmation can be obtained, it will often be invaluable. Common reasons for lack of a clear diagnosis include the following:

- The affected individual may have lived a considerable time ago, when relevant diagnostic investigations were not available. There is little that can be done about this, but it is surprising how much detailed information may be obtained by questioning close relatives who were involved in caring for the patient. Even if an exact diagnosis cannot be established, it may be possible to exclude a disorder. Thus, a man with muscular dystrophy who lived to the age of 40 years clearly would not have had the Duchenne type. Old photographs may show typical facial features of a condition (e.g. myotonic dystrophy).
- The affected individual may have died without essential investigations having been done, or without autopsy being performed. This is all too often the case and is inexcusable. Reasons usually offered are reluctance to trouble the parents in distressing circumstances, or the fact that investigations would not have altered the patient's management; but frequently the real reason is that those involved have not taken the trouble to undertake the studies, or to make arrangements with those who can undertake them. In Britain, a scandal arising from improper consent procedures and other factors brought pathology into some disrepute; the hostile media attention and then the practical difficulties of complying with the Human Tissue Act have led to a sharp reduction in the frequency of autopsy. The potentially tragic consequences of such developments only become apparent when the question of risk to further family members arises. Even when a family is reluctant to permit a full autopsy, a limited examination may be feasible, and careful postmortem imaging by photography and magnetic resonance imaging (MRI) scan may also be very informative. The results of a 'molecular autopsy' may also sometimes be available after a sudden cardiac death.
- A firm diagnosis cannot be reached, even with the affected individual living. This is inevitable in some cases, since our knowledge of many disorders (genetic and non-genetic) remains very incomplete, but a considerable degree of help can be obtained by enlisting the efforts of colleagues, even at a distance. Photographs, radiographs and samples of urine, blood, DNA and cultured skin fibroblasts can all be sent to distant parts of the world for experts to study, and developments in 'telemedicine' now extend greatly the scope of what can be done in this way, especially for imaging. Presentation of puzzling cases at clinical meetings, notably national or international groups for malformation syndromes and bone dysplasias, may often result in a diagnosis being provided. Even if it does not, one can feel happier that one is not overlooking a recognisable disorder if one has sought the advice of those most likely to know, and families also appreciate these efforts. Wherever possible, one should store (with consent) appropriate samples for future biochemical or DNA analysis.
- The diagnosis may be wrong. This is a much more dangerous situation than when the diagnosis is uncertain, as it may lead to false confidence. It is extremely difficult to know how far to rely on other people's diagnoses and how far to insist on confirming them oneself. Clearly, neither a medical geneticist nor any other clinician can be an expert diagnostician in every speciality, and one will frequently have to rely on colleagues' advice. Nevertheless, it is essential for all clinicians involved in genetic counselling to have a wide range of diagnostic ability, to know their own limitations – and those of their colleagues – and to develop a healthy scepticism in diagnostic matters and a sensitivity for where error may lie. For non-medical genetic counsellors, it is essential to work in the closest cooperation with clinical geneticists if major problems are to be avoided.

Bearing in mind the foregoing problems, how can one ensure that diagnostic information is as extensive and accurate as possible? There is no simple answer, but the following points may be helpful:

- Always arrange to see the affected individual or individuals if at all possible, even when they have already been fully investigated. How detailed an examination should be made will depend on the circumstances.
- Always examine asymptomatic members at risk (after careful explanation of why this is important and of the potential consequences), to exclude mild or early disease. This is especially important with variable, dominantly inherited disorders or where there is a possibility of a new mutation. Beware of persons who insist that there is no need for them to be examined because they know they are normal.
- Warn families in advance that the full answers to their questions may not be possible on the initial visit, and ask them to bring as much relevant information as possible about affected individuals, especially those not in the same household as themselves. A preliminary home visit, or at least telephone contact, by a co-worker will be extremely valuable in this respect, as well as giving a general preparation for the clinic visit, as discussed further in Chapter 11.
- Be prepared to interview older or more distant relatives who may have valuable information on deceased individuals. A home visit may be very useful here. Such relatives will almost always be happy to help, but the part of the family requesting advice should be asked beforehand if other branches are going to be approached and enquiry made as to whether any members are likely to be upset by this. It is preferable for initial contact to be made by family members themselves.
- When arranging a follow-up appointment for genetic counselling, allow adequate time for obtaining records and other information. Specific written permission should always be sought before requesting medical records of living relatives.
- A variety of special investigations may prove necessary, including radiological, biochemical and genetic studies, and sometimes biopsy diagnosis. Most studies can be performed on an outpatient basis, but occasionally it is extremely helpful to have facilities for inpatient investigation. It frequently happens that the affected individual on whom investigations are needed is already under the care of a clinical colleague; obviously, careful liaison prior to seeing such a person is essential if confusion or duplication of investigations is to be avoided and good working relationships with colleagues maintained.

GENETIC RISK ESTIMATION

Having taken a careful pedigree, documented the various details of affected individuals and examined relevant family members, one is now in a position to attempt to answer the questions that gave rise to the request for genetic counselling. Then one can estimate and transmit to the family concerned the risks of particular members, born or unborn, developing the particular disorder. The fact that the process of recording information will probably have taken a considerable time is in some ways an advantage, particularly if the family is not under one's regular care but is being seen specifically for genetic counselling. From the way in which information is given (or not given) and from the reaction to questions, much can be learned about the general attitude of the individuals being counselled to the family disorder.

- Did they themselves initiate the request for genetic counselling, or did someone else?
- Is there an unspoken and perhaps exaggerated fear of the disorder?

- Do feelings of guilt, blame or hostility exist between parents?
- Is the rest of the family supportive, or are there tensions between the generations?
- Is an affected child valued and loved, or regarded as a burden?

Much information on these and other important issues can be obtained by a person who is sensitive and observant, without the need for direct questioning.

It is also possible during this preliminary stage to assess the way in which information is to be most suitably transmitted. Some couples will be unable to grasp more than the simplest concepts of 'high risk' or 'low risk', while others will require a precise risk figure and even a detailed explanation of the mode of inheritance. It is common for those undertaking genetic counselling to overestimate the complexity and amount of information that can be absorbed in a single consultation; this is something for us all to guard against in our practice.

Information on genetic risks is rarely an absolute 'yes' or 'no' and in medical genetics, more perhaps than in any other branch of medicine, one thinks and works almost entirely in terms of probabilities or odds. Colleagues in other specialties frequently find this unsatisfactory, preferring to accept only a 'definite' conclusion. Yet when examined closely, there is often as much, if not more, uncertainty in the apparently 'definite' specialities than there is in medical genetics. Thus, the chance that a definite acute appendicitis will be found at appendicectomy is far from 100%, while the entire process of clinical diagnosis is based on the combination of numerous pieces of information, each with a degree of uncertainty, although this is often unappreciated by those involved. The same applies to the 'normal ranges' of most laboratory investigations. It is perhaps only because uncertainty is well recognised in genetics that methods of measuring it and defining its limits have been generally used, as exemplified in genetic counselling. More recently, other areas of medicine have started to use these approaches.

Risk figures in genetic counselling may be given as fractions, as percentages or as an odds ratio. Some people prefer to use fractions and to quote risks as 1 in 2, 1 in 4, 1 in 50, etc. Others prefer to use percentages such as 50%, 25%, 2% or, if they prefer odds, to talk of 1:1 (evens), 3:1 against or 49:1 against. The author admits to inconsistency in this, both in practice and in this book, although not often using an odds ratio except in the context of conditional probability calculations. For this reason, and because others are equally inconsistent, a selection of conversions is given (Table 1.1), which should allow ready exchange between these approaches. It is often necessary to adapt whichever is used to a particular situation, for some people simply do not understand odds, while others are more confused with percentages. Fewer people seem to use odds ratios in daily life except, perhaps, for inveterate gamblers. It also needs to be borne in mind that the margins of error for many risk figures are very high and that using precise figures can give a spurious impression of exact knowledge. In such a situation, the author often prefers not to give a precise figure at all.

Whatever method is used, there are pitfalls in interpretation that must be avoided, described as follows, and this may require much patience.

- Probabilities and odds refer to the future, not the past. Thus, a one in four risk, as seen with autosomal recessive inheritance, does not mean that because the previous child was affected the next three will be guaranteed to be normal. Nor does having two affected children in succession make it less (or more) likely for a Mendelian disorder that the next will be affected. That each conception is an independent event, so that 'chance has no memory', may require repeated explanation, since couples may accept the correct situation intellectually, yet retain an emotionally powerful view based on erroneous ideas.

Table 1.1 Conversion between proportions, fractions, percentages and odds

Proportion	Fraction	Percentage equivalent to	Odds (ratio)	Odds (in words)
1 in 1	1	100%	1:0	Certain
1 in 2	1/2	50%	1:1	Evens
1 in 3	1/3	33.3%	1:2	2 to 1 against
1 in 4	1/4	25%	1:3	3 to 1 against
1 in 5	1/5	20%	1:4	4 to 1 against
1 in 6	1/6	16.7%	1:5	5 to 1 against
1 in 7	1/7	14.3%	1:6	6 to 1 against
1 in 8	1/8	12.5%	1:7	7 to 1 against
1 in 9	1/9	11%	1:8	8 to 1 against
1 in 10	1/10	10%	1:9	9 to 1 against
1 in 11	1/11	9%	1:10	10 to 1 against
1 in 12	1/12	8.3%	1:11	11 to 1 against
1 in 13	1/13	7.7%	1:12	12 to 1 against
1 in 15	1/15	6.7%	1:14	14 to 1 against
1 in 16	1/16	6.25%	1:15	15 to 1 against
1 in 20	1/20	5%	1:19	19 to 1 against
1 in 25	1/25	4%	1:24	24 to 1 against
1 in 30	1/30	3.3%	1:29	29 to 1 against
1 in 33.3	1/33.3	3%	3:97	97 to 3 against
1 in 40	1/40	2.5%	1:39	39 to 1 against
1 in 50	1/50	2%	1:49	49 to 1 against
1 in 60	1/60	1.7%	1:59	59 to 1 against
1 in 66.7	1/66.7	1.5%	3:197	197 to 3 against
1 in 70	1/70	1.4%	1:69	69 to 1 against
1 in 80	1/80	1.25%	1:79	79 to 1 against
1 in 90	1/90	1.1%	1:89	89 to 1 against
1 in 100	1/100	1%	1:99	99 to 1 against
1 in 1,000	1/1,000	0.1%	1:999	999 to 1 against

- It is embarrassingly easy for odds to be reversed. Thus, a patient seen with one child affected by spina bifida, having been correctly advised by her obstetrician that there was a 1 in 20 recurrence risk, at a place and time when that was 'correct', came seeking termination of her next pregnancy because she considered that 'a chance of 1 in 20 of a normal child was far too low'.
- A risk of one in two (i.e. one-half, 1/2 or 50%) given as a fraction is not the same as 1 to 2 (1:2) given as an odds ratio, which is equivalent to a fraction of one in three (one-third) or a percentage of 33.3%. This may be misinterpreted by those unfamiliar with betting. (I should explain that I am not here meaning to condone the undoubted vice of gambling.)
- Many people do not have a clear idea of what constitutes a high or low risk. Thus, some couples who are given a risk that would be deemed low by many people (e.g. 1 in 200) express the view that this is far too high to be acceptable, whereas others may be greatly relieved by a risk of 50% (one in two, or 1:1) if they had thought that every child they had would necessarily be affected.

BOX 1.2: Risk of abnormalities in the 'normal' population (approximate)

Risk of a child being born with some congenital abnormality	1 in 30
Risk of child being born with a serious physical or mental impairment or disability	1 in 50
Risk of a recognised pregnancy ending in a spontaneous abortion	1 in 8
Risk of perinatal death[a]	1 in 120
Risk of a child dying in the first year of life after the first week[a]	1 in 300
Risk that a couple will be infertile	1 in 10

[a] Figure for 'developed' countries; there is great geographical variation.

Clearly, the nature and severity of the disorder will determine what risk is acceptable, but it is helpful to be able to give some kind of reference point for comparison, such as the fact that one child in 50 in the population is born with a significant congenital defect or disability of some sort, or that the population frequency of the disorder in question is, say, 1 in 2,000. Some useful (but very approximate) data of this type are summarised in Box 1.2.

BASIS OF RISK ESTIMATION

The ways in which risks can be estimated and the results of these estimates constitute a major aspect of this book and are considered in detail in later chapters. It is important from the outset, though, to recognise that not all risk estimates are of the same type. They may be based on different sorts of information and may be of greater or lesser reliability. The main categories discussed in the following sections can be distinguished.

Empirical risks

Here the estimate is based on observed data rather than theoretical predictions (Figure 1.3; see also Chapter 3). This is the form of risk estimate available for most of the more common non-Mendelian or chromosomal disorders. The information is usually reliable provided it has been collected in an unbiased manner (which is often not easy), and provided the population from which the consultand (the individual seeking genetic counselling) comes is comparable to the one in which the data were established. Sadly, there is a great dearth of recent empirical

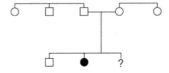

Figure 1.3 Empirical risk estimate: one child is affected with spina bifida. The risk of a subsequent child being affected by a neural tube defect is around 3% in an area of high risk (e.g. South Wales) and with no other affected family members. The risk estimate would be different in an area of low incidence and would be altered by the presence of other affected relatives. It has also changed with time, being less than in earlier surveys decades ago.

risk studies, and the use of older ones is often made more complex as the result of changes in classification following recognition of genetic heterogeneity or the identification of specific genes, as well as by genuine biological changes in disease frequency (e.g. the decrease in frequency of neural tube defects in the United Kingdom over the past half-century). An empirical risk based on old data, or data from a different population, may still be used but the figures will need to be interpreted with care, to give a figure more likely to apply to the particular family being seen in clinic.

Mendelian risks

Mendelian risk estimates can be given only when a clear basis of single gene inheritance can be recognised for a disorder (Figure 1.4; see also Chapter 2). They are perhaps the most satisfactory form of risk estimate because they commonly allow a clear differentiation into categories of negligible risk (e.g. offspring of healthy sibs for a rare autosomal recessive disorder in a family without recognised consanguinity) and high risk (e.g. offspring of an individual affected with an autosomal dominant disorder). It must be remembered that it is the genotype that follows Mendelian inheritance, which will not necessarily give the same risk for the actual disease phenotype if the penetrance is not complete, or if it is age dependent. There often remains the problem of achieving greater certainty in the individual at high risk (e.g. a person at 50% risk of developing Huntington's disease), and information from the next two risk categories may be helpful in this situation.

Modified genetic risks

Non-geneticists may find modified genetic risk estimates (Figure 1.5) difficult to use initially; they are particularly applicable in X-linked recessive inheritance and late-onset autosomal dominant disorders. Fully worked-out examples are given later (see Chapters 2 and 15). The essential feature is that a 'prior' genetic risk, based usually on Mendelian inheritance, may be modified by 'conditional' information, usually genetic, but sometimes from other sources. Thus, the modified risk of a healthy (unaffected) man developing Huntington's disease, whose grandparent was affected, is not the same as the prior risk of one in four, but is reduced by the fact that the intervening parent is or was unaffected, and it may also be reduced by his own age. The fact that the intervening parent (and perhaps the at-risk

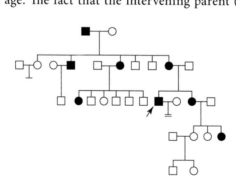

Figure 1.4 Mendelian risk estimate: a family with myotonic dystrophy (an autosomal dominant disorder). The risk for the offspring of affected individuals is 50% regardless of the incidence of the disorder and the number of affected individuals in the family. See Chapter 13 for the relevance of genetic instability to this disorder.

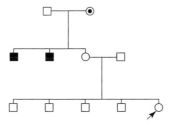

Figure 1.5 Modified risk estimate: Duchenne muscular dystrophy. The grandmother of the individual seeking advice (consultand) is an obligatory carrier; prior risks of the mother and the consultand being carriers are thus 50% and 25%, respectively. These risks are, however, greatly reduced by the fact that the mother has had four healthy sons and no affected sons. See Chapter 2 for further details.

grandson) has 'lived through' a good part of their risk without developing the condition can be used in calculations to modify the individual's residual risk. It may also be reduced by the number of unaffected sibs, if these have reached an advanced age. Such modifying information may drastically alter the risk estimate and should always be used when available, especially if presymptomatic or prenatal genetic tests are being considered, where it may have a considerable influence on decisions.

Another important context in which modified genetic risks are used is when the available mutation testing cannot detect all mutations causing a particular disease but only a proportion (even if that is high, perhaps 95% or 98%). In that case, the failure to find a mutation does not mean that no mutation is present, so that the prior risk of a person being a carrier (e.g. of a recessive disorder, or of a dominant disorder of incomplete or age-dependent penetrance) will be reduced but not to zero.

Risk estimates from independent evidence

Where special investigations can be utilised, these may greatly alter the risk estimates. With a known family history of a genetic disorder, the specific mutation/s (pathogenic variant/s) in the family may be known; in that case, direct testing for the relevant variants may be feasible. If neither direct mutation testing nor tests using genetic linkage are feasible, then other information may still be of value. Thus, a normal serum immunoreactive trypsin (IRT) test in an infant who has a sib with cystic fibrosis will considerably reduce the chance of the infant also being affected. If a sweat test can be performed, the measurement of sweat electrolytes may be performed, a more definitive test for cystic fibrosis than serum IRT.

Similar situations can arise with possible female carriers of haemophilia and Duchenne muscular dystrophy. Family-specific genetic testing can give clear, definitive information about carrier status, but if that is not available, then other investigations may still give useful information (serum creatine kinase for DMD, Factor VIII or IX levels for haemophilia A or B). However, a strong caution must be given here: the results of such investigations are rarely so clear-cut that they can be used in isolation; they require combination with the prior genetic risk, along with other modifying information. Failure to appreciate this may lead to serious error, especially when investigations are being applied as screening procedures in situations of low prior risk: information about the context, especially the family history, is crucial.

Composite risks

Most empirical risks really fall into this category, but in some instances it is obvious that one is dealing with a mixed situation that cannot be satisfactorily resolved. Thus, isolated cases of a disorder such as osteogenesis imperfecta congenita are composed of a large number of cases representing new dominant mutations, with a modest risk of recurrence in sibs (the risk of mosaicism, which in this condition is far from remote), and a very small number of autosomal recessive cases, with a recurrence risk of one in four. Because the two situations cannot always be reliably distinguished by clinical examination, one ends up with an intermediate risk depending on the relative frequency of the two groups. Obviously this intermediate risk does not really exist at all: the family must represent one or other of the extreme positions.

Molecular genetic testing may be able to clarify the family situation but only if the mutation causing the disorder has been identified with certainty. An uncritical, excessive readiness to attribute the disease to a possible, even a plausible, genetic variant will lead to erroneous advice if the variant identified is in fact benign.

Such a composite risk estimate is unsatisfactory and should be regarded as a temporary measure until molecular diagnostics is able to resolve all such uncertainties – or until the mode of inheritance becomes clear as the family reproduces. However, even with the birth of a further affected child in the example given of osteogenesis imperfecta, there will still be uncertainty as to whether this reflects autosomal recessive inheritance (the rare situation with one in four recurrence among siblings) or parental mosaicism for a new dominant mutation. The interpretation of such a birth will also be influenced by the presence of consanguinity in the family and in their community. Without molecular diagnostics, one might have to wait another generation, to see the offspring of the affected children, to be more confident about the pattern of inheritance.

The recognition of Mendelian subsets within a disorder generally considered to be 'multifactorial' (e.g. congenital heart disease, breast cancer) has also proved most important, as discussed in Chapter 3.

COMMUNICATION AND GENETIC COUNSELLING

No matter how well one may have confirmed a genetic diagnosis, utilised appropriate genetic tests and established an accurate risk estimate, all this will count for little if one cannot communicate satisfactorily with the family that one is seeing. The constant and unending variety provided by the interactions inherent in genetic counselling is one of the chief reasons why those involved find it such a rewarding activity, but even the most 'natural' communicators need training to optimise their skills, while a basic knowledge of the main theoretical aspects underpinning counselling skills is also of the greatest help. As indicated later in the chapter, these skills can also help to turn what may start out as an essentially information-giving interview into one that may be more therapeutic in nature.

Genetic counselling and non-directiveness

It will have been noted that the emphasis so far has been placed on ensuring that a correct diagnosis and risk estimate have been reached and that those being counselled have correctly understood the situation. Nothing has been said about recommending a particular line of action or of advising couples against having children in high-risk situations, and it may surprise some readers to learn that the author, in common with most professionals involved in genetic counselling, rarely if ever adopts a 'directive' approach, at least in the context of reproduction and prenatal diagnosis or of predictive genetic testing for neurodegenerative disorders. A survey of American genetic counselling centres has shown that a similarly non-directive approach is almost universal, although this has not always been the case in eastern Europe, nor in some other parts of the globe, especially in relation to cultural and population groups accustomed to a more authoritarian style of professional practice.

This may appear all the more surprising since many doctors with little experience of genetics do frequently give directive advice. Remarks such as, 'We were told not to have more children', or 'The doctors said I should have a termination', are still sometimes heard in genetic counselling clinics. In many cases, great distress has been caused to the couples involved, particularly when the advice has not been accompanied by an explanation of why it has been given or how great the risk really is.

Our view is that it is not the duty of a doctor or genetic counsellor to dictate the lives of others, but to ensure that individuals have the facts to enable them to make their own decisions. This includes not simply a knowledge of the genetic risks, but a clear appreciation of the consequences, long term as well as short term, that may result from a particular course of action. In any case, it seems likely (although not proven) that directive counselling may often be counterproductive. Intelligent couples may resent being told what to do in a situation where they have already spent much troubled thought over the alternatives. Many individuals, among both the more and the less privileged, will feel a strong resentment at being dictated to by authority and, in the context of Huntington's disease in particular but also other disorders, our experience suggests that some who have been given such 'instructions' may deliberately embark on a pregnancy as a gesture of defiance.

In contrast, some couples seen for genetic counselling will plead for direction. 'What would you do if you were in my place?' is a question heard from time to time in clinic. It is tempting to give a clear direction in these circumstances, but frequently these are the very couples for whom this may be most inadvisable. Such a plea often indicates an unwillingness to face the consequences of a serious situation, or a significant disagreement between marriage partners, and for the physician to take on the responsibility that can only really be taken by the couple themselves may have serious and unhelpful long-term consequences.

It would be wrong to pretend that those engaged in genetic counselling never give directive advice. One's own views are likely to be expressed in the way one approaches both the patient and the condition in the family, whether the more serious or the milder aspects of a disease have been stressed and whether one holds out the possibility of future treatment. Even the way a risk estimate is phrased can vary. For example, in the case of an autosomal recessive condition with a one in four recurrence risk, it is possible to make it appear quite encouraging if one states that there are three chances out of four that the next child will be healthy. The type of society in which one lives and practises will also inevitably influence the way in which genetic counselling is both 'given' and 'received', and these points are discussed further in later sections of this book. (See Clarke, 1997, in 'Further Reading' for a discussion of non-directiveness.)

The importance of the non-directive ethos of genetic counselling lies especially in the contexts of reproduction and of predictive genetic testing where decisions about medical management are not at stake. In these contexts, it will usually be unhelpful for professionals to give recommendations; we can support patients in the making of their decisions, but they need to take responsibility for the decisions made. As genetic testing enters healthcare more generally, however, there are contexts where it will be reasonable to recommend genetic tests because of their use in guiding medical management, especially in the care of patients affected by or at risk of certain cancers or inherited cardiac disorders (to be discussed further in the appropriate chapters). There are also occasions when we may recommend that patients share information with family members, and this could be seen as going against an unhelpfully narrow conception of 'non-directiveness'.

Since 'non-directiveness' has become a core tenet of genetic counselling, it is important that it should not be used as an excuse for being vague, for appearing detached, or for presenting so many apparent options that it becomes difficult for those seen to reach a clear decision. People will often need support for a tentative decision, as indicated later in this chapter; the importance of non-directiveness lies in allowing the decisions to be taken by the individuals involved, not by the professional providing the genetic counselling.

It is particularly important that couples realise that, in general, there is no 'right' or 'wrong' decision to be made, but that the decision should be the right one for their own particular situation. It is also important that those giving genetic counselling (and those evaluating genetics services) do not judge 'success' or 'failure' in terms of a particular outcome, and that they give support to families whatever their decisions may be. This may raise difficult tensions when a genetic screening programme is introduced with the goal of reducing the burden of disease or the long-term costs of healthcare in a community.

Advice at a distance

The less one is able to verify a situation oneself, the greater is the possibility of error. However, the person who refuses to give any advice unless able to do everything personally is going to be of limited benefit to patients and colleagues. The author is in no doubt that one of the most valuable roles of a medical geneticist – and the same applies to any clinician with a particular interest in genetic counselling – is to act as a focal point and source of information for colleagues in a variety of specialties who need someone to turn to for advice. A high proportion of general enquiries from colleagues do not require actual referral; frequently, one is simply confirming what is already thought to be the case. In other instances, one may be able to advise that prenatal, molecular or other special investigations are available; in a small proportion of enquiries, however, the advice has to be that one cannot give a reliable opinion without seeing the patient oneself. One soon learns to recognise the small number of colleagues who attempt to use indirect or 'casual' advice as a substitute for a proper referral, as well as the enquiries 'on behalf of a friend' that can disguise a serious personal genetic problem requiring a full referral and thorough assessment.

Actual genetic counselling by post or other indirect means is an entirely different matter, and our policy regarding enquiries from patients and relatives is to arrange a clinic appointment, via their family doctor wherever possible. The same policy applies to enquiries from health visitors, social workers and other paramedical personnel. Not only is there a serious risk that erroneous information may be given or risk figures misinterpreted; but without directly seeing those requesting advice, it is often impossible to decide what the real problem leading to their enquiry is and whether there are additional or underlying factors that have not been mentioned. E-mail enquiries, coming directly from patients or family members, are increasingly frequent, particularly if one has expertise in a specific disorder or is closely involved with lay groups. In this case, one can usually help best by directing the enquirer to useful information sources, often web-based, or to their local genetics centre. Although it may be tempting to try to provide detailed help, especially if there seems to be no local facility, this is – in our opinion – almost always unwise. In contrast, carefully organised and appropriately selected remote video-conferencing consultations may be of real value in difficult geographical situations.

BACKUP TO GENETIC COUNSELLING

It has already been emphasised that genetic counselling does not simply consist of giving risk figures, and that it must often be preceded by a considerable diagnostic effort, in comparison with which the estimation of risks may be a relatively simple matter. Similarly, genetic counselling does not stop with the giving of risks but must include a variety of other actions if it is to be fully effective.

In the first instance, it must be established as clearly as possible that the individuals counselled have really understood what they have been told. This includes not only the risk estimate, but the nature of the disorder and what other measures are available for prevention and treatment. It is often possible to get an approximate idea of how well information has been understood at the time of the interview, but it is well worthwhile, and often a salutary experience, to have this checked by an independent observer. A follow-up appointment may be useful both to check on this and to support the genetic counselling that has been given at the initial interview. For the same reason, it is important to provide a letter summarizing the main points of the consultation, including the risk estimates. It is my practice, in most cases, for the principal letter written after clinic to be the letter to the patient or family; this is then copied to the referring clinician and other professionals involved, with a brief covering note to the referrer if there are additional details to be included that would be too technical for the letter to the family. This approach works for most cases as the referrer can see exactly what the family has been told and is also given any additional information that may help with their assessment of the situation, but it is not suitable for all circumstances. Thus, where it is the referring physician who is asking the questions and not the patient, the principal letter will be written back to the physician.

Where information has been seriously misinterpreted or forgotten, this may be for various reasons. Some individuals have genuinely poor memories, while others may have been seen at an inappropriate time, such as soon after the death of a child; yet others may have come to the clinic encumbered with small and active children and been preoccupied in restraining their activities, rather than in listening to what has been said. Most commonly, one has probably not taken sufficient time and effort to ensure that the information has really been absorbed, and it is important to be aware of one's failures in this respect. We have on several occasions seen couples who have acquired grossly erroneous ideas of risk and have wondered who could possibly have misinformed them so completely, only to find that it was one of us who had seen them some years previously.

An essential accompaniment to genetic counselling is that both those being counselled, and also those delivering the counselling, should have full and accurate knowledge of the various other measures that may be available. In many cases, these require application as an integral part of the counselling process. Thus, an assessment of the risk of a woman having a child affected by Duchenne muscular dystrophy or haemophilia is likely to be incomplete without carrier detection tests being integrated into the process (see Chapter 7). In other cases, the risk may not be altered, but the consequences may be. Thus, where prenatal diagnosis is available (see Chapter 9), many couples will be prepared to embark on a high-risk pregnancy when they would not have considered doing so in the absence of such diagnostic possibilities. Similarly, the development of treatment fundamentally alters attitudes to genetic counselling. Most couples with a child diagnosed with phenylketonuria (PKU) in the newborn period and developing normally with treatment are happy to risk another affected child; where treatment is less satisfactory and the outcome less certain, the attitude may be very different.

There is now a danger that unrealistic optimism about the pace of medical progress could lead some families to risk having affected children in the strong expectation that the child will be 'cured' by progress that has not yet materialised. Such ideas can be discussed explicitly in order to help maintain a realistic sense of hope but without promoting an excessively optimistic faith in progress, that could all too easily lead to disappointment and regrets.

Further 'back-up' measures that may be required are contraception and sterilisation, as well as the exploration of other possible options such as adoption, artificial insemination by donor, or ovum donation. These aspects are discussed later (see Chapter 11), but it cannot be too strongly emphasised that their consideration is an integral part of genetic counselling.

SUPPORT IN THE CONTEXT OF GENETIC COUNSELLING

Many couples coming for genetic counselling require active support in one way or another. Sometimes the actual information given in genetic counselling may be of such grave consequence as to require support if serious problems are not to arise. Huntington's disease (see Chapter 15) is perhaps the most striking example, but a severe depressive reaction is not uncommon in women who have recently lost a child after a chronic illness and who have to be told that the risk for other children is high. A sympathetic family doctor to whom the couple can turn is probably the best safeguard in this situation, but a skilled genetic counsellor can often accurately judge those families particularly in need of support.

Support may also be required for problems quite unrelated to the genetic aspects. Thus, in genetic counselling for a chronic disease, it is frequently found that an affected individual is receiving no medical attention at all, that practical aids such as wheelchairs are not being provided, or that social service benefits of various kinds are not being claimed. It is sometimes argued that such matters are not part of genetic counselling; this may in some theoretical sense be so but, as physicians, we feel strongly that genetic counselling is an integral part of the overall management of patients and their families, that basic supportive measures may be as important as, or even more important than, the actual information regarding genetic risks, and that it is one's duty to see that the necessary measures are taken, if not by oneself then by an appropriate colleague.

Finally, while genetic counselling is largely distinct from psychotherapeutic counselling and does not have therapy as a specific aim, there is no doubt that it does have the potential for containing a strong therapeutic element. Most medical staff, some trained genetic counsellors and other staff involved in genetic counselling have until recently had relatively little specific training in counselling, psychotherapy or related fields. However, from working closely with such colleagues, we have learned not only how counselling skills and a psychotherapeutic orientation can contribute to managing the interview and the handling of family dynamics, but also how much of the 'ordinary' activity of genetic counselling can be therapeutic for those seen, if the interview is undertaken with gentleness and sensitivity and with the benefit of clinical experience.

There is little doubt that the time taken in genetic counselling is an important factor, as is the need for empathy with those being seen, but it is reassuring to know that it is possible for a person not fully trained in psychological aspects to make a contribution of this nature. It is also immensely helpful to have a colleague who is expert in this area for referral of those with serious psychological problems. Such a colleague may also be able to provide 'clinical supervision' not of the medical and diagnostic aspects of the service but of the psychological aspects of the family's situation. This can address the emotional responses in the family or among the professionals to any genetic information that is provided. The need for such psychological supervision is generally appreciated among genetic counsellors and is a part of their professional identity; its importance for clinical geneticists is as great but is less generally acknowledged.

2

Genetic counselling in Mendelian disorders

INTRODUCTION

When assessing the clinical and genetic information available for a family with a particular disorder, the primary question requiring an answer is often: does the disorder follow Mendelian inheritance?

- If the answer is 'yes', it is likely that precise and well-established risks can be given regarding its occurrence in other family members.
- If the answer is 'no', then the information that can be given is usually much less certain, although fortunately for the family the risks are also likely to be lower than for Mendelian inheritance.
- If, as is often the case, the answer is not clear, the correct initial course may be to attempt to obtain further evidence rather than to give risks that may require radical revision. This is particularly the case for those common disorders known to have a significant Mendelian subset (see Chapter 3).

Mendelian inheritance may be established in several ways and the more independent evidence one has supporting the same conclusion, the more confident one can be that the risks one has given are correct. In some cases, the pattern of transmission of the disorder in the family may be conclusive, even if the diagnosis is unknown or proves to be erroneous. Thus the pedigrees shown in Figures 2.1 and 2.2 could hardly be anything other than autosomal dominant and X-linked recessive, respectively. Nevertheless, one can be mistaken, even in what appears to be a classic pattern, as in Figure 2.3, where the inclusion of data from both parental lines in a disorder not known to follow regular Mendelian inheritance makes a polygenic or complex, multifactorial origin more likely.

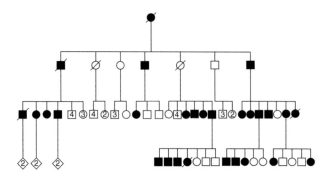

Figure 2.1 Typical autosomal dominant inheritance (a South Wales kindred with Huntington's disease). The disorder is transmitted by affected individuals to around half of their offspring. Both sexes transmit and develop the condition equally. The only unaffected individual to transmit the disorder died young and would presumably have developed it herself at a later date. (From Harper PS. 1976. *J R Coll Phys Lond* 10: 321–332.)

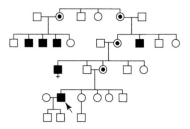

Figure 2.2 Typical X-linked recessive inheritance in a South Wales kindred with Becker (late-onset X-linked) muscular dystrophy. In each generation the disorder has been transmitted by healthy females, but only males are affected. The propositus has not transmitted the disorder to his sons.

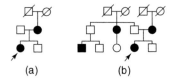

(a)   (b)

Figure 2.3 Polygenic inheritance simulating a Mendelian pattern: manic-depressive illness. (a) The superficial pedigree, with two generations affected, suggests dominant inheritance (autosomal or X-linked). (b) The recognition of affected individuals in both parental lines makes polygenic inheritance more likely than Mendelian. Pedigree details have been modified for illustrative purposes.

More commonly, Mendelian inheritance is established by a combination of clinical diagnosis with a compatible (but not in itself conclusive) pedigree pattern. The pedigree shown in Figure 2.4 is suggestive of autosomal dominant inheritance but could be a chance concentration of cases of a non-Mendelian – or even non-genetic – disorder. (One should recall that pellagra, often affecting multiple members of the same family, was considered to be a genetic disorder until its nature as a vitamin deficiency was established.) The knowledge that the diagnosis in the family in Figure 2.4 was Huntington's disease would remove all doubt and allow genetic counselling to be given accordingly.

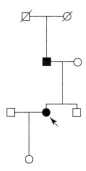

Figure 2.4 Pedigree pattern compatible with, but not conclusive of, autosomal dominant inheritance. Without a specific diagnosis it would be difficult to give more than approximate risks in this situation. In fact the pedigree is of a family with proven Huntington's disease, so confident advice as for autosomal dominant inheritance is possible.

Not infrequently, the pedigree information is entirely unhelpful and one is completely dependent on the clinical diagnosis. Nowhere is this seen more clearly than in the 'sporadic case', as shown in Figure 2.5, where there are the following possibilities:

- The disorder is largely or entirely non-genetic, with insignificant recurrence risk.
- The disorder is polygenic or chromosomal in basis, with a definite (usually low to moderate) recurrence risk, depending on the disorder.
- Inheritance may be autosomal recessive, with a one in four recurrence risk to further children of either sex.
- The disorder may represent a new dominant mutation, with very small recurrence risk to sibs (perhaps 1%–2%, from germ-line mosaicism) but a high (50%) risk for offspring of the affected individual.
- Inheritance might be X-linked recessive, with a risk of recurrence in future sons of the healthy sister.

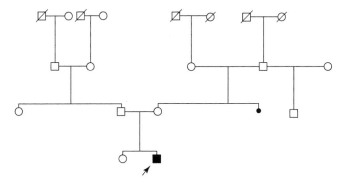

Figure 2.5 A 'sporadic case' of a disorder, the most common form of pedigree seen in genetic counselling. The affected individual could be the result of a non-genetic process, the family could represent autosomal dominant, autosomal recessive or X-linked inheritance, or a chromosomal or polygenic disorder. The absence of other affected family members does not mean that the disorder is not genetic.

Clearly, the conclusion reached (if any) will depend on the accuracy of diagnosis and whether it is known that the disorder consistently follows a mode of Mendelian inheritance. Thus, if the diagnosis were classic achondroplasia, one could confidently predict that the case represented a new dominant mutation, whereas with some complex and atypical malformation syndromes, no definite conclusion might be possible despite the most thorough (including genomic) investigation.

Although such an example may be regarded as extreme, reduction in family size means that the 'isolated case' is rapidly becoming the typical one for genetic counselling in many societies, a trend that will certainly continue. It is no more logical in genetic counselling to await the occurrence of a classic pedigree pattern in a family than it would be in general medicine to delay the diagnosis of a treatable disorder by waiting until the full clinical picture had developed.

A warning should be given at this point not to regard Mendelian inheritance as a rigid and unvarying mechanism following a fixed set of rules. As seen in the following pages, variability and exceptions are frequently found, often resulting in difficulties for genetic counselling. One of the most fascinating developments of recent years has been the discovery of the biological mechanisms underlying these variations and the increased understanding that this has brought to the field of genetics as a whole. As a result, we now have a much more flexible concept of genes and of Mendelian inheritance than was the case even a few years ago. These complicating factors account for why it is so much simpler to identify the genotype (i.e. the gene involved) from the phenotype than to predict the phenotype from knowledge of the genotype or even the whole genome sequence.

AUTOSOMAL DOMINANT INHERITANCE

Although, in theory, autosomal dominant inheritance is the simplest mode for genetic counselling, in practice it provides some of the most difficult problems, with traps for the unwary that require special mention.

An autosomal dominant disorder or trait can be defined either by the observed pattern of transmission between generations in families or as one that is largely or completely expressed in the heterozygote. The homozygous state is either unknown or excessively rare in dominantly inherited disorders, but when it does occur it is usually much more severe than the normal heterozygous form (e.g. familial hypercholesterolaemia) or lethal (e.g. achondroplasia). In Huntington's disease, however, the homozygote appears to be little different from the heterozygote, so this is one of the few cases known to fit both definitions.

In its fully developed form, the pattern of autosomal dominant inheritance is characteristic (see Figure 2.1) and allows precise risks to be given, as illustrated in Figure 2.6. The risk to offspring of affected members will be one half (i.e. 50%, one in two, or with an odds ratio of

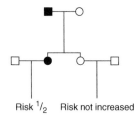

Risk $^1/_2$ Risk not increased

Figure 2.6 Genetic risks in classic autosomal dominant inheritance.

1:1), regardless of sex and regardless of whether the disease is fully developed or sub- or pre-clinical. The risk for offspring and more distant descendants of unaffected family members is not increased over the general population risk, provided that the individual really is unaffected (and is not an example of non-penetrance: see later in this chapter).

Problems arise from the variability of gene expression that is seen in many dominantly inherited disorders and which, until recently, has not been understood to any significant extent. The uncovering of the molecular basis of some of this variability is proving to be one of the most interesting fields of human genetics, as well as helping to resolve the practical problems encountered in genetic counselling.

Late or variable onset

Late or variable onset of a disorder such as Huntington's disease or adult polycystic kidney disease can be a major problem. Here genetic counselling for an affected person provides no problems in risk estimation, but the question of how old family members have to be before they can be certain of not developing the disorder may be extremely difficult to answer. The best approach is to use a 'life table' (Figure 15.1) such as that for Huntington's disease given in Chapter 15. Unfortunately, for most disorders there is either insufficient information or too much variation within families and sometimes between populations; while for others, such as myotonic dystrophy, the discrepancy between age at onset and first detection of the disease may be extreme. More prospective data need to be collected to answer this question for other late-onset autosomal dominant disorders, preferably specific to the gene or even the mutation causing the disorder in that family.

Incomplete penetrance

In a small but important group of dominantly inherited disorders, individuals known to carry the relevant gene – obligate carriers, because they have an affected parent and affected offspring – may show no evidence of disease, even at an advanced age. This is termed 'incomplete penetrance' of the gene. Figure 2.7 shows an example of lack of penetrance in one such disorder, hereditary pancreatitis. In part, this is determined by how hard one looks for minor or subclinical signs, and what biochemical or other diagnostic tests are available. Thus, careful biochemical study of family members in the acute porphyrias will show some who are biochemically affected but who have never had clinical features. Age is also a relevant factor; thus the mutation for Huntington's disease, once middle-aged adults have been affected in a family, has been close

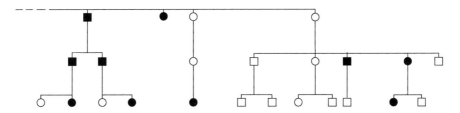

Figure 2.7 Lack of penetrance in autosomal dominant inheritance. Part of a large kindred with hereditary pancreatitis. Three apparently normal individuals have transmitted the disorder to their descendants. A specific mutation in cationic trypsinogen is now known in this kindred. (Courtesy of Dr J. Sibert.)

to 100% penetrant at age 70 years, but only about 50% or so at age ~50 years (see Chapter 15). Ageing of the population, however, may lead to greater numbers of very late-onset disease, so that estimates of penetrance by age 70 may have to be revised downwards. It should be noted that, as molecular analysis becomes possible, many dominantly inherited disorders are proving to show a higher frequency of asymptomatic mutation carriers than expected, raising so-far unresolved questions as to the proportion of these who will eventually develop disease. Conversely, penetrance may decrease with age, as with petit mal epilepsy, where the proportion of family members that can be shown to be affected clinically or by electroencephalography (EEG) decreases after adolescence. Some disorders, of which retinoblastoma is the most notable, show lack of penetrance unrelated to age or other detectable factors and may result from truly random processes.

As our understanding of gene expression increases, the different mechanisms underlying lack of penetrance are becoming clearer. In the case of familial retinoblastoma, it is now clear that a mutation inherited in the heterozygous state must be accompanied by a loss of function of the remaining normal allele in developing retinal tissue if a tumour is to occur (Knudson's 'second-hit' hypothesis). How this occurs will vary, and may involve loss of a part or the whole of the normal copy of chromosome 8, a somatic mutation in the *Rb* locus, or an epistatic process suppressing gene expression. Other important tumour-suppressor genes, where the same phenomenon applies, are the *BRCA1* and *BRCA2* genes, where there may be a genuinely random element in the relevant mutational processes (see the next section).

It is possible to relate in a general way the degree of penetrance to risks for the offspring of an apparently healthy relative; the risk for children of a healthy sib never exceeds 10%, even at the peak of risk when penetrance is 60% (see Pauli and Motulsky, 1981). The basis for this is that, when penetrance is high, it is unlikely that a healthy relative will have the mutant gene; when penetrance is low, the chance of actually being affected will be small, even though the mutation may be present.

Variation in expression

Variation in expression refers to the manner or degree to which the disorder is expressed in an individual (unlike penetrance, which is an index of the proportion of individuals with the mutated gene who show the condition in any way). Although some disorders (e.g. achondroplasia) are expressed with little variation, this is the exception rather than the rule for dominantly inherited disorders, so that it is wise never to assume a family member is unaffected without careful examination. In some disorders, variability is so marked that special care is needed and radiological or other tests may be required; tuberous sclerosis and myotonic dystrophy are notable examples. Apparent inconsistencies such as 'skipped generations' may be explained in this way. Molecular analysis is often helpful or even crucial in resolving such problems.

Variation in expression also produces another problem in genetic counselling for many disorders. Because those individuals who reproduce tend to be the least severely affected, the severity of a variable condition is likely to be greater in the child than in the parent, and this must be made clear to potential parents. Tuberous sclerosis provides a striking example of this. In addition, one may have to consider specific parent-of-origin effects, with severity in the children dependent on the sex of the transmitting parent, especially in Huntington's disease and myotonic dystrophy, and also in relation to imprinting. Genomic imprinting may provide a molecular explanation for some parental influences, while 'anticipation' due to unstable mutations is now recognised as a true phenomenon, as discussed later in this chapter, and is very much involved in the two disorders mentioned.

Mosaicism in a mildly affected parent may also contribute to a greater severity in affected children than their parents, as in tuberous sclerosis and in some skeletal dysplasias resulting from collagen gene mutations.

Basis of variability in Mendelian disorders

The variability that is characteristic of so many genetic disorders, notably but not exclusively those following autosomal dominant inheritance, has so far been discussed as a practical problem encountered in genetic counselling, without attempts to explain its basis. Until recently, we have had no direct evidence as to what the factors involved might be, but this is now changing rapidly, and we already have a series of specific 'epigenetic' mechanisms that have been shown to operate in different situations, and which must be considered when unexplained variability is encountered. Table 2.1 summarises those most clearly identified so far.

This field of 'epigenetics', dealing with those genetic changes not directly involving the DNA sequence itself, is developing rapidly. As we progressively understand the nature and role of the various chromosomal proteins in meiosis and in the structure of chromatin, the different forms of RNA, the role of DNA methylation, and an increasing number of other factors, it is becoming clear that changes in actual DNA sequence are only part of the complexity of the mechanisms underlying genetic disorders. Epigenetic processes mediated by DNA methylation and factors modifying chromatin configuration may account for the effects of early life experiences, both before birth and in infancy, on the development of the common, complex, degenerative disorders of adult life. These effects have often been known collectively as the 'Barker effect' or 'fetal programming'. A more general and more satisfactory term is 'predictive adaptive response'.

GENOMIC IMPRINTING

This term has been given to the process underlying differences in expression of a gene or genetic disorder according to which parent has transmitted it. On the basis of classical Mendelian inheritance, it should make no difference which parent transmits a disease-related gene, but several striking instances exist where a disorder apparently following autosomal dominant inheritance is only fully expressed when transmitted by the parent of one particular sex.

Table 2.1 Factors underlying variability in Mendelian disorders (see text for details)

Genomic imprinting	Phenotype varies according to parent of origin
Anticipation due to unstable DNA	More severe phenotype in successive generations
Mosaicism	Mild or non-penetrant phenotype in a parent
Modifying alleles	Influence of unaffected parent
Somatic mutation also required (e.g. familial cancers)	Variable penetrance
X chromosome inactivation (in females)	For sex-linked loci only (which excludes the pseudoautosomal regions on the X chromosome)

Note: The phenotype may be mild or non-penetrant in the mutation-carrying parent.

Examples include Beckwith-Wiedemann syndrome (paternal transmission), Angelman syndrome (maternal transmission) and one form of familial glomus tumour (only clinically expressed if paternally transmitted).

These observations would not necessarily imply a special and similar underlying mechanism were it not for the fact that the genes involved lie in regions where experimental studies (mostly in mice) show a marked difference between paternal and maternal gene expression. This 'imprinting' influence of the parental genome is reversible and is related to the degree of methylation of the DNA, something that can provide a practical test of whether this effect is operating in the human examples. To what extent imprinting is also involved in more minor variation remains to be seen, since parental effects have often not been looked for carefully in family studies of other disorders.

Imprinting is important not only in Mendelian disorders but also in chromosome abnormalities, since it is only if the parental origin of a chromosome or chromosomal region is significant that the phenomenon of uniparental disomy, in which both copies of a particular chromosome or chromosomal segment are received from the same parent, will be clinically relevant. This important and increasingly recognised occurrence is discussed further in Chapter 4 and is another example of how our concepts of Mendelian inheritance are becoming more flexible.

Recent concern has arisen over whether there may be an increase in disorders related to genetic imprinting in children born as a result of assisted reproduction techniques, such as intra-cytoplasmic sperm injection (ICSI). In animals created by cloning of adult cells there are clear problems related to this. There is perhaps a 3–4× increase in imprinting disorders in children conceived through artificial reproductive technologies but substantial uncertainty remains about which reproductive technologies give rise to what degree of risk.

ANTICIPATION AND UNSTABLE DNA

The concept of a genetic disease worsening with successive generations is far from new and, indeed, was used by the early eugenicists as an argument for preventing reproduction of those with mental illness and mental handicap. While the basis for this was soon discredited, the phenomenon of anticipation persisted in relation to variable dominantly inherited disorders, notably myotonic dystrophy, where a striking progression through the generations in both age at onset and severity was noted as early as 1918 and was difficult to explain without a special mechanism. It was over half a century until the true biological explanation emerged, which is that the myotonic dystrophy mutation is an unstable DNA triplet repeat sequence that expands in successive meioses, and whose size correlates closely with the severity of the disorder. A comparable unstable sequence had already been found to underlie fragile X mental retardation, and the same has now been shown for Huntington's disease and several types of dominant spinocerebellar ataxia. These disorders fall into two rather different groups of 'trinucleotide repeat disorders', mainly neurological in nature, with one group involving an enlarged polyglutamine repeat within the protein and the other group consisting of conditions where the expansion does not code for protein at all.

The details relevant to these diseases are described in Chapters 13–15; so far no other diseases have been found to have such striking instability underlying their variation, but the discovery of this previously unknown and unsuspected mechanism shows how careful one must be before dismissing phenomena for which one has no ready explanation.

Within an individual family, the appearance of anticipation can be produced by parental mosaicism (see later in this chapter), as well as by the natural tendency for more mildly affected parents to reproduce and for more severely affected offspring to be ascertained.

DIGENIC INHERITANCE AND GENE-GENE INTERACTIONS

With the mass of information emerging from exome studies and whole genome sequencing, the importance of variation at more than one locus to disease phenotypes is becoming ever more apparent. Sometimes this is so marked that the pattern of inheritance is described as digenic, but this is the tip of an iceberg of gene-gene interactions. While mutation searching was being conducted by Sanger sequencing, the search for mutations in a patient would often stop once a mutation had been found. With the advent of next-generation sequencing that enables the simultaneous analysis of many loci implicated in the pathogenesis of any particular disorder, it has become much more feasible to recognise the disease-modifying effect of variants at one locus on disease associated with mutations at another locus. Such effects are now recognised as of major importance in a number of disease entities, including hypertrophic cardiomyopathy, primary open-angle glaucoma, the ciliopathies and many genetic cancers.

OTHER MODIFYING INFLUENCES

If variations in penetrance and expression reach more than a certain level, it becomes meaningless to consider the disorder as following Mendelian inheritance. Nevertheless, there are numerous influences that can modify a basic autosomal dominant pattern, including sex (as in familial breast cancer), exposure to drugs (as in the acute porphyrias) and diet (as in familial hypercholesterolaemia). Variations in the 'other' allele – the 'normal' allele – may also exert an effect.

New mutation

The dangers of assuming that an isolated case of a dominantly inherited disorder represents a new mutation have already been mentioned. It is important to establish this accurately because, if it is a new mutation, the risk of recurrence in a sib is generally low or very low (Figure 2.8). The proportion of cases of a disorder resulting from new mutations will be directly related to the degree to which the disease interferes with reproduction, that is, its genetic fitness. Thus, almost all cases of Apert syndrome, where reproduction is rare, are new mutations, whereas in adult polycystic kidney disease, with clinical features presenting most commonly in later life, the proportion is small; this has obvious consequences for the disease incidence.

Evidence from observations and experiments conducted on simpler species used as model organisms has for many years indicated the range of alterations in DNA that might underlie human disease mutations but, visible chromosomal rearrangements apart, it is only recently that we have begun to gain insight into this for many of the important genetic disorders

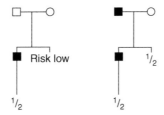

Figure 2.8 Autosomal dominant inheritance. Genetic risks for a new mutation and for a transmitted case.

considered in this book. The practical importance of this new information, considered more fully in Chapter 5, is twofold:

1. It is often possible to correlate the nature and site of the mutation with the severity or characteristic clinical features of the disease. This allelic or mutational heterogeneity is proving to underlie much of the phenotypic variation encountered in Mendelian disorders, recessive as well as dominant, while the identification of a specific mutation in a family often makes it possible to predict, at least within broad limits, the range and severity of disease features that might occur in those at risk.
2. The detection of a specific mutation in a patient whose condition appears to have arisen *de novo* (i.e. as a new mutation) allows this to be tested directly. If neither parent shows the defect, then the presumption of a new mutation having occurred is confirmed. Clearly, this is especially relevant for those variable disorders where it is difficult to rule out the gene being present in one or other apparently healthy parent as a result of the phenomena described previously.

However, before the low or minimal risks already indicated as appropriate to the new dominant mutation can be given confidently, one further factor, mosaicism, must be considered.

Mosaicism and mutation

Mosaicism denotes the occurrence in a single individual of cells or tissue of more than one genetic constitution. The term is confined to differences that have originated after fertilisation (the term chimaera is used for those rare situations where a single individual originates from more than one fertilised egg). Mosaicism results from mutations occurring in early development so that a significant part of the body cells or germ line (or both) carries the mutation. Visible chromosomal mosaicism has been recognised for many years (see Chapter 4), but only since the development of molecular analysis has the importance of its occurrence for other types of mutation been demonstrated.

Somatic mutation of later life, while of the greatest importance in relation to cancer and other degenerative disorders, is not relevant here to genetic risks. The importance of mosaicism from early embryonic mutation is that it may involve the germ line (gonadal or germinal mosaicism) in an individual who is otherwise healthy. If an affected child is born to such a person, there is a serious risk of this being attributed to a new mutation, when a significant proportion of eggs or sperm is in fact carrying the mutation, with a considerable risk of recurrence.

Such a possibility has long been recognised to occur in exceptional situations, but it has now become clear that it is a widespread phenomenon, and one that is far from rare in both dominant and X-linked disorders. For some conditions (e.g. Duchenne muscular dystrophy, tuberous sclerosis), it may give an appreciable risk of recurrence in a situation that would otherwise have been attributed to an isolated new mutation. For other conditions (e.g. osteogenesis imperfecta, achondroplasia), it is well documented but infrequent. For practical purposes, it is probably wise to regard a recurrence risk of around 1% to be likely for any apparent new dominant mutation, unless a more specific estimate is available. In some disorders that result from point mutations, there is a definite paternal age effect. This applies most especially to mutations in certain growth factor receptor genes, such as gain-of-function mutations in *FGFR2* in some of the craniosynostosis syndromes, where there is active selection for cells carrying the mutation within the testis. There will then be a predominantly paternal origin of mutations, a pronounced paternal age effect, and a higher risk of recurrence.

Gonadal mosaicism must be considered as an alternative to autosomal recessive inheritance where two affected offspring have been born to healthy parents, especially where the disorder is usually transmitted as a dominant trait. A number of cases of osteogenesis imperfecta and other disorders of collagen, previously thought to represent families with autosomal recessive inheritance, have now been shown to be the result of previously unsuspected mosaicism for dominant disorders.

Homozygosity in autosomal dominant disease

Almost all patients seen with autosomal dominant conditions will be heterozygotes, having inherited their disorder from only one side of the family or representing new mutations. Homozygosity requires both parents to have transmitted the mutated gene; this is most unlikely to happen unless one of the following is the case:

- The gene is common and relatively mild or late onset in its effects.
- Two affected individuals have married one another.

Familial hypercholesterolaemia provides an example of the first situation; the heterozygote frequency may be as high as 1 in 500, so one might expect chance marriages between such individuals to occur with a frequency of 1 in 250,000. Since only a quarter of the offspring of such a couple would be homozygous, one would expect the frequency of homozygotes to be only one in a million, and they are indeed exceedingly rare. Consanguinity would, of course, increase the chance of homozygosity, exactly as in autosomal recessive inheritance.

The situation more likely to be met in a genetic counselling clinic is where two individuals with the same disorder marry preferentially. This is seen not infrequently in achondroplasia (Figure 2.9); the risks for the offspring in such a situation will be one-quarter homozygous affected, one-half heterozygous achondroplasia, and one-quarter unaffected.

In achondroplasia, the affected homozygote usually dies rapidly after birth owing to the constricted chest; in most other dominant disorders the homozygous condition is likewise very severe or lethal. In the case of Huntington's disease, no such differences have been observed, even though a number of marriages between heterozygotes are recorded; molecular analysis of the offspring has now confirmed that the homozygote may be indistinguishable from the heterozygote.

A somewhat similar (though rare) situation may occur when marriage partners have different, but allelic, disorders. The child may then receive both abnormal alleles and will appear as a 'genetic compound'. This has been recorded with achondroplasia and the milder dysplasia

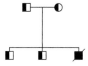

Figure 2.9 Homozygosity for an autosomal dominant disorder, achondroplasia. The parents and the two surviving children all have classic achondroplasia; they are represented by half shading to indicate that they are heterozygotes. The third child received the achondroplasia gene from both parents and had the lethal homozygous form of the disease, dying from respiratory insufficiency soon after birth. The pedigree is analogous to that commonly seen with autosomal recessive inheritance except that the heterozygotes are affected, not the carriers.

hypochondroplasia. The resulting child was more severely affected than either parent, but less severely affected than the homozygote for achondroplasia.

AUTOSOMAL RECESSIVE INHERITANCE

The principal difficulty with autosomal recessive inheritance is to be sure that this is indeed the mode of inheritance in a particular family. The great majority of cases of an autosomal recessive disorder are born to healthy but heterozygous parents, with no other affected relatives. Vertical transmission, so characteristic of dominant inheritance, is rarely seen (Figure 2.10), and with the small families of the present time in many Western, industrial countries, it is unusual to see more than one (at most two) affected sibs. Thus, autosomal recessive disorders, even more than autosomal dominant disorders, usually have to be distinguished from the isolated case, with little or no genetic information to help.

Where the diagnosis makes this mode of inheritance certain, or in the minority of families where the genetic pattern is clear, risk prediction is relatively simple (Figure 2.11). In the great majority of instances, the only significant increase in risk is for sibs of the affected individual, for whom the risk is one in four. Unless the disorder is especially common or there is consanguinity, the risks for half-sibs and children, and in particular for children of healthy sibs, is only slightly increased over that for the general population. The precise risk will depend on the frequency of heterozygotes in the population, since it will be necessary for both partners to contribute the abnormal gene for a child to be affected. It is thus important to know how to estimate the chance of being a carrier for an autosomal recessive disorder, both for family members and for the general population, and this is outlined in the next section.

Risk of being a carrier

The parents and children of a patient with an autosomal recessive disorder are obligatory carriers, while second-degree relatives (uncles, aunts, nephews, nieces, half-sibs, grandparents) will have a 50% chance of being a carrier (Figure 2.12). Each further step will reduce the risk by 50%, so that it is relatively simple to estimate the chance of any relative being a carrier if their closeness to the patient is known (see also Tables 10.1 and 10.2). The risks will be higher in the presence of consanguinity, which can arise when there is an increased background degree of relatedness within a population group as well as situations when the parents are closely related as cousins, often first cousins (see Chapter 10).

Sibs provide a special case: although the chance that the child of two carrier parents will be a carrier is two out of four, the chance of a healthy sib being a carrier is two out of three, because the affected category of individuals would be recognised and would be excluded from consideration.

When calculating the risks for a family member being a carrier, the possibility of new mutation can be ignored because it is excessively rare in relation to the other risks. Likewise, although the general population risk must in theory be added, this is usually insignificant except for the most common disorders.

Population risk

It is rare for the population frequency of carriers for an autosomal recessive disease to be known by direct observation, although this information will become available as more genome sequence information accumulates and as our ability to predict the effect of a gene variant

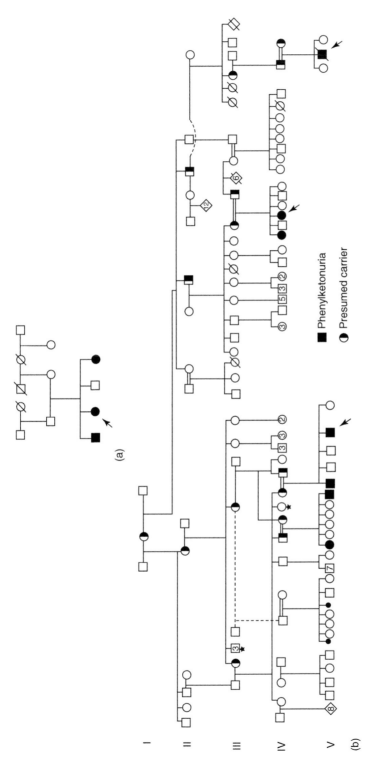

Figure 2.10 Patterns of autosomal recessive inheritance. Although many cases of autosomal recessive disease are isolated ones, a characteristic pedigree pattern is seen with large or inbred families. (a) A family with cystic fibrosis. The disorder is confined to a single sibship, with parents and more distant relatives entirely healthy. Both sexes are affected. (b) Phenylketonuria in an inbred Welsh gypsy kindred. The affected individuals have been born to healthy but heterozygous parents in this highly inbred kindred. The gene can be traced back to a single ancestral heterozygote. The origin of the gene has subsequently been confirmed by use of the phenylalanine hydroxylase gene probe.

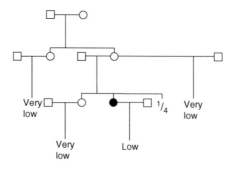

Figure 2.11 Genetic risks in autosomal recessive inheritance.

improves. Fortunately, however, the carrier frequency can be estimated directly from the disease frequency through the relationship known as the Hardy-Weinberg equilibrium. This has the advantage over genome sequence data in that no assumptions or dubious predictions need to be made about the effect of variants found within or close to relevant genes. In the few cases where direct observations are available, they agree closely with the predicted frequencies, so it seems reasonable to rely on them, at least as an approximation.

The basis of the Hardy-Weinberg equilibrium and the possible reasons for deviation from it are covered fully in genetics textbooks and are not given here. What the clinician or genetic counsellor needs to know is that the gene frequency and heterozygote frequency can be predicted, provided that the frequency of the affected homozygote is known. For the usual situation where an individual has two alleles, the more common 'normal' allele with frequency p, and the rarer 'disease' allele with frequency q (the combined frequency of the two must equal one), the frequencies of the different categories, which must sum to one, are as follows:

q^2 Abnormal homozygotes (disease frequency)
p^2 Normal homozygotes
$2pq$ Heterozygotes (carriers)

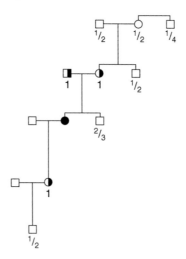

Figure 2.12 Risks of being a carrier in autosomal recessive inheritance (obligatory carriers are half-shaded).

Table 2.2 Risk of transmitting an autosomal recessive disorder in relation to disease incidence (the spouse is assumed to be healthy and unrelated)

Disease frequency (q^2) (per 10,000)	Gene frequency (q) (%)	Carrier frequency ($2pq$) (%)	Risk for offspring of affected homozygote (%)	Risk for offspring of healthy sib (%)
100	10.0	18.0	9.0	3.0
50	7.1	13.2	6.6	2.2
20	4.5	8.6	4.3	1.4
10	3.2	6.2	3.1	1.0
8	2.8	5.4	2.7	0.9
6	2.4	4.7	2.3	0.78
5	2.2	4.3	2.1	0.72
4	2.0	3.9	2.0	0.65
2	1.4	2.8	1.4	0.46
1	1.0	2.0	1.0	0.33
0.5	0.71	1.4	0.70	0.23
0.1	0.32	0.64	0.32	0.11
0.05	0.22	0.44	0.22	0.07
0.01	0.10	0.20	0.10	0.03

The starting point is usually the disease frequency, q^2, which is often known. The square root of this gives the 'abnormal' gene frequency q. From this one can obtain p, which must be (1 minus q). This allows one to work out the carrier frequency, $2pq$.

In practice, p (the 'normal' gene frequency) is close to 1 except for exceedingly common diseases, so $2pq$ differs little from $2q$; that is, for rare recessive disorders, the carrier frequency is approximately twice the square root of the disease frequency.

If this oversimplification helps the non-mathematically minded, it will be more than worth any criticism or retribution the author receives from his fellow geneticists.

Returning to the practicalities of genetic counselling, the risk for offspring of patients with a recessively inherited disease, and for their sibs and other relatives, can now readily be estimated. Table 2.2 gives the risks for a range of gene frequencies. It can be seen that only for the most common of recessive disorders do the risks become considerable, so that whether a relative is or is not a carrier is not of critical importance unless they are themselves marrying a close relation or the close relation of another affected person (see also Chapter 10).

Consanguinity

The estimation of genetic risks in relation to consanguinity is discussed more fully in Chapter 10, but it needs a mention here in relation to autosomal recessive inheritance because it is this category of disorders that is principally influenced by it. Several points need to be emphasised:

- Consanguinity is relevant to genetic risks only if it involves both parental lines, not just one, as shown in Figure 2.13.
- Two brothers marrying two sisters (or similar combinations), as shown in Figure 2.14, does not constitute consanguinity.

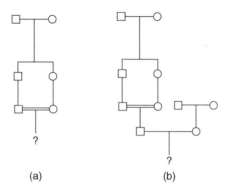

(a) (b)

Figure 2.13 (a) Consanguinity involving both parental lines is relevant to the genetic risk. (b) Consanguinity not relevant to offspring of the marriage in question.

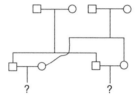

Figure 2.14 Marriage of two brothers to two sisters does not constitute consanguinity.

- The rarer the disorder, the higher will be the proportion of affected individuals resulting from consanguineous marriages.
- The presence of consanguinity in relation to a syndrome of uncertain inheritance favours, but does not prove, autosomal recessive inheritance.
- Consanguinity must be seen in the context of the particular community. Thus, in a population where 30% of marriages are between cousins, the observation that several affected children have consanguineous parents carries much less force than if the same observation were made in a community where there is only 1% of cousin marriages.
- Extensive consanguinity can give the appearance of autosomal dominant inheritance (pseudodominant inheritance), with vertical transmission resulting from an affected person marrying a carrier, as shown in Figure 2.15.

Other problems with autosomal recessive disease

Once one is confident that the mode of inheritance is indeed autosomal recessive, the difficulties in genetic counselling are much less than those encountered in autosomal dominant disorders. In particular, lack of penetrance is rarely encountered, and variation in expression within a sibship is (usually) much less. Genetic heterogeneity in either of two different senses – of multiple loci being involved, or multiple alleles at a single locus – is probably the major cause of variation within an apparently single entity. This can sometimes be recognised biochemically, as in many of the inborn errors of metabolism, while in other conditions it must be inferred from family data or be demonstrated directly by genetic testing.

An example of the practical importance of recognising such heterogeneity is seen in the different types of recessively inherited polycystic kidney disease, in which sibs show close

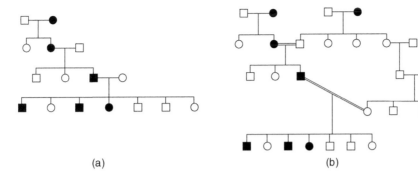

(a)   (b)

Figure 2.15 (a) An incomplete pedigree showing quasi-dominant inheritance of alkaptonuria. (b) The complete pedigree showing that consanguinity accounts for the pedigree pattern simulating autosomal dominant inheritance.

concordance in age of onset and of death (see Chapter 24); similarly in the spinal muscular atrophies (see Chapter 13), where the classic Werdnig-Hoffmann disease will often show close similarity between sibs, whereas the later-onset forms show a much broader scatter. Information of this type, which may influence the likely prognosis, is just as important for parents contemplating another pregnancy as is the actual risk of recurrence.

A further factor of particular relevance for autosomal recessive disorders is the availability of prenatal diagnosis in many cases, especially those where the underlying biochemical or molecular defect is known. This is discussed in Chapter 9. The use of donor insemination, or more rarely donor ovum *in vitro* fertilisation (IVF), is also relevant in recessive disorders, because the risk of an unrelated donor being a carrier for the same gene is small.

A final factor, again related to the fact that an autosomal recessive disorder necessitates both parents being carriers, is the outlook for parents remarrying. With the frequency of divorce at its current level in most of Europe and North America, this must be a serious consideration when sterilisation is being considered in either parent. It is, however, a difficult subject to discuss with parents, particularly when the burden of caring for an affected child is likely to be a major factor in the breakup of a marriage.

In cultures where the status of women is low, and where the recognition of the genetic risks for a particular marriage partnership could have major implications, considerable sensitivity is needed in addressing the issues.

Conversely, the necessary contribution of both parents to an autosomal recessive disorder in a child can be a positive feature in genetic counselling. It is frequently found that one parent (commonly the mother) is assuming the burden of guilt for the occurrence of the disorder, and this may be reinforced by the views (spoken or tacit) of other relatives. The realisation that neither side of the family is solely 'to blame', and that everyone carries at least one harmful genetic factor, is frequently a great relief to couples to whom a child with an autosomal recessive disorder has been born.

Marriages between affected individuals

Marriage between two affected individuals has already been discussed for autosomal dominant disorders and is seen rather more frequently with those showing autosomal recessive inheritance. The usual reason is preferential marriage between similarly affected people, particularly those

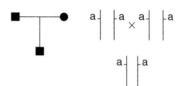

Figure 2.16 Marriage of two individuals with the same disorder; all offspring must be affected since the parents can only transmit the abnormal gene 'a'.

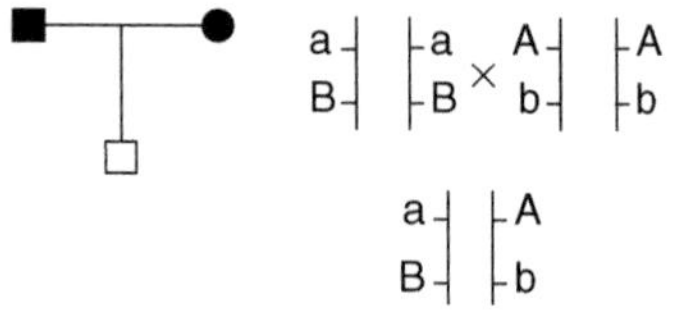

Figure 2.17 Marriage of two individuals with the same disorder; here the abnormal genes occur at different loci so the offspring are unaffected.

with blindness or deafness, who may be educated together and have a common social bond. Albinism and severe congenital deafness provide the two best-documented examples.

If two individuals with the same clinical disorder (e.g. a severe form of oculocutaneous albinism) have children together, their children will either all be affected or none will be affected. If the condition is caused by mutations in the same gene in both the parents, then all their children must be affected, since each parent can only transmit one of their two abnormal copies of the same gene, as shown in Figure 2.16. On the other hand, if their condition is caused by mutations in different genes, then their children will be unaffected but will certainly carry one abnormal copy of each gene.

It is crucial, however, to be sure about whether genetic (locus) heterogeneity is present, because if the parents' disorders are controlled by different loci, all offspring will be unaffected, although they will all be carriers of the abnormal gene allele at both loci (Figure 2.17); a greater potential for erroneous counselling cannot be imagined.

In the case of albinism, careful clinical study will usually distinguish the different forms (see Chapter 18). In severe congenital deafness, however, this is often impossible, except with the use of molecular genetic diagnostics. If such testing is not available, then advice must be based on knowledge of the number and relative frequency of the different types, and on whether the couple concerned has already had affected or normal children. This situation is one of many in genetic counselling where the recognition of genetic heterogeneity is of extreme importance. These problems are being resolved as identification of the specific molecular defects in the different types of both albinism and congenital deafness becomes more readily available (see Chapters 18 and 20, respectively).

X-LINKED DISORDERS

Since virtually no serious human diseases are known to be borne on the Y chromosome, sex linkage is equivalent to X linkage, so far as genetic counselling is concerned. (An example of a disorder that can be transmitted on the Y chromosome is the Leri-Weill dysostosis caused by mutation in the *SHOX* gene on the pseudoautosomal portions of the two sex chromosome short arms: see later discussion.) Microdeletions of the Y chromosome are implicated in male infertility but, except through the use of ICSI (see the discussion on infertility treatments), are not usually transmitted to the next generation.

X linkage produces some unusual problems that are of considerable practical importance, and as a result X-linked disorders occupy a much more prominent place in a genetic counselling clinic than would be expected from the relative contribution of the X chromosome to the human genome.

Several hundred definitely X-linked human disorders or traits have been recognised, and a list of some of the more important ones is given in Box 2.1. The list of disease loci on the X chromosome has of course been known fairly thoroughly for many years, long before the entire DNA sequence of the human X chromosome was known and even longer before the whole genome sequence had been achieved, but of course the availability of the X chromosome DNA sequence has refined this list of disease loci. This has existed for decades, although the relative contribution of the different loci to disease phenotypes is still not yet entirely clear, especially for X-linked cognitive impairment (often termed *intellectual disability* or, at the time when particular gene loci were being named, mental retardation) (see Chapter 14).

McKusick's Mendelian Inheritance in Man, now accessed in its online version (OMIM) (see 'Further Reading'), is the most complete single source for rare conditions. The database contains over 1,800 entries in its X-linked catalogue, although not all these will prove to be separate disease-related loci. The great majority are classed as X-linked recessive, with a much smaller number as dominant and a few as dominant but lethal in the hemizygous male.

The terms 'dominant' and 'recessive' must be used with caution in X-linked disease, because a high degree of variability is seen in disease expression in the heterozygous female. The factors that lead to a heterozygous variant of an autosomal gene manifesting in the phenotype – that is, that make it dominant or recessive – may still apply to loci on the X chromosome but, in addition, there are also the effects of the random nature of X-chromosome inactivation (Mary Lyon's hypothesis). This process applies to a large majority of the loci on the X chromosome in the human female. One of the two X chromosomes is randomly inactivated in each cell in the early embryo and becomes visible cytogenetically as the 'sex chromatin' or 'Barr body' under the nuclear membrane. Because the clonal descendants of each cell retain the same inactivated X chromosome, it follows that a female heterozygous for an X-linked disorder or trait will be mosaic, with two populations of cells, one of which has the 'normal' and the other the 'abnormal' X chromosome functioning.

Whether and how a female will manifest signs of an X-linked disorder for which she is heterozygous will depend upon two principal factors: (1) the proportion of cells in the relevant tissue(s) in which the mutated copy of the gene is on the cell's active X chromosome, and (2) the biology of the gene product (e.g. whether the encoded protein is an enzyme, a structural protein, a membrane component or a signalling pathway component, and whether it functions in a cell autonomous fashion or is secreted and active extra-cellularly).

There is a considerable amount of direct evidence for X-chromosome inactivation in human diseases, which may be expressed in several ways. Some disorders show 'mosaic' or 'patchy' changes in heterozygotes; thus, patchy retinal changes are seen in carriers for X-linked retinitis pigmentosa and choroideraemia, and patchy muscle biopsy changes may be found in carriers for Duchenne muscular dystrophy. More commonly, variability in X inactivation can result in a milder and more variable expression of clinical and biochemical changes. Thus, in X-linked hypophosphataemic rickets, generally considered to be an X-linked *dominant* condition, affected females can have milder disease than their affected male relatives; conversely, in haemophilia A, usually classed as an X-linked *recessive* condition, some carriers show a mild bleeding tendency in addition to reduced levels of factor VIII. The implications for tests of carrier detection in X-linked diseases are discussed in Chapter 7.

BOX 2.1: Important Mendelian disorders following X-linked inheritance

Aarskog syndrome (faciogenital dysplasia)
Addison disease with cerebral sclerosis
Adrenal hypoplasia (one type)
Agammaglobulinaemia, Bruton type
   (sometimes also Swiss type)
Albinism, ocular
Albinism-deafness syndrome
Alport syndrome (many cases)
Amelogenesis imperfecta (two types)
Anaemia, hereditary hypochromic
Cataract, congenital (one type)
Cerebellar ataxia (one type)
Cerebral sclerosis, diffuse
Charcot-Marie-Tooth peroneal muscular
   atrophy (one type)
Choroideraemia
Choroidoretinal degeneration
   (one rare type)
Coffin-Lowry syndrome
Colour-blindness (several types)
Chronic granulomatous disease
Deafness, perceptive (several types)
Diabetes insipidus, nephrogenic
Diabetes insipidus, neurohypophyseal
   (some families)
Dyskeratosis congenita
Ectodermal dysplasia, hypohidrotic (also
   known as anhidrotic) (gene *EDA*)
Ehlers-Danlos syndrome, type V
Fabry disease (angiokeratoma)
Focal dermal hypoplasia (Goltz syndrome)[a]
Fragile X syndrome (FRAXA)
Glucose-6-phosphate dehydrogenase
   deficiency
Glycogen storage disease, type VIII
Gonadal dysgenesis (XY female type)
Haemophilia A
Haemophilia B
Hydrocephalus (aqueduct stenosis type,
   sometimes known as MASA syndrome)
   (gene *L1CAM*)
Hypophosphataemic rickets

Ichthyosis (steroid sulphatase deficiency)
Incontinentia pigmenti[a]
Kallmann syndrome
Keratosis follicularis spinulosa
Lesch-Nyhan syndrome (hypoxanthine-
   guanine-phosphoribosyl transferase
   deficiency)
Lowe (oculocerebrorenal) syndrome
Macular dystrophy of the retina (one type)
Menkes syndrome
Mental retardation, without fragile site
   (numerous specific types)
Microphthalmia with multiple anomalies
   (Lenz syndrome)
Mucopolysaccharidosis II (Hunter
   syndrome)
Muscular dystrophy (Becker, Duchenne
   and Emery-Dreifuss types)
Myotubular (centronuclear) myopathy
   (one type)
Night blindness, congenital stationary
Norrie disease (pseudoglioma)
Nystagmus, oculomotor or 'jerky'
Ornithine carbamoyltransferase
   (transcarbamylase) deficiency (type I
   hyperammonaemia)
Orofaciodigital syndrome (type 1)[a]
Phosphoglycerate kinase deficiency
Phosphoribosylpyrophosphate (PRPP)
   synthetase deficiency
Reifenstein syndrome
Retinitis pigmentosa (can also be AR or AD)
Retinoschisis
Rett syndrome
Spastic paraplegia (one type)
Spinal muscular atrophy (one type)
Spondyloepiphyseal dysplasia tarda
Testicular feminisation syndrome
Thrombocytopenia, hereditary (one type)
Thyroxine-binding globulin, absence
Wiskott-Aldrich syndrome
Xg blood group system

---

[a] X-linked dominant, male lethal.

Although X-chromosome inactivation applies to most of the human X chromosome, there are loci where it does not apply. Such inactivation-exempt loci include those for the Xg blood group, steroid sulphatase and the *SHOX* gene, located in the terminal region of the X chromosome short arm, the pseudoautosomal region of Xp. Such loci are exempt from X-chromosome inactivation in females and have functioning Y homologues; they do not show 'dosage compensation' and are implicated as contributing to the phenotypes of the disorders of sex chromosome number, such as Turner (X0) syndrome, XXY and XXX, as there is no mechanism of dosage compensation.

The pseudoautosomal region of Xp has homology with part of the Y chromosome and is involved in pairing between the sex chromosomes at meiosis. The process of X inactivation is itself controlled by a different region of the X chromosome, the X-inactivation centre including the *Xist* locus on the proximal long arm. The Xist transcript does not encode a protein but functions as a large, non-coding RNA molecule.

Recognition of X-linked inheritance

Recognition of an X-linked pedigree pattern is crucial to correct genetic counselling and is surprisingly often overlooked. The following criteria apply regardless of whether the disorder is recessive, dominant or intermediate in expression (some examples are given in Figures 2.18–2.23). (Note that fragile X syndrome is an exception to some of these rules.)

- Male-to-male transmission never occurs, because a man does not pass his X chromosome to his son.
- All daughters of an affected male will receive the abnormal gene, i.e. they will all carry the disorder and some may show signs or be frankly affected.
- Unaffected males never transmit the disease to descendants of either sex. A notable but so far solitary exception to this is fragile X mental retardation (FRAXA) (see Chapter 15), where so-called normal transmitting (or 'carrier') males can carry a triplet repeat premutation.
- The risk to sons of women who are definite carriers (or affected in the case of an X-linked dominant) is one in two.
- Half the daughters of carrier women will themselves be carriers. In the case of an X-linked dominant, half the daughters of affected women will be affected and – in the general population – twice as many females as males will usually be affected.
- Fully affected females are unusual in X-linked recessive disorders but may occur (1) with a heavily skewed pattern of X inactivation, (2) in the presence of a cytogenetic anomaly, or (3) in a 'common' disorder, when an affected male marries a carrier female (see later section 'Common X-Linked Disorders').

These simple guidelines will cover most genetic counselling situations and will allow a definite decision to be made in most instances as to whether the disorder is X-linked or not. It can be seen that the situation is essentially similar for X-linked recessive and X-linked dominant disorders, the heterozygous women in the latter group being affected rather than simply 'carriers'. Apparent anomalies may be the result of chromosome disorders, (e.g. occurrence of the disease in a 45,X female [see Figure 2.18] or a female who carries an X;autosome translocation), or of non-paternity. Very few disease-related genes are located on the pairing (pseudoautosomal) parts of the X and Y chromosomes, giving an autosomal inheritance pattern in families. Some particular problems are shown in the following examples.

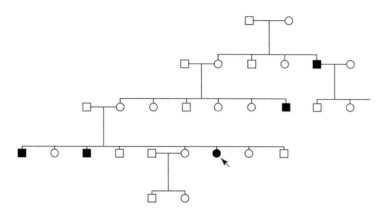

Figure 2.18 Where an affected girl is found to have a rare and clearly X-linked disorder, a sex chromosome abnormality such as Turner (45,X) syndrome should be considered. This proved to be the case in this family with X-linked cerebellar ataxia reported by Shokeir (1970). (I Complete trisomy 22. *Clin Genet* 1: 225–231.)

CLASSIC X-LINKED RECESSIVE PATTERN

Figure 2.19 shows this in a family with haemophilia A.

DISORDERS WHERE AFFECTED MALES DO NOT REPRODUCE

Figure 2.20 shows an example. This may result from the severity of the disease (e.g. Duchenne muscular dystrophy) or from infertility (e.g. Kallmann syndrome). Here the test of male-to-male transmission cannot be applied, so, unless one has other genetic data (e.g. the results of linkage analysis with nearby markers such as single nucleotide polymorphisms or occurrence in a 45,X female), X linkage is presumed rather than proven. The recognition of specific mutations or deletions in genes on the X chromosome is now providing direct proof in such cases.

X-LINKED DOMINANT INHERITANCE

Figure 2.21 shows an example. The pattern may at first glance be mistaken for autosomal dominant inheritance but, if the offspring of affected males are considered, all sons are unaffected and all daughters are affected. The excess of affected females can also be seen.

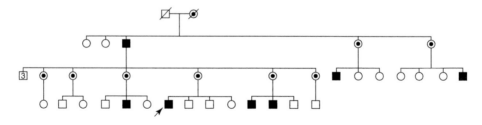

Figure 2.19 Typical X-linked recessive inheritance (haemophilia A). Note that all sons of an affected male are healthy, while all daughters are carriers. The disorder is transmitted by healthy females and is confined to males, but these features are less critical than the lack of male-to-male transmission in establishing or disproving X linkage.

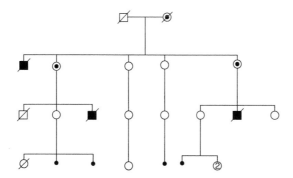

Figure 2.20 Presumed X-linked inheritance: Duchenne muscular dystrophy in a South Wales kindred. Although the disorder is confined to males and is transmitted by healthy females, as expected with X-linked recessive inheritance, the lack of reproduction by affected males means that the crucial test of lack of male-to-male transmission cannot be seen. Genetic linkage data and isolation of the gene have now confirmed X linkage.

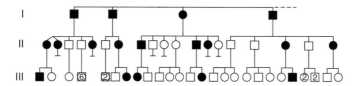

Figure 2.21 X-linked dominant inheritance in a family with familial hypophosphataemia (vitamin D-resistant rickets). The pattern is superficially similar to autosomal dominant inheritance; but when the offspring of affected males are considered it becomes clear that all daughters are affected, but that the disorder is never transmitted from father to son. (After McKusick VA. 1969. *Human Genetics*. London: Prentice Hall.)

'INTERMEDIATE' X-LINKED INHERITANCE

The blurred distinction between dominant and recessive in X-linked disease has already been mentioned. In a few conditions, heterozygotes may show the disease in one branch of a family, but not in another. Figure 2.22 shows an example of this. Although at first sight the pattern appears confusing, the situation is soon clarified if the offspring of affected males are considered – all sons are unaffected, while the females are either affected or carriers.

X-LINKED DOMINANT INHERITANCE WITH THE ABSENCE OF AFFECTED MALES

In a number of disorders, the condition is seen only in the heterozygous females, the affected (hemizygous) males being undetected or appearing as an excess of spontaneous abortions. It is difficult to prove this situation, but it has now been confirmed for several disorders, including focal dermal hypoplasia and incontinentia pigmenti but (in contrast to earlier ideas) does not apply to Rett syndrome.

Genetic counselling risk estimates in these circumstances require some care. Leaving aside spontaneous abortions, one-third of the offspring of an affected woman will be affected; all the live-born males will be unaffected, as will half of the females. Two-thirds of all offspring will be female. If the pattern of inheritance is clear but the mutation unknown, fetal sexing with termination of female pregnancies may be a possibility, at least in theory. Where an affected

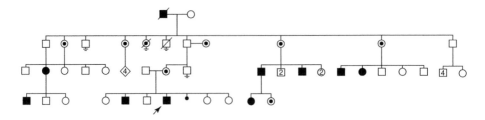

Figure 2.22 Intermediate X-linked inheritance: a South Wales kindred with hereditary oculomotor nystagmus. The pattern is recognised by examining the offspring of affected males. All sons are unaffected, but all daughters are either affected or proved to be carriers.

child has been born to healthy parents, this is likely to represent a new mutation and the recurrence risk is likely to be low (most such patients will be female).

Another reason for the absence of males in a disorder caused by dominant mutations in a gene on the X chromosome is when affected females do not reproduce and the mutational origin of the disease is predominantly at spermatogenesis, so that it almost always manifests in an affected female. This is the case in Rett syndrome, although males can be affected by this if they have Klinefelter syndrome (47,XXY) or if they are somatic mosaics for the causal *MECP2* mutation. A male with a *MECP2* gene mutation that would cause Rett syndrome in a female is usually affected by a substantially more severe, neonatal-onset encephalopathy without the period of apparently normal development for 6 months or more that is found in Rett syndrome. A similar but less marked preponderance of affected females can arise in other sex-linked disorders if the fertility of affected females is reduced and the origin of mutations is predominantly at spermatogenesis (as in craniofrontonasal dysplasia) but may also be postzygotic in mosaic females.

COMMON X-LINKED DISORDERS

Where an X-linked gene is common in a particular population, confusing pedigree patterns may be produced. This may be seen with red-green colour-blindness in European populations and with glucose-6-phosphate dehydrogenase deficiency in the Middle East and many parts of Asia. The marriage of affected males to heterozygous females is not infrequent and will result in homozygous females (see Figure 2.23), all of whose sons will be affected. A similar pattern can occasionally be seen with less common disorders when there is consanguinity.

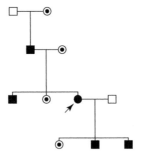

Figure 2.23 Occurrence of an affected homozygous female in a common X-linked recessive trait, red-green colour-blindness.

Risk of being a carrier for an X-linked disorder

Methods of carrier detection in X-linked disorders are discussed in Chapter 7, but it is clearly important to estimate the genetic risk of a female relative being a carrier, so that information from carrier testing (if any) can be appropriately combined with the risk from family structure (i.e. the risk from the pedigree). The estimation of these risks is not always easy and is one of the situations where a mathematical approach is needed in genetic counselling. Young's *Introduction to Risk Calculation* (see 'Further Reading') is strongly recommended for this and other areas of risk estimation.

Leaving aside the problems of new mutations, the situation can be approached as follows, using Figure 2.24 (the pedigree of a family with Duchenne muscular dystrophy) as an example:

1. Obligatory carriers should be identified – these are I-1 and II-2.
2. The prior genetic risk of the individual requiring advice, sometimes referred to as the 'consultand' (arrowed), should be estimated. Here it is one in four, since her mother's risk is one in two.
3. Other relevant information must be incorporated. Here the relevant fact is that the consultand has had two normal sons. Common sense tells us that this makes it less likely that she is a carrier – the question is, how much less likely? In fact, it can be estimated and combined with other information simply (using what is sometimes termed Bayes theorem) by multiplying it with the corresponding prior risk. This is best done by constructing a table, which gives the chances of the two possibilities, as shown in Table 2.3.

The prior risks are clearly one in four and three in four, respectively. The 'conditional' information resulting from the normal sons will give a chance of one in two for this happening once, if she is a carrier, and one in four (1/2 multiplied by 1/2 = 1/4) for both sons being normal if she is a carrier (three sons would give a risk of one in eight, and so on). The corresponding chance of two sons being normal if she is not a carrier is clearly one (100%) as the rate of new mutations is small and can be ignored.

The joint risk is then obtained by multiplying vertically 'down' the two columns. The two figures so obtained now give the relative risks for the two situations (the woman is or is not a carrier). These relative risks (also known as an 'odds ratio') are not the same as probabilities, as they do not sum to one; they must therefore be placed over the same denominator (giving 1/16 and 12/16), which means that she is 12 times more likely not to be a carrier than to be a carrier. This odds ratio (1:12) can be converted into true probabilities (that do add up to one) as she now has a 1 in 13 chance of being a carrier and a 12 in 13 chance of not being a carrier.

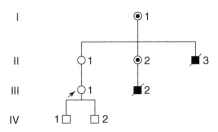

Figure 2.24 A family with Duchenne muscular dystrophy.

Table 2.3 A working table to combine risk information for the pedigree shown in Figure 2.24

	Consultand a carrier		Consultand not a carrier
Prior risk	1/4		3/4
Conditional risk (two normal sons)	$1/2 \times 1/2 (= 1/4)$		1
Joint risk	1/16		3/4 (= 12/16)
Relative risk (odds ratio)	1	:	12
Final risk	1/13		12/13

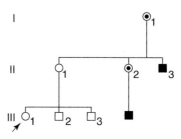

Figure 2.25 Carrier risks with an X-linked recessive disorder (Duchenne muscular dystrophy). See Table 2.4 for calculations.

Care must be taken to relate the 'conditional' information to the correct person. Thus, in Figure 2.25, showing another Duchenne family, the normal sons affect the chances of the mother of the consultand (II-1) being a carrier, and the risk must be worked out for her before proceeding to the daughter (III-1), whose prior risk (1 in 10) is half her mother's risk (one in five) (Table 2.4). If the daughter herself had normal sons, one could proceed as in the previous example but using the new prior risk of 1 in 10 as the starting point.

It can be seen that the use of genetic information in this way can substantially affect the risks given in genetic counselling, and in general with a methodical approach the estimations are not difficult. Incorporation of data from more distant relationships can become complex (computer programs are available to help), but rarely affects the risks to a great extent. It is important to recognise that not only genetic information may be used in this way, but also phenotypic data relevant to carrier detection, such as may be available in haemophilia and Duchenne muscular dystrophy. Some examples of this are given in Chapters 7 and 13.

Table 2.4 Risk calculations, X-linked recessive disorder

	Carrier		Not a carrier
Risks for II-1:			
Prior risk	1/2		1/2
Conditional risk	$1/2 \times 1/2 (= 1/4)$		1
Joint risk	1/8		1/2 (= 4/8)
Relative risk (odds)	1	:	4
Final risk	1/5		4/5
Prior risk for III-1	1/10		

Note: See also Figure 2.25.

A final caution should be given: because all these estimates are based on uncertainty, they may need to be modified in light of future events. Thus, the birth of an affected child to II-1 in Figure 2.25 would make her an obligatory carrier and all previous estimates would have to be discarded in light of this. Likewise, the increasing feasibility of direct gene analysis may be a reason for reassessment of risks in a family.

Isolated case of an X-linked disorder

In autosomal dominant inheritance, new mutations can usually be clearly distinguished from transmitted cases; in autosomal recessive disorders, mutation plays an insignificant part in relation to transmitted genes and can be ignored in genetic counselling. In X-linked recessive disorders, however, it may be extremely difficult, if not impossible, to tell whether an isolated case represents a new mutation or whether the mother is a carrier. Since an accurate distinction is essential for correct genetic counselling, this situation needs careful consideration.

When direct molecular genetic tests are available, or other reliable methods of carrier detection, then they should of course be used. However, caution may be needed if there is any doubt as to whether an identified genetic variant is responsible for the family's disorder. Furthermore, the resources required to establish the molecular genetic basis of inherited disorders are far from being available universally, so that clinicians will often need to remain familiar with simpler and more widely accessible approaches.

The variability of gene expression in heterozygotes for X-linked disease makes carrier detection difficult in a proportion of women, even when phenotypic tests exist. This is clearly seen in haemophilia A and Duchenne muscular dystrophy, where 20%–30% of known carriers show results of phenotypic carrier tests falling within normal limits (see Chapters 7 and 13).

The example shown in Figure 2.26 shows the practical aspects of the problem. Three possibilities exist to explain the occurrence of this isolated case of Duchenne muscular dystrophy:

- *The case III-1 is the result of a new mutation*: In this case none of the numerous female relatives is at significant risk of being a carrier, although there will be the low risk of maternal mosaicism in any subsequent sons born to II-1.
- *The mother II-1 is a carrier, but she is herself the result of a new mutation*: In this case, the daughters III-2 and III-3 are at 50% risk of being carriers, and their daughters IV-1

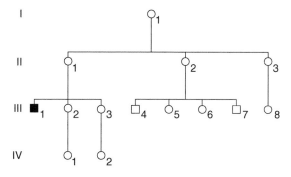

Figure 2.26 An isolated case of a lethal X-linked disorder: Duchenne muscular dystrophy. Is this a new mutation or not? See the text and following figures for the estimation of carrier risks in this difficult situation.

and IV-2 have a carrier risk of 25%. However, the risk for the other female relatives is very small, reflecting the very low risk of germ-line mosaicism in the father of II-1, the maternal grandfather of III-1.

- *The disorder has been transmitted through the mother from the grandmother I-1*: In this case, in addition to those already mentioned as being at risk, II-2 and II-3 are at 50% prior risk, with a carrier risk of 25% for their daughters III-5, III-6 and III-8.

Unfortunately, these three situations cannot always be distinguished with certainty by carrier testing based upon phenotype. In the absence of direct mutation testing, one needs to approach the problem as follows:

1. The prior risk of II-1 and I-1 being carriers as opposed to III-1 resulting from a new mutation must be estimated. From this, the prior risk of other family members such as II-2 and II-3 can be estimated.
2. Conditional information (from normal sons and carrier testing results) can be tabulated as shown in the previous examples.
3. These pieces of information can be combined to give a final risk, as already shown.

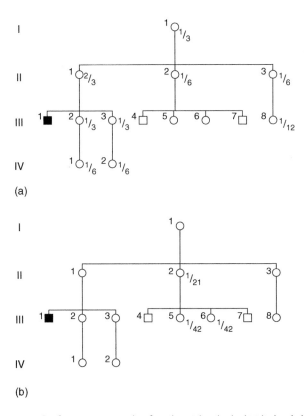

(a)

(b)

Figure 2.27 (a) Carrier risks for women in the family with a lethal X-linked disorder (Duchenne dystrophy) shown in Figure 2.26, assuming that a third of cases are due to a new mutation. (b) The same pedigree showing the modification of risks from the normal sons of II-2.

The difficult problem is to decide what is the prior risk that this isolated case has resulted from mutation or has been transmitted. It has long been assumed that for an isolated case of an X-linked recessive disorder in which affected males do not reproduce and where mutation rates in egg and sperm are equal, the proportions are as follows:

- New mutation (mother not carrier): 1/3
- Transmitted case (mother carrier but not grandmother): 1/3
- Transmitted case (mother and grandmother carriers): 1/3

The derivation of this will not be given here but, using this information, one can readily assign risks to the various women in the family, as shown in Figure 2.27a. In Figure 2.27b the information from the normal sons of II-3 has also been incorporated, and it can be seen that the risks of III-5 and III-6 have been considerably lowered by the normal brothers. Carrier testing results would have produced further information which has been omitted for simplicity.

Unfortunately, there is considerable uncertainty as to whether the formula given earlier is generally applicable; it assumes equal mutation rates in the sexes, and in some disorders a higher proportion of mothers of isolated cases are carriers than the two-thirds expected, as is also the case for disorders where the affected males reproduce, such as in cases of haemophilia and Becker muscular dystrophy. In the absence of other information, it is wise to assume that such a woman is a carrier rather than the reverse. For Duchenne dystrophy, the situation may vary according to whether the change is a deletion or a point mutation. Fortunately, molecular tests are increasingly able to distinguish new mutations, although the relatively frequent occurrence of mosaicism, especially in Duchenne muscular dystrophy, still provides problems for genetic counselling in the isolated case, as noted further in Chapter 13.

MITOCHONDRIAL INHERITANCE

While mitochondrial inheritance cannot be described in any sense as Mendelian, it seems appropriate to describe it in this chapter, since it provides a characteristic pattern of transmission within families that must be compared with the equally distinctive patterns of Mendelian transmission as previously described. The increasing identification of specific mitochondrial mutations makes it especially important to recognise this form of inheritance, which has major implications for genetic counselling.

The mitochondria are the principal cell components outside the nucleus to contain DNA, which is present in the form of a small, circular genome that can replicate and which is quite independent of the mechanisms controlling chromosomal DNA. The usual sequence of the mitochondrial genome is known, as are many disease-associated mutations and the extensive variation within the (rather small) non-coding region, of value in studies on population history (including migration and ancestry). As well as the various RNAs required for protein synthesis, the mitochondrial genome determines the proteins of a series of key enzymes involved in oxidative phosphorylation, although other such enzymes are also produced by genes in the nucleus. Mitochondrial DNA is, for practical purposes, exclusively maternal in origin, with no process involving recombination and a negligible contribution from sperm.

It is most important to maintain a clear distinction between mitochondrial disease and mitochondrial inheritance. The former may result from mutations in the mitochondrial genome but may also be (and more commonly is) the result of gene mutations in the nuclear genome, when they are transmitted as a Mendelian disorder (autosomal recessive, autosomal dominant or sex linked).

It has long been recognised that any disorder following mitochondrial inheritance should be exclusively maternal in its transmission, as shown in Figure 2.28. While a number of individual families with differing disorders have in the past been claimed to fit the pattern, one disorder in particular, Leber hereditary optic neuropathy (LHON) (a.k.a. Leber optic atrophy), has consistently done so and has been predicted to be mitochondrial in origin, a conclusion now fully confirmed by the identification of mutations in the mitochondrial genome. Figure 2.29 shows a typical family with this disorder, and can be used, together with the preceding diagram, to summarise the general risks for family members relevant to genetic counselling, as follows. (Details specific for Leber optic atrophy are given in Chapter 19.)

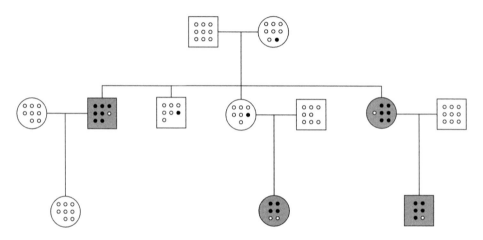

Figure 2.28 Mitochondrial inheritance (schematic pedigree): normal mitochondria, ∘; abnormal mitochondria, •. Since mitochondria are transmitted only through the ovum, not through sperm, affected individuals (shaded) are related through the maternal line. Whether an individual is clinically affected may reflect the proportion of abnormal mitochondria in the relevant tissue.

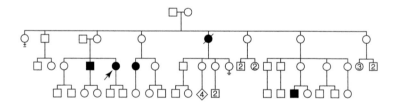

Figure 2.29 A family pedigree of a mitochondrial disorder: Leber optic atrophy. All the affected individuals are related in the maternal line; no male family members, affected or unaffected, have transmitted the disorder. It can be seen that there are numerous females in the pedigree who are potentially at risk of developing or transmitting the disorder, as well as males who can be reassured that they have no significant risk of transmitting it, whether or not they themselves are or become affected.

- No transmission occurs to children or other descendants of males, whether they are affected or not. Nor are such descendants at risk of being gene carriers, a situation that contrasts with X linkage, where all daughters of an affected male are obligatory carriers.
- Both sexes may be affected, the precise sex ratio being dependent on the particular disorder and probably determined by other genetic and environmental factors. In Leber optic atrophy, males are more commonly affected in Europe but not in Japan.
- Females may be symptomless carriers (so may males, but this is irrelevant as they cannot transmit their mitochondria). All daughters of an affected or carrier female are themselves at risk of transmitting the disorder, as well as of becoming affected, while all sons are at risk of becoming affected but not of transmitting the condition.
- The precise proportion of offspring, male or female, who will become affected is variable (in Leber optic atrophy this is around 50% of sons and 30% of daughters) and not determined by any fixed rule.

It can be seen from this summary that the recognition of mitochondrial inheritance is extremely satisfactory for the genetic counselling of males since, whether or not they are affected, a confident reassurance can be given that their descendants will not be. For females the situation is unsatisfactory in the extreme, since there is some degree of risk to all offspring with none of the sharp demarcations and exclusions that are possible in Mendelian inheritance.

The identification of specific defects in mitochondrial DNA, both point mutations and large deletions, and the realisation that such disorders are much more frequent than previously suspected, has been a major advance. Box 2.2 lists some of the more important of these, although they may be thought of more as symptom clusters than distinct diagnostic entities. Not all have a clearly defined phenotype, and the finding that subgroups of such common and heterogeneous disorders as diabetes and deafness may have an underlying mitochondrial defect raises the question as to when a molecular basis for such conditions should be sought. It should be noted, in particular, that there are only genetic implications if the molecular defect is present in the germ line (more likely to be the case if found in DNA from a blood sample), not if the defect is confined to the target organ (e.g. muscle). The distinction between mutations that may be present in essentially all of a patient's mitochondria (homoplasmy), and those that can only be present in a proportion (heteroplasmy), is also important. Substantial deletions of

---

BOX 2.2: Disorders resulting from mutations of the mitochondrial DNA/chromosome

Leber hereditary optic neuropathy (LHON) also known as Leber optic atrophy

MELAS (mitochondrial encephalopathy with lactic acidosis and stroke-like episodes)

MERFF (myoclonic epilepsy with ragged red fibres)

Kearns-Sayre syndrome (large deletions of the mitochondrial chromosome)

Pearson syndrome (lactic acidosis, pancreatic insufficiency, pancytopenia)

Deafness (antibiotic-induced and some forms of progressive nerve deafness)

Leigh syndrome (subacute encephalopathy, often with lactic acidosis; some cases)

Various poorly classified central nervous system degenerations

Diabetes mellitus (some familial types)

the mitochondrial DNA are only found in the heteroplasmic state as they would otherwise be lethal, whereas many point mutations may be heteroplasmic or homoplasmic.

It might be thought that once a molecular mitochondrial defect has been identified in a family, analysis of relatives at risk would help to resolve the genetic counselling problems described. Unfortunately, this is not the case at all, since all those genetically at risk are likely to show at least some degree of the defect, often showing heteroplasmy for the mutation. There is only a weak relationship between the proportion of abnormal mitochondria found (in blood) and the risk of developing or transmitting one of these disorders, though their apparent absence would suggest a low risk.

The proportion of abnormal mitochondria may differ substantially between tissues, and may change over time within one tissue, with the proportion of abnormal mitochondria increasing in some areas more than others, perhaps as a maladaptive response to hypoxic stress. Tests are also inconclusive in prenatal diagnosis for a similar reason, with an added element of randomness from the effect of a bottleneck phase followed by a subsequent expansion in the mitochondria of the ovum leading to marked differences in the proportion of abnormal mitochondria between generations. The absence of the mutant line in a prenatal sample also seems likely to indicate a lower risk, but experience is too limited to give accurate figures (including confidence intervals) that would apply to specific circumstances.

The conclusion at present must therefore be that, while the recognition of mitochondrial inheritance by pedigree pattern and molecular analysis is important in identifying genetic risks and in removing risk from descendants in the male line, it is unhelpful in resolving the situation for those known to be at risk. Caution is required before molecular tests are offered to asymptomatic relatives, who should understand the limitations of testing. Experimental methods using IVF-based technologies have been developed in several countries that promise to enable a female carrier of a disorder of the mitochondrial genome to transmit her egg's nucleus to a child without her mitochondria, using a donor's oocyte cytoplasm instead. Such methods may turn out to be effective but will have the usual disadvantage of IVF procedures including the poor chance of success in each cycle; the physical, emotional and financial burdens; and perhaps the small extra risk of imprinting disorders in the child.

Looking to the future, the hope must be that effective therapeutic agents enhancing mitochondrial function will be developed that can be applied to those at risk before serious and irreversible clinical problems occur.

The final point to be re-emphasised is that many mitochondrial enzymes are determined by nuclear genes. Thus, a mitochondrial disorder does not necessarily imply mitochondrial inheritance. Confusingly, some families demonstrate autosomal dominant inheritance of a disorder of replication of the mitochondrial genome, leading to variable deletions in the mitochondrial DNA. As a result, there do exist nuclear-encoded disorders of the mitochondrial genome (e.g. *POLG*).

3

Common disorders and genetic counselling

INTRODUCTION

The disorders to be considered here, in contrast to most Mendelian conditions, will be encountered frequently by those working in all branches of medicine and in primary care. The common European definition of a rare disease is given, arbitrarily, as a population frequency of those affected being no greater than 1 in 2,000 (i.e. a prevalence of no greater than 0.05%, or 5 in 10,000). There can be some debate as to which disorders this includes, especially with late-onset disorders or those of reduced penetrance, but in general the distinction is clear enough for practical purposes. Any disorder with a higher prevalence, or a higher incidence at birth, will be regarded as 'common'.

Most common disorders do not follow any of the clear patterns of Mendelian inheritance outlined in Chapter 2. This applies not only to the more common birth defects (e.g. neural tube defects, congenital heart disease) but also to most common chronic disorders of later life (e.g. asthma, diabetes, hypertension, coronary heart disease, stroke, the common cancers). Yet it has long been recognised that, to some degree, these conditions show a familial tendency, which may occasionally be striking. As a result, families in which such common disorders occur often seek genetic counselling, especially if multiple members have been affected. The recent general increase in awareness of genetic factors, often heightened by media attention, has increased this tendency, notably in the case of cancer. We consider chromosome disorders elsewhere, although some (especially Down syndrome and some of the sex chromosome anomalies) have a higher birth incidence, in the absence of prenatal screening programmes.

The fact that many of these disorders are so common, at least by comparison with the Mendelian disorders that form the basis of activity for most specialists in medical genetics, creates special challenges. It is quite clear that most genetic counselling for this group must, of necessity, be provided by workers in primary care or those involved directly in disease management, since the sheer numbers would swamp the small number of available specialist clinical geneticists and genetic counsellors.

Until recently, this has proved in practice to be much less of a problem than might have been expected, partly because the risk figures are often simple and approximate, partly because for most common diseases the demand for genetic counselling is very much less in proportion to their frequency than is the case for single gene disorders. There has been a recent change in this, however, as it is becoming both clinically important and practically feasible to identify Mendelian genes that contribute to important subsets of patients among those with common disorders. Clinical genetics services operate on much too small a scale to take on the task of first identifying and then addressing the needs of these Mendelian subsets within the common disease groups, where the application of molecular genetic investigations has such a lot to offer.

As discussed further later in this chapter, important examples of Mendelian subsets 'concealed' within much larger groups of patients are found in those affected by ischaemic heart disease (coronary artery disease, CAD), breast cancer and colorectal cancer. The clinical management of the patient with a relevant, pathogenic mutation (e.g. in *LDLR*, for familial hypercholesterolaemia, or in *BRCA1* or *BRCA2* for a patient with breast cancer) may be altered by this knowledge, and the active management of (so far) healthy family members becomes possible, so that cascade testing of family members at risk can be very helpful in either disease prevention or the early diagnosis and better treatment of disease complications. More is said about these possibilities later and in the relevant disease-related chapters.

This ability to dissect out high-risk Mendelian subsets from the larger group of those with 'common' disorders is a recent development and presents real challenges for the organisation of health services. The range of medical specialties impacted by these developments is widening; it began with oncology and now includes cardiology, endocrinology/diabetes and other specialties. (Neurology has long had a close relationship with genetics, but this has, until recently, largely involved rare diseases.) 'Mainstreaming' of the genetic aspects of the common conditions – the application of genetics to disease management not by genetic specialists but by a general physician or the relevant organ specialist – is inevitable. However, clinical genetics services can promote good practice through collaboration with these specialties. Support for the nongenetics specialist may take many forms such as education, multidisciplinary team meetings to discuss cases and genetic testing (even when the patients or family members are not seen together by the different specialists) and the holding of joint clinics. Each of these approaches will be appropriate in different circumstances, but limited resources may restrict the intensity of joint working.

Genetic testing for Mendelian subsets of the common disorders has proved fruitful in clinical practice, both for the high-risk Mendelian contexts and also for reassurance and the avoidance of unnecessary interventions in family members at low (i.e. population) risk. Apart from this search for genes of major effect, however, genetic testing to produce a 'polygenic risk score' to estimate a person's degree of susceptibility to common disorders has – so far – little or no clinical utility and has not been taken up by health services. It has been suggested that this could be useful in risk stratification within population screening programmes (e.g. screening by mammography for breast cancer), but this is based on a very selective interpretation of the available data (Janssens and Joyner, 2019). An important recent paper argues persuasively that these attempts to over-interpret the potential applicability of polygenic risk scores based on genome-wide association studies (GWAS) are grounded in a persistent but fundamental misunderstanding of the distribution of genetic risk (Wald and Old, 2019).

The available evidence suggests that there is little if any utility in assessing a person's genetic susceptibility to common disease in making lifestyle choices and adopting healthier habits and behaviours; there is even a potential for paradoxical behavioural responses, based on unwarranted feelings of invulnerability if one's risk is said to be below average or fatalism if one's risk is graded as above the population average.

GENETIC BASIS OF COMMON DISORDERS

The terms 'multifactorial' or 'polygenic' are frequently used to describe the genetic basis underlying the great majority of common disorders where there is no clear Mendelian pattern. Of the two terms, multifactorial is the more appropriate since it recognises that these disorders are the result of both environmental and genetic factors and does not prejudge the relative role of either category. 'Polygenic' means that many different genetic loci are involved, and usually implies that there is a very large number of such factors involved, each being of very small effect, and that their influences combine in a straightforward fashion. In fact, for many diseases where the 'genetic architecture' of disease susceptibility has been examined, there is rather a spectrum of genetic factors ranging from rare genetic variants of large effect, through a moderate number of genetic variants of lesser but still substantial effect (sometimes known as 'oligogenes'), to a multitude of genetic variants of small or very small effect. Very little is known about the way these factors interact. It is often simply assumed that they interact in regular, predictable patterns (with relative risks being combined multiplicatively, as if they were independent) because the research that would be needed to measure the complex interactions between the different factors would be so demanding.

Another approach to discussing these disorders, that usefully emphasises the likely complexity of the interactions among the genetic factors and between the genetic and the environmental factors, is to use the term 'common, complex disorder'. The relevant genetic variants involved can include specific alleles of known loci, variation within the non-coding or even non-genic DNA, and larger-scale phenomena such as deletions or duplications, collectively known as copy number variants (CNVs).

The term 'heritability' is often encountered in relation to common disorders and refers to the proportion of variation of all types, familial and other, that is determined by genetic factors, regardless of any pattern of inheritance. This can be assessed by a number of approaches, notably the comparison of monozygotic and dizygotic twin pairs where at least one twin has the disorder. The heritability will be one of the factors influencing recurrence risk in a family, along with the extent to which family members share their environment as well as their genes.

The general principles of the genetics of common disease were worked out more than 50 years ago by pioneers such as Haldane, Penrose and Edwards, and remain relevant today, but our growing ability to recognise specific genes and genetic variants involved with common disorders, described later in this and the next chapter, has allowed two main categories to be defined, as follows:

- Common disorders containing a significant Mendelian subset, resulting from the action of a single major gene in a family.
- Common disorders where a number of genetic (and usually also environmental) factors are involved, each usually being of small or, at most, modest influence.

From the viewpoint of genetic counselling it is essential, whenever possible, to distinguish between these two situations, which are often completely different in terms of the risk estimates involved.

Mendelian subsets

This group is of particular importance in genetic counselling because the recognition of a Mendelian (usually dominant) subset of cases gives extremely high risks for family members (or very low risk if the particular gene variant can be excluded). The familial cancers provide a striking example, becoming increasingly recognised over the past 15 years. Although rare familial cancer syndromes have been recognised for many years (e.g. familial adenomatous polyposis coli as a cause of colon cancer), the identification of Mendelian forms of breast and colon cancer that are not phenotypically distinct from the non-Mendelian majority has had a major influence on both research and genetic counselling practice in these disorders, influences now extending to most common cancers (see Part 3 for details). It is no longer sufficient in assessing risks to derive overall theoretical risks, as was done in early editions of this book, since the separation of the Mendelian forms will affect the recurrence risks for those remaining. This dissection of the multifactorial basis of common diseases is not confined to cancer but has become relevant to a wide range of conditions where previously unsuspected or undefined Mendelian families are proving to account for a significant proportion of recurrent cases. Where those affected are less likely to reproduce, as in many neurodevelopmental and psychiatric disorders, de novo mutations within single genes, or de novo CNVs, can account for a substantial proportion of cases.

The distinction between these categories of common disorders, those with and without substantial Mendelian subsets, is of course not always clear. Two disorders in which variants at an autosomal recessive locus contribute susceptibility to a disease without 'causing' it are discussed later: both haemochromatosis (the *HFE* gene) and the lung disease associated with α-1-antitrypsin (A1AT) deficiency (the *SERPINA1* gene). These can be regarded as autosomal recessive susceptibility states for iron overload and for chronic lung disease, respectively.

Genetic contribution to multifactorial disorders

In the second group, where clear Mendelian forms are absent or very rare, some of the genetic factors primarily responsible for the genetic influence on the disorders are now also beginning to be identified. Much research originally focussed on the HLA region of chromosome 6, long known to be a susceptibility locus for a variety of disorders with an immunological basis, and it remains much the strongest and best-documented susceptibility locus, even after more than two decades of analysing wider genetic markers.

The past two decades have seen intense research efforts into identifying other genetic components, utilising the existence of DNA markers across the whole genome and building on the striking success in mapping genes for Mendelian disorders. Unfortunately, this important but difficult procedure was initially often approached with considerable naïveté and many of the early claims were not substantiated. In the last decade, the use of GWAS based on single nucleotide polymorphism (SNP) microarray and, more recently, high-throughput sequencing techniques has proved more fruitful in identifying genes, chromosomal regions and functional molecular pathways likely to be involved, but it must be emphasised that these remain mostly at the research stage, and that there may be substantial variation in the frequency and effects of specific variants between populations. At present, virtually none of the identified factors is sufficiently strong or reproducible for use in clinical practice or genetic counselling, although tests based on weak evidence have been made available commercially where the regulatory authorities have failed to demand proof of test validity or clinical utility. While for some common disorders (and, indeed, for variation in many quantitative traits within the normal range), the genetic component results from a large number of individually small genetic effects, for other disorders (and traits) there will be a spectrum from rare variants of major effect through the oligogenes of substantial effect size to the many variants of individually small effect.

A third type of genetic involvement in common disease requires a mention, although its importance outside the field of common cancers is not clear. This is where a specific gene variant, relatively rare in the population, has a moderate effect, insufficient to cause much familial clustering but still significant in its contribution to the overall causation of the disorder. Examples are seen in some types of cancer and in some congenital malformations, such as Hirschsprung disease. So far, we know of few such cases where testing has clinical utility.

It must be emphasised strongly that the finding that a particular gene is involved in a common disorder does not convert the disorder (or even a subset of it) into a Mendelian disorder. There are many examples of DNA sequence variants that are highly significantly associated with disease but where the effect is actually very weak (e.g. giving a relative risk of disease of 1:1.01 or 1:1.02). Of course, the gene itself will show Mendelian segregation at the DNA level (it cannot do otherwise), but it is the disease phenotype that is relevant in terms of Mendelian inheritance. This may seem an obvious point, but it continues to be ignored by many who should know much better.

Perception and genetic basis of common disease

For clear-cut single gene disorders, there is rarely much doubt in the minds of professionals or the public that one is dealing with a 'genetic disorder', where environmental aspects are subsidiary to the inherited factor. For most common disorders, by contrast, the situation is far less clear, even though studies may have clearly identified an important genetic component. To a considerable extent, the perception of a disorder as 'genetic' or 'environmental' will depend on how successful workers have been in identifying specific contributory factors; new discoveries may result in a radical change in perception – and in demand for genetic counselling.

Consider these two examples:

- Peptic ulcer was regarded for many years as a largely genetic condition, with important familial influences, and with a large body of research on its genetic basis. Once an infective agent was identified, the genetic aspects rapidly became overshadowed and most people would now consider it as having a primarily environmental (indeed, infectious) cause, with relatively little demand for genetic counselling.
- Conversely, in breast cancer, genetic factors were considered of little relevance outside a few striking families until the *BRCA* genes were identified, which produced a rapid change in perception so that this is now often seen as a mainly 'genetic' disorder, despite the fact that these genes are responsible for only a small proportion of cases overall. There has also been an effect of celebrity status; when a celebrity discusses her family history, genetic test result and decision about prophylactic surgery in the media, there can be a substantial impact on demand for genetic counselling and testing. Such instances may disrupt service plans made on the basis of the anticipated demand but, in the long run, probably help to improve access to genetics services for the whole of society.

In both contexts, the underlying facts and the balance between genetic and environmental factors have not changed at all, but there has been a major shift in public and medical perception, reflected in the demand for, and uptake of, genetics services.

BOX 3.1: Common disorders and Mendelian subsets

Mendelian subset frequent (~5% of all cases)
Breast cancer
Colorectal cancer
Prostate cancer (shared origin with breast and ovarian cancer in some families)

Mendelian subset not frequent (~1%) but significant
Coronary heart disease (familial hypercholesterolaemia)
Early-onset Alzheimer's disease
Most other cancers (data still uncertain)

Mendelian subset rare or absent (<1%)
Schizophrenia
Bipolar affective disorder
Asthma
Late-onset Alzheimer's disease
Stroke

Since these perceptions and the underlying science can change so rapidly, as has happened with the familial cancers, it can be asked whether a sudden increase in demand might be seen for other types of common disease. The field where this effect seems to be most substantial is that of cardiovascular disease (see Chapter 21), where the recognition of Mendelian forms of coronary heart disease, the cardiomyopathies and the familial arrhythmias is having a major impact on cardiologists and affected families. By contrast other large groups of disease, such as the major psychoses, asthma and stroke, show few high-risk aggregations and create relatively little demand for genetic counselling (see Box 3.1).

A final factor is that the degree to which a condition is seen as genetic may reflect the frequency of the environmental factors involved, and these may vary over time or between populations. Thus, for rare infectious disorders, contact with the agent itself will be the determining factor in most cases, while, if the infectious agent is ubiquitous, genetic susceptibility will have the most influence.

GENERAL RULES FOR 'MULTIFACTORIAL' INHERITANCE (COMPLEX CAUSATION)

Since research for most common disorders is still at an early stage in resolving the number and nature of the genes involved, it is this second 'multifactorial' group where it is helpful to have some general rules that will influence risk prediction and genetic counselling. These are summarised here, but it must be recognised that they will need to be considerably modified when the specific genes involved become clear, or once Mendelian subgroups are identified.

The essential distinguishing factor from the Mendelian disorders is that a single genetic locus cannot be held responsible for the condition; it is the result of the additive effects or interactions of a number of genetic loci and often a number of external factors. The net result of these factors and interactions determines a person's liability to be affected with the particular disorder, and this liability can be expected to show a more or less 'normal' distribution curve in the population, with most people having an intermediate degree of liability and smaller

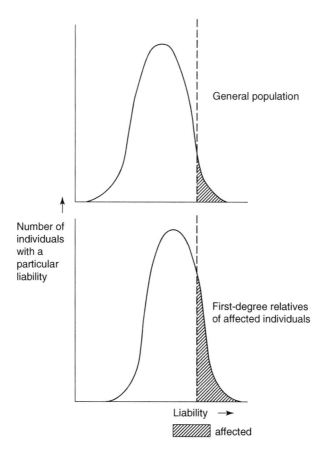

Figure 3.1 Liability and genetic risks in multifactorial inheritance. The distribution of liability to the disorder in the general population follows an approximately normal distribution, with individuals exceeding a certain threshold value being affected. First-degree relatives have a similar normal distribution of liability, but the curve is shifted to the right by the increased genetic component, so a greater proportion will exceed the threshold and be affected.

numbers at each end of the distribution curve having unusually low or unusually high liability (Figure 3.1). The last group comprises those who are actually affected, whose liability is above a postulated 'threshold' for the disorder.

From this concept, it can be seen that even a person with an unusually high genetic liability may not be affected if environmental factors are favourable, and the converse will also apply. The degree to which liability is determined by genetic factors as opposed to environmental factors is often considered as the heritability of a disorder, although in practice familial but non-genetic factors may often be included in this. The liability of relatives of a patient with the disorder will also be normally distributed in a similar way to that of the general population, but the curve will be shifted towards higher liability because of the increased genetic component.

The 'threshold model' is not always required for the operation of multifactorial inheritance; for quantitatively distributed variables such as height or blood pressure, the same principles apply. It should also be noted that only a small number of genetic loci (as few as four or five) are required for the discrete patterns of Mendelian inheritance to be transformed into a relatively smooth curve of distribution of liability.

BOX 3.2: Multifactorial inheritance: Factors increasing risk to relatives

Close relationship to proband
High heritability of disorder
Proband of more rarely affected sex
Severe or early-onset disease in proband
Multiple family members affected

Turning to the practical aspects, the following points are relevant (summarised in Box 3.2):

- Increased risk is greatest among the closest relatives and decreases rapidly with distance of relationship. It is rare to find a significant increase in risk for relatives more distant than second degree; even here risks are usually small.
- The risk of recurrence will depend on the incidence of the disorder, unlike in Mendelian inheritance. A useful approximation where specific figures are not available is that the maximum risk to first-degree relatives is approximately the square root of the incidence; i.e. where the population incidence is 1 in 100, the recurrence risk to the sib or child of an affected individual would be around 1 in 10.
- Dominance and recessivity do not generally apply. Thus, the risk for sibs is comparable to that for offspring. Risks for offspring are not yet available for many serious childhood disorders but can usually be taken as approximately equivalent to the risks for sibs in the absence of further information, unless there is evidence of a significant proportion of isolated cases being the result of new dominant mutations. (We are becoming increasingly aware of parental germ-line mosaicism for a dominant disorder as the reason for recurrence of a Mendelian diagnosis, whereas in the past, the presence of two affected sibs with neither parent affected might have been taken as presumptive evidence of autosomal recessive inheritance.) This is becoming recognised more frequently in autism, schizophrenia and Hirschprung disease. The risk to sibs will be minimal while the risks to offspring will be high (equivalent to half the penetrance). Clearly, it is especially important in this context not to miss a Mendelian subset. Indeed, as more exome and genome sequencing is performed, the number of patients with a 'complex' disorder in whom a plausibly causal new mutation is identified will increase. It will be important to review and revise empiric recurrence risk estimates in light of this emerging information. However, it will also be important to base risk estimates on unbiased estimates of penetrance: the genotype frequency must not be equated with the disease incidence without very good evidence.
- Where there is an unequal sex incidence, the risk is higher for relatives of a patient of the sex in which the condition is less common. For example, in pyloric stenosis (which is more common in males) the risk for brothers of a male index case is 3.8%, but for brothers of a female index case it is 9.2% (see Chapter 23). At first sight this may seem unexpected, but when it is considered that girls require a greater genetic liability to develop the disorder than do boys, it can readily be seen that relatives of an affected girl will also have a greater genetic liability than where the index case is a boy.
- The risk may be greater when the disorder is more severe. This is well shown in Hirschprung disease, where the risk for sibs of patients with long-segment disease is greater than for those with a short segment affected (see Chapter 23). Again, the greater severity reflects greater

liability, part of which will be genetic and thus shared with relatives. For disorders of adult life, early onset in the proband will increase the risk for relatives (as in breast cancer). In part, this effect may result from inclusion of unrecognized Mendelian cases in these severe or early-onset groups.

- The risk is increased when multiple family members are affected. This again results from the concentration of genetic liability in the particular family and is in contrast to the Mendelian situation where the number of affected family members (leaving aside new mutation) is irrelevant. The influence of more distant relatives is less easy to determine, although computer programs have been developed to combine the information. In general, one close (first-degree) relative outweighs several distant ones. Particular care must be taken in such families to be as certain as possible that one is not dealing with a Mendelian subtype of the disorder.

EMPIRICAL RISK DATA

This term, already mentioned in Chapter 1, is merely a statement of the fact that someone has actually looked at what happens in a particular (and recurrent) situation. Data on the risks to relatives are available for a large number of non-Mendelian disorders and, provided the study has been careful and as far as possible unbiased, such information provides the most satisfactory basis for counselling until the genetic basis can be resolved further. It has to be remembered, however, as stated in Chapter 1, that such risk figures are not universal in their application in the same way as Mendelian ratios. In particular:

- Data collected on one population may not be applicable to others where the incidence, and perhaps aetiology, of the disorder in terms of both genetic and environmental factors are different.
- Improved classification of disorders, in particular the resolution of heterogeneity, identification of single gene subsets, or identification of specific causative factors, may require radical revision of risk estimates (especially for some categories of patients).
- Risk estimates may need to be revised when the incidence of disease in a population changes. Ideally, the empiric studies that established the original empiric risk figures will be repeated, but this may not happen often enough, so that revised estimates have to be used with caution as they may lack a firm foundation. The incidence of neural tube defects in South Wales has fallen very substantially (from the 1% of some decades ago) and so a lower recurrence risk figure is now used.
- Risks may depend not only on the diagnosis but also on individual factors such as sex, severity of disease and number of affected family members.

Empirical risk figures are given for as many disorders as possible in the specific chapters of this book. Most are based on old, though thorough, studies, so there is a need for new data of this type using revised diagnostic criteria. In particular, molecular advances have removed or reclassified some cases as Mendelian, so it is difficult to know how this may have affected the risk estimates for those cases where no molecular defect can be detected. Unfortunately, empirical risk studies are now regarded as 'old-fashioned', so there is both a need for and a lack of new data.

As we become more familiar with the results of genome-wide diagnostic studies, both the need for, and the difficulty of, phenotypic studies of penetrance and expressivity will be increasingly recognised: the new, molecularly informed phenotyping will incorporate the new science of molecular genomics as well as epigenetics and the analysis of gene-environment and gene-gene interaction in humans.

MOLECULAR BASIS OF GENETIC SUSCEPTIBILITY

The way in which isolation of specific genes has increased our understanding of Mendelian disease has already been mentioned. The effects on our understanding of common disorders are now also having a major impact, especially where single gene subsets are identified, and this forms one of the most exciting areas of current medical research. It has to be conceded that epidemiological and other approaches to detecting the environmental components have, for most disorders (with a few exceptions such as neural tube defects), been disappointing; thus the value of current genetic research is not so much that it shows a greater importance of genetic factors in common disorders but that it is starting to provide knowledge of their pathogenesis, which is equally relevant to the external factors. Colorectal cancer again provides an excellent example, with the series of tumour suppressor genes identified providing defined points on which environmental carcinogens can act. In diabetes mellitus, the identification of different susceptibility genes in types 1 and 2 reinforces the role of different external factors – predominantly infective and immunological in type 1 and nutritional in type 2. In contrast, the identification of many of the same genetic factors as increasing susceptibility to schizophrenia and bipolar disease on the one hand, and schizophrenia and autism on the other hand, are leading to the generation of theories that seek to unify our understanding of these conditions.

These advances are likely to have major consequences for how we classify diseases and, in the future, how we approach therapy, which may well need different agents according to the underlying genetic changes.

When it comes to using genetic susceptibility tests in risk prediction and genetic counselling, however, their use is at present of minimal value and potentially of considerable harm. Unfortunately, this has not deterred unscrupulous commercial interests from promoting the use of such tests, increasingly via the internet, in situations where the factual basis is minimal or non-existent. However, some efforts have been made by the U.S. Food and Drug Administration to enforce appropriate standards, and European bodies are looking at the scope for regulation or legislation to play a helpful role. Regulators should require that the basis on which risk estimates are derived from molecular results is explicit and defensible. The scientific basis of risk estimates applied to individuals, as opposed to large series, is generally very uncertain, with wide margins of error. Furthermore, the mechanisms through which the impact of specific genetic variants is modified by interaction with other genetic variants, environmental factors and population differences, remain largely obscure, so that any attempted calculation to assess these effects is likely to be based upon the unproven assumptions underlying the simplest of models. Even the strongest associations (e.g. between HLA B27 and ankylosing spondylitis) are far from definitive (see Chapter 16); although a normal result in a suspected patient may make the condition very unlikely, an 'abnormal' result in a healthy relative at risk is still much more likely to be associated with normality than with clinical disease. Most associations (e.g. ApoE4 and Alzheimer's disease) are much less strong and consequently of little use in genetic counselling while, as mentioned earlier, the great majority of associations with particular genes or polymorphisms either fail to be confirmed, are of uncertain significance or give only slight risk alteration.

The harm that can result from the misapplication to particular individuals of such population-based research tools is of two broad types. First, in general terms, they are likely to create needless worry without being able to resolve it. Second, and more specifically, some of those who seek out such tests are likely to have a family history of affected relatives and will unwittingly be using the commercial test they access as a substitute for a thorough clinical genetic assessment. This reliance on an inappropriate technology may give highly misleading results because these tests will often not detect many of the dominant mutations in relevant genes but only SNPs of small, very small or no effect at all. An individual could have a 'somewhat low' (i.e. mildly reassuring) risk of disease on a SNP panel while carrying a mutation known to be pathogenic in a Mendelian gene that would only be detected by full sequencing of that gene. Such false reassurance could lead individuals who are actually at high risk to decide not to seek a thorough assessment, and so they will be denied the opportunity to identify their actual, greatly increased, risk of disease which might have prompted them, if they had known it, to consider effective disease prophylaxis or surveillance.

In summary, the main aims of genetic counselling for common disorders at present remain the identification (and exclusion) of the high-risk genetic subsets, along with the provision of risk estimates based on empirical studies and the general principles given previously. With these points in mind, primary and secondary care clinicians should be able themselves to handle most of the requests for information that they encounter and be able to refer on the relatively small number where unusual family patterns or clinical features point to a high-risk situation, where a specialist in clinical genetics may be of real additional help. In those fields where Mendelian subsets are frequent, a close partnership between clinical geneticists and the relevant specialist (e.g. oncologists, breast or colorectal cancer surgeons, cardiologists or neurologists) is undoubtedly the best way to ensure that the increased workload and the different levels of risk are handled appropriately. Specialist genetic counsellors are also an increasingly important element in such a system, in which the diagnostic aspects have already been dealt with by others.

4

Chromosome abnormalities

INTRODUCTION

Although chromosomes have been recognised as the structures responsible for inheritance for over a century, it was only in 1956 that the normal human chromosome number was found to be 46, not 48 as thought for many years previously. The first chromosome abnormalities were discovered in 1959 and since that time human cytogenetics has formed an important part of medical genetics. Those interested in the history of the field will enjoy TC Hsu's informative and readable book *Human Cytogenetics: An Historical Approach*, while Peter Harper's book *First Years of Human Chromosomes* takes a more clinical approach, based largely on interviews with the early pioneers (see Appendix 1). Over the past half-century the field has been greatly extended and changed by a series of technological developments that have not only had diagnostic implications, but have given important insights into how chromosomes actually function. Although this book does not attempt to cover the area of chromosome biology, it is important to recognise that chromosomes are not simply linear aggregations of genes or passive carriers for them, but that they powerfully influence normal and abnormal inheritance in a much wider way.

Increasing understanding of the molecular basis of meiosis and DNA repair, of the function of histones and other protein components of the chromosome, and the importance of methylation in particular chromosome regions and the spatial organisation of chromatin between cell divisions (i.e. in interphase), are a few examples of how cytogenetics has become part of the wider fields of genomics and epigenetics.

Chromosome disorders are relatively common as the cause of serious childhood malformations and rank high in the requests for genetic counselling, but before describing the risks in specific groups, there are three points worthy of mention that the clinician and genetic counsellor should bear in mind from the outset:

- The great majority of disorders following Mendelian inheritance, especially those of adult life, show no visible chromosomal abnormality.
- The great majority of chromosomal disorders have a low risk of recurrence in a family, especially where no abnormality (including a balanced carrier state) is present in either parent.
- Some chromosome rearrangements will be detected more readily on a karyotype than by array comparative genomic hybridisation (CGH).

Thus, not all patients with a genetic disorder need chromosomal investigation, whether by karyotype or array CGH; to request these uncritically is unnecessary, expensive and will prevent the laboratory from concentrating its resources on samples for which a detailed analysis may be essential. Furthermore, a karyotype may be required to assess reproductive risks, even when a chromosomal deletion or duplication has been recognised by array CGH.

The first-line investigation required when a chromosomal disorder is suspected has changed in many countries from a karyotype to array CGH (see Chapter 5), at least in paediatric genetics and now usually also for prenatal investigations. However, array CGH may fail to detect some cytogenetic anomalies that have significant repercussions for reproduction. Furthermore, performing a karyotype is cheaper for detecting some rearrangements than is array CGH and has the possible advantage of failing to detect copy number variants (CNVs) of uncertain significance.

The judgement as to when an array should be performed and when a karyotype would be more appropriate is dependent upon local experience and resources, both clinically and in the laboratory. Practice is still evolving and may take some years to settle, as methods of genomic analysis continue in flux. In principle, whole genome sequencing 'should' provide all the information yielded by a karyotype as well as array CGH, in addition to much else besides. However, once a chromosome rearrangement, such as a balanced translocation or inversion, has been identified in a family, it may be evident that a karyotype will be the best method for the cascade testing of relatives to identify carriers.

Unbalanced chromosome rearrangements are often more readily detected by array CGH than by karyotype but the reproductive implications – determining the risk of recurrence or the risk of a different but related disorder – may be clarified more readily by karyotype. Therefore, the failure to consider the possibility of a chromosome disorder more complex than a simple CNV may lead to a family being given a falsely low genetic risk on the grounds that a simple deletion or duplication is likely to be a sporadic event, so that a karyotype is not requested. Equally, a normal array CGH result may be understood – mistakenly – to indicate that a genetic cause for a problem has been excluded when, in fact, the genetic pathology may be either of smaller scale and require sequencing to be detected or may reflect a balanced structural rearrangement not detected by array. It remains important to distinguish the small number of cases of chromosome abnormality giving high risks to relatives from the much larger number where these risks are low.

The previously clear distinction between Mendelian and chromosomal disorders has become blurred as the laboratory methods in general use have become better able to reveal the whole spectrum of genetic pathology from single base changes through to structural chromosome rearrangements. It has long been known that some important malformation syndromes appearing to follow Mendelian inheritance are usually caused by small chromosome deletions. Working from the other direction, molecular geneticists have shown that the mutational event involved in some cases of Mendelian disorder is a large deletion – of one or more exons, or of whole genes – rather than a specific single base change. Additional recent developments include the recognition that parent-of-origin effects due to genetic imprinting and uniparental disomy, already mentioned in Chapter 2, are relevant to disorders of whole chromosomes or chromosomal regions.

We need to regard the laboratory methods in current use in most diagnostic laboratories as being in a state of permanent transition. While we expect stability to be reached at some point in the future, once the whole genome sequence (WGS) can be determined rapidly and interpreted reliably, so that a single investigation will reveal both small sequence alterations and structural chromosome rearrangements, that is not imminent in most parts of the world. Until WGS is performed as the single, routine genetic investigation, however, we need to retain an ability to interpret cytogenetic as well as molecular genetic laboratory reports. Even at that future moment, it will still be of great importance to be able to think in terms of chromosomes, in terms of three-dimensional geometry. This is a very different skill from the interpretation of sequence data. For the present, the well-tested techniques of classical cytogenetics remain essential for many of the diagnostic situations described in this chapter.

CHROMOSOME TERMINOLOGY

All 23 pairs of human chromosomes can be distinguished microscopically from each other, and much fine detail within each chromosome can also be recognised (Figure 4.1). An agreed international system of nomenclature (Figure 4.2), reviewed at regular intervals (most recently 2016 – see McGowan-Jordan, Simons and Schmid, 2016), forms the basis of reports from laboratories. Although these reports will usually include an explanatory text or be accompanied by an explanatory letter, clinicians may be deterred by the terminology itself, so some brief notes are given here.

Take the following example:

$$46,XY,t(4;22)(q32;q12)$$

This denotes the fact that the individual has a balanced translocation between the long arms of chromosomes 4 and 22. Several points can be noted:

- The total chromosome number is given first. In this example there is the normal number of 46.
- The sex chromosome constitution comes next. Here the patient is chromosomally male (XY) as opposed to female (XX).
- A translocation is indicated by the letter 't' with details of the chromosomes involved in brackets. In this example, chromosomes 4 and 22 are involved.
- The arms of a chromosome are indicated by the letters 'p' for the short arm and 'q' for the long arm ('p' is for *petit*, reflecting the strong French influence in early cytogenetics). In our example, the long arms of the two chromosomes are involved in the translocation. The breakpoints are given in the second brackets, indicated by numbers corresponding to band designations at points of exchange, in this case bands q32 and q12 on chromosomes 4 and 22, respectively.

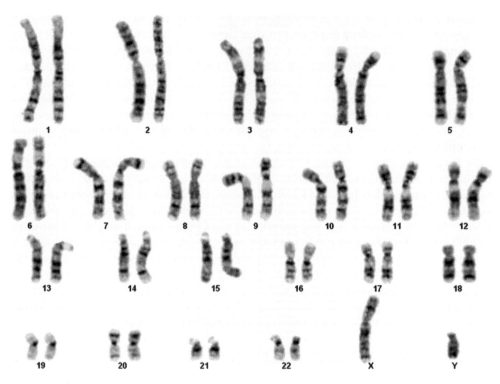

Figure 4.1 The normal human karyotype (male); trypsin-Giemsa preparation to show the G-banding pattern. (Kindly provided by Selwyn Roberts and Merle Vaughan.)

Gain or loss of an entire autosome is indicated by a + or −, so trisomic Down syndrome is represented by 47, XY, +21 (in a male). The sex chromosomes present are simply recorded without + or −, so monosomy X, a cause of Turner syndrome, is given as 45,X.

For gain or loss of part of a chromosome, the terms 'add' (a terminal addition), ins (an interstitial insertion) or 'del' (deletion) are used. An example is 46,XY,del(5)(p15) (deletion of part of the short arm of chromosome 5), as seen in the cri du chat syndrome.

Further details in chromosome reports may deal with mosaicism (the presence of more than one cell line), inversions, ring chromosomes, the identification of particular bands on a chromosome, and the use of fluorescence *in situ* hybridisation (FISH) and other molecular cytogenetic techniques. If in any doubt, the clinician should make personal contact with the cytogenetics laboratory. This will provide a more meaningful idea of the problem and will allow a better assessment of risks by discussion with cytogeneticist colleagues. Most laboratory cytogeneticists will be delighted by the opportunity to learn more specific details from the referring clinician and may in turn be able to suggest further clinical investigations from their knowledge of the phenotype associated with particular chromosomal defects.

Cytogenetic techniques are not described here but are covered by suggestions in Appendix 1. It has already been noted that techniques are evolving rapidly, and that a fusion of molecular and cytogenetic methods is allowing molecular applications to chromosomal disorders, as well as identifying changes in disorders not conventionally thought of as being 'chromosomal' in nature. For rapid or preliminary diagnosis, particularly in urgent prenatal situations, molecular

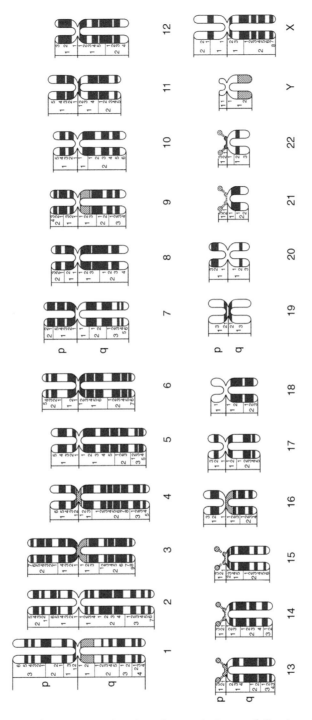

Figure 4.2 The human karyotype using banding techniques, following the international cytogenetic nomenclature (ISCN). The most recent revision (ISCN 2016) should be consulted for details.

techniques such as quantitative fluorescence polymerase chain reaction (QF-PCR) have become part of regular diagnostic practice in the prenatal detection of trisomies.

FREQUENCY OF CHROMOSOMAL ABNORMALITIES IN THE POPULATION

Four sources of information are available:

- Studies of newborn populations
- Studies of particular chromosomal disorders
- Studies of abortions and stillbirths
- Prenatal diagnosis series

Studies of unselected newborn populations

Table 4.1 summarises the principal findings, based on cytogenetic studies that revised earlier estimates by using banding techniques. It can be seen that 9.2 per 1,000 infants (or approaching 1%) had recognisable chromosomal abnormalities, of which around three-quarters had autosomal abnormalities and a quarter had sex chromosome abnormalities. Although the numbers were insufficient to give accurate data on individual rare disorders, these newborn figures are a useful reference point with which to compare any increased risk. Table 4.2 gives data collected on the major specific chromosome disorders; these prevalence data do not exactly correspond with Table 4.1 because of mortality and ascertainment differences. Once large and unselected population figures are available based upon array CGH and genome sequence data and combined with careful phenotypic assessments, these estimates will need to be revised again.

In Tables 4.3 and 4.4, data on spontaneous abortions are summarised. It can be seen that live-born infants with chromosomal disorders represent only a fraction of those conceived with such abnormalities. Indeed, spontaneous abortion is the rule rather than the exception for most serious autosomal disorders, some of which (e.g. trisomy 16) are extremely common in abortuses but never reach full term. The same is true for Turner syndrome. The incidence of chromosomal abnormalities in abortions declines with increasing gestation, and studies of stillborn infants have shown a frequency of around 5%. Identification of a chromosomal abnormality in a stillbirth is of considerable practical importance, especially when multiple

Table 4.1 Chromosomal abnormalities in unselected newborns

Abnormality	Frequency (per 1,000 births)
All abnormalities	9.2
Autosomal trisomies	1.4
Balanced autosomal rearrangements	5.2
Unbalanced autosomal abnormalities	0.6
Sex chromosome abnormalities:	
In phenotypic males	1.2
In phenotypic females	0.75

Source: Based on Jacobs PA et al. 1992. *J Med Genet* 29: 103–108.

Table 4.2 Population frequency of specific chromosomal disorders

	Per 1,000 live births[a]
Trisomy 21	1.5
Trisomy 18	0.12
Trisomy 13	0.07
XXY (Klinefelter syndrome)	1.5
45,X (Turner syndrome)	0.4
XYY syndrome	1.5
XXX syndrome	0.65

[a] Births of appropriate sex only for sex chromosome abnormalities.

Table 4.3 Chromosome abnormalities in spontaneous abortions and stillbirths

	Percentage
All spontaneous abortions	50
Up to 12 weeks	60
12–20 weeks	20
Stillbirths	5

Table 4.4 Major types of chromosome abnormality in spontaneous abortions

	Percentage
Trisomies	52
45,X	18
Triploidy	17
Translocations	2–4

malformations are present, because it allows a possible rare Mendelian disorder to be ruled out and may also identify a familial translocation.

TRISOMIES

Trisomy 21

Most cases of Down syndrome, the most important chromosome disorder, result from free trisomy of chromosome 21, and the overall population incidence (in the absence of prenatal diagnosis) is around 1 in 650 live births. It may have increased in recent years in countries where women have delayed pregnancy to a later age. Early and rapid chromosome analysis is important in all clinically suspected cases, since the clinical diagnosis, though usually clear, is not always so and the risk of potential complications is considerable.

There is a well-recognised (but often misinterpreted) relationship of trisomy 21 with maternal age, as shown in Tables 4.5 and 4.6. Paternal age is of little significance, an observation that fits

Table 4.5 Risk of Down syndrome by maternal age at delivery (years)

Maternal age at delivery (years)	Frequency of Down syndrome (from the model of Morris et al., 2002)
15	1:1,513
16	1:1,509
17	1:1,504
18	1:1,497
19	1:1,488
20	1:1,476
21	1:1,461
22	1:1,441
23	1:1,415
24	1:1,381
25	1:1,339
26	1:1,285
27	1:1,219
28	1:1,139
29	1:1,045
30	1:937
31	1:819
32	1:695
33	1:571
34	1:455
35	1:352
36	1:266
37	1:199
38	1:148
39	1:111
40	1:85
41	1:67
42	1:54
43	1:45
44	1:39
45	1:35
46	1:31
47	1:29
48	1:27
49	1:26
50	1:25
51	1:25
52	1:24

Source: Frequency of Down syndrome figures are taken from the model of Morris JK et al. 2002. J Med Screen 9: 2–6.

Table 4.6 Maternal age and chromosome abnormalities found at amniocentesis (rate per 1,000)

Maternal age (years)	Trisomy 21	Trisomy 18	Trisomy 13	XXY	All chromosome anomalies
35	3.9	0.5	0.2	0.5	8.7
36	5.0	0.7	0.3	0.6	10.1
37	6.4	1.0	0.4	0.8	12.2
38	8.1	1.4	0.5	1.1	14.8
39	10.4	2.0	0.8	1.4	18.4
40	13.3	2.8	1.1	1.8	23.0
41	16.9	3.9	1.5	2.4	29.0
42	21.6	5.5	2.1	3.1	37.0
43	27.4	7.6		4.1	45.0
44	34.8			5.4	50.0
45	44.2			7.0	62.0
46	55.9			9.1	77.0
47	70.4			11.9	96.0

Source: Based on Ferguson-Smith MA. 1983. Br Med Bull 39: 355–64.

with the confirmation by molecular studies that over 90% of cases of the major trisomies are of maternal origin. Parental chromosome analysis is not necessary (though often requested) in an isolated and uncomplicated case of trisomy 21.

It can be seen from the two tables that the estimate varies according to whether live-birth or amniocentesis data are used. Which is most appropriate will depend on the circumstances. In making a decision on whether or not to request amniocentesis when the chance is relatively low, Table 4.5 is usually most helpful. Where a decision has already been made in favour of testing, Table 4.6 may be more relevant. In any event, it should be made clear which criteria are being used. We would not usually suggest invasive testing for a risk based only on maternal age.

It is important to note the following points:

- The incidence in offspring of young women (25 years and under) is very low at 1 in 1,000. It may rise again slightly in the youngest mothers.
- The chance does not rise above that of the overall population incidence until a maternal age of around 30 years.
- The chance of a Down syndrome child reaches 1% at a maternal age of about 40 years and rises steeply thereafter, with a slight fall possible in the few births to women in their late 40s. Increasing use of *in vitro* fertilisation (IVF) procedures in older women points to the need for more accurate data for this group.

RECURRENT TRISOMY 21

The risk of another affected child being born to a couple who have had one child with trisomic Down syndrome is increased over the normal risk, but the increase does not show a simple relation to maternal age. Confirmation of a low overall recurrence risk comes from combined amniocentesis data, which show a risk of 1 in 200 (0.5%) for trisomic Down syndrome and of 1% for all chromosomal abnormalities in pregnancies where the indication was a previous child with trisomy 21. Because live-birth and amniocentesis data are similar here, an appropriate risk for non-translocational Down syndrome recurring is 1 in 200 under the age of 35 years. Above this age the risk appears to be little different from the general population age-specific risks given in Tables 4.5 and 4.6. There is no detectable increase in risk for second-degree or more distant relatives.

RISK FOR OFFSPRING OF DOWN SYNDROME PATIENTS

Risks would be expected to be high, but data are scanty since affected males or females rarely reproduce. A risk of around one in three for offspring of female patients seems likely. There is no satisfactory information for mosaics. Males with Down syndrome are affected by hypogonadism and are likely to be of reduced fertility.

Other viable autosomal trisomies (13, 18 and 22)

Other trisomies are rare (as live births) in comparison with trisomy 21. Recurrence is uncommon except for translocation cases but data are few; most age-related recurrence risks will be for the more common Down syndrome, for which the risks given earlier should be used. Maternal age is also a factor; Table 4.6 gives the age-specific risks for trisomies 18 and 13 at amniocentesis. The live-birth risks are considerably lower because of the frequency of spontaneous abortion, being around one-third the rate at amniocentesis for trisomy 18 and one-sixth that for trisomy 13. Since trisomy 13 can be due to a translocation (either Robertsonian or reciprocal), and both conditions may also be mimicked by non-chromosomal (often autosomal recessive) disorders, cytogenetic analysis (a karyotype) is essential in any suspected case.

Non-viable autosomal trisomies (e.g. trisomy 16) are extremely common in spontaneous miscarriages, and it is questionable whether amniocentesis in a subsequent pregnancy is warranted when such an abnormality is detected; non-invasive prenatal testing (NIPT) has altered practice in this area. How far risks for a future live-born child are increased by a previous chromosomally abnormal miscarriage or stillbirth is still uncertain; if the abnormality was a late miscarriage or stillbirth, then it seems prudent to use the same risk figures as for a live birth until better figures are available.

In *triploidy* there is a complete additional set of chromosomes. It is frequent as a cause of spontaneous pregnancy loss but is usually sporadic. Live birth is exceptional. There are phenotypic differences between the two different types of triploidies, in the fetus and the placenta, depending upon whether there is a 2:1 or 1:2 ratio of paternally derived to maternally derived chromosomes, with the molar changes of a partial hydatidiform mole indicating that the paternally derived chromosomes are present in excess.

SEX CHROMOSOME ABNORMALITIES

Recurrence in a family is exceptional for any of the sex chromosome abnormalities (Table 4.7). Even among the offspring of affected fertile individuals, transmission is rare, for reasons not fully understood.

The 45,X (Turner) syndrome is very common at conception, but most cases miscarry spontaneously. It is frequently associated with aortic coarctation and almost invariably with

Table 4.7 The more common sex chromosome disorders: Clinical features

Clinical features	Klinefelter syndrome	XYY syndrome	Turner syndrome (non-mosaic)	Triple X syndrome
Chromosome constitution	XXY	XYY	45,X	XXX
Phenotypic sex	Male	Male	Female	Female
Gonads	Atrophic testes	Normal	Streak ovaries	Often normal
Fertile	No	Yes	No	Yes
Intelligence	Normal/slightly reduced	Usually normal	Usually normal	Usually reduced
Behavioural problems	May occur	May occur	Minimal	May occur
Other features	Hypogonadal features	Tall; severe acne	Short; neck webbing; aortic coarctation	Few

streak gonads, primary amenorrhoea and short stature. Despite the apparent mildness of phenotype in most children with Turner syndrome, a wide range of clinical problems may occur in later life, most notably cardiovascular disease. Mosaic patients or those with partial deletions of the X chromosome (see later) may show streak gonads without the full phenotypic features, as may isochromosomes (see later). During pregnancy, oedema may be reflected in abnormal nuchal thickness on prenatal ultrasound testing.

The phenotypic effects of these conditions are largely the result of dosage differences for the pseudoautosomal regions of the X (and Y) chromosomes and other loci on the X that escape X chromosome inactivation.

Hypogonadism is likewise a primary feature of the XXY (Klinefelter) syndrome, but not of the XYY syndrome. Both conditions are associated with tall stature and XXY with some behavioural problems. The association of XYY with behavioural problems is substantially less strong and specific than originally believed.

Information on the long-term outlook for individuals with sex chromosome abnormalities is now available from studies of infants detected at birth by population studies. In general the phenotypic effects in XXY, XYY and 45,X individuals are mild; in particular, serious mental retardation is exceptional, although there is a slight reduction in mean intelligence quotient (IQ), along with an increased incidence of learning disability, often correctable with support. This may be more marked in XXX individuals. It is important that parents of a newly diagnosed child, as well as couples in whom such a condition has been detected by amniocentesis, are given an accurate picture of the likely situation, rather than one biased by the more serious problems of the minority attending hospital clinics.

Chromosome abnormalities in recurrent abortion and infertility

This topic is covered in Chapter 25.

CHROMOSOME TRANSLOCATIONS

Translocation Down syndrome

The great majority of cases of Down syndrome have 47 chromosomes owing to trisomy 21, but in about 5% of cases the chromosome number is normal (i.e. 46) and the extra chromosomal material is translocated onto another chromosome. This type of rearrangement is known as a *Robertsonian translocation*. Most commonly, the second chromosome involved is chromosome 14, and less commonly chromosome 22, 13, 15 or even another chromosome 21.

The genetic risks in such a situation depend entirely on whether there is an abnormality in the parental chromosomes. If parental chromosomes are normal, as in 75% of cases, the risk to further offspring is minimal, probably similar to that following a trisomic child at the same maternal age, and under 1% in younger women. If one parent has an abnormal karyotype, the situation is entirely different.

If there is a parental abnormality, it is usually a balanced Robertsonian translocation, in which the chromosome number is 45 but the total amount of chromosomal material is normal; one 'normal' chromosome 21 will be absent, and an abnormal chromosome will be seen, composed of the 'missing' 21 and the chromosome onto which it has been translocated. Banding techniques will allow precise identification. The lost material is likely to consist of centromeric heterochromatin and some (redundant) ribosomal RNA genes, so there is no associated phenotype and the rearrangement will not be detected on array CGH as there is no loss or gain of unique euchromatic material.

The possibilities for offspring of such a parent are shown in Figure 4.3. If segregation were random, one might expect all the categories to occur in equal proportions; but since trisomy 14 or the absence of one chromosome 14 or 21 (monosomy) is lethal and rarely results in an identified pregnancy, the risk of a child with translocation Down syndrome 'should' be one in three. In fact it is considerably lower, particularly when the father is carrying the balanced translocation. Table 4.8 summarises the risks.

Three cautions should be given regarding these risks:

1. The risk of an abnormality detected at amniocentesis is higher than given in Table 4.8 for live births, probably around one in eight for pregnancies of a woman who is a balanced 14/21 translocation carrier.

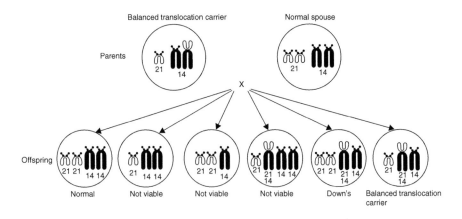

Figure 4.3 Possibilities for offspring in families with translocation Down syndrome.

Table 4.8 Possibilities for offspring in families with translocation Down syndrome

Type of translocation	Parent carrying balanced translocation	Risk to offspring (%)
14/21	Mother	10
	Father	2.5
	Neither parent	>1
21/22	One parent	Data scanty, risks probable as for 14/21 translocation
	Neither parent	Low (probability >1)
21/21	One parent (either sex)	100
	Neither parent	Low (probability >1)

2. Data have been obtained principally from women who have already had an abnormal child. Where the balanced chromosomal abnormality is detected incidentally, the risk may be lower.
3. Do not forget the (low) risk in the 'balanced carrier' offspring of a parent carrying a Robertsonian translocation involving chromosome 14 or 15 of uniparental disomy of chromosome 14 or 15 with their associated phenotypes. See later in this chapter.

Data for the rarer 21/22 translocation are much less extensive than for 14/21, but risks are similar. However, in the case of the very rare 21/21 balanced translocation, all pregnancies will be abnormal because the only possible outcomes are the unbalanced translocation Down syndrome and the lethal monosomy. However, most unbalanced 21/21 cases are *de novo* isochromosomes (one chromosome with two copies of the same arm – usually the long arm – either side of the centromere), with no abnormality in the parents and with minimal recurrence risk.

Once a case of translocation Down syndrome has been identified, it is essential to test the parents. If one of them proves chromosomally abnormal, carrying the rearrangement in balanced form, other relatives should also be offered testing in order to identify unsuspected balanced translocation carriers (of either sex), who can then be offered prenatal diagnosis in any future pregnancy. It is rare now for a case of Down syndrome not to be karyotyped, but clearly this is especially important in the infants of younger mothers, in whom trisomy is less frequent (although it is much more common than translocation at all ages). A register of both translocations and trisomies, with advance parental consent to release information when it could be relevant to relatives, may help to avoid unnecessary amniocentesis in relatives at a later date.

Data are available on the likelihood of an unstudied case of Down syndrome being the result of an inherited translocation at various maternal ages (Table 4.9). It can be seen that risks for offspring of healthy relatives are extremely small and rarely warrant amniocentesis.

Reciprocal and Robertsonian translocations

Down syndrome is not the only disorder that may result from autosomal translocations. Some may be responsible for other multiple malformation syndromes, or parental abnormalities may be discovered as a result of chromosomal studies for recurrent abortion or infertility (see Chapter 25).

Table 4.9 Figures for the approximate likelihood of a chromosomally unstudied Down patient representing an inherited translocation

Age of mother (years)	Likelihood of being inherited translocation (%)	Risk for offspring of a healthy sib (%)	
		Female	Male
>20	2.8	0.14	0.035
20–24	2.7	0.135	0.03
25–29	1.8	0.09	0.02
30–34	1.3	0.065	0.015
35–39	0.4	0.02	0.005
40–44	0.1	0.005	0.001
45–49	0.04	0.002	0.0005
<30	2.3	0.12	0.03
>30	0.5	0.025	0.006
Totals	1.2	0.06	0.15

Source: Based on the data of Albright GG, Hook EB. 1980. *J Med Genet* 17: 273–276.

The principal form of rearrangement is a reciprocal translocation, where there is an exchange of chromosome material between chromosomes but no change in total chromosome number. It can be appreciated that such changes, especially if small, may be difficult to recognise on karyotype; it may occasionally also be difficult to be sure whether the rearrangement is balanced or unbalanced. Array CGH is helpful in such situations.

The risk to offspring will depend on whether and how the rearrangement interferes with the normal process of meiosis. The individual situation will need careful study, and it is possible to work out the specific risks from the breakpoints or from diagrams of meiosis involving the abnormal segments, as shown by Gardner and Amor and by Young (see Appendix 1). It is wise to consult closely with the genetics laboratory, but the following general points can be made:

- The recurrence risk of an abnormality is very low if neither parent is a balanced carrier for the translocation.
- If the rearrangement in the affected individual appears balanced, it should be questioned whether it is related to the condition concerned or could be coincidental. Study of the family may help by showing healthy members with the same chromosome 'abnormality'. Array CGH can be helpful in detecting a minor imbalance in the affected individual.
- As array CGH detects the unbalanced state but not a balanced translocation, the clinician should always consider the possibility that a deletion or duplication (or especially both) may result from a structural rearrangement (a translocation or, if a deletion and duplication affect the same chromosome, an inversion), and consider whether a karyotype should be performed. This will be especially likely if the regions involved are terminal (if they each include the end of a chromosome arm).
- Reciprocal translocations involving certain chromosomal segments – for example the short arm of chromosome 9 and the distal part of the short arms of chromosomes 4 and 5 – have a high risk of an unbalanced defect (possibly as high as 30%). Otherwise, recurrence risks where one parent is a carrier will often be approximately 20%.

- X-autosome translocations may impair fertility as well as result in unbalanced abnormalities in offspring. If the rearrangement has disrupted a specific gene, it may result in a female balanced X-autosome translocation carrier showing marked signs of an X-linked disease, such as Duchenne muscular dystrophy or hypohidrotic ectodermal dysplasia.
- Balanced Robertsonian translocations of chromosomes other than 21 (most often 13 and 14) are usually phenotypically normal despite the overall chromosome number being 45. They are relatively common and are not usually associated with unbalanced chromosome defects in the offspring, but there is a (low) risk of abnormality associated with uniparental disomy for chromosome 14 or 15, which can occasionally occur in the offspring of a parent with a Robertsonian translocation involving either of those chromosomes.

Figure 4.4 shows the arrangement of the two pairs of chromosomes involved in a reciprocal translocation – the quadrivalent – in early meiosis. Having this diagram available (in the mind if not on paper) can be very helpful when explaining the possible outcomes of a pregnancy when one parent is the balanced carrier of a reciprocal translocation.

INVERSIONS

Rearrangement of genetic material within a chromosome is usually recognised by chromosome banding techniques but is also revealed by whole genome sequencing. When the rearrangement is confined to one arm of a chromosome (paracentric inversion), the risk of abnormality in the offspring is small (3% has been suggested). However, if the centromere is involved (pericentric inversion) in an autosome, this may cause problems in pairing with the homologous chromosome at meiosis, so that gametes with an unbalanced chromosome complement may be formed. This may be discovered in a parent after a child with an unbalanced chromosome abnormality has been born, or it may be an incidental finding.

Once again, figures are scanty as to the risks of abnormality. Where an abnormal child has been born and the inversion is familial, the risk is probably comparable to that seen for translocations, and amniocentesis is advisable in future pregnancies. Where it is an incidental discovery, it is much less certain whether there is a significant increase in risk. The situation should be discussed carefully with the diagnostic genetics laboratory. Pericentric inversion of chromosome 9 is common and, when the breakpoints lie in the pericentromeric heterochromatin, is a normal variant.

Figure 4.5 shows the arrangement of chromosomes with either a pericentric or a paracentric inversion at meiosis. Having this diagram 'available' to you is, again, helpful in explaining the outcomes of chiasma formation at meiosis in the offspring of those who carry such inversions.

MOSAICISM

A chromosomal mosaic is an individual whose organs contain more than one chromosomally distinct line of cells. When one of the cell lines is normal (e.g. 45,X/46,XX Turner mosaicism), the phenotype of the individual will usually be intermediate between the full disorder and normal. Some chromosome disorders are only known in mosaic form (e.g. mosaic trisomy 8, and mosaic 12p tetrasomy or Pallister-Killian syndrome), the full condition probably being lethal.

Mosaicism may be undetected in blood chromosome preparations, and skin biopsy should be performed for culture if it is seriously suspected or array CGH may be performed on endothelial cells from the mouth. Mosaicism confined to placental tissue (as studied in chorionic villus samples) may occur when the fetus is normal (see Chapter 9). Accurate risk figures for the

(i) Original arrangement and the exchange of chromosome segments

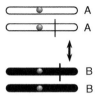

A
A

B
B

(ii) The established balanced rearrangement

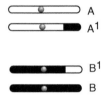

A
A^1

B^1
B

(iii) The quadrivalent at meiosis, enabling homologous pairing of all chromosome segments

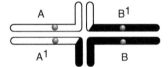

A   B^1

A^1 B

(iv) Three of the more common patterns of segregation of the quadrivalent from meiosis:

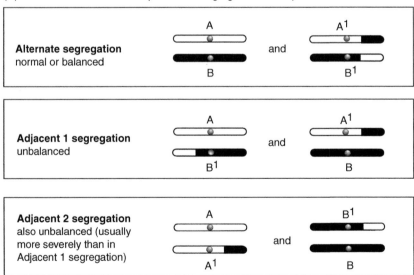

Alternate segregation
normal or balanced

A   and   A^1

B   B^1

Adjacent 1 segregation
unbalanced

A   and   A^1

B^1 B

Adjacent 2 segregation
also unbalanced (usually
more severely than in
Adjacent 1 segregation)

A   and   B^1

A^1 B

Figure 4.4 The arrangement of the two pairs of chromosomes involved in a reciprocal translocation at meiosis.

(a)

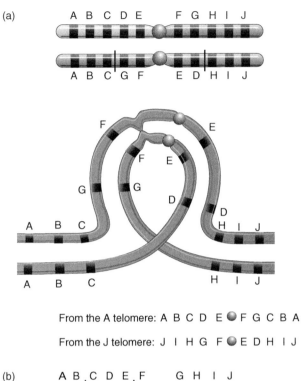

From the A telomere: A B C D E ⬤ F G C B A

From the J telomere: J I H G F ⬤ E D H I J

(b)

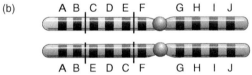

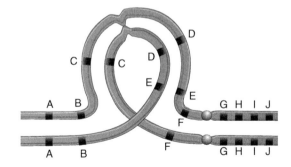

From the A telomere: A B C D E B A (acentric fragment)

From the J telemere: J I H G ⬤ F C D E F ⬤ G H I J (dicentric fragment)

Figure 4.5 The arrangement of chromosomes with either (a) a pericentric or (b) a paracentric inversion at meiosis, and the outcomes of chiasma formation in the inverted segment.

offspring of patients showing chromosomal mosaicism are not available, but prenatal diagnosis for their pregnancies should be offered, even though likely risks of abnormality are small.

Chromosomal mosaicism has been found to underlie some cases of malformation syndromes characterised by striped or whorled skin lesions that have in the past sometimes been confused with incontinentia pigmenti (see Chapter 18). The increasing recognition by molecular techniques of mosaicism in single gene disorders was already described in Chapter 2. Buccal swabs may be used to give access without trauma to a tissue other than blood.

Mosaicism should be distinguished from *chimaerism*, where an individual is composed of cell lines from more than one zygote, which may rarely occur in a twin pregnancy.

DELETIONS

Deletions involve visible loss of a part of a chromosome (under the microscope). Phenotypic features are less severe than when an entire chromosome is lost, so they are seen involving chromosomes where complete loss is incompatible with a full-term pregnancy. Some of the increasing number of abnormalities that give relatively specific clinical features are included in Table 4.10.

Risks of recurrence for sibs will be minimal in the absence of a rearrangement in a parent. Where chromosome studies are normal despite a distinctive phenotype, it is worth considering array CGH and further molecular studies (e.g. sequencing of genes within the relevant chromosomal region), likely to be much more sensitive than the karyotype.

Ring chromosomes are essentially deletions in which the deleted ends of the abnormal chromosome have joined together. Parental chromosomes should be checked, but recurrence is rare if these are normal.

MICRODELETION SYNDROMES

Several techniques can now be used to identify small chromosomal deletions that would usually not be identified when performing a standard karyotype. These include sophisticated banding techniques, often carried out early in mitosis when the chromosomes are in a relatively elongated phase. Microdeletions can also be readily detected through the use of FISH or multiplex ligation-dependent probe amplification (MLPA) (if a specific microdeletion is suspected) or with array CGH (see Chapter 5). Some of these disorders follow Mendelian inheritance; Table 4.10 lists some of these.

It is important to recognise that not all patients with the clinical disorders typical of well-known microdeletion syndromes show the chromosomal abnormality; conversely, it is important to ensure that the laboratory knows if the suspected disorder is one of the small and difficult to detect abnormalities that are now being recognised more frequently as experience accumulates with array CGH. Indeed, array CGH is much more sensitive than conventional cytogenetics in detecting these variants, although other methods (e.g. FISH, MLPA or quantitative PCR) can be used to confirm them if they are detected on karyotype. These techniques may also be used to confirm a finding on array CGH, when the specific disorder may not have been suspected at all; clinical acumen then has less opportunity to contribute to the laboratory investigation. Indeed, since the advent of array CGH studies, some additional, recurrent chromosomal deletions are being recognised whose phenotypes are variable and of incomplete penetrance. Genetic variants at other sites, both CNVs and sequence variants, may interact with environmental factors to influence their expression. Examples include the deletions of 15q13.3 and of 16p11.2, both associated with a range of phenotypes including autistic spectrum disorders, intellectual disability, epilepsy and schizophrenia.

Table 4.10 Eponymous syndromes associated with chromosomal deletions recognised by conventional cytogenetics and some other recurrent Copy Number Variant (CNV) microdeletion and microduplication syndromes.

Chromosome disorder	Associated clinical disorder
1p36 deletion	1p36 deletion syndrome
1q21.1 microdeletion	Neurosusceptibility locus[a]
4p16 deletion	Wolf–Hirschhorn syndrome
5p15 deletion	Cri du chat syndrome
7q11.23 microdeletion	Williams (Williams-Beuren) syndrome
Trisomy 8 mosaicism	Developmental problems and dysmorphism
8q24 deletion	Langer-Giedion syndrome
11p13 deletion	Wilm's tumour, aniridia and other anomalies (WAGR)
11p15 (paternal) duplication	Beckwith-Wiedemann syndrome
12p tetrasomy	Pallister-Killian syndrome
13q14 deletion	Retinoblastoma-plus syndrome
15q11 microdeletion	Neurosusceptibility locus[a]
15q11-13 deletion	Prader-Willi and Angelman syndromes (see text)
15q13.3 microdeletion	Neurosusceptibility locus[a]
16p11.2 microdeletion	Neurosusceptibility locus[a]
16p12.2 microdeletion	Neurosusceptibility locus[a]
16p13.3 deletion	Rubinstein-Taybi syndrome
17p11.2 deletion	Smith-Magenis syndrome
17p13.3 deletion	Miller-Dieker lissencephaly syndrome
17p11.2 duplication	Charcot-Marie-Tooth disease type1A
18q deletion (distal 18q-)	de Grouchy syndrome (very variable)
20p12 deletion	Alagille syndrome
22q11.2 deletion	DiGeorge//Shprintzen//Velocardiofacial syndrome (see Chapter 19)
22q11.2 duplication	Developmental problems and dysmorphism
22q13 microdeletion	Distal 22q deletion syndrome with neurodevelopmental disorder
inv dup(22)(q11)	Cat eye syndrome

[a] Neurosusceptibility variants are associated with a range of disorders including neuro-developmental disorders, psychiatric disorders, micro- or macro-cephaly and sometimes other congenital anomalies. The penetrance of the associated phenotypes is often reduced, with these variants acting in conjunction with other genetic factors or adverse antenatal or perinatal exposures as susceptibility factors to developmental problems.

While deletions of 22q are frequent in specific forms of congenital heart disease, smaller deletions within the area of the common, large deletion are being recognised. While the associated phenotypes are also very variable, they are generally less marked and still in the process of being clarified. In Prader-Willi and Angelman syndromes, the same region of chromosome 15 (15q11-13) has long been implicated; because of genomic imprinting, a different phenotype will result, depending on which parental region is lost. When the loss is from the paternal chromosome, the child will have Prader-Willi syndrome, when the loss is from the maternal chromosome, the child will have Angelman syndrome. Smaller deletions within this region of 15q, and the corresponding duplications, are now being identified with array CGH. The phenotypes associated with these smaller rearrangements are being clarified but include autistic spectrum disorders, intellectual disability, schizophrenia and epilepsy.

There are often at least two possible breakpoints at either end of the larger common, recurrent deletions, as with deletions of 15q11-13 or 22q11. Mispairing at meiosis can then lead to micro-deletions or -duplications between these adjacent potential breakpoints, which will not lead to the large recurrent deletion but will generate a loss (or a reciprocal gain) of a much lesser bulk of chromatin. However, this can still lead to problems with development. Such microdeletions and -duplications may be associated with developmental problems, autistic spectrum phenotypes, dysmorphism, malformation and psychiatric disorders. They often increase the probability of such problems in conjunction with other genetic factors or an adverse environment, without necessarily being causal in a strong sense, and are often termed 'neurosusceptibility loci' as they impact on similar processes of development and psychological function.

Other recurrent microdeletion disorders are being recognised although the phenotypes are variable, and some carriers may be unaffected. The chance of such conditions giving rise to a clinical phenotype may be increased by adverse experiences *in utero* or by coexisting CNVs or point mutations (the 'two-hit' model of developmental disorders: Girirajan et al., 2010).

For all chromosome microdeletion syndromes, the recurrence risk in sibs will be low if parents are clinically normal and do not show the chromosomal or molecular defect present in the affected child.

UNIPARENTAL DISOMY

It is a fundamental fact of genetics that a child usually receives one copy of each chromosome pair from each parent (i.e. one of each autosome and one sex chromosome), but occasionally this does not happen; when both copies originate from one parent, this is termed *uniparental disomy*. This may have no harmful effects, in which case it will usually be unrecognised, but problems may arise if either of the following is true:

- The transmitted copies both carry a recessive mutated gene present in heterozygous state in the parent. (This has occurred in rare cases of cystic fibrosis.)
- Part of the chromosome shows 'genetic imprinting' (see Chapter 2), so that either two inactivated chromosome regions or two functioning copies are transmitted when we usually have only a single functioning copy.

Prader-Willi and Angelman syndromes provide the clearest examples of uniparental disomy in conjunction with imprinting, although this is less common than microdeletions. Recurrence is very unlikely with any form of uniparental disomy.

Now that responsible genes have been identified in the critical region of chromosome 15, it is usually possible to determine the genetic basis of Prader-Willi syndrome or of Angelman syndrome. The causes of Angelman syndrome are more complex and varied: mutation in the maternally inherited *UBE3A* gene will lead to Angelman syndrome, just as with a deletion of the maternal 15q, paternal disomy 15 or a disturbance of the local imprinting mechanism.

Uniparental disomy for chromosome 14 is also associated with disorders of fetal growth and development, whether the disomy is paternal or maternal, and can very occasionally arise in association with a Robertsonian translocation involving chromosome 14.

When a Robertsonian translocation carrier is identified with involvement of chromosome 14 or 15, and her or his fetus appears to be an unaffected carrier of the translocation, prenatal molecular studies may be indicated to exclude the small risk of pathogenic uniparental disomy (UPD).

ISOCHROMOSOMES

Isochromosomes are most commonly seen for the X chromosome. The majority result from breakage in the short or long arm so that a symmetrical chromosome consisting of either two long arms, or rarely two short arms, is formed. Patients show varying degrees of the Turner phenotype. In general, deletions of Xp are likely to lead to somatic features of Turner syndrome, while deletions of Xq will more often result in infertility.

HEREDITARY FRAGILE SITES

Fragile sites occur on several chromosomes, giving the appearance of breakage at a specific point. On the autosomes they are entirely harmless, being seen usually only in the heterozygous state. On the X chromosome, the occurrence of a fragile site near the end of the long arm (at Xq27.3) is generally associated in males with the important form of X-linked mental retardation, the fragile X syndrome. This is discussed in more detail in Chapter 15. Note that there are two other X-chromosome fragile sites (FRAXE and FRAXF) close to the FRAXA site at Xq27.3. FRAXE has much less association with cognitive impairment, and the FRAXF site may be without any phenotypic association.

Fragile sites may be of considerable importance in relation to sites of translocation, and to the somatic genetic changes involved in neoplasia, but there is no evidence that carriers of autosomal fragile sites are especially prone to cancer or to other diseases.

NORMAL VARIATIONS

Human chromosomes vary considerably in their morphology, and clinicians may be concerned by a report of a minor variant and uncertain of its significance. Since for the most part it is people with a disorder who have their chromosomes examined, these variations are frequently reported in association with clinical problems that later prove unrelated. Studies of the rest of the family may resolve the issue by showing the variant in healthy members; close discussion with the laboratory should avoid problems in most instances. Relatively frequent changes of this kind are especially seen in the heterochromatic regions of chromosomes 1, 9 and 16, and variable length of the long arm of the Y chromosome. Most laboratories no longer include the finding of such normal variants in their reports. At a molecular level, array CGH has shown a large amount of normal variation in copy numbers of DNA sequences.

5

Genetic and genomic investigations

INTRODUCTION

The analysis of individual genes and the detection of specific changes (mutations) responsible for human genetic disorders has been an integral part of medical genetics services for some three decades, since the recognition of deletions within the dystrophin gene as causing Duchenne muscular dystrophy. While technical progress in this area continues, the development of genome-wide technologies – in contrast to targeted, single-gene investigations – is extending the scope of application of genetic testing. This is allowing the contribution of genetic variation to disease to be recognised much more widely and to enter mainstream medical practice.

Those using genetic investigations in their medical practice should understand what can be learned from genetic laboratory investigations. This need not involve a detailed knowledge of laboratory practices but rather an understanding of the basic principles. For those involved as specialists in clinical genetics services, it is also helpful to have some appreciation of the historical sequence of technical developments as this can assist the interpretation of patient records and family files.

One should make a mention here of terminology. The word 'mutation' can refer here either to the process of change in the genome (a mutational event) or to that which is thereby produced (the mutated copy of the gene). The first sense of the word continues as a useful term. The second sense has become entangled in an unhelpful assumption: it has often been assumed, in the past, that the mutant version of the gene you have sequenced, in a patient affected by the corresponding disease, will of course be the cause of their disease. Given the introduction of exome and genome sequencing, however, many variant sequences are now discovered that may be quite unrelated to the disease in question. They may be completely benign, or they may indicate a risk of a different, (co)incidental disease. For the second sense of the word 'mutation', therefore, it is good practice to use the word 'variant' instead and to specify a variant as being pathogenic if there is good evidence of that (see Richards et al., 2015). The point is to avoid the inadvertent drawing of false conclusions from unwarranted assumptions.

The first genetic investigation used in clinical practice was the karyotype, as already described in Chapter 4. The visual inspection of the full set of Giemsa-stained (banded) chromosomes from cells caught in an arrested mitosis, using the light microscope, allows the recognition of (large) deletions or duplications and other structural rearrangements. When the microscope image is photographed, so that the chromosomes can be neatly arranged into their pairs, we describe this display as the karyotype. This is likely to remain a standard investigation in genetics for many years but only for a restricted set of contexts, where a structural rearrangement of the chromosomes is likely or where such a rearrangement is known to be present in the family and a relative seeks cascade testing, to see if they have inherited the rearrangement. Other applications of the karyotype are being superseded by molecular investigations; in fact, the distinction between the cytogenetics and the molecular genetics laboratory is disappearing as 'molecular' methods are now often used to answer 'cytogenetic' questions.

The karyotype can be seen as the first 'genomic' investigation, because the entire set of chromosomes is examined, if rather crudely. There has been debate over whether the term 'genomic' brings any added value to the perfectly satisfactory term 'genetic'. I would argue that it does, because it conveys a shift in approach – a shift in thinking about what constitutes a genetic test. In historical terms, after the karyotype, the introduction of molecular genetic methods led to a focussing in progressively greater detail on ever smaller chromosome regions and eventually – in DNA sequencing – the single nucleotide base pair. The advent of genomic methods entailed a reversal of this process of focussing; genomic methods allow the simultaneous examination in great detail of all areas of the genome. The phrase 'genome-wide' conveys this shift in paradigm. There remain circumstances, however, where a focussed genetic test is the most appropriate investigation.

COPY NUMBER VARIANTS

The ability to detect chromosomal deletions and duplications through the microscope has been limited: only the larger deletions or duplications have been detected. Several approaches have been developed to improve our recognition of such copy number variants (CNVs). Three approaches are mentioned here:

1.   Fluorescence *in situ* hybridisation (FISH)

This uses fluorescent-labelled DNA probes complementary to specific sequences of interest, such as those from within regions commonly deleted or duplicated in particular syndromic disorders. Deviations from the normal two copies of an autosomal sequence can be detected in this way with much greater sensitivity than when using light microscopy unaided. This method gives information about the number of copies of the sequence of interest and shows on which chromosomes they are found.

2.   Multiplex ligation-dependent probe amplification

Multiplex ligation-dependent probe amplification (MLPA) is an application of the polymerase chain reaction (PCR) in which it is not the patient's DNA that is amplified by PCR but, instead, carefully designed probe sequences. Two DNA probes are designed to recognise and anneal to immediately adjacent sequences in a gene of interest; once in place, they are ligated together by a DNA ligase. The two probes carry an additional sequence, not complementary to human DNA sequences, including PCR primer binding sites and additional 'stuffer sequences' designed so that the PCR product is of a very specific size. The PCR reaction of the probe sequence, not human sequence, can then proceed, yielding a quantity of product that relates directly to the number of copies of the target DNA in the patient's genome (Figure 5.1).

Because the MLPA amplicons (the sequences being amplified by PCR) can be designed to be of different sizes, it is possible to amplify many such pairs of ligated probes in the same reaction and with the same primers and primer sites for each of the different target sites of interest: the length of the product obtained from each site is distinct. While the PCR primer sites used are the same for all probes, the site specificity derives from the sequence of the hybridising probes initially used and not from the PCR primers that are located on the sections of the probes that are not complementary to human DNA. It is possible to use several MLPA sites within a commonly deleted region so as to define the extent of the deletion more precisely, such as for the

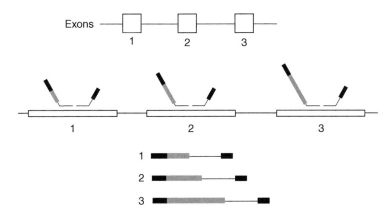

Figure 5.1 Multiplex ligation-dependent probe amplification (MLPA). The MLPA reaction is a method used to detect the relative dosage of different target sequences in the human genome, indicating the dosage (the presence of deletions or duplications) simultaneously across many sites (e.g. a panel of recurrent microdeletions or other CNVs, or the exons of the dystrophin gene). The MLPA probe recognises the unique human sequence of interest. It is introduced as two halves, each of which has one end complementary to adjacent portions of the target sequence and another end that is a primer for a PCR reaction. When annealed to the target, the two molecules are immediately adjacent and can be joined together by the enzyme ligase. This creates the intact MLPA probe with a PCR primer at each end that can then be amplified.

Key:

- *The broad black portion of the MLPA molecule probe*: Primer for PCR amplification of MLPA probe (contains no human sequence).
- *The broad grey portion of the MLPA probe*: 'Stuffer' sequence, whose sole function is to alter the length of the MLPA probe so that the different probes, each amplifying a different human target in the same reaction, can be distinguished by their length from all the other probes that correspond to different target sites (e.g. the other exons in the same gene).
- *The narrower, black portion of the MLPA probe*: Sequence complementary to target DNA (consists of normal human sequence).

22q11 deletion region, or within a large, multi-exonic gene in which deletions (or duplications) are a common cause of disease (e.g. the dystrophin gene locus). MLPA is very sensitive in detecting altered copy number, although it does not show the chromosomal location of any additional copies.

3. Array comparative genomic hybridisation or chromosomal microarray

Single-stranded sequences of DNA from across the genome (or from specific areas of the genome of particular interest) are laid out in a structured array of microdots. The length of these sequences has become shorter with each new generation of the technology: originally consisting of bacterial artificial chromosomes (BACs) with many kilobases of human DNA inserted, they now usually consist of oligonucleotides (oligos) of some 20+ bases. DNA from two sources, each labelled with a different fluorescent dye, is allowed to anneal with the array. One source will be the patient under investigation and the other a control. The ratio of the two different light emissions from each dot on the array then indicates the relative number of copies of the corresponding sequence in the two sources of DNA.

If the patient has a deletion of one sequence, the ratio of signal between the two fluorescent dyes will be 1:2 (patient:control) instead of the usual 2:2; if there is a duplication in the patient, the ratio will be 3:2.

The resolution of array comparative genomic hybridisation (aCGH) depends upon the number, size and spacing of the sequences chosen to be included on the array; it will far exceed the resolution of light microscopy. It can be thought of as if FISH or MLPA were being applied to every region of every chromosome at the same time.

The difficulty with high-resolution aCGH is that it detects more variation than we currently know how to interpret with confidence. There is extensive variation in CNVs among healthy individuals, although finding a variant in a healthy individual does not prove that the CNV has no pathogenic significance: penetrance of the disease phenotype may be incomplete and interactions with environmental factors, other CNVs or other genetic variants may be required for its pathological effects to manifest. Therefore, diagnostic laboratories will often restrict the sensitivity of the aCGH they employ, or will choose to disregard small deletions or duplications, especially if they are identified at only a single site on the array, as this could be artifactual. Only if at least two or three contiguous sites are deleted or duplicated, and if these span a minimum size specific for that array, will a diagnostic laboratory report that CNV with confidence. Laboratories often use different criteria in reporting the results of an aCGH if it is performed on a prenatal, fetal sample (e.g. a chorionic villus biopsy or amniocytes) in contrast to a sample obtained after delivery from an infant (or child, or adult). This is to avoid excessive uncertainties of interpretation in the prenatal context. Practices are evolving as confidence in interpreting prenatal aCGH results increases, as our collective experience accumulates.

Array CGH is the first genomic investigation to have been introduced into clinical practice on a wide scale since the karyotype, which it has largely replaced in many laboratories. The karyotype is still required for studies of specific chromosome rearrangements, such as inversions and reciprocal translocations, but array CGH is also replacing FISH and related investigations, such as searches for subtelomeric deletions.

Array CGH itself must be regarded as a provisional or transitional technology, however, as it will become feasible to replace it with whole genome sequencing (WGS), as the junction fragments resulting from each site of a chromosome breakpoint will reveal even complex cytogenetic rearrangements. For now, however, the combination of cost and ease of interpretation still favours the use of the karyotype to assess structural chromosomal rearrangements.

DNA SEQUENCING

Although in some Mendelian disorders a high proportion of mutations result from large deletions or duplications, as in Duchenne muscular dystrophy where at least two-thirds of cases arise as CNVs (deletions, or sometimes duplications) of one or more exons, this situation is the exception. For most conditions the majority of gene defects are the result of smaller point mutations detectable only by sequencing.

Genetic laboratories have used several methods to determine the DNA sequence of specific genes. Most have depended upon the PCR to amplify the specific fragment of DNA that is of interest, from among the rest of the patient's DNA obtained from their blood or other tissues. DNA primers are constructed to flank the stretches of sequence in which mutations are often found and then these are amplified using PCR to generate a sufficient quantity of 'pure' (or at least 'clean') material for analysis. Amplification of DNA by cloning can also be used. The DNA from one or a few PCRs will then be sequenced by the conventional (Sanger) method. The amplified DNA is copied by a DNA polymerase in four separate reactions with a small proportion of dideoxynucleotides (ddNTPs) present in the standard mix of nucleotides, and with a fluorescent label attached to one of the four ddNTPs. When a ddNTP is incorporated, that molecule can no longer be extended and so the length of the molecule with the ddNTP at its end identifies the nucleotide at that specific position in the gene.

The Sanger method of DNA sequencing was originally performed manually. Automated methods were developed, which still depended upon a prior amplification step of the sample DNA. Newer methods, often known as 'next-generation' or 'high-throughput' sequencing, have been developed that determine the sequence of very large numbers of single DNA molecules in parallel, without any amplification. These methods differ in the length of sequence that they can determine and the chance of introducing error. Some methods detect charge differences as large molecules move across a boundary; others depend upon changes associated with DNA synthesis. Methods include pyrosequencing, nanopore sequencing and ion semiconductor sequencing. The cost per base of sequencing has fallen dramatically, so that applications of sequencing that would have been inconceivable 20 years ago are now commonplace both in research and, increasingly, in diagnostics.

An important choice is made as to whether an enrichment step is used prior to sequencing, that selects for the sequences to be determined. This makes the difference between WGS, when there is no enrichment step or, for example, whole exome sequencing (WES) in which only the transcribed portions of protein-coding genes are sequenced. With exome sequencing, there is another choice to be made as to whether all transcribed regions are to be included in the analysis or a subset of the exome, such as all genes known to be associated with disease of any sort (the ~5,000 genes included in the 'clinical exome' of Online Mendelian Inheritance in Man [OMIM] Morbid Genes) or all the genes known to be associated with a specific class of disease (e.g. all genes associated with cardiomyopathy).

For diagnostic purposes, a laboratory will report its depth and breadth of coverage in the sequencing achieved: the depth refers to how many times each section of the genome is sequenced, and the breadth refers to how much of the genome (or the exome, or the specific panel of genes being reported) is covered to the specified depth. These figures are crucial to the confidence that a clinician can place in the findings reported.

HUMAN GENOME PROJECT AND THE 'OMICS'

The more-or-less complete sequence of the human genome took more than a decade to determine, from 1990 to 2003. This both stimulated and was enabled by rapid improvements in DNA sequencing technology and in bioinformatic analysis. Subsequent improvements have greatly reduced the cost of sequencing, and this knowledge of the usual human genome sequence – including the more common variants – enables human genome sequencing to be performed much more readily.

Prior knowledge of the human genome sequence is used not only to permit the more straightforward task of *resequencing* a patient's genome (i.e. determining the sequence not 'from scratch' but by comparison with the reference genome sequence) but also to enable a number of derivative, high-throughput investigations. These include the characterisation of the protein content of a tissue at any particular stage of development (the proteome), the pattern of CpG methylation in the genome (the methylome) and the pattern of intermediary metabolism (the metabolome). Collectively, these high-throughput investigations are known as 'the omics'. They are being used within the research setting to develop a systems biology approach to human physiology and the study of disease.

ASSOCIATION, CAUSATION AND LINKAGE

Finding altered sequence in a plausibly relevant gene is not at all the same as finding the cause for a patient's disease. When a disease is already known to be strongly associated with mutations in a particular gene, and a patient with that disease is found to have a pathogenic variant in that gene, which has previously been found in numerous other cases of the disease, then it may indeed be reasonable to conclude that we have identified the cause of that patient's disease. However, the situation is often much more complex.

We must distinguish between pathogenic (disease-causing) variants, alleles that are more loosely associated with a disease, common population variants (polymorphisms) that are thought to be benign, and rare variants of uncertain significance. This is best appreciated through an awareness of the different technologies involved. This requires an awareness of the principles involved and does not demand detailed technical knowledge.

Historically, two different approaches have been taken towards the identification of important genetic contributions to disease: linkage and association. Both depend upon the recognition of widespread sites of normal variation within the genome, sites of polymorphism, that can be used to identify factors that contribute to disease causation.

Linkage

With clearly inherited diseases – Mendelian genetic disorders of high penetrance – a set of widely scattered (genome-wide) polymorphisms can be tracked through families to see if, within any one family, any polymorphisms might co-segregate with the disease. Such a polymorphism need not itself be the disease-causing mutation (that would be most unlikely) but might lie nearby on the same chromosome, and this knowledge could be used to locate and then identify the gene in which mutations would cause the disease. In different families with the same disease, the allele of the linked marker associated with the disease is likely to be different and the disease-causing mutation is also often likely to be different (except in triplet-repeat disorders and disorders where there has been one or a few important founder effects in the relevant population).

Linkage studies to identify the gene responsible for a specific disease are now used only infrequently, such as in the context of locus heterogeneity, when there may be several loci potentially involved in a disease but in only one of these loci would a mutation cause the disease in any particular family. The methods of linkage analysis may also be used to track a variant of uncertain significance (a VUS or VoUS) in a gene, to determine whether it tracks with the disease through a family, either to exclude the variant as being pathogenic or to gain support for its pathogenicity (using an appropriate Bayesian calculation of that conditional probability).

The polymorphisms used in these studies have varied with the development of technology. Restriction enzyme sites were often used in the 1980s, in conjunction with DNA electrophoresis, to separate DNA fragments of different sizes in a gel, followed by Southern blotting of the DNA onto a membrane (initially made from nitrocellulose, then nylon), but these restriction sites are often uninformative and were superseded by (usually benign) sequence variants: at first by CA repeat microsatellites, and then by single nucleotide polymorphisms (SNPs). Polymorphisms that were initially detected by protein-based or immunological methods are sometimes still in use, especially among the HLA loci on chromosome 6p, but with the alleles now usually being distinguished by molecular (DNA) methods rather than immunologically. See Appendix 5.1 for information on linkage analysis and Appendix 5.2 for information on the isolation of DNA from human cells and on Southern blotting.

Association

Association between a polymorphism and a disease is very different from linkage. Association can be sought even among sporadic cases. It is the particular allele of the polymorphism that is examined. This has to be approached statistically: 'is allele A at locus L more or less frequently found, in this population, in patients with the relevant disease than in healthy controls?' Many associations have been found between specific SNP alleles and disease, often using large case-control series and employing thousands of SNPs from around the genome in genome-wide association studies (GWAS). The associations found through GWAS are mostly rather weak, with relative risks such as 1:1.01 or 1:1.02, although they can be very robust (i.e. with high statistical significance). Such findings can be of research interest – indicating pathogenetic mechanisms underlying disease – but are not of direct application in the clinic. Even cumulatively, using a large basket of such SNP associations for the same disease, there is usually no clinically useful information that can be applied to the individual patient. Indeed, even when summed together these associations typically account for only a rather modest fraction of the heritability of most conditions.

The contribution of such common SNPs to disease is usually weak, as the SNPs are by definition not rare and must be ancient (many thousands of years old) to have been dispersed widely throughout humankind. If the SNPs had been strongly pathogenic, then they would probably be much less common and much less widely dispersed, being unlikely to have persisted for so many generations, unless the pathogenicity has only appeared recently with changes in the environment and in life expectancy.

It may be noted that the degree of association between a SNP and a disease will be an average effect that might mask very substantial differences, depending upon other genetic and environmental factors, sex and the stage of the life cycle at which the effect operates. Even alleles that appear not to be associated with a disease at all could have strong but contrary effects in the different sexes or in different environments or at different stages of life, including embryonic versus fetal or antenatal versus postnatal effects. In humans, as opposed to laboratory model organisms, it requires very sophisticated research in order to detect and quantify such phenomena, where a polymorphism may be maintained either through heterozygote advantage or by disruptive selection (favouring the two homozygotes) or by antagonistic selection, with contrary effects under different circumstances or in the different sexes or at different stages of the life cycle. As these effects are well known in *Drosophila*, for example, we have no reason to believe that they are less widespread among our own species – just more difficult to demonstrate and quantify.

VARIANTS OF UNCERTAIN SIGNIFICANCE: IS A VARIANT A DISEASE-CAUSING MUTATION?

Once a Mendelian gene has been identified, in which mutation will often cause disease, the question may arise as to whether any particular variant in that gene is likely to be pathogenic (see Box 5.1). This question is often asked when a new variant, previously unreported, has been identified. There are several factors to consider in thinking through this question. It will usually be the diagnostic laboratory that has primary responsibility for deciding whether a new variant is pathogenic, or how likely that is, but a clinician or counsellor should have some familiarity with the relevant considerations and may need to discuss individual cases with the laboratory team or a specialist in bioinformatics or perhaps bring the case to a multidisciplinary forum. These questions – of whether a sequence variant is likely to be disease-causing, and whether it is likely to lead to a distinct phenotype in the heterozygous state (i.e. as a dominant disorder) or only as a homozygote (i.e. a recessive disorder) – are important and need to be understood by the clinician and genetic counsellor. This is for at least three reasons:

1. To assess whether a genetic variant is or is not the cause of a patient's disease phenotype may lead to grave consequences for the patient if practical decisions are based on erroneous advice (in predictive testing within a family and decisions about continuing disease surveillance or disease prevention, or in reproductive decisions, perhaps influencing decisions about continuing or terminating a pregnancy).
2. In attempting to clarify the effects of a VUS, it may be helpful to obtain samples for analysis from other members of the family. The counsellor should understand from whom samples would be helpful and why, and whether these further studies may have repercussions for the health or reproduction of the relatives who donate a blood sample 'to help my sister' (for example).
3. Rational approaches to treatment depend upon an understanding of the molecular mechanisms underlying disease. Thus, approaches to treatment for a recessive disease, or for a dominant disease resulting from haploinsufficiency, may focus on protein replacement or on boosting gene expression, whereas such approaches will not work for a disease that develops through a 'dominant negative' disease process, where removal or repression or inactivation of the disease-associated allele or gene product may be required.

EXPRESSION OF X-LINKED DISEASE IN FEMALES

For genes on the X chromosome, the question of VUSs (that *may* be pathogenic mutations) is especially complex, as pathogenic mutations will usually manifest in a male, but many factors will influence their phenotypic expression in females. The pattern of X-chromosome inactivation (XCI) in the relevant tissue(s) may be of central importance but is often difficult to study, while the pattern of XCI in white blood cells may not correspond at all closely to XCI in the relevant tissue.

BOX 5.1: Is this VUS a pathogenic mutation?

Has this variant been reported before, in either a ('normal', 'healthy') population database or a disease-specific database?

In how many healthy individuals, and from which populations, has it (*not*) been found?

In an apparently *de novo* case of disease, has the variant also arisen *de novo* or has it been inherited through the family?

It will often be helpful to investigate samples from the patient's parents, if available, and sometimes other family members.

Is the genetic variant expected (predicted) to lead to a change in amino acid sequence in the protein?

Further, is the amino acid change substantial or minor? (Is there a stop mutation and/or frameshift, or is it a missense mutation? If a nonsense mutation, is the mRNA likely to decay? With a missense mutation, is there a major difference in size or polarity between the original and the new amino acids?)

Is the genetic variant likely to impact on splicing? There is a range of programmes available to assess whether this is likely, but they do not always agree. Functional studies may sometimes be required to assess this.

Does the mutation occur within a domain of the protein that is known to be of critical importance (e.g. the active site of an enzyme, a protein-protein interaction site)?

Has the corresponding protein domain or the particular amino acid been highly conserved in evolution?

Are benign (well-tolerated) changes in the DNA found at this point in the protein or does there appear to be strong constraint on variation?

What is the nature of the gene product?

Does the gene encode an enzyme? If so, is it likely to be haplosufficient? Or is there reason to think that it may be a critical or rate-determining step and perhaps haploinsufficient?

Is the gene function to encode a structural protein? If so, is it multimeric or does it contribute to a multicomponent structure? Might the function of the protein assembly be disrupted by altered components?

Is the phenotype caused by a loss of control of the cell cycle? If so, could the phenotype develop from a Knudson-like, two-hit process? (The second hit to the other allele may be a second-point mutation, a gene deletion, chromosome loss at mitosis, an epigenetic process, or mitotic recombination leading to homozygosity for an allele knocked out by an inherited recessive mutation or a parent-of-origin, imprinting [epigenetic] effect).

Is the variant likely to affect promoter function, or influence transcription in some other way? (This may require functional studies *in vitro* to obtain a satisfactory resolution.)

Finally, if this has not already become clear, is the key question of whether the variant is likely to manifest in the heterozygous state:

Is gene function haplosufficient or haploinsufficient?

Might there be scope for a dominant negative effect, as with critical components in a complex structure or a novel function of the mutant protein?

Might there be increased or constitutive protein activity? (Especially relevant in receptors for cell-signalling pathways and proteins regulating the cell cycle.)

Does the mutation lead to a 'leak' (e.g. of an ion) across a membrane, whether a cell membrane or an epithelium? (Might this lead to altered cell excitability, or renal loss of an ion?)

Apart from XCI, other factors that affect expression of an X-linked disease phenotype in females include the tissue of expression of the gene product, and its biology, and whether the gene's protein product functions within the cell (in which case half the cells will usually function normally and half not) or in the extracellular compartment, such as the blood (as in haemophilia A, where circulating levels of factor VIII will on average be one-half of the normal, which is usually sufficient to avoid serious problems with bleeding). Thus, genes that are expressed within the cells of epithelia that are visible to inspection, such as the skin or retina, may manifest with a patchy or streaky phenotype. Similarly, mutations that lead to a leak across a membrane (e.g. the renal tubular epithelium) will often have a dominant pattern of expression, as a leak across only half the epithelial surface is still a substantial leak.

Females may manifest full expression of a mutation, as if they were male, under particular circumstances, including genes in which mutations cause disease through a dominant negative mechanism; marked skewing of X-chromosome inactivation towards inactivation of the intact allele (perhaps by chance); homozygosity for mutation in an X-chromosome gene (e.g. where the mutant allele is common, or in the context of consanguinity); Turner syndrome; and disruption of the gene by a balanced translocation between the X chromosome and an autosome.

In most sex-linked disorders, finding a healthy, unaffected male with the variant in question provides strong evidence that it is not pathogenic. There are exceptions even to this rule, however, in such special contexts as FRAXA. Apparently healthy males carrying a premutation in the triplet repeat of the *FMR1* gene provide an instance of transmitting but unaffected males, although they may develop FXTAS when older (see Chapter 14).

MOLECULAR BASIS OF MUTATION IN GENETIC DISEASES

The different types of mutation that may produce genetic disorders have already been mentioned briefly; many of these mechanisms were already known from studies on *Drosophila* and other experimental organisms and from work on much studied molecules such as human haemoglobin. Now that information is available on numerous human genes and diseases, the wide variety of mutations is even more apparent. In some disorders, such as cystic fibrosis, a single common mutation may predominate in at least some populations while, in other diseases, dozens or hundreds of mutations may occur with a relatively even frequency. There may be particular 'hot spots' in the gene where most mutations occur, as in Duchenne muscular dystrophy, while the full range of disease-associated mutations may include deletions of varying sizes, duplications or insertions of DNA, and point mutations in different parts of the gene, including the promoter and more remote regulatory sequences.

The phenotypic effects of a mutation depend on many factors, but size is often not the most important: a large deletion of many exons that conserves the downstream reading frame in the dystrophin (Xp21 muscular dystrophy) gene may cause much milder disease than a single base-pair nonsense mutation (to give a stop codon) or a single base-pair deletion or insertion (that will disrupt the reading frame 3' from the mutation, towards the C-terminus of the protein).

Frameshift mutations, as well as nonsense mutations that terminate translation, often have more severe effects than missense mutations. However, the complete absence of some proteins may cause fewer problems than a simple amino acid substitution, especially in protein molecules that are subunits contributing to large, macromolecular assemblies that can be disrupted more by a missense mutation in one component than by a heterozygous deletion.

For many genetic disorders, we are only just beginning to gain a clear picture of the correlation (if any) between the type, extent and site of a mutation and its clinical effects, but already this is beginning to be useful in giving an approximate guide to likely prognosis, as in myotonic dystrophy, Gaucher disease and cystic fibrosis. Computer-based mutation databases can help to synthesise this information and to make it available to the clinical and scientific communities.

Experience and observation have led to some important, although not universally valid, conclusions about the inheritance of disease:

- *Genetic heterogeneity*: This has proved to be the rule rather than the exception, with more than one locus responsible for a clinical disorder in most instances (e.g. adult polycystic kidney disease, hypertrophic cardiomyopathy, familial colorectal cancer). Sometimes, subtle clinical and other differences can be recognised once it is possible to separate the different genetic forms.
- *Multiple phenotypes from a single locus*: This has been a more surprising finding, with some widely different disorders proving to result from mutations in the same gene (e.g. *RET* oncogene mutations in both multiple endocrine neoplasia and Hirschsprung disease, or muscular dystrophy, lipodystrophy and progeria resulting from different mutations in the *lamin A/C* gene).
- *Extensive homology of genes and mutations across different species*: Even those only distantly related, such as insects and mammals: this has been of immense importance in allowing the use of model organisms in research and in understanding developmental processes and defects (see Chapter 6).
- *Recognition of subsets of common disorders*: Following Mendelian inheritance within a much larger 'multifactorial' group (see Chapter 3).
- *With a few exceptions, human genetic diseases seem to be rather randomly scattered around the different chromosomes,* with genes involving similar pathways or diseases often widely separated. However, there has been considerable conservation during evolution, so that areas of the mouse genome, for example, can be shown to correspond to specific human regions. This is proving important in showing homology between human disorders and the numerous well-studied mouse mutants. The X chromosome shows the highest degree of homology among mammalian species ('Ohno's law').

CLINICAL APPLICATION OF LABORATORY GENETIC DIAGNOSTICS

Most regional medical genetics centres have diagnostic genetics laboratories alongside their clinical genetics services, although the shape of these genetics laboratories is changing. There are contrary forces at work. To achieve economies of scale and to pool sequence data that will help interpret future findings, there are pressures to reduce the number of genetics laboratories and instead provide efficient transport of samples and transfer of results between clinical sites and large, centralised laboratories with associated bioinformatics teams. However, these economies may be better obtained *within* an institution because molecular methods are becoming ever more widely applied in pathology services, including haematology, biochemistry, and microbiology, and previously distinct laboratories within the same institutions may reduce costs by sharing expensive equipment internally and adopting common practices and procedures.

At the same time, new technologies hold the promise of close-to-patient testing, less centralisation and improved access for all health professionals as genetic approaches to health enter the mainstream of medical practice. While the provision of certain laboratory and/or bioinformatic facilities may be best centralised, at least in some countries, both the equipment and the expertise required are becoming widely dispersed. Doubtless, the competition between the centripetal (centralising) and the centrifugal (dispersing) forces will result in different service configurations in different countries. The optimal balance between these forces is also likely to change repeatedly over the coming decades, with different solutions being adopted in different healthcare systems.

Close links between clinical and laboratory geneticists in the past have led to supportive and collegial links between centres that have been productive of good research and have often given access to the latest diagnostic tests for families affected by rare diseases. The context is now changing as genomic methods are introduced, so that the benefits of testing in a particular laboratory are becoming less clear. It is now the interpretation rather than the generation of specific sequence information that requires expertise, as all human genetics laboratories move towards the same, standard investigations to tackle diagnostic challenges: aCGH, exome sequencing and WGS. There will remain a role for more targeted testing, and for the use of the karyotype, in specific circumstances such as cascade testing for a known disorder in the family.

Given the pace of change in what is technically feasible, the onus is now very much on clinicians to ensure that families under their care are aware of what can and cannot be delivered in terms of molecular diagnosis and prediction, and to recommend that they keep in close contact with their local genetics service. They should also ensure that DNA is banked on those patients with a genetic disorder where information from DNA analysis may be essential if accurate information is to be available to relatives in the future.

There can be few fields of medicine where what is possible is changing so rapidly. The available databases and internet sites – only some of which are indicated in Appendix 1 – are probably the best route for anyone to learn the current situation.

Unfortunately, there is a serious gap between what is known (i.e. what has been discovered) and what is available through regular medical genetics services. In part this is because, once initial research interest has faded, the disorder may be 'dropped' as research workers move on to other fields. In addition, however, and especially for rare disorders, it may prove difficult to set up systematic funding for detailed clinical assessment, patient management and phenotype-related studies even when genetic diagnostics could be provided through the new genomic approaches. There is an urgent need for a comprehensive network that will cover a wide range of the less common genetic disorders on a national or international basis. In the United Kingdom, the genetic diagnostic aspects have been addressed through the Deciphering Developmental

Disorders (DDD) project, and since then (especially in England) the 100,000 Genomes Project (100KGP) and the Genomic Medicine Service that has emerged from it. There are diagnostic initiatives for Europe as a whole (EuroGenTest and the European Rare Disease Framework), for North America, within Australia and for numerous other countries, often involving close links with industry.

The adoption of genome-based technologies within healthcare may overcome some of the difficulties, at least in countries that can afford them. Probably the last problem to be addressed satisfactorily will be that of funding and the associated (in)equities of access. While state funding and research projects may promote rare disease diagnosis, the problems of supporting rare disease management are likely to prove much more enduring and socially divisive, as the costs of good quality chronic care for those with physical limitations and cognitive impairments are greater than most societies seem willing to tackle in a socially coherent and equitable manner.

Mutation analysis

Whatever the specific mutation that has caused the disease in a family, its recognition allows a specific test to be applied to relatives at risk, regardless of pedigree structure. This is particularly helpful in the sporadic (isolated) case. This emphasises the point already made (but all too often ignored) that DNA should be isolated and stored from such cases (with appropriate consent), to allow future mutation tests that can help family members who may be at risk.

If mutations can be detected in most or all affected individuals, this raises the possibility of the test being used as part of primary diagnosis, rather than solely for cascade testing within established families. This may be extremely helpful in clinically variable disorders (e.g. myotonic dystrophy, where detection of the specific expansion can confirm or exclude the diagnosis), or where a particular genetic disorder is part of a range of possible diagnoses. However, it must be borne in mind that the possible personal and familial implications of a genetic diagnosis may not have been explained to patients and relatives (see later).

A further note of caution in interpreting the finding of an apparently specific mutation is the need for firm proof, or at least strong evidence, of cause and effect, already mentioned earlier in connection with DNA sequencing. In the early stages of research after a gene is identified, it may be far from clear whether a particular change is a causative mutation or a harmless normal variant unrelated to the disease state. This emphasises the need for a clear body of peer-reviewed evidence before a test is accepted as the basis for delivery of molecular genetic diagnostic services.

A final point to be emphasised here is that the detection of a mutation in a person at risk does not make the diagnosis of a clinical disorder. Many mutations are proving to have much lower penetrance than was initially thought likely; while tracking the mutation in a family will of course show a Mendelian pattern of inheritance, this does not necessarily mean that the related disorder will do so. This obvious point is often overlooked, and many healthy individuals with a predisposing mutation are, as a consequence, falsely (and harmfully) labelled as having a 'disease' when they are (and may remain) perfectly healthy instances of non-penetrance (see 'Presymptomatic [Predictive] Testing' later in this chapter).

Carrier detection

Molecular techniques have revolutionised carrier detection for many genetic disorders, as described in more detail in Chapter 7. Molecular investigations can identify carriers unambiguously, as long as the mutation is known: dominance and recessiveness reflect the relationship between genotype and phenotype while molecular tests reveal the genotype directly. This has its greatest advantage in X-linked disorders, because one avoids the problems produced by X-chromosome inactivation, a process that has often made other attempts at carrier detection in these disorders fraught with uncertainty. With these accurate molecular approaches, reliable carrier detection is available for such disorders as the haemophilias and Duchenne muscular dystrophy, although previous carrier test results should not be ignored.

Genomic approaches utilising next-generation sequencing can make carrier screening available for many recessive disorders in a single step, whether by targeted sequencing of many recessive disease loci (readily available commercially), by exome sequencing or by WGS. Many countries are beginning to embrace carrier screening programmes with enthusiasm as recessive diseases are individually rare while being collectively common and often severe. Such screening programmes are being welcomed especially in wealthy countries with a high level of customary consanguinity. The details of these programmes are evolving rapidly; some will need to utilise exome analysis if they are to address the concerns of their communities because of the multiplicity of rare recessive diseases that are found within particular kinship groups. The introduction of such comprehensive carrier screening programmes also raises social and ethical challenges that are discussed further in Part 4 (especially Chapter 34).

Prenatal diagnosis

DNA does not usually alter during embryonic development (with the possible exception of unstable trinucleotide repeat mutations), so a further advantage of the molecular approach is that it can be used in early prenatal diagnosis (see Chapter 9), in particular in material from chorion biopsy at the end of the first trimester.

Molecular prenatal diagnosis has been practised for some three decades and is usually based on direct mutational detection; the range of disorders involved includes most serious Mendelian disorders where the gene has been isolated or accurately mapped. Chapter 9 gives further details.

Chorion villus sampling (CVS) provides a sample that can be analysed directly without the need for cell culture, and the DNA yield of CVS is generally superior to that of amniocentesis. Since the risk of an affected pregnancy in prenatal diagnosis of Mendelian disorders is usually high, the possible extra miscarriage rate is not usually such a critical factor as it may be in the context of amniocentesis often made available later in pregnancy and for much lower risks of cytogenetic disorders. The potential use of molecular techniques in pre-implantation diagnosis, together with the need for caution, is also discussed in Chapter 9. The ability to analyse fetal DNA present within maternal plasma (non-invasive prenatal testing, NIPT) is a recent development that promises major changes in the clinical practice of prenatal diagnosis and antenatal screening programmes. This is also discussed in Chapter 9.

Presymptomatic (predictive) testing

The fact that tests based on DNA are essentially independent of disease onset and other phenotypic features makes it possible to use them in a wide variety of late-onset disorders where clinical features of the condition may not be detectable for many years. Although this has obvious advantages where earlier treatment or preventive measures are possible, such interventions are often not feasible. Even where there are such options, as in some of the familial cancers, important issues are raised that need detailed discussion before testing is performed. Depending on the individual disorder, a variable proportion of individuals at risk will decline the offer of testing when fully informed. This proportion ranges from around 5%–10% in familial adenomatous polyposis coli, where effective surgical treatment exists, through around 50% in familial breast cancer, where the outcome of early treatment is much less clear, to perhaps 80%–85% in Huntington's disease, where no effective therapy exists (at the time of writing, in 2019) and where the reasons for people wishing to be tested relate more to relief of uncertainty, to reproductive decisions and other personal factors than to medical measures.

There has been a general consensus within the 'clinical genetics and genetic counselling community' that presymptomatic testing should not be considered as a purely laboratory activity, but that it should be closely linked to genetic counselling, so that fully informed consent can be based on a proper foundation of information, preparation and support. Precisely how this can be ensured will vary according to the disorder; its complexity will reflect the difficulties inherent in the condition and there is no need for an identical model of 'counselling-plus-testing' to be applied universally. There is, however, a range of issues that are common to most disorders of late onset, and some of these issues are relevant to all genetic disorders. These include the implications of an abnormal result for future employment and insurance; family and reproductive issues, including the genetic implications for relatives; strategies for coping with an abnormal result and likely support from family and friends; and the more general issue of whether the consequences of all these aspects should lead to a decision to proceed with testing or to decide against it (at least to defer testing).

Most experience so far has come from Huntington's disease (see Chapter 15), which represents an extreme situation on account of its severity and the lack of therapy. At least a 'two-stage' approach has been generally adopted here and found to be necessary, both to allow the complex issues to be fully discussed and to give a 'pause for reflection' that permits individuals to withdraw from the testing process should they so wish. Testing protocols for other neurodegenerative disorders have followed a comparable line. For the familial cancers, practice has varied and is likely to continue evolving for some time. An opportunity for patients to pause and reflect before having a test is becoming appreciated by many clinicians but the use of test results for management of the condition – influencing the type of chemotherapy and perhaps surgery used for treating an established cancer – may lead to decisions being made more rapidly by those who have already become affected by their family's condition.

Diagnostic genetic testing

The term 'diagnostic' is often used rather loosely and inaccurately in relation to genetic testing. While it is reasonable to use the term molecular diagnostics for this whole field, it must be remembered that most of the analyses relate to determination of genotype, which may or may not provide a definite diagnosis, while many of the individuals tested are healthy individuals rather than 'patients' with symptoms requiring a diagnosis. This distinction may seem pedantic, but there are very real differences in the approach that is needed depending upon context. A person who has manifest symptoms and needs an explanation and a diagnosis will often have very different needs from someone else who is healthy but anxious in case he or she develops symptoms in the future. The contextual differences have a great influence on the individual's questions and concerns and, therefore, on any genetic counselling that may be appropriate.

Increasingly, true molecular genetic diagnosis is possible when a patient is being investigated whose clinical features suggest a particular genetic disorder. Such testing may make unnecessary other more invasive (and often more expensive) tests such as muscle biopsy or electrophysiology, or the different approaches may be used in conjunction or sequentially. In the setting of a patient with a likely clinical diagnosis of a genetic condition, detailed genetic counselling, as practised in relation to presymptomatic testing, may often not be necessary, and a simpler explanation is frequently adequate. Likewise, diagnostic genetic testing is something increasingly being arranged for their patients by a wide range of clinicians as part of their practice, without involvement of a specialist clinical genetics service; again, this is in contrast to the presymptomatic testing of a healthy individual, where such specialist involvement is usually important.

Before it is concluded, though, that diagnostic genetic testing can be handled just as any other medical test, several important points need to be considered. First (but often omitted) is the need to inform the patient that a genetic disorder is under consideration, and that an abnormal result may have a major impact on the wider family. This is especially relevant for those disorders with a small genetic subset (e.g. motor neurone disease, the prion dementias), where the individual and family concerned may have no appreciation that the disorder could be inherited. Second, it is essential that any symptoms are related to the disorder being tested for; this is especially so if a family history has been recognised. Thus, to take the example of Huntington's disease given in Chapter 15, genetic testing for an individual whose complaint is headache (unrelated to the disorder) would really be presymptomatic (predictive), not diagnostic, and should be handled accordingly.

As the practice of genetic testing becomes more widespread, many clinicians requesting such tests may not have thought about these important issues until they encounter them in practice: there will be a 'learning curve' that could be improved by appropriate liaison with clinical genetics services. To continue with a different metaphor, there should be no need to 'reinvent the wheel'.

GENOMIC DIAGNOSTICS

The development of genome-wide diagnostic tests is reshaping the process of clinical investigation and, therefore, clinical thinking. Those working in clinical genetics continue to approach the question of a diagnosis with the aim of making a clinical diagnosis of an affected individual that can be confirmed by a specific, targeted investigation. This is intellectually elegant and professionally satisfying. Furthermore, it is usually much cheaper than requesting a wide range of expensive investigations; it is therefore encouraged by the professionals' institutional base and/or the funding agency, such as their hospital or the patient's insurance company. However, professional practice is changing with the developments in technology and funding; where they lead, expectations of the professional are likely to follow. Nevertheless, it will be important that professionals ensure that their professional standards are maintained; they must not allow themselves to be coerced into bad practices because of constraints or pressure on healthcare budgets.

Whereas conventional (traditional), focussed investigations depend upon clinical acumen and experience to pinpoint the most likely diagnosis (or at least a limited differential diagnosis) ahead of investigation, genomic investigations do not require much thought in advance of the result. They merely require the recognition that the particular case fits into a category of 'quite possibly genetic in origin' and the precise test then requested will depend upon what is available locally. A detailed clinical assessment, and hard thinking with the aim of making a diagnosis, may seem only to be needed in those cases in which genomic testing fails to identify a single diagnosis plausibly relevant to the patient's symptoms and signs, that is, when either no diagnosis emerges or when too many potentially pathogenic variants are identified, none of which is entirely convincing. There is a danger that clinicians will defer thought until the genomic test results have returned, when it becomes apparent that clear clinical thinking might have been helpful at an earlier stage.

There are several tiers of high-throughput, genome-based diagnosis, to be accessed in rather different circumstances:

1. *Array CGH*, described previously, is used to detect chromosomal aneuploidy and, in particular, small deletions and duplications that cannot be detected by chromosome analysis.

2. *Targeted next-generation sequencing* of genes associated with a particular condition or phenotype, or at least of their exons (targeted exon sequencing), entails sequencing all the genes in which mutations are known to have been implicated as potential causes of a disease category, such as 'pigmentary retinopathy' or 'hypertrophic cardiomyopathy' or 'epileptic encephalopathies of infancy' or 'deafness'. These are not single diseases but rather clusters of related phenotypes, in which many different genes can be involved. It is both much faster and much cheaper to analyse all the genes in one of these 'panels', 'clusters' or 'baskets' simultaneously (in parallel) rather than attempting to sequence them by conventional (Sanger) technologies one at a time (sequentially, in series). There are many such clusters of genes linked by their common clinical features. Indeed, the clinician will no longer need to know the precise phenotypic features that distinguish the disorders caused by mutation in the different genes; it will only be necessary to recognise the 'diagnostic ballpark'.

   Strongly in favour of this approach, of course, is that there often are no clear and consistent phenotypic differences between the effects of mutations in many of the genes within a cluster, so this approach yields diagnostic clarity much more rapidly than any other method. However, there are also unfortunate consequences of such shortcuts to a diagnosis, such as the loss of an expert knowledge of the relevant disease phenotypes where these may be or become important. Despite any such drawbacks, however, we may expect the introduction of genomic methods to genetics laboratory diagnostics to have at least as great and beneficial an effect as brain imaging by magnetic resonance imaging (MRI) scan on clinical neurology.

3. *SNP-based arrays*, as used in GWAS, utilise an array of SNPs from across the whole genome and indicate the pattern of SNPs in an individual, which can yield information about identity, family relationship, common ancestry and population of origin. Longer stretches of homozygosity than usual for the SNPs along a single chromosome indicate the possibility of complete or partial uniparental disomy (UPD). UPD may be present from conception or, more usually, may arise from the loss of one chromosome from a trisomic embryo ('trisomy rescue') or (usually in mosaic form) from a mitotic recombination event.

   As discussed earlier, GWAS may also give some incomplete information about susceptibility to disease and pharmacogenetic responses and about quantitative traits (e.g. height), but they usually account for only a modest fraction of the genetic contribution to such quantitative traits, and this is not usually of clinical value.

   When the extent of SNP homozygosity affects all the autosomes, this suggests the possibility of consanguinity; if the degree and extent of homozygosity are especially marked, it may raise the question of whether the child was conceived in an incestuous relationship. This in turn may raise the question of the rape of the mother, perhaps as a minor. The legal implications will vary between jurisdictions.

4. *Whole exome sequencing (WES)*, if the coverage of protein-coding regions has achieved sufficient depth, will identify the large majority of disease-associated mutations, especially those that lead to an altered amino acid sequence in the corresponding protein, although some remote ('trans') effects on transcription may not be recognised (e.g. the effects of a sequence variant deep within an intron or in a remote regulatory region, perhaps in *trans*). The ability of exome sequencing to detect low-level mosaicism for a mutation is limited unless very high read depths are achieved, but most constitutional mutations will be detected.

5. *Whole genome sequencing (WGS)* will detect the vast majority of disease-causing mutations, although epigenetic 'second hits' will not be detected, and the interpretation of the findings will be constrained by the coverage of sequencing, the read depth obtained and the (rapidly changing)

limits of current knowledge. A high-quality WGS will also identify structural chromosome rearrangements from the resulting 'junction fragments' (where sequencing a single molecule moves from sequence appropriate to one chromosome to sequence appropriate to another).

Genomic difficulties

Both exome sequencing and WGS are powerful techniques that will generate highly accurate data. The problems that arise in their application are of three principal categories:

1. *Errors and omissions*: Although NGS is highly accurate, the number of bases to be sequenced is also enormous, so that occasional errors and omissions will inevitably arise. This is especially true when the *coverage* of the genome at appropriate *depth* is limited. For confidence in the results to be high, we need to know that both copies of any particular stretch of DNA sequence have been determined and that it is more likely to be achieved the greater the overall average 'read depth' (the number of times each section of genome has been sequenced). These problems will lessen over time as the technology continues to improve.

2. *Variants of uncertain significance (VUSs)*: These were previously discussed, but the volume (number) of VUSs will be much greater in WGS than in the targeted sequencing of single genes or gene panels, or even WES, as there are far fewer variants in exons than in introns or intergenic regions: the evolutionary constraints on variation are much more intense for those sequences that are translated into protein. The frequency of VUSs is set to fall over time as our collective ability to interpret genome data improves, and as more variants are definitively assigned to the categories of either a benign polymorphism or a pathogenic mutation.

   Progress is rapid but the challenge of interpreting gene-gene interactions, let alone gene-environment interactions, is enormous. It seems most unlikely for an entire WGS to be readily and clearly 'interpretable' in health terms, without substantial residual uncertainties, within the next decade.

3. *Incidental findings (IFs)*: These are more likely to arise as more information is generated in any investigation. IFs are therefore less likely to arise in sequencing a single gene than in a panel of phenotypically related genes, are more likely to arise in WES and even more likely in WGS than in WES.

   The essence of an IF is that it is a potentially important finding but unrelated to the reason for performing the investigation. If a child is being investigated to account for dysmorphic features and neurodevelopmental difficulties, then a small deletion within the *BRCA1* gene is unlikely to be relevant to the indications for investigation but may nevertheless be very important to the child (when older) and also perhaps to other members of the child's family (e.g. the child's mother, to whom it may be important now). It is an IF.

   It can be seen that if WES or WGS are performed without a specific indication but simply 'out of interest' or 'in case it proves useful', then *every* finding will be an *incidental* finding (IF). This amounts to genome analysis as a form of genetic health screening, which may sound futuristic but which is in reality already with us although, so far, only for modest numbers of individuals.

This discussion raises the question of how a WES or WGS should be reported, once the initial questions (that the analysis was designed to address) have been answered. What additional information should be generated and disclosed?

This question is vast in scope and the field is developing rapidly, so this section cannot give answers. However, some points may be suggested:

1. Whether the sequence is to be stored permanently (at least 'for the long term') is a real question and a positive answer ('Yes, of course') should not simply be assumed. There is a cost to storing genome data, including necessary updates to the information technology (software and hardware), the protection of confidential patient information from inappropriate access, and the likely obsolescence of the data as the repetition of the analysis with newer methods would not only be much cheaper but would be likely to generate much more useful information in one or two decades (with the interpretation of methylation and other epigenetic markers, for example, and improvements in read depth, giving a WGS+ or WGS 2.0). It would be all too easy to commit resources to long-term data storage and then to find that the stored data are worthless and the patient's genome has to be reanalysed anyway for a contemporary interpretation of the new WGS+.

2. If the data are stored, decisions will have to be taken as to how often the interpretation of the WES or WGS should be updated, who has the responsibility to do this, and who should act on the re-interpretation.

   It can be argued that a policy of 'analyse, interpret, report and destroy' might be more appropriate, with a complete reanalysis being conducted when required. Different policies are likely to be adopted in different healthcare systems, and policies may also change with the accumulation of data and of experience.

3. There should be a process for deciding what potentially disease-associated information should be generated and disclosed to the patient, in addition to the answers to the specific questions that originally triggered the analysis. The American College of Medical Genetics and Genomics (ACMG) has made a very helpful contribution to this discussion by suggesting a list of genes in which mutations likely to be pathogenic should usually be analysed and reported to the patient's physician. Rather than IFs, these may be thought of as 'additional, sought findings'. This list has already been modified (Kalia et al.), and it will doubtless change again over time, but it has proved to be a very helpful starting point. It has already given a major push towards establishing a professional consensus. It is helping to focus discussion on important questions, and it is helping laboratories to resist pressure to report interpretations on other areas of the genome, where results would be provisional and of uncertain benefit.

'The ACMG List' of genes consists mostly of genes in which variants are known sometimes to be associated with a dominant inherited predisposition to cancer or cardiac disease. From a European perspective, the list seems to include genes where the benefits of identifying a sequence variant are not always immediately apparent. The list of Additional Findings, to which participants in the 100KGP (the 100,000 Genomes Project of Genomics England) can sign up, is much more conservative (i.e. much shorter).

There will be other dominant loci at which it may be helpful to report pathogenic variants and, in addition, recessive loci where disclosure of an abnormal result would often also be helpful. For example, being homozygous (or a compound heterozygote) for known pathogenic variants at either of the haemoglobin loci, the α-1 anti-trypsin locus or the haemochromatosis (*HFE*) locus is information that should be passed to the person concerned, perhaps via their primary healthcare professionals.

The ACMG has taken the position that such tests for additional, sought findings should be carried out on children, with the results being reported to the child's parents, as well as adults. This runs counter to the habits of many clinicians, who regard it (vey reasonably) as better not to test a child for a late-onset disorder for which the child is known to be at risk. The present circumstance, however, is very different as the parents may not be aware of their risk so that the information could be of great importance to the carrier parent as well as (in the future) to the child. It will be important for individual circumstances to be considered, but the habit of neither generating nor disclosing such information about children should not be regarded as automatically applying to these new and different contexts.

There is the additional question of whether an individual should, as a matter of course, be offered information of largely reproductive significance, especially about the autosomal recessive loci for which they are (or at least appear to be) heterozygous carriers. There are many hundreds of such autosomal recessive, disease-associated loci, in which many variants will be of uncertain significance: there may be very substantial and long-lasting problems of interpretation, although the common alleles known to be associated with disease will usually be interpreted more readily.

Genetic and genomic testing: The wider process

The previous paragraphs on the applications of genetic testing have illustrated how important it is for this to be regarded not purely as a laboratory activity (although laboratory quality issues are vital) or as a process of data interpretation (although bioinformatic analysis is now a vital component of any genomic investigation) but as part of a more general, societal process. In some cases, the associated aspects are relatively simple and can readily be handled by whoever initiates the test. In other settings, however, notably in presymptomatic testing for serious late-onset disorders and in testing related to reproduction, the issues can be exceedingly complex and may need the time and skills of a specialist in this area. Part 4 of this volume discusses some of these aspects further. Deciding what the particular clinical situation requires is going to be an increasingly important skill to be developed in the training of the clinicians and others involved, with implications just as great as deciding on the criteria for complex interventions and specialist referrals in other fields of medicine.

APPENDIX 5.1 GENETIC LINKAGE ANALYSIS

There remain some conditions that have been mapped but where the gene remains unknown, or where it has not proved possible to identify a specific, disease-causing mutation. In this situation, linked DNA markers may be the only possible approach to predictive genetic testing. This may be extremely valuable, especially now that highly informative SNP-based markers have been developed. However, the use of linked markers raises numerous possibilities for error and misinterpretation, some of which are considered here. While the use of genetic linkage studies will usually be replaced by mutation-specific tests when available, their use may prove helpful in assessing the pathogenicity of VUSs encountered in clinical practice. Segregation studies may be required within families to help determine the clinical significance of their unique VUSs: do they track with the disorder in question? If the family is large enough, a small linkage study may be undertaken. It is therefore important that the use and limitations of linked markers are appreciated. The main issues are as follows:

- *What is the recombination rate between marker and disease?* This will represent the minimal error rate. Bear in mind that, until data are abundant, this figure may have wide confidence limits, and that recombination may vary between male and female meioses. Now that most markers used are within the relevant gene, these error rates are normally very low.
- *What is the penetrance of the pathogenic variant being studied?* This is vital information for any interpretation of the molecular results within a family to be helpful.

- *Are there flanking markers?* If two close marker loci on either side of a disease locus can be shown not to have recombined, it will be most unlikely that error from recombination will have occurred in relation to the disease, because that would require either a double recombination or a gene conversion event. If a set of closely linked markers is used as a haplotype, with the spread of markers both within and flanking the gene of interest, then the risk of such an error (i.e. a misleading result) will be even smaller.

- *Is there evidence for genetic heterogeneity in terms of more than one locus?* Since most families seen for counselling are relatively small, this is a particularly important point; again, the answer may not be clear until much information has been collected, as seen in disorders such as adult polycystic kidney disease and tuberous sclerosis, where two loci exist for each clinical diagnosis and phenotypic differences are subtle. Several types of cardiac disease show much more marked locus heterogeneity, such as hypertrophic cardiomyopathy and the long QT syndrome.

- *Is the 'phase' known?* (Do we *know* which marker allele is on the same chromosome as the disease allele in the potentially transmitting parent, or is this only inferred?) This is important in assessing the reliability of predictive or prenatal genetic testing. For phase to be known, testing will need to be performed on three generations. A related question is whether the pattern of marker alleles allows testing to be fully or only partially informative. This is looked at in more detail in Chapter 9.

- *Is the family structure suitable for linkage prediction?* This overlaps with the last question and requires consideration before tests are offered; where parents or affected members are dead or unavailable, it may be impossible to make a prediction. And even when a missing person's genotype can be inferred, this inference gives some (usually only small) scope for error.

APPENDIX 5.2 OTHER LABORATORY PROCESSES

DNA isolation

It is surprisingly easy to isolate pure DNA from human cells: DNA is much more stable than RNA or most proteins, and a series of fairly simple steps allows it to be isolated from any cell type that has a nucleus, including white blood cells, buccal cells, amniotic cells, chorionic tissue and skin fibroblasts. The DNA will be essentially the same whatever its tissue of origin, except for tumours where it may be important to identify the specific differences between the patient's constitutional DNA and their tumour DNA. A sample of only 5–10 mL of whole blood (often less) gives ample DNA for multiple diagnostic procedures; what is more, it is very stable and can be stored for years if necessary. Techniques of DNA amplification, such as the PCR, can utilize and amplify minute quantities of DNA, allowing material such as mouthwashes, stored filter-paper screening blood samples and hair roots to be used for the detection of specific mutations. While blood remains the choice for most diagnostic testing, many laboratories are able to utilise the DNA present in saliva.

DNA hybridisation (Southern blotting)

The types of molecular abnormality detected by this approach are principally those altering the length of a DNA fragment, so that fragments of different size can be separated by electrophoresis through a gel. The differences in size arise from deletion, duplication, variation in the number of tandem repeats (e.g. of a di- or tri-nucleotide repeat) or from altering the site at which a restriction enzyme works. The band corresponding to a fragment may be absent, or its size (as shown by its position) may be altered. Most point mutations in a gene will not be detected. While this was a common method of linkage analysis, its applications in the genetic diagnostic laboratory are now very few. It may be used where a mutation is unstable and fragment sizes may become both too large for reliable amplification by PCR and too variable to give a single discrete band; this sometimes occurs in fragile X syndrome and myotonic dystrophy.

6

Dysmorphology and genetic syndromes

INTRODUCTION

Congenital malformations represent one of the most frequent and important reasons for seeking a clinical genetics evaluation and genetic counselling, with 2%–3% of births in most populations affected by a condition that falls into the category of 'congenital malformation and/or genetic disorder presenting at birth, in infancy or in early childhood'. Dysmorphology is the study of these congenital malformations, but its subject is broader than this term may indicate, as it includes any prenatal influences that alter physical appearance, even when this does not amount to a malformation and when the cause is not primarily genetic. Furthermore, the dysmorphic features associated with some conditions may be very variable and sometimes very subtle.

In the past, clinicians had to rely almost entirely on their own skills and experience to make an accurate diagnosis. With the accumulation of experience in specific centres and by particular individuals, regular meetings of interested physicians refined this knowledge, and valuable books and databases were produced that helped to disseminate the knowledge and wisdom of this craft. The clinical delineation of dysmorphic syndromes interacted most productively with mammalian developmental biology and the study of mouse (and other animal) models of the disorders found in human patients. This interaction led to the recognition of the underlying genetic basis of many of these disorders and to the realisation that disorders with similar features often resulted from mutation in functionally related genes (genes involved in the same developmental or biochemical pathway or the same physiological process). The most clearly established pathway of this type is the Ras pathway of functionally interacting proteins involved in inter- and intra-cellular signalling. Mutations that affect these proteins lead to a number of related phenotypes, including Noonan syndrome, Costello syndrome, cardio-facio-cutaneous syndrome and neurofibromatosis type 1.

BOX 6.1: Laboratory investigations in the diagnosis of congenital malformations

Autopsy (including imaging by X-ray or magnetic resonance imaging [MRI], photography, DNA extraction from liver or spleen, fibroblast culture from skin)

Biochemistry (from serum, urine or fibroblasts): Especially useful in the peroxisomal disorders

Genetic investigations: DNA extraction from blood or tissue for (1) array CGH, and perhaps (2) specific gene analysis, next-generation sequencing gene panel targeted on a developmental pathway, exome or whole genome sequencing (WGS)

With the identification of the genetic basis of many dysmorphic syndromes, it has become clear that the range of phenotypes associated with mutation in the relevant gene is often much broader than had been appreciated. Previously, when no tests were available, the physical features had to be very clear for confidence in a diagnosis to be high. The broadening phenotype of many disorders has made the purely clinical recognition of conditions more difficult and has reinforced the necessity of turning to laboratory investigations to answer many of the clinical challenges we face.

A range of different laboratory approaches can be used to assist in the clinical genetic assessment of children (or, indeed, adults) with dysmorphic features (Box 6.1), but the key recent development is the application to this field of high-throughput genomics, both array comparative genomic hybridisation (CGH) and next-generation sequencing (a term that will have a limited life expectancy and may be replaced by 'massively parallel sequencing'). In the United Kingdom, the field has been substantially advanced by two ground-breaking projects based at the Wellcome Trust Sanger Centre: the DECIPHER database and the Deciphering Developmental Disorders (DDD) research project. High-throughput biology generates a mass of unselected data, so the mental effort required to understand the pathobiology now follows the laboratory investigation rather than lying in the selection of which test it would be most helpful to perform (i.e. which gene to sequence).

The situation is now comparable to that reached some years ago for inborn errors of metabolism. Garrod himself foresaw this a century ago and the available information has been brought together in a book, *Epstein's Inborn Errors of Development* (see Appendix 1). This has been a key reference source for the scientific analysis of congenital malformations.

In case any reader should think that these scientific developments make clinical skills redundant, it should be emphasised that the reverse is the case. It is only possible to use the new laboratory approaches effectively by using an effective combination of (1) targeting appropriate panels of genes for analysis, where this is most likely to yield a diagnosis without generating too many distracting variants of uncertain significance (VUSs) and incidental findings (IFs) and (2) whole exome or whole genome approaches (array comparative genomic hybridisation [aCGH], whole exome sequencing [WES], WGS) where targeted analyses are unlikely to be fruitful. Furthermore, familiarity with the clinical features of many disorders and a careful clinical examination conducted with sensitivity will often be needed to come to a judgement as to whether a specific genetic variant is likely to have led to the particular phenotype observed. However, the contribution of the clinical geneticist to the care of patients with dysmorphic features is certainly changing as more children have molecular investigations performed before being referred for a clinical genetics assessment.

In the United Kingdom, such children will often have an array CGH test performed before referral for genetic assessment, so that the clinical geneticist's role will sometimes be to discuss the findings of an aCGH test that has already been performed. The clinical geneticist will still often make diagnoses on clinical grounds or adjudicate on the likely significance of an aCGH result of uncertain significance. Once paediatricians have ready access to exome sequencing, and even more so once they can access WGS, the geneticist's contribution will lie especially in five areas:

1. Making a clinical diagnosis when WGS has failed to identify the cause of a patient's physical features or malformation
2. Interpreting genetic laboratory results of uncertain significance
3. Assessing the severity of a patient's clinical features on the spectrum of those with a particular diagnosis, and advising on practical aspects of management and care, often drawing on his or her personal experience with other, similarly affected, patients
4. Addressing the 'genetic counselling' issues of reproductive risk, reproductive options and family communication
5. Guiding the patient or family towards clinical research and, especially, clinical trials of new, rational treatments that may be of interest to them

The clinical geneticist has a special advantage in the clinical diagnosis of malformation syndromes, partly as the result of providing a service for a large population – often a million or more – enabling considerable experience to be gained of even the rarest disorders, which a paediatrician or obstetrician may encounter only a few times during their career and a family doctor is unlikely ever to encounter. The 'genetic approach' of placing emphasis on an accurate and specific diagnosis, of keeping long-term records and registers that allow comparison of old material with new cases, along with the dysmorphology groups that have grown up to discuss difficult cases and exchange information, have all placed the clinical geneticist at the centre of this field; but others will usually be involved first and will have to make the principal decisions concerning long-term management.

DEFINITIONS

Confusion of terminology abounds in the study of congenital malformations. The very term *dysmorphology* is disliked by some but has the advantage of clearly identifying the field as the study of disordered development, without specifying the causes or limiting the subject to genetic influences. In general, the field covers what are broadly known as congenital abnormalities or birth defects – abnormalities that are apparent at or before the time of birth and where there are recognisable structural anomalies. Thus, most inborn errors of metabolism do not fall into this area, except for those few where visible defects are present at birth, such as maternal phenylketonuria and some of the peroxisomal defects. Likewise, many other progressive Mendelian disorders are excluded, such as Duchenne muscular dystrophy and Tay-Sachs disease, even though histological or biochemical study may show clear changes before birth.

The term *syndrome* is used to denote a combination of clinical features occurring together consistently, usually causally related but not necessarily developmental. It is also widely used outside the birth defects field, often with variable and inconsistent meanings.

The term *malformation* is now generally restricted to a specific primary abnormality of development, such as a congenital heart or neural tube defect. A *malformation syndrome* is the occurrence together as an entity of several such defects as primary events, the cause being unknown in many but clear-cut in some; examples are the occurrence of central nervous system defects, congenital heart disease and cleft palate due to trisomy 13. A *malformation sequence* occurs when a primary malformation itself determines additional defects, such as foot deformity and hydrocephalus secondary to spina bifida, or posterior urethral valves leading to oligohydramnios and thence to pulmonary hypoplasia and fetal compression (Potter so-called 'syndrome' that is more correctly regarded as a sequence). Some defects in organs already normally developed can be clearly identified as the result of compression, constriction or immobility; such abnormalities are best termed *deformities or deformations*. The term *disruption* is used when there is a process that destroys or damages a structure already formed, such as amputation due to amniotic bands or the effects of fetal exposure to alcohol or a teratogenic drug.

Such distinctions of nomenclature may seem pedantic, but agreement and consistency are essential if confusion is to be avoided. These basic groupings also largely determine our thoughts and investigations into the causes of such defects, as well as are important for the estimation of genetic risks and for the prognosis and management of the affected individual.

Unfortunately, not all syndrome names are based on a scientific approach. It is not uncommon to be faced with referral of a family with a 'syndrome' that one has never heard of, only to find that the diagnosis is really something quite familiar masquerading under a strange name. Problems can also arise from the use of inappropriate eponyms that either celebrate cruel and unethical researchers or cause offence and distress to the patient or their parents through the generation of inappropriate acronyms.

DIAGNOSTIC APPROACH TO THE DYSMORPHIC CHILD

Although many aspects of the diagnostic approach to the dysmorphic child are similar to those already outlined more generally for genetic disorders, there are differences of emphasis. *Pregnancy history* is of crucial importance, because it may reveal a non-genetic cause: specific drugs, alcohol or teratogenic infection; mechanical uterine factors causing deformation or disruption (increasingly identifiable with widespread early use of ultrasound); or features such as hydramnios or lack of fetal movements may be a clue to the cause of abnormalities only apparent after delivery.

A *full pedigree and information on relevant family members* are essential, as in any other situation where genetic counselling will be needed, and may show a clear genetic cause in a phenotypic category where recurrence risk would otherwise be low (e.g. congenital contractures). In examination of the affected infant, careful measurements are essential, while vague terms should be avoided. Precise measurement not only avoids confusion as to whether the characteristic is really abnormal (adequate reference ranges are now available; see Appendix 1), but also allows serial evaluations to be made. As in any clinical situation, the extent and direction of the examination will be influenced by pointers given in the history and pedigree. Thus, if a syndrome known regularly to involve the eye is suspected, then a full ophthalmic assessment may need to be undertaken, even in the absence of any obvious eye defect.

A special note should be made of the importance of *photography* in the investigation of the dysmorphic infant. Not only does it supply an accurate means of documenting structural defects, but it also allows evaluation of serial changes much better than reported descriptions or even measurements can. Most valuable of all is the ability of a good photograph to convey an overall impression of a defect to a group of people who may never have seen the patient. Despite this, photography is unfortunately often still regarded as a hobby rather than a serious medical investigation. One should be aware of the sensitivity that patients and families may feel about photography but, as with most procedures, people are usually willing to help provided that the trouble is taken to explain why photographs are important and that full consent is obtained and recorded.

Imaging is another technique that is too often neglected, especially in the abnormal stillbirth or fetus. It is remarkable how an investigation with potentially harmful effects on the living is so seldom performed on the dead, to whom it can do no harm, but where a specific diagnosis may be immediately apparent. Lethal bone dysplasias and osteogenesis imperfecta are particular examples, but the value of a normal skeletal X-ray of a stillbirth should not be underestimated in excluding particular disorders. MRI may also be a very helpful plan B when a fetal or paediatric autopsy would be appropriate but the parents are unwilling to permit this.

Studies of the chromosomes should be undertaken in all dysmorphic infants with multiple defects, whether by aCGH (the preferred method) or by conventional cytogenetics (to give a karyotype). Skin biopsy has the advantage of potentially revealing mosaicism and may also yield a result from a foetus postmortem, when growth of leucocytes is more likely to fail. Where aCGH is not available, close liaison between clinical and laboratory staff will help to select any additional investigations that may be appropriate, such as fluorescence *in situ* hybridisation (FISH) for specific microdeletions suspected on clinical grounds. Doubtless, aCGH will in time be superseded by WGS once this is more widely available and more readily interpretable.

Although *biochemical studies* currently prove helpful in only a small proportion of dysmorphic infants (e.g. peroxisomal disorders such as Zellweger syndrome and chondrodysplasia punctata, and some lysosomal storage diseases), consideration should also be given to storing tissue for future analysis. Cultured fibroblasts may be saved after chromosome analysis while, in fatal cases, skin and liver tissue can be deep-frozen.

Molecular analysis is of major importance in the diagnosis of malformation syndromes and is increasing rapidly in its applications. The progressive understanding of the molecular basis of malformation syndromes is probably the most exciting area of dysmorphology and is considered later in the chapter. A sample of DNA, or tissue from which it can be isolated, should be kept for future analysis.

Autopsy by an experienced paediatric pathologist is of great value in any infant death or pregnancy loss associated with malformation. It may show unsuspected internal defects (e.g. renal abnormalities) that are related to the dysmorphic features. However, a careful external examination with photographic and radiological or MRI images can still be of great value, even if autopsy is not permitted or not available.

Finally, careful literature search, discussion with and presentation to colleagues, and the use of computer databases are all important diagnostic measures, as mentioned later. In particular, the recognition of relatively unusual diagnostic features may provide a useful 'handle' that can distinguish a specific syndrome from other related conditions.

SYNDROME DIAGNOSIS AND CLINICAL MANAGEMENT

The accurate diagnosis of malformations is sometimes disparaged by clinicians as an exercise in classification that contributes little to the welfare of the affected child. Nothing could be further from the truth, and it is surprising how often clinical geneticists have to point out to their paediatric and obstetric colleagues the existence of some major complication, the possibility of which they were unaware of because a precise diagnosis had not been made. Quite apart from affecting the risks of recurrence on which genetic counselling is based, management of the individual case may be critically affected. A few examples among many encountered are as follows:

- *Holt-Oram syndrome*: An atrial septal defect in an infant with limb defects may be missed if the possibility of cardiac involvement is not considered.
- *Thrombocytopenia with absent radius (TAR) syndrome*: Lack of awareness of this disorder can lead to a misdiagnosis of Fanconi anaemia, with a prediction of probable mental retardation and high risk for malignancy (both of which are absent in TAR).
- *Exomphalos*: Prenatal detection by ultrasound led to caesarean section. The infant had multiple other defects due to a major chromosome anomaly; if recognised antenatally, such interventional obstetric management may not have been undertaken.

Now that highly sophisticated (and often successful) neonatal intensive care and surgery are available, it is all the more important that a full and accurate diagnosis of any genetic syndrome is made rapidly, even prenatally if possible. While laboratory tests, in particular chromosome analysis, are often a vital part of this, the diagnostic skill of a clinical geneticist experienced in dysmorphology may be of even greater value in ensuring the appropriate management of many of these difficult problems.

AETIOLOGICAL BASIS OF MALFORMATION SYNDROMES

Many of the important syndromes are described in the individual chapters of Part 2 of this book and can be located using the index. Here an outline is given of some of the aetiological groups that are increasingly becoming defined. Not only is it important to establish aetiology, where possible, for practical reasons of genetic counselling, but some of these disorders are proving to be of great importance in basic research, particularly where specific genes are involved. As the techniques of molecular genetics are applied to dysmorphology, many more syndromes will prove useful as models for disordered developmental processes that can be analysed at the molecular level and for which new, rational treatments may be on the horizon.

Chromosomal syndromes

While the major chromosomal disorders (see Chapter 4) have been recognised for many years (e.g. trisomy 21, trisomy 13), clinical cytogenetics has delineated many others that involve parts of specific chromosomes (e.g. 22q11.2, 22q13.3 or 1p36 deletion syndromes), or mosaicism for entire chromosomes (e.g. mosaic trisomy 8). Syndromes of this type involving an autosome are usually accompanied by mental retardation, but in many cases the combination of physical abnormalities is sufficiently specific to allow a presumptive diagnosis before the chromosome constitution is known. While most cases are sporadic, it is important to recognise the small proportion where an unaffected parent is the balanced carrier of a structural rearrangement, is mosaic for an anomaly or manifests the condition very mildly.

Microdeletion syndromes

In the microdeletion syndromes, individual components may be the result of deletion of a single gene or of several, contiguous genes; the combination of clinical features has been a most valuable clue to the localisation and relative ordering of the loci involved. The deletions involved may be visible, especially if high-resolution cytogenetic analysis is used, but will often only be apparent if more sensitive, molecular techniques are employed, such as aCGH, quantitative polymerase chain reaction (qPCR), FISH or multiplex ligation-dependent probe amplification (MLPA) (see Chapter 5). Some such microdeletion syndromes are listed in Table 4.11.

Examples of particular importance are those involving chromosome 11p and giving various combinations of Wilms tumour, aniridia, genital defects and mental retardation (the WAGR complex), and the complementary paternal and maternal deletions of 15q resulting in Prader-Willi and Angelman syndromes, respectively. About one-third of those with these conditions have no detectable deletion. These results from uniparental disomy or (especially with Angelman syndrome) mutation in specific genes or disruption of the control of imprinting in this region.

A development of considerable importance is the recognition that a significant proportion of cases of congenital heart disease result from microdeletions of 22q11.2, with a considerably broader and often more subtle range of features by comparison with the originally recognised categories of the DiGeorge and velocardiofacial syndromes (see Chapter 21).

Since the phenotype in some microdeletions can vary, sometimes being relatively mild and compatible with reproduction, the study of parents (clinical as well as chromosomal) is of particular importance. When a parent is affected, the child will often be affected more severely. This can be for two reasons: (1) more mildly affected cases are more likely to become parents, and (2) the affected parent may be mosaic for the disorder, with the child being fully affected.

Teratogenic syndromes

In teratogenic syndromes (see Chapter 28), the factor may be infective (e.g. rubella), drug related (e.g. anticonvulsants) or metabolic (e.g. maternal phenylketonuria). The number of well-documented and specific syndromes in the group (e.g. maternal warfarin) remains small. Some may closely mimic genetic syndromes, so it is important not to assume a teratogenic cause without good evidence. Conversely, some genetic syndromes may easily be mistaken for intrauterine infections (e.g. recessively inherited microcephaly with calcification of the basal ganglia).

Syndromes due to disordered function of specific genes in development

The possibility of identifying the specific genes responsible for individual malformation syndromes has become one of the most important and rapidly evolving fields of medical genetics and has immediate practical consequences. It clearly reinforces the need for an accurate clinical classification of dysmorphic syndromes, as well as provides the possibility of early prenatal diagnosis for families. In the past, the identification of disease loci was principally achieved by gene mapping, positional cloning and mutation searches in plausible candidate loci already known to be important in development. Now, the genetic factors underlying developmental defects are sought more often by genome-wide methods as outlined in Chapter 5.

Work with a variety of model organisms, especially *Mus, Drosophila*, and even simpler organisms such as the flatworm *Caenorhabditis* and yeast *Candida*, has led to

Table 6.1 Molecular basis of congenital malformations (specific examples)

Disorder	Gene
Apert syndrome	Fibroblast growth factor receptor (FGFR 2)
Campomelic dysplasia	SOX 9 (SRY-related developmental gene)
Hirschsprung disease	RET oncogene (also involved in MEN 2)
Holt-Oram syndrome	TBX5 (transcription factor)
Opitz syndrome (X-linked)	MID 1 (midline developmental gene)
Rubinstein-Taybi syndrome	CREB binding protein (16p) and other genes
Saethre-Chotzen craniosynostosis	TWIST (Drosophila homologue)
Thanatophoric dysplasia	Fibroblast growth factor receptor (FGFR 3)
Treacher Collins syndrome	TCOF1 gene (involved in branchial arch development)
Waardenburg syndrome	PAX 3 (important in embryonic migration of some neural crest-derived cells)

an understanding of human phenotypes associated with defects of cell-signalling, segmentation of the body plan, and defects in cell cycle control and in cell signalling. These developments allow us to consider the basic science known as 'evo-devo' as interacting most constructively with dysmorphology; dysmorphology has both contributed to and drawn from the underlying biology in a most fruitful synergy that led to the concept of 'inborn errors of development'.

Many of the relevant genes are strongly conserved between species, so that the human counterparts can be isolated and tested for abnormalities in various syndromes. In addition, at a more clinical level, clear homologies exist between a number of mouse mutants and human malformations, so that if a molecular defect is found in the mouse model, it is likely to be relevant also to the human condition. Table 6.1 gives a selection of examples; others will be found in the specific chapters. Interestingly, some of the genes involved in developmental defects are proving to be involved in neoplasia as well (e.g. the RET oncogene in both Hirschsprung disease and multiple endocrine neoplasia type 2).

These exciting developments offer the possibility of matching human developmental defects with the individual genetic steps in embryonic development. The possibility of constructing transgenic mouse models in addition to those occurring naturally further strengthens this approach. Malformation syndromes can now be seen as the equivalent of inborn errors of metabolism, specific defects that will eventually tell us as much about normal embryonic development as rare inborn errors have told us about metabolic pathways. *Epstein's Inborn Errors of Development* (see Appendix 1) gives an authoritative source for defects in different developmental pathways, although numerous changes have accumulated since then.

GENETIC RECURRENCE RISKS IN MALFORMATION SYNDROMES

For some of the more common disorders, empirical recurrence risks exist and are mentioned in the appropriate chapters in Part 2 of this book. Frequently, however, such data are inadequate or non-existent, and the clinician is faced with giving genetic counselling without a secure basis on which to estimate the risk of recurrence.

BOX 6.2: Malformation syndromes following autosomal recessive inheritance

Bardet-Biedl syndrome
Campomelic dysplasia
Carpenter syndrome (acrocephalopolysyndactyly)
Cerebro-oculo-facio-skeletal (Pena-Shokeir) syndrome (some families)
Chondrodysplasia punctata (rhizomelic type)
Cockayne syndrome
Cohen syndrome
Cryptophthalmos (Fraser) syndrome
Dubowitz syndrome
Ellis-van Creveld syndrome
Fanconi pancytopenia
Fryns syndrome
Holoprosencephaly (some families)
Hydrolethalus syndrome
Jarcho-Levin syndrome
Johanson-Blizzard syndrome
Leprechaunism (Donohue syndrome)
Marden-Walker syndrome
Meckel syndrome
Multiple pterygium syndrome
Neu Laxova syndrome
Orofaciodigital syndrome type II (Mohr syndrome)
Roberts syndrome
Rothmund-Thomson syndrome
Seckel syndrome
Seip lipodystrophy syndrome
Smith-Lemli-Opitz syndrome
Thrombocytopenia with absent radius (TAR) syndrome

The greatest potential for error in such a situation lies in mistaking a disorder following Mendelian (particularly autosomal recessive) inheritance for a similar but non-genetic or polygenic condition. In the absence of a positive family history, and especially if full documentation is not available, such a mistake is all too easy. For this reason, lists are given in Boxes 6.2–6.4 of some of the disorders where Mendelian inheritance is probable.

While the potential for recurrence in sibs is greatest for the autosomal recessive (see Box 6.2) and X-linked disorders (see Box 6.4), variability of expression can be a trap with autosomal dominant inheritance, and this group is listed in Box 6.3. As a counterbalance, a list is given of disorders where recurrence is unusual, often (where the reason is known) because they usually result from *de novo* dominant or post-zygotic mutations (Box 6.5).

It must be borne in mind that an increasing range of malformations with specific developmental molecular defects are proving to be new and genetically lethal dominant mutations. Chromosomal disorders, craniofacial syndromes and skeletal dysplasias are considered in the relevant chapters.

BOX 6.3: Malformation syndromes following autosomal dominant inheritance

Beckwith-Wiedemann syndrome (often sporadic but with parent-of-origin effects in some families)
Craniosynostoses (including Crouzon disease and Saethre-Chotzen syndrome but excluding Carpenter syndrome)
EEC syndrome (ectrodactyly, ectodermal dysplasia, clefting)
Freeman-Sheldon (whistling face) syndrome[a]
Greig cephalopolysyndactyly
Holt-Oram syndrome
Larsen syndrome
Multiple lentigines with deafness (LEOPARD) syndrome
Nail-patella syndrome
Noonan syndrome[a]
Oculodentodigital syndrome
Opitz hypertelorism with hypospadias (G) syndrome (some families)
Popliteal pterygium syndrome (some families)
Rieger syndrome
Robinow (fetal face) syndrome
Stickler syndrome[a]
Townes-Brocks syndrome
Treacher Collins syndrome (Mandibulofacial dysostosis)[a]
Trichorhinophalangeal syndrome (type I)
Van der Woude syndrome
Waardenburg syndrome

[a] Expression variable and sometimes minimal.

BOX 6.4: Malformation syndromes following X-linked inheritance (not exhaustive)

Aarskog syndrome (faciogenital dysplasia)
Börjeson-Forssman-Lehmann syndrome
Coffin-Lowry syndrome
Corpus callosum agenesis with retinal defects (Aicardi syndrome) (dominant, lethal in male)
Ectodermal dysplasia, hypohidrotic
FG syndrome (Opitz)
Focal dermal hypoplasia (Goltz syndrome) (dominant, lethal in male)
KBG syndrome
Lenz microphthalmos syndrome
Menkes syndrome
Opitz G/BBB syndrome
Orofaciodigital syndrome, type I (dominant, lethal in male)
Otopalatodigital syndrome
X-linked α-thalassaemia mental retardation (ATRX) syndrome

> ## BOX 6.5: Malformation syndromes in which recurrence in siblings is most uncommon (although there is often a genetic basis)
>
> Amniotic bands disruption syndrome
> CHARGE: Often a de novo mutation in CHD7
> de Lange syndrome (severe form: See Chapter 16)
> Goldenhar syndrome (now also known as hemifacial microsomia or oculoauriculovertebral dysplasia)
> Klippel-Feil syndrome (although autosomal dominant and autosomal recessive inheritance is known, with locus heterogeneity)
> [a]Klippel-Trenauny-Weber syndrome
> [a]McCune-Albright (fibrous dysplasia) syndrome – caused by somatic mosaicism for activating mutation in GNAS)
> Möbius syndrome
> Poland syndrome
> [a]Proteus syndromes – caused by somatic mutations in AKT1
> Rubinstein-Taybi syndrome (usually caused by de novo microdeletions at 16p13 or mutations in CREBBP)
> Russell-Silver syndrome (sometimes the result of UPD7[mat] or methylation abnormality at 11p)
> Sacral agenesis (caudal regression syndrome): Consider maternal diabetes
> Sotos (often caused by mutation, usually de novo, in NSD1)
> VATER (or VACTERL) association
> Weaver (often caused by mutation, usually de novo, in EZH2)
>
> ---
>
> [a] Indicates that this usually arises as a disorder of somatic mosaicism.

COMPUTERISED DATABASES

The recognition and delineation of new syndromes has benefited immensely from the development of computerised databases of known and unknown disorders. Several systems are now available that are regularly updated and are becoming essential tools of the clinical geneticist and others involved with dysmorphic children. These systems not only provide help to the non-expert but give a framework through which new entities can be worked out (or 'deciphered'). By including information published or presented all over the world, they are especially helpful in rare or atypical disorders; by suggesting various alternative diagnoses and giving key references, they also stimulate the clinician to think in new directions. Molecular details and available tests are coming to be included in these databases.

Three main systems currently exist: the London Dysmorphology Database, POSSUM and Decipher. They all have illustrations of patients and are regularly updated. It must be emphasised that they do not normally make the diagnosis for the clinician but rather give a series of possibilities; they require practice and knowledge for their optimal use. The Decipher database originally linked reports of array CGH anomalies from laboratories in many countries with the associated clinical features but now also covers point mutations; it thereby greatly facilitates the recognition of new diagnostic entities.

Two additional databases of more general information available on the internet are the Orphanet database and that provided by the National Organization for Rare Disorders (NORD) (see Appendix 1).

7

Carrier testing

INTRODUCTION

One of the major tasks in genetic counselling is to clarify reproductive risk in families with genetic disorders. This includes identifying those individuals who, while themselves healthy, have a high risk of transmitting a genetic disorder. Recognition of a particular mode of inheritance will often allow the risk to be estimated and, in some cases, excluded; but where the risk is high, it may often be impossible to tell with certainty on clinical grounds alone whether or not a particular family member possesses the abnormal gene. For this reason, tests that will identify the correct genotype of a person are of great importance and in many instances form an integral part of the overall process of genetic counselling.

This chapter explores the range and limitations of tests of carrier status and attempts to show how the information can be used in conjunction with other genetic and clinical data to make as accurate a determination as possible.

WHAT DO WE MEAN BY 'CARRIER'?

The term 'carrier' is widely used in medicine. It is often applied to those harbouring an infective agent but not overtly sick because of it, quite apart from its use in medical genetics. The term may be used by different people with entirely different connotations, and a precise definition is important if confusion is not to arise. A working definition of the carrier state in inherited disease is as follows:

> A carrier is an individual who possesses in heterozygous state the mutation determining an inherited disorder, and who is essentially healthy at the time of study.

Table 7.1 Genetic risks for carriers of Mendelian disorders

Inheritance	Risk to offspring of carrier
Autosomal recessive	Very low unless the disorder is extremely common, consanguinity is present or the same disorder is present in the spouse's family
Autosomal dominant	50% (risk of overt disease will vary with disorder)
X-linked recessive	50% of male offspring affected; variable expression of disorder possible in female offspring

From this definition, several important points follow:

- A carrier is a heterozygote, so the term can be applied satisfactorily only to Mendelian disorders determined by a single locus. It is logical to talk of a carrier for cystic fibrosis or for haemophilia, but not of a carrier for spina bifida, where the genetic determination is poorly understood and non-Mendelian.
- The definition of 'carrier' can be stretched to individuals with a balanced chromosomal abnormality such as a translocation, where the inheritance is essentially Mendelian (see Chapter 4), and to asymptomatic individuals with a mitochondrial mutation. Perhaps it should also include a healthy male with a premutation for FRAXA, whether or not he goes on to become affected by FXTAS.
- Although a carrier is heterozygous, this does not necessarily imply that the affected individual must be homozygous. This will be the case only in autosomal recessive disorders; in autosomal dominant disorders, almost all individuals with the abnormal gene, whether affected or carriers, will be heterozygous. In sex-linked disorders, the situation is more complicated with the hemizygous males usually being affected and heterozygous females who 'carry' the disorder often being healthy or if affected often to a lesser degree than is usual for males.
- Although the risk of a carrier transmitting the abnormal gene is high (normally 50%), it does not always follow that there is a high risk of having an affected child. The risk may in fact be extremely low and will depend on the mode of inheritance (Table 7.1).
- The fact that a carrier is 'essentially healthy' at the time of study does not mean that minor clinical features may not be discernable, nor does it mean that the individual will necessarily remain healthy. Those carrying the mutation for Huntington's disease provide an example of the latter point.

It is clear from these considerations that carrier detection has to be approached in light of the natural history of the particular genetic disorder and its mode of inheritance.

OBLIGATORY AND POSSIBLE CARRIERS

When the testing of carriers is being considered, it is often not recognised that, in addition to individuals at a higher or lower risk of being a carrier, there are those who, on genetic grounds, must be carriers (Figure 7.1). Recognition of these 'obligatory' carriers is important for several reasons: it may save complex and unnecessary testing procedures, it allows much more definite genetic counselling to be given and it also provides a reference population against which any new or improved carrier test can be evaluated.

Obligatory carriers for autosomal recessive disorders include all children and parents of an affected individual (mutation as an alternative is too rare to be a practical problem). In X-linked

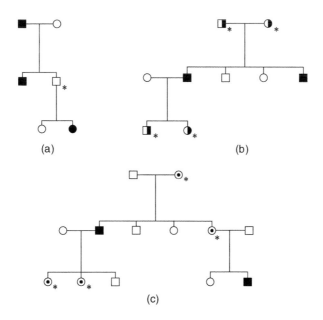

Figure 7.1 Obligatory carriers in Mendelian inheritance. Obligatory carriers for the three major modes of inheritance are marked with an asterisk (*). By convention, carriers for autosomal recessive disorders are half shaded, and those for X-linked disorders dotted. (a) Autosomal dominant inheritance: any individual having both an affected parent and affected offspring must be a carrier. (b) Autosomal recessive inheritance: both parents and all offspring of an affected individual are obligatory carriers. (c) X-linked recessive inheritance: obligatory carriers include all daughters of an affected male and all women who have an affected son and at least one other affected male relative.

recessive inheritance, all daughters of an affected male will be obligatory carriers, as will those females who have an affected brother and an affected son; in autosomal dominant inheritance, obligatory carriers are people who have both a parent and a child affected but who show (or showed when alive) no abnormalities themselves. This situation is commonly seen in Huntington's disease and other late-onset disorders when an individual has died young of an unrelated cause but is later shown to have transmitted the disorder. It may also occur if the gene concerned is not fully penetrant (see later in this chapter), which molecular analysis has shown to be a more frequent occurrence than was formerly thought to be the case.

PRINCIPAL TYPES OF 'CARRIERS'

There are two key questions that help to decide what type of carrier a person is:

1. If a carrier has a child, does the child's chance of being affected depend essentially upon their genetic inheritance from one parent alone or equally upon their inheritance from both parents?

In terms of risk to offspring, there are two types of carriers: those whose children are at risk from that one parent alone, with the other parent's contribution effectively 'irrelevant', and those who are only at risk if both parents carry and transmit the disorder to the child.

The first category comprises the sons of female carriers of sex-linked disorders, the children of the healthy, 'balanced' carriers of chromosome rearrangements, and the children of those carrying but so far unaffected by autosomal dominant disorders. In these conditions, the genetic constitution of the other parent is largely irrelevant to the risk of the child being affected.

The second category consists of the usual type of autosomal recessive disease, where a child has to inherit mutations from both parents to be affected.

2. If a person carries the mutation in question, will they be affected or not? These two categories are very different, not only biologically but also in terms of the personal and emotional consequences of testing.

The question of whether the apparently healthy carrier of a mutation will become affected distinguishes dominant from recessive disorders, although with some more complicated factors to consider, especially sex-linked inheritance (and the variation in X-chromosome inactivation in heterozygous females) and variable penetrance, sometimes related to the chance of a 'second hit' mechanism.

All carriers can transmit 'their' disorder to their children, but in the context of a dominant disorder, the carriers are also themselves at risk. The impact of carrier testing is therefore often much greater when performing predictive, or presymptomatic, testing for a dominant disorder, because concern for the risk of disease and the welfare of the person being tested are important in addition to any question of risk to their offspring or future generations. This situation is considered in Chapter 8. We consider the question of prenatal diagnosis in an established pregnancy in Chapter 9.

CARRIER DETECTION IN AUTOSOMAL RECESSIVE DISEASE

Autosomal recessive disorders provide by far the largest number of carriers numerically but are by no means the most important in genetic counselling in terms of giving high risks. We are all likely to be carriers for at least one serious recessive disorder and several lethal ones, quite apart from numerous polymorphisms such as blood groups where heterozygosity is normal and may have been beneficial in the past, if not now.

From the standpoint of genetic counselling for autosomal recessive disorders, there are three main situations that are encountered:

- An individual is, or is likely to be, a carrier for a rare autosomal recessive disorder.
- An individual is, or is likely to be, a carrier for a common autosomal recessive disorder.
- The situation is complicated by consanguinity or by marriage to an individual whose family may be affected by the same disorder.

The importance or lack of importance of the carrier state in these three situations is directly related to the principles of autosomal recessive inheritance, which are discussed in Chapter 2.

Rare autosomal recessive disorders

Rare autosomal recessive disorders are the ones about which advice is most commonly sought, and family members may be greatly worried and alarmed by having been told they may be carriers. Such worry (usually induced by doctors in the first place) is entirely unnecessary but is often extremely difficult to allay. Some individuals may believe that being a carrier means they have the disease in a mild form or are in some way not entirely healthy. Others believe that, even though they are healthy themselves, their children will inevitably be affected.

Neither situation is, of course, the case. Heterozygotes for autosomal recessive disorders are almost always entirely healthy and will remain so, even when minor distinguishing biochemical or haematological features can be found. Those most commonly seeking advice are the sibs of affected individuals, who have a two-thirds chance of carrying the condition, but their risk of having affected children is exceptionally low, in the absence of consanguinity. A confident reassurance can be given that this is the case for all rare autosomal recessive disorders. Some family members may request carrier testing for themselves and their spouses, if this is feasible, 'just to be sure'. It is becoming increasingly simple to identify family members who carry one of the disease-causing mutations found in the patient but, with a rare disease, it may be much more difficult to give categorical carrier/non-carrier results to those marrying into the family. If carrier testing has to rely on older, metabolic investigations, then we would discourage testing because the margin of error of the test will often make misclassification a real possibility in a situation of low prior risk. Prenatal diagnosis on the basis of unsatisfactory genetic tests or metabolic assays is rarely justified.

The advent of molecular testing for many rare autosomal recessive disorders has increased the likelihood of inappropriate carrier testing. While it is often possible to distinguish the heterozygous carrier within a family having such a disorder, it may be difficult or impossible to do so in the population as a whole, particularly where a disorder may be due to any one of a large number of mutations. The unsatisfactory situation can thus be created where worry is increased by the sib of an affected individual being shown to be a carrier, without it being possible to resolve the situation by testing the unrelated partner. Even if a specific mutation has been detected in the family, there is no guarantee that a carrier partner would have the same mutation, so an extensive search for all possible mutations may be needed if one has embarked on this course, often leaving the situation inconclusive, though the availability of complete gene sequencing may somewhat improve matters.

The application of high-throughput genetic technologies to genetic screening programmes, to identify carriers of autosomal recessive disease, can be very helpful. A number of schemes have been developed to identify the rare recessive mutations found in specific population groups in North Africa and the Gulf. These schemes often involve cooperation between an Arab state and a European or North American genetics centre. The way in which these schemes operate in practice can tell us much about the social organisation of the particular community. These 'rare' mutations are often not at all rare within the relevant community, especially where endogamy is usual or consanguinity preferred.

To conclude, it can be seen that for most rare autosomal recessive disorders, the time and energy of the person involved in genetic counselling should normally be employed to give a clear explanation of the risks, usually very low, and the lack of importance to one's health of being a carrier, rather than indiscriminately recommending what may be difficult, expensive and often unnecessary tests of carrier detection. The limitations and inaccuracy of any testing situation should be clearly understood and explained, before testing is carried out.

Common autosomal recessive disorders

The common autosomal recessive disorders provide a much more important indication for carrier detection, although the disorders have to be extremely common to present a significant risk to individual couples. Even for a disorder as relatively common as phenylketonuria (1 in 10,000 births in the United Kingdom), the risk for offspring of a healthy sib is only 1 in 300. Very few of the classic enzyme deficiencies for which carrier testing is available are as common as this, except for special concentrations such as Tay-Sachs disease in Ashkenazi Jewish populations.

The haemoglobinopathies and thalassaemias provide the most important group on a worldwide basis, and carrier detection is fortunately feasible in most of these; population screening for the carrier state in these disorders is now widespread and is discussed later and in Chapter 34. Particular countries or regions (e.g. Finland, Quebec), geographically isolated populations or endogamous (reproductively isolated) communities may have high frequencies of other disorders, making carrier detection important for them. Laboratories and clinical genetics services both need to ensure that ethnic origins and the local pattern of genetic disorders and mutations are taken into account in the analyses and risk estimates undertaken.

When carrier testing for one of the common autosomal recessive disorders is being undertaken, it is logical to test both the family member at risk and the spouse (or prospective partner) at the same time. If only one proves to be a carrier, the couple can confidently be reassured; if not all mutations are detectable in the testing of an unrelated partner, this should be pointed out before any testing is embarked upon, as it may make the whole exercise meaningless. Where an individual affected with an autosomal recessive disorder is concerned, it is the testing of the partner that is the critical factor, since the affected person will inevitably transmit one copy of their mutation.

DNA mutation analysis has progressively replaced biochemical and haematological tests, though these may still be useful as first-line or screening tests, especially in the haemoglobinopathies. Cystic fibrosis is a good example of a disorder where all phenotypic tests for the carrier state proved unreliable but where testing for mutations now allows determination of which close relatives are carriers. This is made easier by the predominance of one common pathogenic variant in the *CFTR* gene (delta F508, now more correctly known as c.1521_1523 del CTT; p.Phe508del) in most northern European populations; excluding the carrier state in an unrelated partner may require testing for a much wider range of less frequent variants. The implications of this for population screening in cystic fibrosis are discussed in Chapter 34.

Consanguinity (see also Chapter 10) may occasionally produce the need for carrier testing in a rare autosomal recessive disorder where the risks would otherwise be negligible; even less often, the same disorder may be present in the families of two unrelated partners. The heterozygote can be distinguished in the case of numerous rare inborn errors of metabolism, but it should be noted that, with biochemical assays, there is often considerable overlap between the normal and heterozygote ranges, so that a clear indication of the likely margin of error should be obtained from the laboratory involved. Molecular testing is often easier when consanguinity is present since, if mutation analysis is being used, one is looking for the same mutation in both partners.

CARRIER DETECTION IN X-LINKED DISEASE

A relatively small number of X-linked recessive disorders provide the most important of all applications of carrier detection. The reason for this is simple: the carriers are generally healthy and so will be likely to reproduce, but in contrast to autosomal recessive inheritance, they will be at risk of having fully affected male offspring regardless of whom they marry. In such a situation, the availability of carrier detection for women at high risk is a major contribution and forms such an integral part of genetic counselling that it is often unwise to give a definitive risk estimate until information from testing is available.

The haemophilias and X-linked muscular dystrophies (principally Duchenne dystrophy) are overwhelmingly the most important disorders that have to be considered in this group, and the approaches to carrier detection and the problems of interpretation are remarkably similar in each and apply also to most other X-linked disorders. For this reason, although details are given with the individual disorders, they will be used here as examples of carrier detection in X-linked recessive disease generally. Fragile X syndrome is also a frequent indication for carrier detection, but its unusual genetic features, especially with 'normal transmitting males' who carry an unstable triplet repeat pre-mutation, make it different from most other X-linked disorders in terms of carrier detection.

In both haemophilia and Duchenne muscular dystrophy, a few carriers may be detectable clinically, probably as the result of X-chromosome inactivation having resulted, randomly, in a higher than usual proportion of those X chromosomes that bear the abnormal gene functioning in the particular tissue of importance. This process will also, inevitably, result in the opposite – namely, carriers in whom, principally, the normal X chromosome is functioning, and who will thus be difficult or impossible to identify as carriers even by the most sensitive tests of phenotype. This variability of X-linked carriers is characteristic and must always be borne in mind. Tests based on DNA are not affected by X inactivation, and this property is one of the most important reasons for their use being greatly preferable in the detection of X-linked heterozygotes.

The phenotypic test still sometimes used for Duchenne muscular dystrophy, the elevation of serum creatine kinase levels, is considerably further removed from the basic molecular defect than the assays for factor VIII in haemophilia, with consequently less precision in detecting carriers. In both disorders, however, there is a considerable overlap between normal and carrier ranges, which makes it impossible to classify most individuals as definitely 'normal' or 'abnormal'. Instead, a series of likelihood ratios must be used that will give odds for or against the carrier state for any particular result of the test. By using these odds, one can arrive at a much more precise separation of carriers and non-carriers than would otherwise be possible, especially if the results are integrated with other genetic information, as described in Chapter 2. Although phenotypic tests in these and other X-linked disorders have been progressively replaced by molecular analysis, they retain a place in both Duchenne muscular dystrophy and the haemophilias. These methods are cheap and rapid, and a clearly abnormal result will rarely be outweighed or contradicted by molecular evidence.

The isolated male case of an X-linked disorder presents major problems in carrier detection. There is considerable variation between diseases as to the proportion of such cases likely to represent new mutations and, correspondingly, the proportion of mothers who are carriers. The prior risk of such a mother being a carrier will be somewhere between 50% and 100%, depending on the relative mutation rates in the two sexes, and the interpretation of carrier testing will clearly be influenced by this figure. Even the recognition of gene deletion in such an isolated case does not always allow exclusion of the carrier state, because some mothers show gonadal mosaicism. This may be a further factor in the apparent lack of phenotypic features in carrier women and seems to be especially frequent in Duchenne muscular dystrophy.

All daughters of a man with an X-linked recessive disease must be carriers, and so (assuming paternity is correct) tests of carrier detection are irrelevant for such people. Despite this, they are often referred for 'genetic counselling and carrier detection' under the misapprehension that a normal result will somehow make a definite carrier less definite. False reassurance is a real danger in such a situation. Equally, it should be made clear to such a carrier that a mutation test is essentially a paternity test.

In X-linked disorders that regularly manifest in females, such as hypophosphataemic rickets or Rett syndrome, the question of whether the mother will be a carrier also arises. In Rett syndrome, in which mutations usually occur at spermatogenesis, the mother will usually not be a carrier and the risk of recurrence from parental mosaicism applies as much to the father

Table 7.2 Phenotypic changes in carrier detection for X-linked disorders

Disorder	Abnormality in carrier
Adrenal leucodystrophy	Long-chain fatty acid synthesis
Alport syndrome	Microscopic haematuria
Amelogenesis imperfecta	Patchy enamel hypoplasia (heterogeneous)
Becker muscular dystrophy	Serum creatine kinase (less discriminating than in Duchenne)
Centronuclear (myotubular) myopathy (lethal type)	Muscle biopsy changes
Choroideraemia	Pigmentary retinal changes
Chronic granulomatous disease	Partial NADPH oxidase deficiency; discoid lupus-like skin lesions
Duchenne muscular dystrophy	Serum creatine kinase
Fabry disease	Skin lesions; α-galactosidase assay
Fragile X syndrome type A (FRAXA)	Variable cognitive impairment; may show chromosomal fragile site
Glucose-6-phosphate dehydrogenase deficiency	Quantitative enzyme assay and electrophoresis
Haemophilia A	Factor VIII assay
Haemophilia B	Factor IX assay
Hunter syndrome (MPS II)	Enzyme assay on hair bulbs and serum (variable)
Hypogammaglobinaemia (Bruton type)	Reduced IgG (some individuals only)
Immune deficiency (SCID)	X-inactivation analysis on leucocytes
Lesch-Nyhan syndrome	HGPRT assay on hair bulbs
Lowe syndrome	Amino aciduria, lens opacities
Ocular albinism	Patchy fundal depigmentation
Retinoschisis	Cystic retinal changes
Vitamin D-resistant rickets	Serum phosphate (may be clinical features)
Wiskott-Aldrich syndrome	X-inactivation studies; in white blood cells; IgA levels
X-linked congenital cataract	Lens opacities
X-linked ichthyosis	Corneal opacities, reduced steroid sulphatase
X-linked hypohidrotic ectodermal dysplasia	Patchy sweating, dental defects (number or shape of teeth), sparse hair
X-linked retinitis pigmentosa	Pigmentary changes; abnormality of electroretinogram, more than one locus

as to the mother. In the male-lethal disorders, such as incontinentia pigmenti, there is little information about whether the mutation usually arises first in the egg or the sperm.

Table 7.2 shows some of the X-linked recessive disorders where phenotype-based carrier detection can be helpful. The range of approaches is wide and may be morphological, functional, biochemical or molecular. The last of these approaches is the definitive one, which is preferred whenever it is possible. Taken as a group, X-linked disorders are probably the most satisfactory and the most satisfying in terms of our ability to detect the carrier state and its applicability in allowing families to avoid recurrence of the disease.

METHODS OF CARRIER DETECTION

The techniques available for detecting the carrier state vary greatly according to the nature of the particular disease and our understanding of its metabolic basis. It is impossible to give all the details here, and available approaches are mentioned as far as possible with individual disorders, but it is worth considering the broad forms of approach and some of the limitations that exist.

Molecular analysis

Molecular analysis has become the approach of choice for carrier detection in most Mendelian disorders (see Chapter 5 for details), but it should not be assumed that the older technologies are necessarily inferior. Molecular analysis can itself have drawbacks – for example, when any one of several different genes might be involved, or when it may be difficult to be certain whether a particular change is pathogenic or simply a harmless variant. These and other potential problems make it essential that only experienced laboratories, subject to regular quality control, and preferably closely linked with clinical genetics services, are used in the molecular analysis of genetic disorders.

The major recent change in the molecular methods used in identifying carriers is the introduction of next-generation sequencing (NGS). This allows screening for mutation in all genes associated with autosomal recessive or sex-linked disease, even without any specific family history. This is in effect population screening of the individual. Panels of genes known to be associated with a specific phenotype can also be tested for mutations in healthy relatives if the index case never had a confirmed genetic diagnosis and has died or is unavailable for testing. This maximises the chance of finding a mutation, if there is one to be found in the at-risk relative. These developments are in the process of transforming the approach to carrier detection.

Measurement of the primary enzyme or other defect

This remains a satisfactory approach, where available, and is feasible for numerous inborn errors of metabolism, mostly following autosomal recessive inheritance, as well as for non-enzymatic defects such as haemophilias and various haemoglobinopathies. DNA analysis will often only be essential if there is a special need to know the specific mutation involved, such as for prenatal diagnosis. However, once the mutations present in a family are known, molecular genetic testing for carrier status may be simpler, cheaper and more robust than the enzyme assays. The range of enzyme results in heterozygotes may show considerable overlap with the normal range, and less commonly with that of the abnormal homozygotes. The appropriate tissue to use will also vary. Serum may be adequate, but more often red or white blood cells or cultured fibroblasts are required, and the techniques may be difficult and specialised. X-linked disorders are particularly variable, as already discussed, making DNA analysis much preferable.

Secondary biochemical changes

The value of these will, in general, be related to how close the abnormality is to the primary defect. Important examples have been the use of creatine kinase measurement in Duchenne muscular dystrophy, elevation of haemoglobin A levels in β-thalassaemia and abnormalities of porphyrin excretion in the acute porphyrias. As our knowledge has increased, however, such tests have tended to be superseded or used largely as preliminary screening tests. Thus, in phenylketonuria, until the gene was isolated, carrier detection was usually achieved by studying the blood phenylalanine-to-tyrosine ratio under standardized conditions, or by performing a phenylalanine loading test, but this approach is now obsolete.

Cytogenetic studies

These remain of obvious importance in families with a balanced translocation or a chromosome inversion, but karyotype or FISH are being used much less often for disorders recognised on aCGH, which is finding application in disorders not previously considered chromosomal. Copy number variants of modest penetrance can be particularly difficult to discuss with families and even with non-genetics health professionals. There are, for example, several newly recognised, small microdeletions that are found within the regions of recurrent, larger and much better recognised chromosome deletion syndromes (e.g. small microdeletions within the well-known 22q11 or 15q11-13 deletion regions, usually resulting from unequal recombination events between two sites of homology at the same end of the larger region prone to unequal exchange). Where a small deletion or translocation is involved (see Table 4.10), the presence or absence of any anomaly in a relative is likely to determine whether the risk is high or low. In the important case of fragile X syndrome (FRAXA), molecular analysis for the mutation is of greater value than cytogenetic study in the identification of asymptomatic gene carriers, whether these are females or normal transmitting males (see Chapter 14).

Physiological tests

Examples include the use of electroretinography in detecting the carriers of X-linked retinitis pigmentosa or sweat testing in heterozygous female carriers of X-linked hypohidrotic ectodermal dysplasia. Such tests have been largely superseded by molecular tests for diagnosis.

Microscopic techniques

These may rely on biopsy, as in Duchenne muscular dystrophy; blood film examination, as with sickle cell anaemia or thalassaemias; or biomicroscopy, as in slit-lamp examination for the lens opacities of myotonic dystrophy or the Lisch nodules of neurofibromatosis. Again, though, specificity of these tests is not always complete, while some are invasive, so their use has diminished as molecular analysis has become possible. Where microscopy can be combined with a technique that enhances specificity, such as immunohistochemistry, then it may retain usefulness under specific circumstances when molecular tests are unavailable.

Imaging (by X-ray, magnetic resonance imaging and ultrasound)

This applies most often in testing for autosomal dominant disorders (see Chapter 8) but may occasionally be relevant in carrier detection, as with the abnormal neuronal migration apparent on MRI in female carriers of X-linked lissencephaly. The same cautions over specificity (see earlier) apply here.

Clinical observation

Many carriers may exhibit clinical features that show their genotype and, although the absence of such evidence rarely excludes an individual being a carrier, their presence provides a strong positive indication. Ophthalmic disorders (e.g. choroideraemia and retinitis pigmentosa) are particularly susceptible to carrier detection in this way, as are skin disorders. Female carriers of an X-linked recessive disorder may show a 'patchy' appearance, as already noted. Again, this is particularly evident in skin, dental and eye disorders where the tissue concerned is open to inspection. However, one must be cautious about the specificity of such minor clinical features. A Bayesian approach can be very helpful. The prior chance that a woman is a carrier may be very important in the interpretation of clinical observations: fine scalp hair and the absence of two deciduous incisors in a girl at 50% prior risk of carrying XHED points to her perhaps being a carrier of XHED much more strongly than if she had no such family history.

Population screening

See Chapter 34 for a discussion of population-based screening for recessive disease carrier status.

8

Predictive genetic testing

INTRODUCTION

In this chapter, we consider the approach to take when counselling individuals who are at risk of developing a genetic condition and who wish to discuss the possibility of predictive genetic testing.

There are sometimes clear medical reasons for testing, in which case we can recommend testing as medically helpful. For instance, if a young person is at 50% risk of familial adenomatous polyposis coli (FAP), we can recommend that they have a genetic test to clarify whether they will or will not develop multiple colorectal polyps and then malignancies. This allows their risk to be managed appropriately. By way of contrast, if we consider the neurodegenerative disorder Huntington's disease (HD), the decision about testing is much more personal and cannot be recommended on medical grounds. However, once a safe and effective intervention has become available that prevents progression of the disease, this situation will change: testing for HD will, in this respect, become much more like testing for FAP.

PROCESS OF 'GENETIC COUNSELLING-PLUS-TESTING' AS A PACKAGE

One of the major tasks in genetic counselling is to take patients through genetic testing with appropriate information, discussion and preparation beforehand and appropriate support afterwards. In the context of those healthy individuals who know they are at risk of a genetic disorder, it is crucial that the testing does not become detached from the process of information, discussion, preparation and support. This is true for any genetic testing, even when the decision to undergo a test is (medically) obvious, because there can still be personal and family consequences that are difficult and may cause distress. These can usually be managed more successfully if the potential problems have been anticipated and considered in advance. When it comes to predictive testing for a (so far) untreatable disorder, such as HD, it is even more important.

There are pressures on health services to promote the testing and cut back on the talking – to let the technology set the pace – but this endangers the welfare and interests of patients and families caught up in the process. In this chapter, we consider the approach to predictive genetic testing for late-onset dominant disorders. In particular, we consider the approach to testing for HD, as this has served as the paradigm for the 'counselling-plus-testing' package for untreatable neurodegenerative disorders. This model of counselling-plus-testing can then be modified so as to become appropriate for the various different contexts of other disorders.

In the setting of predictive genetic testing for non-medical reasons, as with prenatal genetic diagnosis, the genetic counselling element of the integrated counselling-plus-testing package is guided by the principle of non-directiveness. Where the reasons for predictive testing are not clinical but personal, the professionals cannot make firm recommendations about the decision to be taken. Rather, we can support patients through a process of reflection on the decision. The aim is not for professionals to lead their patients to make particular decisions – to be tested, or not – but to support each patient in making their own decision. We can give accurate information, and we can give patients space in which to reflect upon their situation and how the decision will impact on it. We can prompt them to imagine various outcomes of testing and the scenarios that would result. We can help them to reflect on how family relationships would work out in these different scenarios. We can help them imagine being given the different possible test results and how they might respond to each of them.

There will often be no 'right' or 'wrong' decision, but it may be important for those who request testing to pause, reflect and either choose to delay testing (deciding 'not now' rather than 'not ever') or to proceed in the full awareness of the likely social and emotional as well as medical consequences. We hope that this pause and reflection helps those at risk to make decisions they can live with afterwards. It is our responsibility to help people not to walk blind into entirely predictable and avoidable problems but to make better decisions than they otherwise might.

Predictive genetic testing is often sought by people who are healthy but already know they are at risk of developing a late-onset disorder, such as an inherited cardiac condition, a familial cancer disorder or a neurodegenerative condition. Their primary concern may be their own future health or it may be the health of their current or future children. They may feel that they have little or no choice: their continued relationship with their partner and children, especially if the 'children' are now young adults, may depend upon their being tested. They may feel (implicitly) coerced.

This chapter explores the range and limitations of predictive genetic tests and attempts to show how the information can be used in conjunction with other genetic and clinical data to make the assessment of risk as accurate as possible. It also sets out a framework within which patients can be supported through the process, especially where there is no clear medical benefit from testing.

PREDICTIVE GENETIC TESTING ('CARRIER' DETECTION) IN AUTOSOMAL DOMINANT DISEASE

For practical purposes, (almost) all individuals with a dominantly inherited disease are heterozygotes, so the carrier state can only exist where the disorder is mild, variable or late in onset. One cannot be a 'carrier' for achondroplasia – one either has it or one does not (gonadal mosaicism can provide occasional exceptions to this; see Chapter 2). Thus, the number of

Table 8.1 Carrier detection in variable autosomal dominant disorders: Clinical and biochemical approaches

Disorder	Clinical or biochemical feature
Angioedema, hereditary	C1 esterase inhibitor levels
Familial adenomatous polyposis coli	Examination of the retina for CHRPEs (areas of congenital hyperplasia of the retinal pigment epithelium)
Hereditary spherocytosis	Red cell morphology, osmotic fragility
Holt-Oram syndrome	Minor digital abnormalities
Hypercholesterolaemia, familial	Lipoprotein and LDL cholesterol assays
Malignant hyperpyrexia	Elevated creatine kinase, muscle biopsy
Multiple epiphyseal dysplasia	Short stature, premature osteoarthritis
Muscular dystrophy (facioscapulohumeral)	Minimal weakness
Myotonic dystrophy	Minimal weakness, electromyography; lens opacities
Neurofibromatosis (NF1)	Skin lesions, Lisch nodules
Osteogenesis imperfecta	Dental changes, deafness, blue sclerae
Polycystic kidney disease (adult)	Renal ultrasound
Porphyrias (acute intermittent, variegate and coproporphyria)	Specific enzyme assays, urinary metabolites and clinical history; skin photosensitivity in some types
Tuberous sclerosis	Skin lesions (UV light), computed tomography (CT) scan, dental pits
Van der Woude syndrome	Lip pits
Von Hippel-Lindau syndrome	Retinal lesions
Waardenburg syndrome	White forelock, hypertelorism

dominantly inherited disorders where carrier detection is applicable is very small compared with autosomal recessive inheritance, but the importance in terms of risks to offspring is much greater.

Table 8.1 lists some of the major autosomal dominant disorders where predictive testing (or 'carrier detection') is feasible using clinical or biochemical approaches. These disorders fall into three principal categories:

- The first group consists of disorders that frequently remain asymptomatic and which, under normal circumstances, might hardly be considered diseases. Acute intermittent porphyria and malignant hyperpyrexia, both drug-aggravated disorders, are examples.
- The second group consists of those difficult disorders that show variable penetrance and expression, and which are especially important in genetic counselling because of this variability. Tuberous sclerosis, osteogenesis imperfecta and myotonic dystrophy all fall into this class. Now that molecular analysis is possible for mutations causing many dominantly inherited conditions, it is becoming clear that incomplete penetrance is seen in a significant number.
- The final group consists of age-dependent diseases that sooner or later follow regular dominant inheritance, but where the true state of affairs may not be clear at the time individuals at risk wish to have children. Huntington's disease (see Chapter 15) is the most important

and most difficult disorder in this group, but some of the other progressive neurological degenerations are comparable. In this group, tests of carrier detection are essentially tests of presymptomatic diagnosis.

Molecular testing has had a major impact on carrier testing for autosomal dominant conditions, including most of those listed in Table 8.1. It has now very largely replaced more conventional approaches, especially where these are invasive or of limited accuracy. Minor clinical findings have frequently proved to be non-specific, so it must be remembered that results from the past, based solely on these, are not always dependable (e.g. myotonic dystrophy, see Chapter 13). The lack of age dependence in molecular analysis is a considerable advantage, though equally a danger in terms of inappropriate childhood testing (see Chapter 35). The ease of the procedure from the individual's viewpoint, with only a blood sample required, is likewise a double-edged sword, with the danger that samples may arrive in the laboratory without appropriate genetic counselling having been performed.

Gene sequencing techniques have proved particularly valuable in the analysis of dominantly inherited disorders, especially those where the genes involved are small or the mechanism of disease is a trinucleotide repeat expansion, since they are usually able to detect or exclude an abnormality even when this may not be known from a previous family member. It can be assumed that mutation detection is at least potentially feasible for any dominantly inherited disorder where the responsible gene has been identified. Genetic testing within a known family is generally much more satisfactory if the family's mutation has been determined unambiguously in an affected individual. If that is not the case, the feasibility of molecular testing in unaffected family members will depend on the particular family circumstances as well as the range of mutations in the gene, whether there is genetic heterogeneity and, if linked markers rather than mutation analysis are being used, the structure of the particular family pedigree.

In contrast to autosomal recessive disorders, the risk of the offspring of a carrier for an autosomal dominant condition having overt disease at some stage of their life is high. Although in a few cases (e.g. the myopathy underlying malignant hyperpyrexia) the disorder may remain constantly subclinical in successive generations, it is common to find more severely affected offspring born to asymptomatic parents. This in part reflects the natural variability of these disorders, but also results from the fact that the carrier parents will often form the mildest extreme of a range of variability, so that in 'reverting to the mean' the children are more likely to be clinically affected. In some instances, as with myotonic dystrophy and Huntington's disease, there may be parent of origin effects leading to progressively more severe disease in the offspring as the result of special factors producing anticipation, more marked in the children of affected men (in HD) or women (in myotonic dystrophy) (see Chapters 2, 13 and 15).

Autosomal dominant disorders of late onset also produce a special difficulty in carrier detection because, in contrast to those with a static course and those with recessively inherited disease, the carrier is not only at risk of transmitting the disease but also of developing it. Thus, to identify an individual as a carrier of Huntington's disease (apart from those individuals with a subclinical or reduced penetrance mutation – see Chapter 15) is inevitably to mark out that person as being destined to develop the disease at some time in the future. The whole field of presymptomatic detection for late-onset disorders carries serious practical, societal and ethical consequences (see also Chapters 5 and 35). We now have considerable information on the effects of this in Huntington's disease, which has provided a general model for other late-onset disorders, including the familial cancers, although these differ importantly from Huntington's disease in often having preventable and treatable aspects.

METHODS OF PREDICTIVE TESTING AND 'CARRIER DETECTION'

Clinical observation

Many carriers may exhibit clinical features that show their genotype and, although the absence of such evidence rarely excludes an individual being a carrier, their presence provides a strong positive indication. However, one must be cautious about the specificity of minor clinical features, such as blueish sclerae in someone at risk of osteogenesis imperfecta or freckling in a child at risk of NF1 (especially if they have red hair and the accompanying freckle-prone complexion).

Imaging (by ultrasound or X-ray or magnetic resonance imaging)

The presence of a few simple renal cysts detected on ultrasound scan in someone at risk of polycystic kidney disease (PKD) – or even someone with no such family history – may give a strong indication that the patient is affected. The appearance of cysts on renal scans will usually precede any symptoms or physical signs of the condition and can be used as a form of predictive testing, with the proviso that failure to detect cysts on imaging before 30–35 years does not exclude the diagnosis as cysts become evident on imaging in an age-dependent fashion.

Molecular genetic diagnostics

The key question is to identify the disease-causing mutation in the family. Simply knowing the disease will specify the mutation in some cases, most typically the triplet-repeat expansion disorders including HD, myotonic dystrophy, the spinocerebellar ataxias and the sex-linked Kennedy disease (with a triplet expansion in the X-chromosome gene for the androgen receptor).

In most conditions, however, it will be necessary not only to have confirmation of the clinical diagnosis in the family but to have the molecular genetic test results from affected family members. Even when the gene is known, it may be large and the gene may often contain variants of uncertain pathogenicity, as with *BRCA1* and *BRCA2*. One has to be satisfied that *this* variant in *that* gene is the mutation that puts the patient at risk: one has to *both* know what has been found in the affected relative(s) *and* be satisfied that it is the relevant pathogenic factor.

Even in the triplet repeat diseases, it is highly reassuring to see the molecular confirmation of the family diagnosis in at least one relative. However rare, there will often be other genes in which mutations can lead to similar clinical features and which could therefore cause confusion. To test an at-risk patient for mutation in the wrong gene would obviously be most unhelpful, with a high risk of generating a false-negative result as the 'wrong' gene will usually carry no mutation. Further, if a variant in that other gene has been (falsely) identified as disease-causing in the affected parent, then the test result will be irrelevant: there will be a random relationship between the result and the actual risk of disease (if indeed the risk is Mendelian), so that false-positive, false-negative, true-positive and true-negative results will all be equally likely. Thus, testing an individual, who is at risk of dentatorubral-pallidoluysian atrophy (DRPLA), for HD would clearly be both irrelevant and unhelpful.

APPROACH TO GENETIC COUNSELLING FOR PREDICTIVE GENETIC TESTING

Specific issues that arise in predictive testing for Huntington's disease

- Presymptomatic testing for HD should only be done within a framework of adequate preparation, information and support. Almost all centres use a minimum of two separate interviews before giving results.
- Important information needing to be given, and thought through, includes the psycho-emotional and social impact of an abnormal test result (on the individual and their family members), and the broader implications for insurance, employment, driving, etc.); information on the disorder itself (not all those being tested will have had personal experience of HD); sources of support; and approaches to coping with an abnormal result.
- The reasons for requesting testing vary, but commonly involve the wish to resolve uncertainty and to remove risk from children, whether already born or planned for the future.
- It is generally agreed that presymptomatic testing of young children, requested by parents, should not be carried out, the view being that individuals have the right to decide for themselves as adults. Requests from adolescents are few, and these need sensitive discussion before any decision is made.
- One issue in presymptomatic testing that has arisen since specific mutation analysis became possible is the testing of those at 1 in 4 (25%) risk; that is, individuals whose parent is at risk but healthy. If the mutation is detected in the younger generation, then this will imply that the parent also carries it, and will probably be much closer to onset of the disease. How should one respond to such a request if the parent does not wish to be tested themselves, or does not know about their offspring's request? Fortunately, data from both the United Kingdom and elsewhere show that such difficult scenarios are rare, probably because the situation is usually resolved by sensitive genetic counselling. In this area, and many others, HD not only highlights an issue that is relevant to presymptomatic testing in general, but also shows how important it is that presymptomatic testing is not isolated from the general genetic counselling process or regarded as an activity purely for the laboratory.
- It has become generally accepted that presymptomatic testing for HD is something that should be done by clinical geneticists, in contrast to diagnostic testing of symptomatic individuals, which is becoming part of the practice of neurologists, psychiatrists and other involved clinicians. It is important that the difference between these two categories of genetic testing be fully appreciated (see Chapter 5), as there are major practical considerations involved.

The points noted are equally relevant to the increasing number of other late-onset dominantly inherited neurological disorders where presymptomatic testing has become feasible.

Genetic counselling approach to Huntington's disease as a model for predictive genetic testing: Key questions for the practitioner

Is the individual being seen because they wish to find out about their risk of HD and perhaps to consider testing, or because they have spent years weighing up the decision about testing and have now decided to seek testing? The referral letter may not make that clear.

Why have they come now, rather than last year? Or rather than leaving it for another year, or two, or ten? What – or who – is driving the request for testing at this point, today? What are they looking for from testing? [This then needs a careful consideration – an extended discussion over the two or three, or occasionally more, consultations – of whether they are likely to get the benefit they are looking for. If it is 'reassurance' that they seek then, of course, they may be bitterly disappointed.]

How often is the person thinking about HD, and their risk of HD? [If they are subject to frequent, highly intrusive thoughts, so that the primary motivator behind testing is the removal of the uncertainty and the anxiety it causes, then they need to consider how they would cope if they knew that they would go on to develop HD. One set of highly distressing and recurrent images and fears might well give way to another, perhaps even more distressing, although there would be the 50% chance of reassurance.]

Would it be worth the patient losing the hope, that they might escape from the family's disease, in order also to lose the nagging uncertainty? [Some say so, but if there is no other strong motivator – such as the need for the individual or their children to know, so they can make informed decisions about reproduction – then the decision to be tested can be regretted. The decision about testing is about how the person wishes to live their remaining healthy years – either hoping that they will be unaffected or (if the test is positive) knowing that they are destined to develop HD. The younger the age at which the decision is made, the longer the symptom-free interval that the decision will affect. As with the traditional hasty marriage, a quick decision to be tested can be repented (regretted) at leisure.]

When did they find out about HD in the family, and when were they told, or when did they discover or realise, that they were at risk? [We are generally reluctant to test those who have only recently discovered that they are at risk. They may be trying – understandably – to detach themselves from the disease, not yet able to appreciate the 50% risk that this attempt will be unsuccessful. We usually suggest waiting at least a year after someone has found out or acknowledged that they are at risk, before testing.]

How familiar are they with the different ways in which HD can present, and with the evolution of the illness from the vague early signs through to the severe terminal stages? [The variability in presentation and the slow progression of the illness may need to be emphasised. It can be very helpful to hear them describe the illness as they have seen it in their parents, siblings or others in the family.]

Do they know their percentage risk of developing the disease? [How old are they? Have they an intervening at-risk but so far unaffected relative? Are their ages sufficient for this to alter their risk appreciably from one in two or one in four? Might their risk assessment be influenced at all by older, linkage-based test results? If apparently at a one in four risk, might genetic test results on siblings modify their risks, up or down? The ability to perform simple Bayesian calculations 'on the back of an envelope' can be useful.]

Who has come with the at-risk person to the clinic? Who else knows that they are coming to the genetics clinic to discuss the HD and perhaps seek testing? [This throws light upon the pattern of communication about HD within the family, the workplace and the general social context. It can be very helpful to explore this. It may also be helpful to suggest that they should not talk about testing very widely or in very specific detail, except with a few very close friends or family members, so that – when it comes to the point of being given their result, if they proceed with testing – they do not have a wide circle of acquaintances who know precisely when this is going to occur.]

Are they in a long-term relationship? If yes, does their partner know their risk of HD? (Perhaps their partner has accompanied them for testing but, if not, they may be unaware of the situation.) What is at stake for their relationship, in terms of the test result? If they are not in a long-term relationship, will testing make it more difficult to embark upon romantic relationships? How and when would the fact of HD in the family – and their test result – be mentioned to a new boy- or girlfriend? [The fact of HD in the family will of course have to surface at some point in any serious and committed relationship. People differ greatly as to when and how it is mentioned to a prospective partner: this is never easy unless the person has already known them and their family for years and accepts the risk as an intrinsic part of the relationship. While we can recommend openness, and secrecy can be very destructive, the moment of telling can be a fearful moment of threat to a budding romance.]

Do they have (their own, biological) children? Are their children aware of the family history and of their own risk? If not, might the children (if they are mature enough to be discussing these issues) prefer to be told of their risk situation now, when the risk may seem rather modest, rather than once they have perhaps been put at a 50% risk? Might the children resent being kept in the dark? Might they resent having been prevented from offering emotional support to their parent? If the children are aware of their risk, what do they think about their parent clarifying the situation, and perhaps increasing their (the children's) risk from ∼25% to ∼50%? Have they been asked for their opinion on this?

With whom will they share the result of their genetic test, if it is a good/favourable result? Is there anyone, whom they would find it difficult to tell if they had a good result? [Such as an at-risk brother or sister, who has not been tested and may not want to be tested.]

With whom will they share the result of their genetic test, if it is a bad//adverse//unfavourable result? Is there anyone, whom they would find it especially difficult to tell if they had such a result? [Perhaps their parents or their children.] This may be a particular problem if they have inherited the condition through an at-risk but still healthy parent who has not been tested and who does not want to know their own genetic status (the 1 in 4 risk problem), or with whom they have little or no direct communication.

Do they understand the range of possible test results? Most individuals are given a clearly positive ('bad') or negative ('good') result, but some (a few) are given a somewhat indeterminate result. Thus, the number of CAG repeats may be below 40 but still sometimes cause disease (the reduced penetrance range of 36–39) or may be lower (27–35 CAGs) and not associated with disease but potentially unstable at meiosis and, so, potentially able to expand upon transmission to cause disease in future generations. Those who want the test to give them complete certainty may be upset at receiving either of these results, whose interpretation is less than clear.

Do they understand that a positive (adverse) result may generate as many questions as it answers? [Instead of whether a person will develop HD, the question may become when and how will this happen? And the test result will often give little indication of this: for most sizes of the CAG expansion, the range of possible ages of onset is rather broad.]

Are they anxious about possible early signs of HD? Do they think they might already be affected? [If so, is it appropriate to continue with the counselling approach for predictive testing or would it make sense to switch to a more clinical, neurological approach and offer a formal physical examination and a diagnostic molecular test?]

How have they coped with 'bad news' in the past? Have they ever suffered from depression or any other psychiatric disorder? Are they under treatment for a psychiatric disorder? Have they ever – or do they now – drink alcohol to excess? Or use 'street drugs'? Have they ever self-harmed? Have they ever considered or attempted suicide? [Positive answers to such questions do not bar an at-risk patient from access to testing but should trigger contact with their general practitioner (GP) or psychiatrist for an assessment of what extra support could be put in place, in case of an adverse result, and should prompt the question as to when would be the best time for the test to be performed and the result given. There may be other life events – moving house, the ending of a relationship, a likely imminent bereavement, college exams, a likely redundancy or the start of a new job – that may lead all concerned to choose to delay testing, even for just a few months.]

To whom will they turn for support, if they have a bad result? Is this person someone else in the family who is also at risk? [Might that person find it challenging to support them?] Are there people in the family, or at work, whom it will be difficult to face if they have a bad result? [If the person being tested cares for an affected parent or another affected relative, aunt or uncle, brother or sister, then seeing that person can become very painful once the person knows that they will follow the same path. Those who work in nursing or social care can also find it difficult to care for patients with the same or a similar condition, once they have had an adverse predictive test result.]

Is there anything that can be done now – between this clinic appointment and the time they are likely to be given their test result, if they remain committed to testing – to support their coping with an adverse result? This can be separated into what the patient can do in preparation and what those around them can do (partner, family, friends, colleagues at work or other health professionals, e.g. GP, counsellor, community psychiatric nurse).

Do they have any life insurance or health insurance policies, or plans to take out such policies? Or a mortgage on their home? Do they drive? Are they in work? (What work?) [These are some of the practical and legal matters that it is important to mention – especially the need to be honest with the driving authorities and with insurance companies at all times, although discovering that you are at risk of HD after taking out a life insurance policy should not alter that policy, whereas it may well alter a health insurance policy.]

Do they understand the distinction between a diagnostic test and a predictive test? [This is vital for the patient, the insurance company and the employer to appreciate as well as their healthcare professionals. Having a positive predictive result does not mean that the person has the disease – it is not diagnostic – and only a clinical assessment can establish whether someone is currently affected. Neither the patient nor the physician has to inform the relevant authorities as soon as the patient has been given a positive predictive result. Rather, the patient should inform the appropriate authorities once early signs of the disease have appeared, so that their fitness to work or to drive can then be monitored. It is not the genetic test result but the patient's clinical state that is relevant. A physician may have to step in if this does not happen otherwise, but the details of such obligations and who bears them will vary between jurisdictions.]

Are there other major life decisions, including financial planning, that they wish to take, and that will depend upon their test result? This may relate to business decisions, if they are self-employed or run their own business, or to plans for education, savings and pensions, travel, and their general 'approach to life'. [My advice here would be not to accept such hypothetical plans at face value – as very likely to be followed in reality – as many people seem not to make the major changes they had thought in advance that they would. However, it is always difficult – indeed, impossible – to know afterwards how events would have worked out 'otherwise' (counter-factually). For some people, such plans are made and serve a very useful purpose. If nothing else, they give the sense of retaining some control over events that otherwise might feel utterly out of control.]

When a person at risk of HD is struggling to make their decision, or if the counsellor feels that they are rushing into the decision without having engaged with the various hypothetical outcomes that are possible, the counsellor might wish to return to the question, 'How would you want to live your remaining disease-free years, if you are destined to develop HD: in the hope that you might escape or in the certainty that you will not?' [This is a sobering question. I would not always use such words, especially not if the person had clearly agonised over the question. However, it may be appropriate if the person has not known about their risk for very long, if they are insistent upon testing at once, and if they seem to be rushing towards testing as an inadequately considered act of denial.]

Not all these questions would be raised with any one individual, even in the course of several discussions. But these points indicate the type of questions that it can be appropriate to raise with the patient at risk.

Other diseases

The range of questions to be raised and considered can be very similar with other untreatable late-onset neurological disorders. However, in other disease contexts, the relevant factors to consider can be very different.

Inherited cardiac disorders will often raise fears of sudden death and these can have an emotionally devastating impact, especially perhaps on the parents of young children at risk. Striking the right balance can be very difficult: between avoiding trigger factors such as competitive sports, on the one hand, and being dreadfully over-protective and discouraging all activity, on the other hand. What does this do to an adolescent's physical fitness and their emotional state? How do they manage social activities such as dancing? Or romance and sex? While many young people at risk do 'cope', their parents may find it harder even than the young person at risk.

Comparable considerations can arise in the context of susceptibility to neurodevelopmental, behavioural and psychiatric disorders. For example, if one's child has a microdeletion predisposing to behaviour problems or schizophrenia, how should one respond to his or her tantrums as a toddler, or general naughtiness when a bit older? Should one avoid confrontation and always give unconditional positive feedback, or should one provide firm boundaries enforced by parental disapproval? More is said about this in Chapter 21 on inherited cardiac disorders and Chapters 13 and 14 or 14 and 15 on neurodevelopmental and psychiatric disorders.

More generally, when there is a medically straightforward decision to make that invites us to be directive – to make a clear recommendation – how do we respond when a patient makes a decision that one regards as unwise? Just how persuasive or forceful should we be? Will there be implications for other members of the family too? If your patient refuses to accept the implications of their risk of developing FAP or thyroid cancer, for example, will their reluctance mean that their siblings or children remain ignorant of their risk, and therefore also unprotected?

It is important not to assume that patients and their relatives will readily accept the view – and the corresponding course of action – that health professionals may regard as obviously correct. There can be many personal factors that intervene to alter how individuals – or whole families – take a view on such matters. We must remain in discussion with these families and try to appreciate why they adopt the stances they do. This can involve building a long-term, supportive and respectful relationship with several generations of a kindred. Such efforts are important, worthwhile and rewarding. Simply trying to impose the 'obvious' (to you, to us) solution will often be unhelpful and may even be counter-productive.

9

Prenatal diagnosis, antenatal screening and reproductive aspects of medical genetics

INTRODUCTION

The development of techniques for diagnosing genetic disorders *in utero* was a major advance in medical genetics and has so altered the outlook for families at risk of having affected children that it has become one of the main options open to those receiving genetic counselling, especially where there is a high risk of a serious and untreatable disorder. Prenatal diagnostic procedures for many genetic disorders were initially often developed by, or in close association with, those actively involved in genetic counselling and, perhaps as a result of this, have in general been used appropriately and responsibly. As these techniques have diversified, especially with ultrasound, with biochemical screening and now with non-invasive prenatal testing (NIPT), and as they have come to be implemented much more widely, especially by obstetricians, prenatal diagnostic procedures have often been applied as a substitute for genetic counselling, in isolation from the estimation of genetic risks and other relevant factors supporting it. The procedure-driven nature of prenatal diagnosis and screening, with the potential for NIPT to be made available outside the framework of accurate, sensitive and supportive genetic counselling, could then lead to it being a mixed blessing: this will be an area to watch, especially where healthcare providers have a pecuniary interest in maximising the number of procedures performed. The prospect of over-the-counter or direct-to-consumer NIPT raises particularly serious concerns.

One crucial distinction to be emphasised is that between a population screening test (e.g. a test offered to all pregnant women) and a prenatal diagnostic test, offered to those who already know that the chance of their fetus being affected by a genetic disorder is increased. This 'being at increased risk' may arise because of a known family history of a condition or because of the result of a population screening test.

We believe strongly that the separation of genetic investigations of the fetus from the broader context within which they are made available is unfortunate and potentially harmful. Prenatal screening and diagnosis, like other clinical and laboratory techniques, should not be driven by what is possible but must be seen in the context of the entire situation: the risk of a pregnancy being genetically affected, the other measures such as carrier detection which may define that risk more precisely or even eliminate it, the potential for treatment of the disorder in question and, most importantly, the attitude and wishes of the couple concerned. Whether this is undertaken by non-medical genetic counsellors, midwives, clinical geneticists or by obstetricians themselves is of less importance than that it is done well. In many centres the non-medical genetic counsellor now plays an important role.

When a couple is already known, long in advance of any pregnancy, to face an increased risk of a fetal condition, prenatal diagnosis should be considered, discussed and planned before a pregnancy occurs, if at all possible. To begin this process during pregnancy is highly undesirable: not only may procedures have to be hurried, but most pregnant women (and their partners) are not in a state where an objective assessment of the factors for or against prenatal diagnosis and possible termination of pregnancy can easily be undertaken. It is likely that much of the emotional trauma sometimes associated with prenatal diagnosis results from an absence of careful prior planning. The availability of chorion villus sampling (CVS) or NIPT in the first trimester makes it even more important that the situation be planned carefully in advance of a pregnancy.

In the real world, however, it is inevitable that these difficult situations will arise in the course of some pregnancies, and we must have systems in place to do as good a job as we can in the circumstances. A couple may only become aware of the relevant family history during a pregnancy: Indeed, the fact of the pregnancy may trigger the disclosure of the information within the family. Or the index case may have just been diagnosed, and that may be especially important if the disorder is sex-linked or a chromosomal rearrangement.

Most genetic counselling in relation to antenatal screening and prenatal diagnosis will inevitably, and rightly, be carried out by obstetricians and those involved in primary care, with specialists in medical genetics responsible for those cases where the genetic aspects are complex. A welcome development has been the growth of interdisciplinary fetal medicine groups, where obstetrician, radiologist, medical geneticist, non-medical genetic counsellor, neonatal paediatrician and other colleagues can meet regularly to discuss specific cases, but there remain too many instances where skilled genetic advice has been sought too late or not at all.

The widespread use of screening tests in pregnancy now means that most prenatal diagnosis is undertaken where there was no previous risk or expectation of a genetic disorder. The population aspects of this are considered in Chapter 34, but the very real implications this has for individual families are dealt with later in this chapter.

CRITERIA AND INDICATIONS FOR PRENATAL DIAGNOSIS

When prenatal diagnosis is being considered in genetic counselling, several basic factors must be examined (Box 9.1), but the most important is whether the couple concerned actively wish for prenatal diagnosis; all too often it is suggested simply because it may be technically feasible and without adequate information.

Because most prenatal diagnostic procedures involve a large amount of worry to the parents, and a significant morbidity and mortality to the fetus (with 100% mortality if the test proves abnormal and termination is requested), prenatal diagnosis should normally be carried out only if the general criteria summarised in Box 9.1 are fulfilled. These are self-evident but, as in most clinical situations, cases of real doubt may occur. Where the prospects for fetal therapy become realistic – as is now true in just a few, unusual contexts – this situation may change.

Severity of disorder

This is beyond doubt in most of the disorders for which prenatal diagnosis is actively sought, including many chromosomal disorders, open neural tube defects, the lethal skeletal dysplasias and the rare neurodegenerative metabolic disorders. Other conditions may be more questionable, especially those where physical abnormalities (e.g. limb defects, cleft lip and palate) are likely to be accompanied by normal intellect and life expectancy. Albinism, which has few general health implications in northern climates, may, because of the likelihood of skin cancer, be a fatal disorder in tropical countries. Such variable categories are increasing, particularly as molecular analysis increasingly recognises specific mutations with relatively mild clinical effects, and this may present difficult decisions, the outcome of which will vary from family to family and between different societies. Relatively minor but visible defects may be considered unacceptable in some cultures, whereas serious internal disorders may be accepted. Some of the more general problems posed for society by these new developments are discussed in Chapter 35.

Specific mention should be made of Down syndrome in this regard. The lives of many people with Down syndrome are of such a quality that many families with an affected child believe that termination of pregnancy for Down syndrome would usually be inappropriate and that the screening programmes established primarily to detect (and terminate) pregnancies affected by Down syndrome are also inappropriate and may be offensive. However, this does not match the

---

BOX 9.1: Criteria for prenatal diagnosis

Is the disorder sufficiently severe to warrant termination of the pregnancy?

Is treatment absent or unsatisfactory?

Is termination of an affected pregnancy acceptable to the couple concerned?

Is an accurate prenatal diagnostic test available?

Is there a significant genetic risk to the pregnancy?

experiences and wishes of other families and of parents who feel unable to cope well with an affected child. Down syndrome is highly variable in the severity of the physical complications, including especially the cardiac malformations that affect at least 40%, and of the associated cognitive impairment. The outlook for survival is very different in societies where facilities for paediatric cardiac and gastrointestinal surgery are restricted. In developed nations, affected individuals may have a happy childhood and a fulfilling life but may also be well aware that they are 'different', and they may feel the burden of this stigma. This is not the place for a full debate on the ethics of antenatal screening for Down syndrome; suffice it to say here that it is a complex matter and that there is more than one perspective that must be heard with respect.

Another problem that arises from time to time is that clinic staff may make the assumption that the parents of a fetus with a likely lethal or a very severe disorder (e.g. thanatophoric dysplasia, Patau syndrome, severe open neural tube defect) will choose to terminate the pregnancy. It takes a degree of self-confidence, that many people may lack at such a vulnerable time, to resist this assumption and assert a different choice such as to continue the pregnancy and allow the child to be born, be nurtured and then to die. This is undoubtedly the right decision for some couples; staff should ensure that it is made available as a fully supported option for any who might wish to make this choice. Adjustment to the early death of a child who was born and loved may be the course preferred by some to adjustment to a termination of pregnancy for fetal abnormality.

Treatment availability

Treatment may be clear-cut and satisfactory in some disorders that might otherwise be considered for prenatal diagnosis. Thus, in phenylketonuria, now detectable prenatally by molecular analysis, most children treated from birth have near normal health and intelligence, at least in countries where dietary treatment is available, and prenatal diagnosis is hardly ever requested. In contrast, in galactosaemia, liver damage is occasionally present at birth and the long-term outlook for the infant is less clear. Whether prenatal diagnosis is undertaken here will often depend on the attitudes and previous experience of the parents. In congenital adrenal hyperplasia (see Chapter 25), the outlook with treatment for a second affected child is much better than for the firstborn, in whom delayed diagnosis may result in death or serious morbidity from a salt-losing crisis.

Acceptability of termination

The acceptability of termination of pregnancy to a couple must be determined before any prenatal procedures are contemplated. In some cases, it is unacceptable on religious grounds or because of the prevailing attitude of the community; in others, it is a more personal ethical view. Acceptability may be a relative phenomenon. Thus, in the past many couples found fetal sexing by amniocentesis unacceptable, when a future male infant would be at risk of a sex-linked disorder, if the only available intervention was a late termination of a male pregnancy that would be facing a 50:50 chance of being either affected or unaffected. These same individuals often became willing to accept first-trimester termination, following CVS, of a definitely affected male pregnancy. Similarly, in some religious traditions, early termination may be allowable, while late termination is forbidden. It is essential to know the attitude of a couple before pregnancy occurs because this may well affect their decision whether or not to have further children.

The unacceptability of termination to the parents should not be considered as automatically ruling out prenatal diagnosis. Some parents may feel that they will gain by being able to prepare for an affected child, although this is uncommon, especially when the finite risk of miscarriage from invasive prenatal procedures is pointed out. This situation may change with the advent of NIPT for a wide range of disorders, as the risk of miscarriage will no longer be a concern. It is also important not to make the assumption, because a family comes from any specific religious group, ethnicity or population, that termination of pregnancy will automatically be unacceptable. Religious communities are not homogeneous and monolithic in their views, and professionals must not make assumptions about such matters.

Potentially serious ethical problems arise if prenatal diagnosis is undertaken for a late-onset disorder and the pregnancy continues: the predictive testing of an infant for a late-onset and untreatable disease. The need to avoid this difficult situation if at all possible needs to be discussed with the couple while they are making their decision about prenatal diagnosis. About 10% of pregnancies in the United Kingdom in which prenatal diagnosis gives a positive (high-risk) result for Huntington's disease are continued, with often difficult consequences for the families.

Feasibility of prenatal diagnosis

The feasibility of laboratory diagnosis for the disorder in a patient or family is something that continues to change rapidly with scientific advances, so it cannot be too strongly stressed that the person providing the genetic counselling must obtain accurate information on this point before suggesting the possibility to a couple, and must be satisfied that the technique is reliably applicable as a service rather than just as a research procedure. Failure to do this is as reprehensible as submitting a patient to some new surgical procedure without enquiring as to its likely benefit and risk of mortality. This is especially relevant when using new molecular advances, where the boundary between research, the development and refinement of new methods and the use of established techniques can be hard to define, especially for very rare disorders, or where the relevant gene has only recently been identified.

Genetic risk

The final point to be emphasized here is that the risk of the disorder occurring in a particular pregnancy must be estimated accurately before prenatal diagnosis is considered; in other words, the consideration of prenatal diagnosis must be an integral part of genetic counselling. Patients may be referred for prenatal diagnosis inappropriately, when the risk to the pregnancy has not been properly evaluated and where the risk on occasion proves to be so low as to make prenatal procedures unwarranted. Even if prenatal diagnosis were free of risk (which it is not), such a slipshod approach cannot be justified. Even NIPT carries risks to the pregnancy from the generation of unsought information that may influence decisions 'inappropriately'. If the clinician involved cannot accurately evaluate the risk (which will be the case less often after reading this book, it is hoped), then the advice of a colleague who can do so should be sought.

AMNIOCENTESIS

A variety of techniques exist by which a prenatal diagnosis may be achieved for different disorders. The oldest of these, amniocentesis, the procedure by which a sample of amniotic

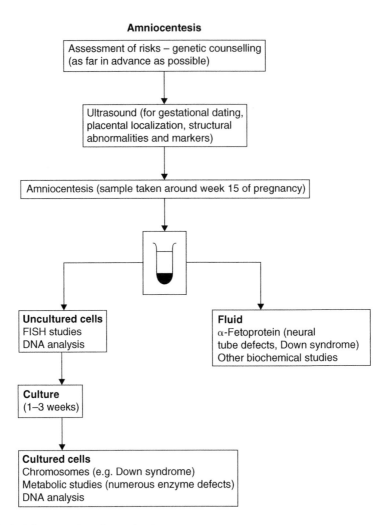

Amniocentesis

Figure 9.1 Amniocentesis – the main steps.

fluid and its cells is obtained from the pregnant uterus, was first used in 1956 in relation to fetal sexing, but it is still a technique with quite wide application, especially for cytogenetic studies on lower-risk pregnancies (Figure 9.1). It is important, however, to recognize that other approaches exist (Box 9.2), which have taken over from amniocentesis in many circumstances.

The amniotic fluid sample should consist of clear fluid, in which are suspended the cells (fetal in origin) that can be cultured for chromosomal, biochemical or molecular studies, or may in some situations be analysed directly. A bloodstained sample usually indicates damage to the placenta; a discoloured fluid may indicate impending or actual fetal death, and is an important factor to note because the subsequent inevitable abortion might otherwise be attributed to the amniocentesis itself. Both of these findings reduce the chance of a successful cell culture.

Once obtained, the sample is usually spun immediately and duplicate cell cultures set up. The supernatant fluid can be used for α-fetoprotein(AFP) estimation and, less frequently, for metabolic studies. Most diagnostic studies, however, if they are cytogenetic or biochemical,

---

> ## BOX 9.2: Approaches to prenatal diagnosis
>
> *Amniocentesis*
> Chromosomal disorders (especially where risk is low)
> Open neural tube defects
>
> *Chorion villus sampling*
> DNA and enzyme analysis
> Chromosomal disorders (especially when risk is high)
>
> *Ultrasound scan*
> Placental localization, gestational dating and exclusion of twins
> Structural malformations, including limb, neural tube, cardiac and other internal defects
> Nuchal thickening and related measurements
>
> *Fetal blood and tissue sampling (now most unusual)*
> Thalassaemias and related disorders (when DNA analysis not feasible)
> Other severe haematological and metabolic disorders detectable from fetal blood
>
> *Maternal blood sampling*
> α-Fetoprotein (AFP) (neural tube defects and Down syndrome)
> β-hCG, oestriol and other biochemical markers (risk of Down syndrome)
> Cell-free DNA analysis (non-invasive prenatal testing that permits inference – but not
>   direct determination – of the fetal genotype)

require cultured amniotic fluid cells and, depending on the number required, it may be 8 days to 3 weeks before a sufficient quantity is available. It is important that cultures be checked regularly to ensure that satisfactory cell growth is occurring; if not, it may be preferable to repeat amniocentesis soon, rather than to wait until it is certain that growth will not occur, by which time it may be too late.

See Box 9.2 'Approaches to Prenatal Diagnosis'.

Practical aspects

It is important that clinicians referring patients for amniocentesis or suggesting its application should realise what is involved and how best to utilise the service that is provided. The need for proper assessment and genetic counselling before a pregnancy is undertaken has already been stressed, but several points are often overlooked.

Timing

The earliest time that a satisfactory sample can reliably be obtained is from ~15 weeks' gestation, so the couple must be prepared to accept the result as late as 18 weeks if they intend to terminate an affected pregnancy. It is not uncommon for a patient's attitude to change during pregnancy, particularly once fetal movement has occurred. Early amniocentesis (at 12–14 weeks) has proved to result in a higher risk of pregnancy loss than conventional amniocentesis; so, if early diagnosis is essential, first-trimester chorion villus sampling (see later in this chapter) should be used.

Who performs the procedure?

There is no doubt that the risks are increased if amniocentesis is performed by an 'occasional operator' and there is much to be said for a centralised service in which skilled amniocentesis, accurate genetic counselling and appropriate laboratory facilities can be combined as an integrated package.

The procedure

Some patients expect amniocentesis to be a painful procedure, but this is not the case. Direct needling, after ultrasound scan has localised the placenta and confirmed the correct gestation, can be done under local anaesthesia without need for hospital admission, although rest afterwards is advisable. It is surprising how many women are referred without a clear picture having been given of what amniocentesis entails, something that is clearly the responsibility of the obstetrician and referring clinician. In larger centres, as noted earlier, a fetal medicine group will usually have been set up, with those involved meeting at least weekly. This allows unexpected findings to be discussed, along with the likely genetic risks and possible diagnoses, something that is especially important in interpreting the findings of ultrasonography in pregnancies not known previously to be at risk.

Results and follow-up

The couple must be warned that a definitive result may take 10 days to 3 weeks (sometimes longer for biochemical and DNA studies) and that there is a possibility that a repeat sample may be needed. Results of rapid trisomy testing on uncultured cells should still be regarded as provisional. The possibility of abnormality unrelated to that primarily being looked for (an 'incidental finding') should be mentioned (e.g. a sex chromosome anomaly in a pregnancy at risk for Down syndrome), and a clear policy must be defined in the event of no definite answer being reached because of culture failure or other reasons.

Follow-up after delivery is important not only to check the accuracy of the diagnosis but also because the outcome may affect the genetic risk to subsequent pregnancies.

Risks of amniocentesis

Amniocentesis is not without risk to the pregnancy. Approximate figures that can be used in discussion with families, based on a number of large studies, are as follows:

- *Abortion*: The added risk is around 0.5%, but repeat amniocentesis carries a much higher risk (5%–10%), as does the performance of the procedure by an inexperienced person. Each centre should audit its own figures and use them in advising patients.
- *Perinatal problems*: These are not significant; an increase in postural orthopaedic deformities was suggested in one early UK study, but this was not confirmed.
- *Maternal risks*: These are minimal, apart from a possibility of Rhesus sensitization. (Rhesus-negative mothers should receive anti-RhD antibody unless it is known that the fetus is also Rhesus negative.)

In general, amniocentesis has proved to be a safe and reliable procedure, but it is essential that it be used selectively and appropriately, and that the risks be carefully explained to couples who may be considering it. Each centre should monitor and make available its own risks and failure rate.

CHORION VILLUS SAMPLING

Prenatal diagnosis towards the end of the first trimester, using tissue from the conception obtained from chorionic villi, is preferable to amniocentesis in many circumstances, especially for molecular diagnoses. However, it has not superseded amniocentesis for low-risk cytogenetic indications or for diagnoses conducted later after the recognition of structural anomalies on ultrasound scan. CVS may also indicate mosaicism for an abnormal cell line (e.g. an autosomal trisomy) that is not present in the fetus, and an amniocentesis may still be required in some circumstances to clarify this.

Samples are usually obtained transabdominally and under ultrasound guidance from around 11 weeks but may be obtained transcervically (depending upon the operator and the location of the placenta, which is in the process of localising at 11–12 weeks). It is difficult to obtain tissue transcervically after 12 weeks, although transabdominal placental biopsy is feasible at a later stage. Maternal tissue is dissected away microscopically, and the remaining villi consist of pure fetal tissue that can be used for a variety of diagnostic approaches, including the following:

- *Molecular studies*: Uncultured chorionic villi are the most satisfactory sample for these and can provide a rapid and accurate prenatal diagnosis requiring fetal DNA (usually for mutation analysis or array comparative genomic hybridisation [aCGH]). The potential for chromosomal mosaicism in the chorion/placenta must be remembered, although this has not proved to be a problem with testing for specific mutations.
- *Enzyme studies*: The normal ranges in this material may differ considerably from amniotic fluid cells, while in X-linked diseases, skewing of X chromosome inactivation may give very low levels in a female heterozygote.
- *Chromosome studies*: A high frequency of chromosomal mosaicism, not present in the fetus itself, may prove misleading, and is one of the reasons why amniocentesis remains preferable to CVS for most chromosomal indications.

Experience with CVS is now extensive. It is likely that the rate of miscarriage after CVS is slightly higher than after amniocentesis (perhaps 1% additional, procedure-related risk compared with 0.5%, perhaps more with transcervical CVS, and considerably more in inexperienced hands. However, recent series from good centres suggest that these may be over-estimates). Reports of an excess of limb defects possibly related to the procedure have been found with biopsies before 10 weeks; these have not been found after later biopsies but, in general, amniocentesis remains the primary approach for pregnancies at lower risk, with CVS used in higher-risk situations and notably for molecular analyses.

CHROMOSOMAL DISORDERS AND PRENATAL DIAGNOSIS

The recurrence risks for the major types of chromosome disorder are discussed in Chapter 4, and the strength of indication for prenatal diagnosis will depend on the magnitude of this risk as well as on the nature of the disorder and the attitude and experience of the couple concerned in relation to it. The relative risks of amniocentesis and CVS will need careful consideration, especially where the risk of abnormality in the pregnancy is low. The main chromosomal indications for prenatal diagnosis are considered individually later in this chapter (see also Box 9.3).

> **BOX 9.3: Principal chromosomal indications for prenatal diagnosis (see Chapter 4 for detailed risk figures)**
>
> One parent carrier of a balanced autosomal translocation or a Robertsonian translocation
> Advanced maternal age
> Increased risk result on screening test for autosomal trisomy
> Ultrasound findings suggestive of Down syndrome or another chromosome disorder
> Previous child with autosomal trisomy or similar abnormality
> Parent mosaic for chromosomal abnormality
> Chromosomal instability syndromes (although molecular diagnosis usually preferred)

Translocation Down syndrome

The rare, but high-risk, group with translocation Down syndrome comprises only 5% of all cases of Down syndrome. The risks for the offspring of balanced carriers of the various forms of translocation are discussed in Chapter 4 and are given in Table 4.8.

It is clearly vital that the precise type be established from study of the index case in a family, and that relatives at risk should be investigated using blood before a pregnancy occurs. CVS may be preferred to amniocentesis in a high-risk situation. If the individual is a chromosomally normal sib or more distant relative, there is no indication for prenatal tests. Where the parents of a child with translocation Down syndrome are both chromosomally normal, the risk of a further affected child is also low, probably similar to that for trisomic Down syndrome (see the next section). Although it may be reasonable to offer prenatal diagnosis to such couples in a subsequent pregnancy, it should not be undertaken under the false assumption that the risk of Down syndrome is high.

Trisomic Down syndrome and other autosomal trisomies

All studies agree that the recurrence risk for the autosomal trisomies is low, with the exception of very rare families in which there appears to be some special factor causing a cluster of chromosomal abnormalities, possibly by predisposing to non-disjunction or as a result of gonadal mosaicism. It is important that the chromosomes of the child, or of both parents if the child is dead, be studied before another pregnancy is considered, and that the age of the mother is considered in estimating the recurrence risk (see Chapter 4).

In practice in the United Kingdom, most couples who have had an affected child elect for prenatal diagnosis in a subsequent pregnancy, even in the full knowledge of the risk from the procedure and the low probability that the abnormality will recur.

For other relatives of a child with isolated trisomic Down syndrome, there is no evidence of an increased risk in their offspring, and this should be made clear at the time of diagnosis of the index case to avoid unnecessary worry. Where the index case is no longer living and no definite chromosomal status has been recognized, it is preferable to undertake an urgent blood karyotype of the at-risk relative rather than perform an unnecessary amniocentesis. Unfortunately, there is still no test – chromosomal or molecular – that will distinguish, prior to conception, the couple particularly likely to have a trisomic child.

Problems with chromosomal prenatal diagnosis

The following problems may complicate prenatal chromosomal diagnosis.

FAULTY DIAGNOSIS IN THE INDEX CASE

Down syndrome said to affect an older relative may prove to be an entirely different disorder, and the records (or the affected individual, if living and available) should be examined wherever possible. A national or regional cytogenetic register of all known cases of Down syndrome, particularly translocation Down syndrome, is most helpful.

CHROMOSOMAL VARIANTS UNRELATED TO THE CLINICAL ABNORMALITY

These may cause confusion, particularly in the investigation of cases of mental retardation, where chromosome studies are commonly performed, and should be treated with particular suspicion if healthy family members show the same chromosomal pattern. They may also be discovered in the amniotic cells of the fetus at amniocentesis. In most cases, there should be little doubt as to whether they are pathological; again, help may come from finding the same pattern in a healthy parent. The findings should always be discussed with the cytogenetic laboratory that has actually performed the analysis.

The introduction of aCGH to the prenatal diagnostic repertoire has increased both the number of cases with a diagnosis and also the number of cases with a variant of uncertain significance or of reduced penetrance, which are difficult for both families and professionals to handle. The consequences of the use of aCGH are discussed in general terms in Chapter 5. The emotional and ethical sensitivity of the situation in prenatal diagnosis will of course make it more difficult for all concerned when variants of uncertain significance or unrelated/unsought/incidental findings are reported. One approach is for the laboratory to apply somewhat different reporting criteria, or even to use different technology, when conducting a prenatal as opposed to a postnatal investigation. In any case, a forum for discussion of difficult cases is most helpful and should be available in any centre applying aCGH to prenatal investigations. Experience is accumulating, but it remains true that practice differs substantially between centres and countries. Particularly difficult to manage are the 'neurosusceptibility' copy number variants that increase the risk of neurodevelopmental and psychiatric disorders, and sometimes of malformation also, but which have a reduced penetrance and will sometimes not lead to any overt problems.

UNRELATED OR UNEXPECTED ABNORMALITIES

These may be chromosomal (e.g. sex chromosome anomalies or, when a karyotype is performed, a balanced translocation) or a raised AFP level (where that is still measured in amniotic fluid) and may suggest a neural tube defect in a pregnancy studied primarily for a chromosomal indication (see Box 9.4). Such findings may lead to a difficult dilemma, and in general one has to discuss the facts with the couple and respect their decision. It is always easier if the possibility of such a situation arising has been explained prior to the amniocentesis.

The principal sex chromosome anomalies, Turner syndrome and the sex chromosome trisomies (47,XXX, 47,XXY, 47,XYY) can cause particular consternation for families. Parents will sometimes misunderstand the significance of a sex chromosome anomaly and think it relates largely to gender orientation or to the external genitalia. While there can be problems associated with these aneuploid conditions, concern about the diagnosis will often be mitigated if misunderstandings about the phenotypes can be removed. There are newer studies that give a much more accurate picture than the early reports that suffered from highly biased ascertainment (see Chapter 4).

MOSAICISM

Interpreting this is often difficult – not only the likely consequences and severity in the child, but also whether it is a genuine reflection of the chromosome state of the fetus. This is especially the case in CVS samples or with NIPT findings, where mosaicism is discovered that is often confined to the placenta; amniocentesis may be needed to check this but (as always) close liaison with the laboratory is wise.

STRUCTURAL MALFORMATIONS

Neural tube defects

A series of factors have combined to reduce the birth frequency of neural tube defects in most populations where these have previously had a high incidence. This is a major achievement which, like Rhesus isoimmunization, is in danger of being overlooked now that major defects of this type no longer represent such an important cause of serious abnormality, disability and death in childhood. The principal factors include the following:

- A natural decline in incidence, especially in high-risk populations such as South Wales, probably related to maternal nutritional status
- Primary prevention in high-risk pregnancies and the wider population by preconceptional use of folic acid, taken as a food supplement
- Increasing resolution of prenatal ultrasonography
- Maternal serum AFP screening

The first step was the discovery that pregnancies ending in an open neural tube defect had elevated amniotic fluid levels of AFP, which provided an accurate prenatal test for pregnancies known to be at high risk. The subsequent development of ultrasonography provided a means of both confirming the diagnosis and detecting most closed lesions. As ultrasound scanning has become more sensitive and is used more routinely, this has allowed detection in pregnancies not known to be at risk. The first true screening approach came from maternal serum AFP analysis. In areas of high incidence, this remains the main screening test, in conjunction with an ultrasound scan. In areas where the incidence is low, high-resolution ultrasonography alone is often preferred, as the proportion of false-positive raised AFP samples will be higher in these areas.

Amniocentesis is usually not performed for confirmation of the diagnosis where a clear abnormality is found on scan, since delay will inevitably result. Where there are doubts, however, this test could be undertaken for confirmation, together with chromosome analysis (e.g. by array-based methods) on the amniotic fluid if there is any suspicion of a complex malformation syndrome.

In general, these methods of prenatal diagnosis of neural tube defects have proved reliable and free from major problems. However, several points need to be borne in mind.

BOX 9.4: Abnormalities other than neural tube defects that may cause a raised amniotic fluid α-fetoprotein level

Spontaneous intrauterine death
Omphalocele and gastroschisis
Bowel and oesophageal atresias
Turner syndrome
Congenital nephrosis (Finnish type)
Sacrococcygeal teratoma
Bladder exstrophy
Focal dermal hypoplasia, aplasia congenita cutis and other skin defects

---

- There are a number of other causes of a raised serum AFP level (Box 9.4), including normal twin pregnancy. These other causes can often be distinguished by the level of acetylcholinesterase in amniotic fluid, which is specifically raised in open neural tube defects.
- Routine obstetric ultrasound scanning is an inadequate substitute for high-resolution ultrasonography performed by an expert, at the optimal gestation (usually at least 18 weeks).
- Pregnancies already known to be at high risk (before screening) must be considered separately from general population screening and the risks estimated appropriately.
- Any pregnancy terminated should have an expert fetal autopsy, since numerous syndromes associated with neural tube defects exist, some Mendelian, others chromosomal (see Chapter 14).

Other structural abnormalities: Ultrasound scanning in prenatal diagnosis

Ultrasonography is now a sensitive, valuable and widely available approach to prenatal diagnosis. Box 9.5 summarises some of the main applications, but a few general points must be made.

- There is an immense difference between the results of expert units specialising in the detection of malformations and the results of radiologists, radiographers and obstetricians using ultrasound as a more general tool. This applies to both false positives and false negatives and to the interpretation of any possibly abnormal results. The rapid spread of ultrasonography outside specialist centres can be actively harmful unless there is a comparable spread of expertise, which is still not always the case and varies within and between countries and regions. Most genetics centres are aware of pregnancies that were terminated because of supposed ultrasonographic abnormality and where the fetus proved to be entirely normal at pathological examination postmortem.
- Although ultrasound is itself apparently risk free, one must also consider the risks of any attendant or consequent investigations resulting from apparently abnormal or uncertain findings. These may be considerable.
- In investigating genetic abnormalities, the prior risk of the situation must be taken into consideration. The ability to detect or exclude an abnormality in the face of a high genetic risk is quite different from doing so when the risk is low or when ultrasound scanning is used as a routine, population screening procedure. This obvious fact is still ignored (or not understood) by some of those using the technique.

BOX 9.5: Ultrasound in prenatal diagnosis of structural malformations

General applications
Accurate gestational dating
Multiple pregnancy
Placental localisation before amniocentesis or chorion biopsy

Central nervous system abnormalities
Anencephaly
Spina bifida (in conjunction with other approaches)
Hydrocephalus and hydranencephaly
Microcephaly (see Chapter 14 for limitations)

Skeletal defects
Severe neonatal bone dysplasia (e.g. achondrogenesis)
Osteogenesis imperfecta (severe congenital forms only)
Limb defects (especially of digits)

Internal abnormalities
Congenital heart defects
Renal agenesis
Infantile polycystic kidney disease
Severe obstructive uropathy
Omphalocoele and gastroschisis
Fetal tumours

- One useful application of NIPT in this setting is to arrive at a precise diagnosis of a malformation or skeletal dysplasia, or at least to exclude some possible diagnoses. A familiar example is the identification on scan of a short-limb skeletal dysplasia, with or without restriction of the thorax, leading to a search for *de novo* mutations in the *FGFR3* gene.
- Many ultrasonographic 'abnormalities' or 'soft markers' may be transient and physiological rather than pathological in nature. Others may indicate abnormality in only a proportion of cases (e.g. nuchal oedema in trisomy 21; choroid plexus cysts in trisomy 18).
- The best results from ultrasound scanning are likely to be when it is used in conjunction with other appropriate investigations. The balance of value of the various tests will change, but they should be considered together for each particular problem. Likewise, the interpretation of puzzling findings is best carried out in conjunction with other specialities, preferably as part of a fetal medicine group, as mentioned earlier.

The diagnosis of congenital heart disease by ultrasonography provides a good example of the uncertainty of the role of this technique. Although severe lesions can be detected in the middle trimester of pregnancy, there is still uncertainty as to how accurately less severe defects can be recognised or excluded, or whether this is a suitable investigation for families with the more common forms of congenital heart defect, especially where the recurrence risk is low. Where a cardiac defect is suspected from routine ultrasound scanning, or when a family is at even slightly increased risk (e.g. when one parent is affected or when a family has had a previous affected child), then referral for expert fetal echocardiography may be very helpful.

Renal anomalies indicating polycystic kidney disease (PKD) are sometimes found 'incidentally' in the mother during a fetal ultrasound scan. This is likely to be the adult, autosomal dominant form of PKD with a risk of the fetus also developing this later (see Chapter 24). The mother may benefit if she had not previously been diagnosed, and it may be helpful for the risk to the child to be indicated. Another possibility is for PKD to be recognised in the fetus. This may either be the infantile form of PKD, usually much more severe, or the adult form presenting at a rather early age. Occasionally, a parent can then be diagnosed with adult PKD after an early presentation *in utero* in the fetus.

ANTENATAL SCREENING FOR DOWN SYNDROME AND THE OTHER AUTOSOMAL TRISOMIES

The chances of having a fetus with an autosomal trisomy increase with maternal age ('advanced' maternal age often defined as maternal age >35 years), especially for Down syndrome, with a lesser chance of other trisomies. The difference in frequency between these conditions found at amniocentesis and at birth has already been emphasised (see Tables 4.5 and 4.6). In some countries, the provision of information about this and the offer of screening tests for fetal trisomy is therefore focused on women aged 35 years or older. This used to be the case in the United Kingdom, where amniocentesis was offered to women aged 35 years or older, so that 'screening' for Down syndrome consisted of asking a woman her age. Now, as in many other countries, screening is offered to women of all ages: biochemical and ultrasound measurements are used to modify the age-related probability of the fetal trisomies.

Although population maternal serum screening was originally started for neural tube defects in areas of high incidence, as indicated earlier, the finding that the distribution of AFP levels was reduced in the case of fetal Down syndrome has led to its use in screening antenatally for this condition, especially since the additional measurement of levels of β-hCG, oestriol and pregnancy-associated plasma protein-A (PAPP-A) has given a greater discrimination than AFP assessment alone. The biochemical measures are integrated with maternal age to calculate the chance that the pregnancy is affected, An additional screening technique for Down syndrome is the fetal nuchal fold thickness as measured by ultrasound scan in the first trimester, which can be used in conjunction with serum screening.

The value of this approach is that – in theory at least – the number of invasive tests such as amniocentesis can be kept constant or even reduced, while the proportion of tests with abnormal results is raised. In practical terms, this can allow mothers of all ages to be offered amniocentesis if the chance of abnormality, taking into account the screening test results, exceeds an agreed threshold (often around 1 in 200 or 0.5%), while other women can avoid amniocentesis (or become ineligible for it) if their risk following serum screening (and perhaps nuchal fold measurement) is reduced to below this level.

In practice, the situation is often less simple. Older women may be reluctant to forego a definitive test (and their obstetricians may fear the legal consequences of not providing a test that their patients request). The greater completeness of coverage may itself increase the amniocentesis rate, overloading the laboratory, while many women (and often their doctors) may be worried by being given a specific risk estimate, however small it is, and request amniocentesis. If the indication for amniocentesis is to test for a trisomy after screening, the laboratory may choose not to perform a full karyotypic analysis and use other methods to look solely for trisomies 21, 18 or 13; this is cheaper and gives much more rapid results. An additional problem, as with all screening, is that an abnormal screening result produces severe distress and anxiety in women who – originally – had not perceived themselves to be at high risk, and who may have been given inadequate information about the test. Many genetics clinics have found themselves having to attempt to resolve such traumatic situations, an almost impossible task. There can be no doubt that, for these particular women at least, screening may have caused more harm than good.

While the uptake of screening varies greatly between countries and regions, this can have different causes. One factor, at least in the past, has often been the failure of maternity services and other professionals to give adequate information about screening, together with geographical variability in the quality of services provided and their accessibility.

Non-invasive prenatal testing (NIPT)

Antenatal screening for the autosomal trisomies, and potentially also for many other genetic conditions, is undergoing major developments as NIPT has been introduced in many areas. In the United Kingdom, NIPT has been approved for use within the National Health Service (NHS) as a second-line screening test for those identified by conventional screening (based on ultrasound and maternal serum markers) as having an increased chance of fetal Down syndrome (or trisomy 18 or 13). The major benefit is that only those with an increased chance of an affected fetus on both tests (conventional serum screening and NIPT) will have amniocentesis, so there will be many fewer procedures – and many fewer procedure-related pregnancy losses.

A different approach is being used in some private clinics in the United Kingdom and in other countries, in North America, Europe and elsewhere. NIPT is being used there as a first-line screening test. However, the performance of NIPT is not as satisfactory as a first-line test, because the prior risk of a trisomy is lower, so that the positive predictive value (PPV) of a 'positive' screening test is around 80% as a first-tier test, whereas it is at least 90% as a second-tier test. Furthermore, if additional testing for a wider range of CNVs is requested as well, then the performance becomes much less satisfactory so that the number of 'unnecessary' invasive tests, to confirm or exclude a potential diagnosis of a microdeletion syndrome, based on the NIPT result, would increase again. However, NIPT on its own is certainly more effective as a screening test than earlier methods.

What must be clearly understood by all concerned is that NIPT is not a diagnostic test in this screening context. Whether screening by NIPT is offered as a first-tier or second-tier screening test for autosomal trisomy, it is not diagnostic. Therefore, a pregnancy should not be terminated in the mistaken belief that a positive screening test based on NIPT has no need for confirmation; any positive NIPT screening test requires confirmation by additional (usually invasive) testing. This is discussed further in the section on NIPT later in this chapter.

The overall issues of population screening are discussed in Chapter 34. If the purpose of antenatal screening for Down syndrome is taken to be the opportunity to avoid having an affected child, the evidence currently suggests that conventional screening approaches will allow this in a considerably greater proportion (60%–70%) of pregnancies than age-related screening alone. Screening that employs NIPT will have a higher sensitivity and higher PPV and could be used to avoid more than 95% of cases. How this can be weighed against any adverse effects on women being screened, on our patients with Down syndrome and other genetic conditions, and on society as a whole, are open questions; more evidence, social as well as scientific, is urgently needed as such screening becomes more comprehensive.

Good practice necessitates the full provision of up-to-date information to allow informed choices by women and their partners. It is therefore most important that professionals understand the use of several key terms in the evaluation of population screening tests. These include the sensitivity, specificity, and the positive and negative predictive values of the test. These are set out in Box 9.6.

BOX 9.6: Performance of a screening test

The best way to look at this is to make a 2 × 2 table of four figures: the true and false positives and the true and false negatives:

		Test result		
		+	−	
True diagnosis	Affected +	TP	FN	Sensitivity = TP/(TP + FN)
	Unaffected −	FP	TN	Specificity = TN/(TN + FP)
		PPV = TP/(TP + FP)	NPV = TN/ (TN + FN)	

The positive predictive value (PPV) and negative predictive value (NPV) are derived from the two different columns, the sensitivity (SENS) and specificity (SPEC) from the two rows thus:

PPV is the chance that a positive result on the test is a real positive, which is TP/(TP + FP). NPV is the chance that a negative result on the test is a real negative, which is TN/ (TN + FN).
SENS is the chance that a case will be detected by the screening test, which is TP/ (TP + FN).
SPEC is the chance that a true negative (unaffected) will not be misidentified as being affected, which is TN/(TN + FP).

Using data from the systematic review of Taylor-Phillips et al. (2016), the performance of NIPT as a first-line screening test for the general obstetric population can be summarised thus:

		Test result		
		+	−	
True diagnosis	Affected +	417	18	SENS
	Unaffected −	94	99,471	SPEC
		PPV	NPV	

PPV = 417/(417 + 94) = 81.6%
NPV = 99,471/(99,471 + 18) = 99.98%
SENS = 417/(417 + 18) = 95.9%
SPEC = 99,471/(99,471 + 94) = 99.9%

The PPV is at least as important as sensitivity in determining how well a screening test is performing, especially when a follow-on diagnostic test or other intervention depends upon the test result.

Focussing on the performance of a screening test may sound rather dull and dry but it is crucial, especially when different providers promote their services in the marketplace. This is because providers will often seek to present their test's performance in terms of its 'accuracy'. This, however, is most unhelpful: if that were applied to Down syndrome screening in the general population, then simply giving every pregnancy a low-risk result (without even bothering to do the test) would score an accuracy of substantially greater than 99%. It is therefore absolutely essential that professionals who provide such services understand how these tests operate as screening tests, how they should be explained to patients and how their performance should be evaluated – and that requires grappling with the 2 × 2 table in Box 9.6 and the concept of the positive predictive value (PPV).

X-LINKED DISORDERS

Where a pregnancy is at high risk for an X-linked disorder, fetal sexing offers the possibility of determining whether the fetus is indeed at risk. However, in most disorders, direct molecular prenatal diagnosis of an affected male is now possible and, even where it is not, linked DNA markers can often be used. First-trimester fetal sexing is now possible and highly accurate with NIPT, which can be used to avoid an invasive CVS of a female conception. Fetal sexing is possible by DNA and cytogenetic methods and should always accompany metabolic studies, which may give variable and misleading results in X-linked conditions if the pattern of X-chromosome inactivation is skewed away from 50:50.

Where a woman is only a possible carrier, not a definite one, it is vital to estimate the risk before fetal sexing is undertaken and to use methods of carrier detection where applicable to resolve any uncertainty (see Chapter 7). The most successful approach to prenatal diagnosis is where no prenatal procedure is required at all, because the carrier state has been excluded. As with any prenatal diagnostic investigation, this should be approached as a planned procedure with the issues for and against resolved, as far as possible, beforehand.

Occasionally, in haemophilia or Becker muscular dystrophy, for example, fetal sexing may be requested for a pregnancy with an affected father, with a view to termination of a female fetus, which would inevitably be a carrier. The author has serious misgivings about the wisdom of this, because such daughters would almost always be healthy and would be very likely to have available the option of direct prenatal diagnosis in their own future children, even in situations where this is not currently possible. The situation is less clear-cut for disorders where heterozygous females frequently show substantial clinical effects, such as sometimes in ornithine carbamoyltransferase (previously known as ornithine transcarbamylase) deficiency (OCT or OTC, respectively) and more often in the fragile X syndrome (FRAXA).

Prenatal sex selection

Fetal sex may be determined by ultrasound, NIPT or amniocentesis. This information is then sometimes used to enable fetal sex selection for parental choice by the selective termination of pregnancies carrying a female fetus. Such prenatal sex selection is currently illegal in many countries, including the United Kingdom, except in the context of a family history of sex-linked disease. However, such fetal sex selection is being grossly abused in some parts of the world, notably India and China, despite its being illegal in both countries, and is almost always applied in favour of a male pregnancy. A form of reproductive tourism has developed to countries, such as the United States, that permit fetal sex determination and do not prohibit sex selection through the termination of (female) fetuses.

Developments in sperm sorting, still less than reliable but likely to become more effective, have raised the issue of whether this should be permitted for non-medical reasons.

The Nuffield Council on Bioethics has examined the issue of prenatal sex selection as a part of its comprehensive report on NIPT. It argues firmly against the use of NIPT for sex determination ahead of the gestational age of the fetal anomaly ultrasound scan at 18–20 weeks (see later section on NIPT). A consistent opposition to fetal sex selection has the virtue of expressing solidarity with the women of countries where they are oppressed and where further distortion of the sex ratio is likely to worsen their collective plight. Furthermore, in the author's opinion, use of the phrase 'family balancing' in the justification of fetal sex selection on social grounds is usually either disingenuous or mischievous: it purports to protect liberty but wilfully ignores those whose liberty needs protection.

INBORN ERRORS OF METABOLISM

The development of prenatal diagnostic techniques for a variety of inherited metabolic disorders has been one of the major achievements of human genetics, even if the number of families at risk for such disorders is small in comparison with the much more frequent chromosomal disorders such as Down syndrome. So many serious inborn errors are now prenatally detectable that this aspect is one of the first to be raised by most couples who have had an affected child.

Chapter 26 covers some of the more important disorders and virtually all of them are now diagnosable prenatally, either biochemically or by DNA analysis or a combination of both.

The following points need to be borne in mind when prenatal diagnosis of a metabolic disorder is being considered.

- The great majority of these disorders follow autosomal recessive inheritance, so that only sibs of affected patients are at high (one in four) risk. Risks for other relatives are rarely high enough to warrant undertaking prenatal diagnosis unless the chance of both parents being carriers is substantial (principally in the setting of consanguinity).
- Many disorders can be diagnosed by molecular genetic (DNA-based) methods and the need for enzyme assays on chorionic villi or cultured amniocytes is much less than it was 20 years ago. The direct metabolic tests (biochemical assays) usually require chorionic villi or cultured amniotic fluid cells for their diagnosis. In general, if a particular enzyme defect can be detected in the cultured skin fibroblast, it can also be detected in villus material or cultured amniotic fluid cells, although normal ranges may differ considerably in the different cell types.
- Large numbers of cells are often required, making direct analysis of chorionic villi especially suitable. The need for cell culture with amniocentesis may add delay and uncertainty, which should be explained beforehand. A late termination may be unacceptable to a couple who would accept termination in early pregnancy.
- Many of the enzymatic techniques are exceptionally specialised and can be undertaken only by a few laboratories. If they are required, therefore, careful advance planning is essential because cells may have to be sent long distances. Fortunately, DNA analysis is generally a much more robust technique, can be conducted successfully in many more centres, and has largely replaced enzyme assays in prenatal diagnosis. Where enzyme assays are required, a remarkable degree of cooperation nationally and internationally exists between laboratories involved in this work, although careful distinction is needed between a centre that 'has an interest' in a disorder and one that has proven experience in its prenatal diagnosis.
- Wherever possible, samples from the affected individual should be studied alongside those at risk. If the affected child is likely to die, every effort should be made to reach

a precise enzymatic or molecular diagnosis beforehand, and to arrange for storage of DNA, cultured cells or postmortem material to be used at a later date. Failure to do this may result in serious problems in relation to a future pregnancy, which could have been avoided.

A few inherited metabolic diseases can be diagnosed directly from amniotic fluid itself, although the use of cultured cells is usually desirable as a backup. These include the organic acidurias (propionic and methylmalonic aciduria), the mucopolysaccharidoses, the 21-hydroxylase form of congenital adrenal hyperplasia and congenital nephrosis (diagnosed by elevated amniotic AFP levels).

MOLECULAR PRENATAL DIAGNOSIS

The impact of molecular genetics has been particularly strong in the area of prenatal diagnosis. There are many reasons for this, including the independence of the techniques from gestational timing and tissue specificity, the lack of variability in heterozygotes (which can make enzymatic diagnoses so difficult), and the suitability of first-trimester or even pre-implantation samples. In short, many of the features of prenatal diagnosis that made pre-molecular methods so difficult are no longer obstacles as the molecular methods are so robust. Most of all, molecular analysis has extended the possibility of prenatal diagnosis to numerous serious disorders, often dominantly inherited, where lack of specific biochemical knowledge previously precluded any attempts at prenatal diagnosis. In any inherited disorder for which the specific gene has been isolated, it can be assumed that prenatal diagnosis is potentially feasible.

The range of molecular approaches available is the same as already indicated in Chapter 5, and also outlined in relation to carrier detection in Chapter 7. Where a mutation has been identified in an affected relative, search for this will avoid the necessity for additional tests. Where this has not proved possible, a wider search for mutations may be needed and this may have limitations, though complete gene sequencing combined with dosage analysis has reduced these. If linked genetic markers are being used, intragenic markers will be reliable provided that other family members can be typed; for recessive disorders a previous affected child is usually the critical sample. The importance of storing a sample from such key individuals for the future must yet again be emphasised.

If linked DNA markers outside the gene are used, the risk of error due to recombination must be carefully estimated and discussed before embarking on prenatal testing. Although in general, linkage analysis is used much less frequently now than formerly, it has a particular application in pre-implantation genetic diagnosis as it helps to overcome the possibility of misleading results from allele drop-out (see later in this chapter). In large genes, where there is a substantial rate of recombination across the gene – such as the dystrophin gene for the Xp21 types of muscular dystrophy, Duchenne and Becker – a set of markers should be studied to give a haplotype along the length of the gene.

Linkage analysis is also used in prenatal exclusion testing, scarcely used except in Huntington's disease (HD), where an at-risk parent neither wishes to transmit the disorder to a child nor to discover their own genetic status. Closely linked markers are used to determine whether the at-risk parent has transmitted to the fetus the copy of the gene she or he has inherited from her (or his) affected or unaffected parent. There are complex issues of counselling to consider because we would wish to avoid a predictive test result for HD on a newborn infant. This is discussed further in Chapter 15.

FETAL BLOOD AND TISSUE SAMPLING

Direct umbilical cord sampling under ultrasonographic control has been used in the past to obtain pure fetal blood, but DNA techniques have made it unnecessary in most situations where it was used before – notably in the haemoglobinopathies and haemophilias. Access to the cord vessels may still be required but that is likely to be for therapeutic purposes (blood transfusion).

Fetal skin biopsy has proved both reliable and safe for a variety of severe conditions, including lethal and dystrophic epidermolysis bullosa, ichthyosiform erythroderma, Sjögren-Larsson syndrome and severe oculocutaneous albinism; there is usually no visible scar. As with fetal blood sampling, though, molecular analysis using DNA from a chorion villus sample has progressively replaced this approach.

PRE-IMPLANTATION GENETIC DIAGNOSIS

For many couples at high risk of transmitting a serious genetic disorder, this could potentially offer the possibility of avoiding both an affected child and the termination of an established pregnancy. It is now possible to undertake molecular analysis of cells from an early embryo (often a blastocyst) produced by *in vitro* fertilisation (IVF), and to implant only an embryo shown to have an unaffected genotype.

Testing the one cell (or sometimes two cells) removed from the embryo at biopsy for a specific mutation at the disease locus can give false-negative results if the abnormal allele fails to amplify at polymerase chain reaction, so a haplotype of marker single nucleotide polymorphisms (SNPs) from in and around the locus of interest is now often used instead, or even a full, genome-wide set of SNPs, that could be used to test for any disorder of known location. This has the advantage that the validation of the laboratory analysis for quality control can be performed in a single step for the genome-wide set of SNPs, rather than locus by locus or mutation by mutation, although samples from other family members may be required for the linkage analysis.

In principle this should allow pre-implantation diagnosis to be offered for any disorder where a specific molecular or chromosomal defect can be identified. In practice there are still several notes of caution to be sounded. These notes of caution include the following:

- The paucity of long-term data on potential harmful effects of the procedure, over and above any problems from the process of IVF.
- The high emotional and often financial cost of the procedure.
- The physical demands placed on the woman, including the potential hazards of ovarian hyperstimulation (for egg collection).
- The limited success rate for IVF in general of successfully establishing a pregnancy, when fertility will usually not be a concern.

In view of these limitations, it is most important that centres should always make such limitations very clear to the referring clinicians and to the patients referred. Their prior experience with that particular disorder should be made clear and whether the investigation they are offering is being made available as research or service. Pre-implantation diagnosis should also always be offered in the context of full genetic counselling: it is disturbing that this is not always the case. Given the complex genetic situations often involved, expert information on the wider genetic aspects is essential if families are to make an informed choice between the possible options open to them. There is a clear need for effective regulation in this field, especially since it is often run as a commercial venture rather than as part of established universal health services. Such regulation is present in some European countries (including the United Kingdom, to some extent), but is largely absent in the rest of the world. Until a uniformly high standard is achieved in practice, it is important that all those involved in genetic counselling maintain a critical and fully informed attitude to pre-implantation diagnosis, have detailed knowledge of the services in their region or country, and try to ensure that families embarking on the procedure are similarly well informed.

FETAL DNA ANALYSIS OF MATERNAL BLOOD

This is another field that is coming into clinical use, though further development of the technology is to be expected, and there is a real danger that the availability of testing may already be driving clinical practice far ahead of the evidence on its outcomes.

It has long been known that a small number of fetal cells are present in maternal blood but more recently free fetal DNA has also been shown to be present. This derives from the chorionic component of the placenta. Sequencing of this cell-free DNA in maternal blood provides a non-invasive approach to prenatal diagnosis. Initially used in relation to Rhesus haemolytic disease and for fetal sexing, current applications include the use of this as part of a primary screening test for Down syndrome and other aneuploidies. A systematic review of its use in prenatal screening is very helpful (Taylor-Phillips et al., 2016), and a report from the Nuffield Council on Bioethics (2017) provides a constructive but critical guide to the issues it raises. Both are freely available (open access); both include useful references for further information.

Other applications that are being explored now include the use of NIPT to look for mutant sequences inherited from the father, especially dominant disorders but also recessive disorders where the parents carry different mutations in the same recessive gene. CNVs can also be detected fairly readily, so that microdeletions can be added to the autosomal trisomies sought in antenatal screening, although the performance of the test – as demonstrated in its sensitivity and its positive predictive value – is not as well studied as for the trisomies and may not be as good. Accordingly, the great advantage of NIPT over conventional antenatal screening for Down syndrome (by ultrasound and maternal serum screening) would be lost. When the test's high PPV is reduced, the reduction in the number of amniocenteses recommended after screening will be reversed, so that the fall in the number of miscarriages will also be reversed, if such tests are simply added in because they are technologically feasible and may enhance the marketability of the test to the inadequately informed.

NIPT can in principle be used to perform any genetic investigation on the fetus, whether or not it has any clinical utility in the pregnancy. Fetal whole genome sequencing can be performed as long as the free DNA in maternal plasma is sequenced to sufficient depth: there are no limits to the genetic information that can (in principle) be obtained about the fetus. In addition to the complexities introduced by placental mosaicism and vanishing twins, the bigger questions that arise concern the limits of what information it is helpful and acceptable to generate about a fetus, a person not yet born. We return to this question in Chapter 34.

NIPT can entail any of three different activities:

1. Detecting pathogenic variants that would not usually be present in the mother's blood (i.e. have been transmitted from the father or arisen *de novo* in the fetus).
2. Measuring the ratio between different alleles of a particular gene or SNP.
3. Detecting the ratio between sequences from different chromosomes and then using the results to make inferences about the genetic constitution of the fetus.

The reliability of the test will vary with the basis of the particular test that has been performed. Detecting a variant that is not present in the mother but is present in the father (e.g. SRY, Rhesus antigen, any dominant or recessive disease-causing allele) will allow very high confidence in the interpretation of the results, whereas evidence of types (2) or (3) give results that are somewhat less certain.

BOX 9.7: Types of non-invasive prenatal testing (NIPT)

Population screening applications:

- Population-risk aneuploidy screening: first tier (as available commercially in the United Kingdom).
- Increased chance aneuploidy screening: second tier (fetus is known to have an increased probability) (as is being made available in the United Kingdom through the NHS, when a pregnancy is at increased risk of trisomy on the basis of other screening tests).
- Population risk screening for microdeletion syndromes, usually of unknown or low PPV (compared to detection of the fetal autosomal trisomies).

Potentially diagnostic applications (sometimes abbreviated to NIPD):

- Panel of mutations given the specific fetal anomalies found on ultrasound scan: looking for a restricted range of possible causes of *de novo* dominant disorders (such as the skeletal dysplasias associated with pathogenic variants in *FGFR3* using targeted analysis of specific gene variants).
- Paternally derived variants (rare disease diagnostics based on family history, where it is the paternal allele that is being sought [when the disorder for which the fetus is at risk is *either* a dominant disorder that may be inherited from the father *or* a recessive disorder, with the mutation that may be inherited from the father being distinct from that present in the mother]).

Diagnostic applications by inference:

- Maternally derived variants (rare disease diagnostics on the basis of family history with an affected mother, or a previous affected child, or a recessive disease with the same mutation present in both parents; involves assessing the relative frequencies of the two different versions of each SNP or allele and then inferring the fetal genetic constitution).
- Genome-wide investigation of fetal anomalies on ultrasound scan with no clear diagnosis, looking for a broader range of genetic disorders (e.g. whole exome or whole genome sequencing of the fetus). (Should be performed as a trio analysis, with samples from both parents.)

Curiosity-driven 'genome scanning' without a clinical indication (usually at parental request):

- Exome or whole genome analysis without a clinical indication (which appears to the author as at best unwise and quite possibly unethical and unprofessional).

The very broad range of tests that may be described as NIPT are listed in Box 9.7. Note that the clinical setting will determine the prior risk of disease being present, so that the clinical setting and the laboratory methods employed will together determine the reliability of the test: (1) the test's positive predictive value (how likely a positive test result is to be true) and, therefore, (2) whether a follow-on invasive test is required to confirm a positive test result, and also (3) how likely it is that unsought 'incidental' or 'additional' findings will emerge.

TWINS AND PRENATAL DIAGNOSIS

The discovery of a twin pregnancy poses obvious practical problems in undertaking amniocentesis, but it also alters the genetic risk figures that would normally be given for a singleton pregnancy. The problems involved in estimating the modified risks are summarised in Table 9.1. It is assumed here that one-third of twin pairs are monozygous.

In general, the risks are considerably higher than for a singleton pregnancy, and they are altered if information is available on one twin from amniocentesis. The figures do not include the increased risk of malformations known to be associated with monozygotic twin pregnancies (see Chapter 10). Clearly, the couple concerned should be informed of these altered risks, and the same is true even when prenatal diagnosis is not being considered.

Table 9.1 Genetic risks in twin pregnancies

	Chromosome abnormality	Neural tube defect	X-linked (fetal sexing only)	X-linked (specific diagnostic test)	Autosomal recessive
Before amniocentesis					
Risk for singleton pregnancy	Y^a	$\dfrac{1}{25}$	$\dfrac{1}{2}$	$\dfrac{1}{4}$	$\dfrac{1}{4}$
Risk of at least one twin being affected	$\dfrac{5}{3}Y$	$\dfrac{2}{25}$	$\dfrac{2}{3}$	$\dfrac{3}{8}$	$\dfrac{3}{8}$
Risk of both twins being affected	$\sim\dfrac{1}{3}Y$	$<\dfrac{1}{100}$	$\dfrac{1}{3}$	$\dfrac{1}{8}$	$\dfrac{1}{8}$
Twin A normal; risk of twin B being abnormal	$\dfrac{2}{3}Y$	$\dfrac{1}{25}$	$\dfrac{1}{3}$	$\dfrac{1}{6}$	$\dfrac{1}{6}$
After amniocentesis (one sac successfully tested)					
Twin A abnormal; risk of twin B being normal	$\dfrac{2}{3}-\dfrac{2}{3}Y$	$\dfrac{9}{10}$	$\dfrac{1}{3}$	$\dfrac{1}{2}$	$\dfrac{1}{2}$
Twin A abnormal; risk of twin B being abnormal	$\dfrac{1}{3}+\dfrac{2}{3}Y$	$\dfrac{1}{10}$	$\dfrac{2}{3}$	$\dfrac{1}{2}$	$\dfrac{1}{2}$

Source: After Hunter AGW, Cox DM (1979), *Clin Genet* 16: 34–42.
[a] Risk (Y) will vary with maternal age, etc.

BOX 9.8: Genetic disorders in pregnancy and maternal health

Maternal health adversely affected by pregnancy
Cystic fibrosis (respiratory decompensation)
Aortic stenosis, cardiomyopathy or other potential cause of cardiac failure
Homocystinuria, sickle cell disease (thrombotic episodes)
Marfan syndrome and other aortopathies (risk of aortic dissection and rupture)
Limb girdle muscular dystrophies (including dystrophin-related dystrophy in a clinically affected female 'carrier')

Obstetric complications increased
Achondroplasia (pelvic disproportion, uterine myomas)
Ehlers-Danlos syndrome (premature rupture of membranes)
Myotonic dystrophy (postpartum haemorrhage, anaesthetic problems)
Steroid sulphatase deficiency (delayed labour, increased risk of stillbirth)

A further point to be noted is that the normal range of maternal serum AFP concentrations is raised in twin pregnancies. Charts of the AFP percentiles in twin pregnancies are available; it should be noted that all twin pregnancies ending in a neural tube defect had a serum AFP concentration at least 75 times the normal singleton median value.

Techniques of selective abortion are possible when only one of a twin pair is found to be abnormal, although if they share a circulation then this may be hazardous also to the unaffected twin. Not only may the unaffected twin be at direct risk from the agent used but, in addition, a common circulation with a dead co-twin (whether this occurs naturally or as an iatrogenic complication) is itself hazardous from the effects of necrotic material that can lead to vascular complications in multiple sites, including the brain. Twin pregnancies remain a difficult field of management. Multiple births are also seen at higher rates following fertility treatment and IVF procedures.

MATERNAL ASPECTS OF GENETIC COUNSELLING IN PREGNANCY

Although prenatal diagnosis is principally concerned with procedures involving the fetus, genetic counselling in pregnancy also needs to look at aspects of health involving the mother, as well as the psychosocial issues. In many dominantly inherited disorders, the mother will be affected by the disorder, which may pose direct risks to her health in pregnancy or give obstetric complications. Prognosis of an affected parent is a further relevant point in relation to any decisions. Examples of the range of problems needing consideration are given in Box 9.8.

10

Special issues in genetic counselling

GENETIC INFORMATION AND CONFIDENTIALITY

It may appear completely redundant, or even insulting, to refer to confidentiality in a book for health professionals, for all of whom respect for confidentiality will surely be second nature. For health professionals who have not yet had much experience of working in clinical genetics, however, some remarks may prove helpful. There are aspects of confidentiality that can easily prove challenging in certain recurrent scenarios that we encounter.

When we take a family history, we are collecting information that will usually be correct in its broad shape although particular details may not be. Medical information about relatives may be incorrect and the details of family relationships may be wrong.

There are a number of reported 'diagnoses' that we have to regard with scepticism until we have definite proof. These include multiple sclerosis (MS), especially when it seems to run in a family, and liver cancer. The awareness of inherited neurodegenerative conditions has increased greatly in the past few decades and so 'MS' in an earlier generation may easily have been the name applied to a very different condition. In a similar way, 'liver cancer' (or 'brain cancer') may refer to liver (or brain) metastases from a primary site elsewhere. In looking for a pattern of inherited susceptibility to cancer, we need to look for the sites of the primary cancers, not where they spread to.

Inaccuracy in such medical details is unfortunate but is usually the result of the simple forgetting of details, whose significance may have been unclear to those involved. Inaccuracies in a family history can be different, in that family members sometimes conceal important facts from each other. These can relate to paternity, abortions, adoption (into or out of the family) and whether an individual was affected by a particular disorder, especially if it is seen within the family as shameful or degrading. The details of a person's death may be obscured or suppressed, if one side of a family does not want to be blamed for transmitting a disease, or if parents choose to 'forget' the sad deaths of infants, or if someone commits suicide. Such information can remain very sensitive within a family but may form a valuable part of the evidence pointing towards a diagnosis and could be very helpful in making a clinical genetic assessment.

Having discovered such information, of possible relevance to others in the wider family, it can be all too easy for professionals to disclose it to those who have not already learned about it through family channels. Such a disclosure of other people's personal information can cause great distress. Those who had tried to conceal the information can be distressed and angry that the information has escaped, or at least that they were not the ones to tell their relatives; those who have now found out can be angry that they have only just now found out. ('Why did they not tell us that years ago?')

Even giving information that a relative has also been seen in the medical genetics service may amount to a breach of confidence. Indeed, we used to list the names of family members referred to the service on the front of 'family files' until it caused upset in more than one family when another branch of the family noticed this. They realised that their relatives had also been referred about the same condition but had not told them.

We are now careful to keep physically separate the information about referrals of individuals within the same family and will often take different family histories from each new referral so that looking at their version of the 'family tree' does not reveal to one family member information that another would not want them to know. Each branch of the family has its own version of the family tree. Of course, when relatives attend clinic together and talk frankly in front of one another, it makes the professional's task much simpler.

It is important that individuals feel that their own personal information is private and treated as such, with full respect for confidentiality. However, some information about the family can be regarded as belonging to the family as a whole. Thus, in a family with a child affected by cystic fibrosis, the fact of the disease will usually be widely known although the precise mutations responsible for the disease may not be. There is a strong case to say that the laboratory has every right to use their knowledge of the responsible mutation(s) to make carrier testing available to other family members. Once knowledge of the disease has been communicated within the family, knowledge of the mutation(s) can perhaps be assumed to belong to the family as a whole and not exclusively to the individual in whom the mutations were first identified.

In the different context of Huntington's disease (HD), the fact that HD is present in the family (and that I am at risk of it) may be known to many, including my brothers and sisters and my children, but my own test result should be treated as private. It would be a breach of my privacy for health professionals to reveal to others whether I have or have not inherited this condition. However, it may be thought that my children have some claim to this personal information about me (my test result), despite my reluctance to tell them, because if I have inherited the HD gene then they will be at high risk. In such a case, respect for my privacy conflicts with a potential set of obligations to other family members. One factor that may be important in determining the strength of the duty to protect an individual's privacy is the medical context: in practice, what is at stake? If others are deprived of the information, will they suffer adverse health consequences? (Is knowledge of the condition 'actionable'? Could it lead to better or earlier treatments or prevention? Might it influence reproductive decisions?)

In such cases of conflict between competing duties, it may be necessary to discuss the case with colleagues to help decide on the ethically correct course of action given the particular circumstances of the case. This could be at an internal departmental meeting, a clinical ethics committee or a forum such as the 'Genethics Forum' in the United Kingdom. It may also be helpful, occasionally, to seek legal advice (see later in this chapter).

CONSANGUINITY

Consanguinity, or marriage between close relatives, is a common and important issue in genetic counselling. Where an inherited disorder is present in the family, consanguinity may significantly influence the risks. Even without a known disorder, couples who are closely related may be concerned about the risks to their offspring.

There are three aspects of consanguinity that need to be considered in relation to genetic counselling:

- What is the exact relationship between the two individuals?
- How is the risk of a genetic disorder in the family influenced by the occurrence of consanguinity?
- How likely is it that any harmful gene might be handed by both members of the couple to a child, i.e. that the child is homozygous by descent for such a pathogenic gene variant (allele)?

An attempt is made here to answer these questions in simple terms, avoiding a complex mathematical approach. These same questions are of more general interest to population geneticists, and detailed accounts of the subject can be found in genetics textbooks (see Appendix 1).

Genetic relationships

An accurate idea of how individuals are related is important in all genetic counselling, regardless of the presence or absence of consanguinity, but when a marriage between close relatives is being considered it becomes essential. Table 10.1 summarises the main categories of relationship, and it is always important to construct a precise pedigree pattern rather than rely on verbal descriptions, which may be confusing. Table 10.2 gives examples.

Marriage between first-degree relatives is almost universally prohibited by law and social custom; but incestuous relationships, usually between father and daughter or between sibs, are

Table 10.1 Degrees of relationship

Degree	Proportion of genes shared
First-degree	1/2
• Sibs	
• Dizygotic twins	
• Parents	
• Children	
Second-degree	1/4
• Half-sibs	
• Uncles, aunts	
• Nephews, nieces	
• Double first cousins	
Third-degree	1/8
• First cousins	
• Half-uncles, aunts	
• Half-nephews, nieces	

Table 10.2 Patterns of relationship

Relationship (between shaded individuals)	Degree of relationship	Proportion of genes shared	Chance of homozygosity by descent (F)
Monozygotic twins	–	1	–
Dizygotic twins	First	1/2	1/4
Sibs	First	1/2	1/4
Parent-child	First	1/2	–
Uncle (aunt)-nephew (niece)	Second	1/4	1/8
Half-sibs	Second	1/4	1/8
Double first cousins	Second	1/4	1/8
First cousins	Third	1/8	1/16
Half-uncle–niece (or similar combination)	Third	1/8	1/16
First cousins once removed	Fourth	1/16	1/32
Second cousins	Fifth	1/32	1/64
Second cousins once removed		1/64	1/128
Third cousins		1/128	1/256

more common than is generally recognised and give rise to particular problems discussed later. Marriage between second-degree relatives is also legally barred in many countries, although uncle-niece marriage is frequent in some Asian communities.

First-cousin marriages are the most common reason for couples seeking genetic advice about consanguinity. These are legal in most Western countries but may be the subject of religious or social restrictions. In many Asian communities they are actively encouraged. The less common half-uncle–niece marriage shown in Table 10.2 is, in genetic terms, identical to a first-cousin marriage.

Among the more distant relationships, the problem of terminology may cause confusion. The term 'removed' refers to a difference in generations between the individuals. Thus, the son of one's first cousin is a first cousin once removed, while the children of one's parents' first cousins are one's second cousins.

It should be noted that the 'degrees' of relationship shown in Table 10.1 are those used in genetic terminology, as well as in English canon and common law, but not in civil law, where a different approach is used. Thus, uncle and niece, who would generally be considered second-degree relatives, would be termed 'third-degree relatives' in civil law.

It is helpful in genetic counselling to be aware of the legal aspects of consanguineous marriages because many couples have unspoken fears about the legality of a relationship as well as the genetic risks. Clearly the situation will vary between countries, and in the United States between individual states. The situation in the United States still provides some remarkable inconsistencies, although others have been amended. First-cousin marriages are illegal in over half the states, while half-niece or half-nephew marriages are prohibited in only a quarter of states. Some states prohibit marriages between first cousins once removed. Eleven states allow marriages between half-sibs. Some European countries have relaxed or removed restrictions on marriage between even the most closely related individuals.

Quite apart from these complexities, there are a number of restrictions on marriages between unrelated individuals. Thus, the wife of an uncle may be considered as a legal aunt even though no genetic relationship exists. In addition, different religions may have specific prohibitions over and above the legal requirement.

Taking all these facts together, it can be seen that there are numerous legal as well as genetic pitfalls confronting those involved in genetic counselling for consanguineous marriages. If there is any doubt, the couple should obtain legal (or, in some settings, ecclesiastical) advice, and this aspect should be clarified before the genetic risks are discussed in detail.

Social aspects of consanguinity

Working in the field of medical genetics, it is easy to regard consanguinity as a 'problem' and something to be discouraged. In fact, it is a preferred pattern of marriage over large parts of the world, something that would not have occurred without good reasons. These are obvious to members of such populations but need to be emphasised for students or professionals unfamiliar with the context. Quite apart from legal and property rights, a consanguineous marriage may greatly strengthen the position of a woman, who is thought less likely to be ill-treated if her husband's family members are bound by ties of kinship. These considerations may apply just as much to immigrant groups in Western countries as in their country of origin, as they are even more dependent on family links to survive and prosper. Consanguinity is a beneficial pattern for many millions of couples, though one with a genetic price to pay in terms of autosomal recessive disorders.

It must be said that the way consanguinity is discussed within clinic consultations is important and can lead to difficulties.

Thus it is not difficult for a professional in the United Kingdom to cause offence by asking those from a minority community about consanguinity in a brusque or insensitive manner, and if the professional is perceived as judgemental, being antagonistic to customary consanguineous marriage, then the offence may be grave and undermine any professional relationship. Such encounters can store up awkwardness and problems for future clinic visits.

Discussion within society at large can also impact on minority groups and on the atmosphere in consultations. There have been examples of very unhelpful, high-profile discussions of consanguinity within the UK Parliament, and outside Parliament by Members of Parliament and by public health officials. This has consequences in the society at large and that includes consultations in the genetics clinic, in which addressing the topic then becomes more delicate and difficult. Continuing to discuss relationships within the family is of course still necessary; approaching these questions in a calm and matter-of-fact manner will usually allay any fears or sensitivity in a consanguineous family.

It must also not be forgotten that shame in consanguinity, and feelings of guilt if a child has a genetic disorder, can be intense among those from the white British majority in the United Kingdom who have married a cousin contrary to the usual cultural expectation. Their needs should not be forgotten.

Risks of consanguinity with a specific genetic disorder in the family

Where a specific genetic disorder occurs in a consanguineous marriage, this may have serious implications for the extended family, who will have to weigh up the social benefits against the genetic risks. It is clearly important that the extended family as well as the immediate family have information on the precise risks involved, as outlined later. Such risks decline rapidly with distance of relationship.

In general, consanguinity will have no effect on risks if the disorder is X-linked recessive or autosomal dominant, unless both partners of the couple actually have the condition or carry the gene concerned. Autosomal recessive inheritance provides the main problem; it is likely that risks are also increased for polygenic disorders, even though these effects are difficult to quantify.

The essential question to be asked for an autosomal recessive disorder is this: what is the chance that the harmful mutant gene will have passed down both sides of the family simultaneously and appear in homozygous state in the child? The situation is best illustrated by the example shown in Figure 10.1. Here, a man having a sister with a rare autosomal recessive disorder has married his first cousin. We can ignore the very small added risk of new mutation or the mutant gene being present by chance.

- The chance of the husband carrying the mutant gene is two in three (not two in four, as is commonly thought, because the homozygous affected category has been excluded). The chance of a child receiving the gene from him is thus one in three.
- The chance of the wife (first cousin) also being a carrier must now be estimated. Both parents of the husband must be carriers and one of the common paternal grandparents also must be, so the chance of their daughter being a carrier is one in two and for their granddaughter (the wife in the couple being considered) it is one in four. The chance of the mutant gene being transmitted to her child will be one in eight. The risk of the child receiving the gene from both sides simultaneously (i.e. of having the disorder) is simply the product: $1/3 \times 1/8 = 1/24$. (We pass over the possibility that both of the paternal grandparents might carry the condition.)

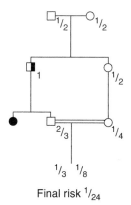

Final risk $^1/_{24}$

Figure 10.1 Genetic risks in a consanguineous marriage (see text for explanation).

A second example is given in Figure 10.2. It is a little more complex, but the approach is the same. Every generation added to the path diminishes the risk by one-half.

Figure 10.3 summarises some of the general risks in this situation. This information could be important for genetic counsellors and others working in isolated areas with little access to specialist advice, as is the case in many parts of the world where consanguinity is the norm. Indeed, there is no reason why community or religious leaders should not use such a table for the most common situations, since they are often involved when marriages are being arranged. A simple computer programme, based on those already widely used in population genetics, could also be readily produced. The figures show clearly how substituting a more distant consanguineous marriage for a closer one could give a more acceptable, lower risk, and thus allow the social benefits of consanguinity to be retained. If the situation is simply presented in

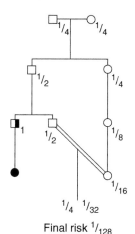

Final risk $^1/_{128}$

Figure 10.2 Genetic risks in a consanguineous marriage (first cousins once removed). The chance of a child being homozygous for (i.e. affected by) the rare autosomal recessive disorder present in the husband's niece is 1 in 128.

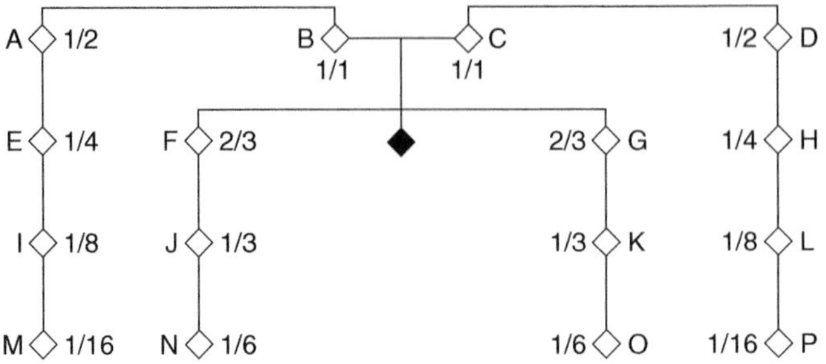

A × D* = 1/16		I × H* = 1/128
A × F = 1/12		I × L* = 1/256
A × H* = 1/32		I × P* = 1/512
E × F = 1/24		J × K = 1/36
E × H* = 1/64		J × H = 1/48
E × K = 1/48		J × L = 1/96
E × L* = 1/128		J × P = 1/192
F × H = 1/24		M × N = 1/384
F × K = 1/18		M × L* = 1/512
F × L = 1/48		M × P* = 1/1024
I × F = 1/48		N × K = 1/72
I × J = 1/96		N × O = 1/144
I × N = 1/192		N × L = 1/192
		N × P = 1/384

Figure 10.3 Genetic risks in consanguineous marriages where a known autosomal recessive disorder is present in the family (sex of individuals not specified for simplicity). The diagram indicates the main categories of marriage for which genetic risk estimates may be sought. In each case, the risk of the disorder will be 1/4 × the product of the two individual carrier risks; for example, for E × L, the risk is 1/4 × 1/4 × 1/8 = 1/132. Selected examples are summarised previously. Note: Some of the relationships are not consanguineous, even though genetic risks are increased. These are indicated by an asterisk (*).

terms of consanguinity being a problem, rather than introducing the concept of a graded risk, social damage could result that might outweigh the potential harm from a genetic disorder.

General risks of consanguinity

Estimates of risk for the offspring of consanguineous marriages when no disorder is known in the family are based on two approaches:

- Information on the probable number of deleterious recessive genes carried by healthy individuals in the population.
- Surveys of the outcome of pregnancies from consanguineous marriages.

Several studies have suggested that everyone carries at least one gene for a harmful recessive disorder, and probably at least two for lethal conditions that would result in a spontaneous abortion or stillbirth. Using this as a basis, risks can easily be estimated if one knows the relationship of the couple concerned.

The simplest approach is to trace the fate of such a harmful mutant gene from the common ancestor or ancestors to the offspring at risk, in a manner similar to that described in the previous section. Figure 10.4 shows this for a first-cousin marriage, where it is clear that the

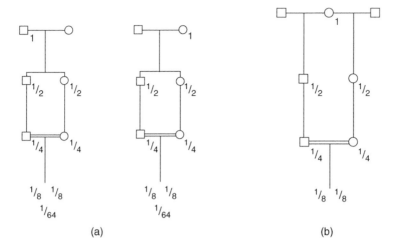

Figure 10.4 (a) First cousin marriage: the chance of a harmful gene in a common ancestor being homozygous by descent in the child is 1 in 64. Because there are two common ancestors, the risk will be twice this (total risk 1 in 32). (b) Marriage between half first cousins: the situation is as for full first cousins but there is only one common ancestor to be considered (total risk 1 in 64).

risk of one harmful recessive gene reaching the offspring through both parents simultaneously is 1 in 64. Because the other common ancestor has to be considered as well, the total risk is 1 in 32. If the two lethal genes carried by each individual are considered in the same way, the risk is 1 in 16. This latter estimate is identical to the risk of any gene being homozygous by descent in the offspring, a figure known as the coefficient of consanguinity (F). This forms the generally used yardstick for measuring closeness of relationship between two individuals (see Table 10.1) and can also be used in connection with populations as well as individuals, as discussed later.

Studies of the actual empirical risks to the offspring of consanguineous marriages are summarised in Table 10.3 but show considerable variation between populations.

It is also difficult to separate an increase in specific genetic disorders from problems with a large environmental contribution. In an extensive early study in Japan, the offspring of first-cousin marriages followed over a 10-year period showed a 3% increase in mortality over those with unrelated parents, but only a small increase in severe malformations (1.7 versus 1%). The offspring of marriages between first cousins once removed and between second cousins showed no increase in malformation rate. The data from different studies are well summarised in Vogel and Motulsky's book (see Appendix 1).

Studies of the offspring of incestuous matings have confirmed the high predicted risk to offspring and show a risk of around one in three of childhood death or severe abnormality. In addition, there appears to be an increased risk of mental retardation without physical

Table 10.3 Observed increase in severe abnormalities and mortality among offspring of consanguineous parents

Parental relationship	Increase (%)
Incestuous matings (first-degree relatives)	30
First cousins	3
First cousins once removed and second cousins	1

abnormality, so that only about half of the children may be fully normal. This poses a special problem because such children are commonly placed for adoption, and adoption agencies and potential adoptive parents will want to know how great is the risk of a (so far) undetected but serious recessive disorder. It seems likely that around three-quarters of such disorders will express themselves in the first 6 months of life, so it may be considered reasonable to wait until around this age before finalising an adoption placement. It is also worth actively testing for the more common autosomal recessive disorders such as cystic fibrosis and phenylketonuria.

There is no clear evidence for a significant effect of consanguinity on intelligence in first-cousin or more distantly related marriages.

Occasionally, there may be a need to resolve uncertainty as to whether a child is indeed the offspring of an incestuous mating. In this situation, information can be obtained from the proportion of DNA polymorphisms for which the individual is homozygous.

In summary, consanguinity without known genetic disease in the family appears to cause an increase in mortality and malformation rate which is extremely marked in the children of incestuous matings, but which is of little significance when the relationship is more distant than that of first cousins. First-cousin marriages, the most common counselling problem, seem to have an added risk of about 3%, so that a total risk of 5% for abnormality or death in early childhood, about double the general population risk, is a reasonable, though approximate, guide. Some immigrant groups of Asian origin in the United Kingdom show an unusually high frequency of recessively inherited disorders, some extremely rare. This may well reflect increased consanguinity due to isolation and restriction of marriage partners.

Multiple consanguinity

Individuals may be related to each other in more than one way. This causes difficulty in drawing the pedigree as well as in calculating the precise degree of relationship. The simplest approach is to deal with each mode of relationship separately, work out the coefficient of consanguinity for each, and then add them.

More complex situations may need the help of a colleague expert in population genetics, but this method should be sufficient for most counselling situations. Figure 10.5 gives an example. The couple are first cousins by one set of parents, but also second cousins by the other set. Their coefficient of consanguinity (F) is thus that for first cousins (1/16) plus that for second cousins (1/64), giving a total of 5/64. The risk of a serious recessive disorder, assuming one harmful recessive gene per person, would be about half this, i.e. 5/128 or about 4%.

Alternatively, the route of a harmful gene can be plotted as in Figure 10.5, taking the 'inner loop' (first cousin) first and then the outer (second cousin) loop. The two pathways give risks of 1/32 and 1/128, respectively (each path must be gone over twice for the two common ancestors), giving a combined risk of 5/128, as did the first approach.

Inbred populations

It is possible for a couple to be closely related simply because they are both members of an inbred population which has many of its genes in common. Such populations, particularly when isolated or derived from a small founding population, such as the Amish of North America, are often notable for the rare recessively inherited diseases occurring in them, and for many of them estimates of the coefficient of consanguinity (F) for the population as a whole are available. Even in the most inbred, the level of consanguinity rarely approaches the first-cousin level.

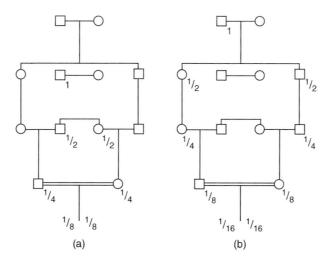

Figure 10.5 Estimation of risks with multiple consanguinity. One harmful recessive allele is assumed for each individual. (a) Risk is $2 \times 1/8 \times 1/8 = 1/32$. (b) Risk is $2 \times 1/16 \times 1/16 = 1/128$. Total risk is $1/32 + 1/128$ (about 4%).

In some cases, the frequency of carriers of a harmful gene in the population may be known, and this may be used in counselling. Thus, for a healthy man whose sister had Tay-Sachs disease, the risk of marrying a carrier would be 1 in 20 if he married someone of Ashkenazi Jewish descent, but only 1 in 400 if he married a non-Jewish person.

In the absence of such information, the risks are similar to those where the partners are known relatives with a particular coefficient of consanguinity. Thus, a couple from the highly inbred Canadian Hutterite community (F = 0.03 or 1/67) would be predicted to have a risk of recessively inherited disorders in the offspring similar to that of second cousins (F = 1/64). Practical proof of these risks is rarely available, however.

Where a known consanguineous marriage occurs in an already inbred population, the two contributions must be added. Thus, the risk of homozygosity by descent (F) for a first-cousin marriage in a traditional Welsh traveller population would be 1/16 (F for a first-cousin marriage) plus 1/50 (F for the whole population), a total of 1/12. The risk for a serious recessive disorder would be half this, i.e. 1/24 (as discussed earlier).

PATERNITY AND RELATIONSHIP TESTING

The uncertainty of paternity is a subject that has always concerned people, more for legal and social reasons than for any connections with genetic disease. Indeed, some societies in the past have not recognised the existence of paternity at all, while only in comparatively recent times has it been accepted that the paternal and maternal contributions to the child are approximately equal. The possibility of non-paternity must always be considered when trying to explain a puzzling pedigree pattern; non-maternity, by contrast, is an exceptionally rare problem – it is seen chiefly when resolving possible cases of the confused identity of infants in maternity hospitals and in instances where a woman claims a kidnapped baby to be her own.

The testing of paternity depends almost entirely on the use of genetic polymorphisms. Clearly, the more polymorphic a system is, the greater the chance of it distinguishing between

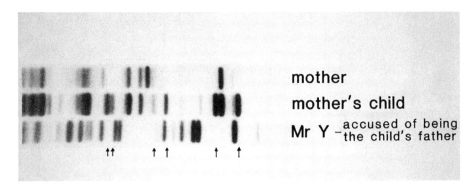

Figure 10.6 Use of the hypervariable mini-satellite DNA approach in paternity testing ('genetic fingerprinting'). The arrows indicate bands present in the child but not in the mother, which should thus be present in the biological father. The putative father can here be seen to lack these and is readily excluded. (Example kindly provided by Professor Alec Jeffreys, University of Leicester.)

two individuals, which is the object of the exercise. This took great steps forward with the technique of 'DNA fingerprinting', resulting from the discovery by Jeffreys and colleagues of hypervariable mini-satellite DNA sequences giving a pattern unique to each individual, apart from identical twins (Figure 10.6). (Other polymorphic systems may also be used, including genome-wide panels of SNPs.)

The difference between individuals results from the existence of a variable number tandem repeat (VNTR) polymorphism, which can detect a considerable number of genetic loci, and which can be thought of as a large number of separate polymorphisms combined into a single test. The end result is a large number (30–40) of distinct bands, half of which come from the father, and half from the mother. Provided that one parent and the child are known, the bands inherited from the other parent can be determined and matched against any proposed candidate for paternity.

This technique is in widespread use for paternity testing (in animals as well as in humans), for immigration procedures involving kinship, and in forensic investigations such as rape and murder cases. The growth of forensic DNA databases has serious potential for abuse, however, particularly if disease-related, behaviour-related or population-related (ancestry) genotypes were to be used. Regulatory bodies need to monitor this area closely.

Modification of the techniques and the development of locus-specific markers have increased stability and reliability, so that this is now an exceptionally powerful and legally acceptable tool for use in a wide variety of medicolegal situations. Nevertheless, it is not infallible, like any technique, and can be misinterpreted and misused. There are important issues of consent involved. The same approach can also be used, though with less certainty, in establishing or excluding less close relationships.

TWINS

Studies of twins have played an important part in human genetics but most of the available data are neither suitable nor relevant to genetic counselling. Only a few of the more important areas are discussed here; some Further Reading is given in Appendix 1. Twinning in relation to prenatal diagnosis is discussed in Chapter 9. Multiple births frequently arise as the result of *in vitro* fertilisation procedures.

Determination of zygosity

Determination of zygosity may be simple; for example, twins of unlike sex must be dizygotic. Triplets and other multiple pregnancies resulting from fertility drugs are likewise usually not monozygotic. In a like-sex twin pair, the most reliable clinical information comes from whether the twins consider themselves identical and are confused by others. This has been shown to correspond closely with detailed genotyping. Reported placentation is not a reliable guide. DNA testing – either 'fingerprinting' or a panel of SNPs – now gives a definitive method of confirming zygosity.

Risks of monozygotic twin pairs

For a fully penetrant Mendelian disease, there should be complete concordance – both twins should either have or not have the disorder. There is often remarkable similarity in clinical features and age at onset.

For dominantly inherited disorders, an affected pair of monozygotic (MZ) twins with normal parents is compatible with a new mutation (unlike dizygotic twins), and there is no increased risk of the disease in subsequent children of the normal parents, so it is important to confirm that the twins are indeed monozygous.

For X-linked disorders in female MZ twins, there is a suggestion that the carrier state is more likely to manifest – to cause signs of disease – in at least one of the twins than is usual in carriers who are singletons.

For non-Mendelian disorders, the risk to a co-twin will vary with the degree of genetic causation of the disease, being very high where genetic factors are predominant (as seen also in normal facial features and dermatoglyphics).

Risks of dizygotic twin pairs

Since dizygotic twins are genetically no more alike than sibs, risks for Mendelian disorders are essentially the same as for sibs. For non-Mendelian conditions, the shared intrauterine (and to some extent postnatal) environment gives a somewhat higher risk than that seen in sibs, but few accurate figures are available. In some instances, concordance may be less than expected. For example, in neural tube defects, affected co-twins are exceptional, and it is possible that such pregnancies are lost, a point of relevance when one twin is found to be abnormal in prenatal diagnosis.

Twinning in families

Monozygotic twins are rarely familial and have a rather constant incidence of around 4 in 1,000 pregnancies. Dizygotic twinning, by contrast, shows marked geographical variation and is frequently around 6 in 1,000 in European and white American populations, but it occurs in about 1% of pregnancies in American blacks, and up to 4% of pregnancies in parts of Nigeria. The recurrence risk for dizygotic twins is about 1.7% for Europeans.

Malformations in twins

Monozygotic (but not dizygotic) twins have an increased overall malformation rate of around 5%, twice that for a singleton pregnancy, a fact of considerably greater importance in genetic counselling than the twinning itself. The increase is for a variety of structural malformations, including neural tube defects and congenital heart disease.

Conjoined twins

The phenomenon of conjoined twins can be regarded as an extreme example of monozygotic twinning and is most unlikely to recur in a family. Ultrasonography should now give early warning of the problem. A partially developed co-twin may cause confusion on ultrasound scan.

Twin risks in common disorders

Twins have played an important role in determining the relative importance of heredity and environment in common non-Mendelian disorders. The critical point is not the absolute concordance in twins but the difference between monozygotic and dizygotic twin concordance rates. Unaffected monozygotic co-twins are of special importance; thus, the demonstration that the increased risk of schizophrenia in the children of the unaffected co-twins is similar to that in the children of the affected monozygotic twins provides strong evidence for a primary genetic basis of the disorder. (But note that concordant MZ twins may arise from an effectively Mendelian new mutation of high penetrance. If this is not recognised, it may inflate the apparent heredity of a disorder of usually complex causation).

Estimates for the risk of monozygotic co-twins are available for a number of common disorders and are mentioned in the relevant chapters; however, it is not always certain that these data are representative.

A final point of caution concerning monozygotic twins relates to DNA testing. Should such a twin request presymptomatic testing (e.g. for Huntington's disease), the result would automatically apply also to the co-twin. Obviously, testing in such a situation needs handling with the greatest care.

LEGAL PROBLEMS IN MEDICAL GENETICS

Few areas of medical practice can avoid serious consideration of the legal aspects; medical genetics, involving many controversial and relatively new situations, might be expected to be especially vulnerable. Yet it is surprising (in the United Kingdom anyway) how rarely serious medicolegal problems do arise. The author suspects that this probably speaks more for the tolerance and goodwill of our patients than for the skills of the medical profession. The fact that in medical genetics we spend a great deal of time with our patients is also relevant, as is the practice of providing families with a written letter to summarise our consultations and the results of any tests.

There are some areas that are bound to be difficult in legal terms, especially relating to reproductive technologies such as artificial insemination and IVF (discussed in Chapter 11), the identification of relatively mild disorders such as the sex chromosome aneuploidies in pregnancy, and the demand for fetal sexing for non-medical reasons. However, these are not the issues likely to involve the clinician with the law: the main problem is that of 'negligence', as in other areas of medical practice.

Negligence in this respect is not likely to mean giving an imprecise recurrence risk in genetic counselling, but rather giving no information at all when it could have been given, by a colleague if not by oneself. Thus, the obstetrician or other clinician who fails to give genetic counselling, or to inform the patient that particular tests are available, is indeed likely to be held negligent if this is felt to fall short of what might reasonably be expected from a person in that position, while a specialist in medical genetics might be expected to have provided information of greater detail and accuracy. The laboratory is more likely to face problems from misidentification of samples than from the misinterpretation of results, though both are important. It is important to note that a screening test, with a significant false-positive and false-negative rate, may be regarded by the family as a definitive test, unless this is carefully explained.

In the United States, the situation is probably not radically different from Europe, although the climate is much more litigious.

Among the broader legal issues that need consideration, most link closely with the social and ethical problems discussed in the final section of this book. Few are unique to genetics, but genetic situations often highlight them or bring them up in a new form.

We have already discussed some aspects of maintaining confidentiality within the family and also refer to this question later. Here, we turn to address the broad topic of consent.

Consent

This is probably the most important general issue. It arises when genetic testing is being undertaken, especially in the case of children and others unable to consent fully, in the scope and nature of research studies on genetic disorders, the long-term storage of samples, and in the use and transfer of laboratory or clinical information for third parties, such as insurance companies or employers. Different standards of consent may apply in different contexts: a superior quality of understanding and consent may be expected for participation in some research studies than in diagnostic testing of direct benefit to the individual. One would not want their difficulty in grasping some specific details to prevent a patient benefiting from a thoroughly appropriate healthcare intervention.

Since genetic information is often relevant and necessary for family members, particular issues arise as to how far consent is necessary to share information within the context of genetic counselling for family members. This has been addressed briefly at the beginning of this chapter. This and related areas raise both ethical and legal issues. In general, there is little legal precedent, so that it is unlikely that a person following ethical guidelines and accepted standards of good practice will be exposed to unexpected legal challenges. However, episodes arising outside medical genetics in which good practice has not been followed have resulted in a sharp change of attitudes, making it essential that practice in all areas involving consent be clarified.

This area of potential dispute – the tension between respect for the privacy of sensitive information about a patient (their right to confidentiality) and the need for family members to be given important and relevant information – is attracting more attention, internationally, than in the past. For example, there is the ongoing ABC legal case in England which might lead to serious changes in professional practice. In England and Wales, a professional failure to pass important information of therapeutic relevance to the appropriate relatives would most likely be treated as potentially a question of negligence. A second example is the recent legislation in France that requires patients to pass information to their relatives if it is important and relevant to them. However, professionals may be required to transmit information without the patient's consent if the patient refuses to do so. There is helpful guidance from the UK's General Medical Council about when it may be permissible to breach patient confidentiality, and how a practitioner should set about preparing to do this if he or she believes it to be necessary.

Finally, it is most important to remember the contrast between family-based genetic testing and population screening for genetic disorders of one sort or another. Most of our patients in clinical genetics services are being seen in relation to their pre-existing concern over a specific family or personal history of a genetic disorder. In population screening, there may be no pre-existing concern, and it is we health professionals who generate concern through raising the spectre of a possible genetic condition. It is therefore incumbent upon us to ensure that those who are caught up in a screening programme, perhaps with a positive screening test result, have high-quality information and decision support if they need to decide whether to proceed with further investigations.

11

Clinical genetics services

INTRODUCTION

A primary aim of this book from its beginning nearly 40 years ago has been to encourage clinicians to regard genetic counselling as an integral part of the management of patients and their families, and to dispel the view that all genetic problems must of necessity be referred to a specialist clinic. Nevertheless, the organisational aspects of genetic counselling require careful consideration, whoever is doing it, and the following notes are intended to cover some of the practical aspects needing close attention if a satisfactory and efficient service is to be provided for patients.

Adequate time is essential if genetic counselling is to be at all worthwhile, and it may be argued that the main advantage of a patient or family being seen in a specialist genetic clinic is the greater amount of time that a medical geneticist or non-medical genetic counsellor is likely to be able to devote to the problem, compared with a busy clinician. All too often patients complain not that their doctor advised them incorrectly, but that he or she was too busy to answer their questions adequately or even to appreciate the problem that existed for them.

Clearly the first duty of any professional interested in a patient's genetic problems is to ensure that this time is provided. The author finds an hour to be the usual time required to establish what are the main issues, take full pedigree details, undertake examination of the patient and discuss the genetic risks and possible measures of support. A follow-up visit is frequently required to interpret the results of investigations or records that have been obtained on relatives, and half an hour is usually allowed for this. Investigation of an extended family may take considerably longer, and it is wise to attempt this in stages. The arrival of a complete kindred of people can create consternation in a clinic, while the conflicting views of several branches of a family are also best dealt with separately.

THE SETTING

The necessity of adequate time usually means that a specific session is best set aside for genetic counselling, whether this be in a medical genetics centre, a family doctor's office or surgery, or in a hospital clinician's outpatient department. Whatever the precise location, several needs must be borne in mind.

Quiet and freedom from disturbance are essential. The design of many hospital outpatient departments makes this almost impossible, while the rumpus associated with most children's clinics is also a distraction. The absence of a telephone is an advantage (they can usually be unplugged or switched off), and the coming and going of well-meaning nurses or other clinical staff must be discouraged. The author, until he was fortunate enough to have his own genetic counselling area, found it necessary to place a sign on the door, reading 'Genetic Counselling: Do Not Disturb'.

The number of people present must be small if patients are not to be inhibited in discussing personal details – usually not more than one medical colleague and a genetic counsellor or co-worker. A single student could perhaps be added, but pressure to accommodate large student or postgraduate groups should be resisted. One-way screens are sometimes advocated to avoid this problem, but the author dislikes them.

If the clinic is held in a paediatric setting, there must be facilities for examining adults as well. The unexpected emergence of a large, undressed adult in the midst of a paediatric clinic may cause anxiety. Legal requirements now exist in the United Kingdom regarding clinical facilities for children.

EQUIPMENT

Very little equipment is needed. It is a pleasure in these days of expensive technology and centralisation to be able to provide a high-class service to people in relatively remote areas without the need for cumbersome equipment or excessive cost to the community (or to the patient). A full set of examination equipment is essential, for many patients sent for counselling will prove to be really in need of diagnosis. Facilities for taking blood and for radiography (especially skeletal X-rays) are essential, as is a good camera or access to a medical illustration department. Blood samples for most laboratory tests, including genetic investigations as well as biochemical and haematological tests, can be taken at a distance if necessary, and brought back or even mailed to the central laboratory for analysis.

PEDIGREES AND RECORDS

The number of families seen increases with a remarkable rapidity, and unless a clear and simple system is decided on from the outset, the clinician will soon be unable to find relevant information. The keeping of systematic records is also the basis for much of the research on inherited disorders, and should allow for follow-up and long-term preventive measures, where appropriate.

A clear and detailed pedigree is the foundation of good genetic counselling, and a simple lined sheet is useful to keep it neat and orderly. The temptation to construct a rough pedigree for later improvement should be resisted – time and energy are rarely enough for this to happen and with practice a clear pedigree can be produced quickly using the method and symbols described in Chapter 1. Relevant information can be recorded at the foot of the page using letters to identify the particular individuals. Figure 1.2 shows typical examples on the original author's pedigree chart.

Other medical details will also need recording in the patient's hospital notes, and in the author's clinic the policy is to write a brief summary of the more detailed record that is kept separately in the genetics family file and to place a copy of the subsequent correspondence. This is our usual practice unless it contains details that might adversely affect other individuals. A copy of all notes and letters, along with the pedigree, is kept in the medical genetics department, where it is immediately available for consultation, in contrast to the main hospital case-record, which may be in use elsewhere or missing. These practices will of course need to change once our institution introduces electronic medical records.

An easily workable index system is vital, especially in regions like Wales where many unrelated people share the same few surnames. It can be embarrassing to discover that the Mrs Davies whom one thought had a child with Duchenne muscular dystrophy is, in fact, a different Mrs Davies who is at risk for Huntington's disease. Computerised systems are now almost universal in medical genetics clinics and other medical record systems for indexing and organising records and appointments, even where the clinical notes themselves exist only on paper. Some of these systems allow integration of clinical genetics records with molecular and cytogenetic laboratory information. A clear diagnostic index system is also essential. In addition, registers exist in some clinics for specific disorders.

STRUCTURE OF THE MEDICAL GENETICS SERVICE

Much genetic counselling, especially for common disorders, will be provided by clinicians who are not specialists in medical genetics. There will always be patients who require a specialist referral, however, and at present the awareness of genetic problems and consequent need for genetic counselling is still growing faster than the ability of general clinicians to provide it. Many countries, including the United Kingdom, have evolved a system of regional genetic counselling centres to provide a specialist service and, since resources are limited and potential demand very large, it is important to consider how these are best utilised by doctors and other referring personnel.

In the United Kingdom, there is a genetic counselling and clinical genetics centres in every healthcare region, usually based in the medical teaching centre of the region concerned and commonly staffed by, or closely associated with, an academic medical genetics unit. There is usually a close link with the genetics and other laboratory services. There used to be a sharp distinction between molecular genetics and cytogenetics laboratories and their staff and their training programmes. Both the science and the techniques and technology have moved on, however, so that there would be no purpose in maintaining this distinction. It will be important to ensure that a karyotype can still be examined and interpreted, at least until whole genome sequencing replaces even the occasional use of the karyotype in patients or families with translocations, inversions or more complex rearrangements. For the most part, however, genome-based technologies provide the most effective ways to locate and identify a pathology while the choice of method to confirm this and then to track the pathology in other members of the family can be decided by what is likely to be the cheapest and most convenient in the circumstances.

Hospital regions in Britain commonly serve a population of two to five million people and vary greatly in their geography. The service of the author and his colleagues covers Wales, a country that functions as equivalent in size to a single region within the UK National Health Service (NHS), with a population of three million and a maximum distance of 300 kilometres from the teaching centre. Here, as in some other parts of the United Kingdom, a series of regular district-based clinics has been established to serve more distant parts of the region, which are serviced from the main unit in the medical teaching centre, originally on a 'hub and spoke' basis, but now with two sub-centres. In addition to this service, a number of specialist clinics have been set up in the main centre, often jointly with relevant clinicians, to deal with particular problems such as Marfan syndrome, neuromuscular disease and Rett syndrome, often combining diagnostic and genetic aspects of the condition with disease management.

Genetic counselling services in the United Kingdom have evolved historically within the framework of the NHS and thus differ in many ways from the pattern seen in much of continental Europe and the United States. It may well prove to be one of the major and lasting achievements of the NHS that the development of medical genetics has been able to take place relatively painlessly inside the service, without the necessity for charging fees to patients or relatives. This applies equally to the provision of clinical, laboratory and prenatal diagnostic services. Whether the existing structure of the services will prove adequate to cope with the widening scope of genetics within medicine and the increasing demand placed on our clinical services remains to be seen. It will depend partly on how clinical geneticists, genetic counsellors and clinicians in hospital practice and primary care can jointly develop appropriate and mutually supportive roles in providing genetics services, as well as on whether the government is prepared to provide adequate funding.

The pressure from an earlier administration in the United Kingdom to commercialise public services and to disband or fragment regional services and healthcare planning mechanisms seriously harmed the development of medical genetics services and similar problems have occurred in other countries. Since then, the UK central government has recognised the potential importance of genetics and chosen to make investments in the provision of genomic laboratories by imposing a top-down model of change. In the context of a decade of austerity, with most medical services struggling to cope, this has created many difficulties as well as presenting positive opportunities. The emphasis on investment in genomic laboratories has been accompanied by the neglect of the clinical services required to support the implementation of widespread genome-based diagnostics. The mainstreaming of genetics services is an important goal but requires strong clinical genetics services if other specialties are to be able to respond to the opportunities without a slow reinvention of the wheel through repeating the mistakes of the past.

Most clinical genetics services around the world are led by medically qualified staff with specialist training in genetics. Many countries, including the United Kingdom, many other countries in the European Union, the United States, Canada and Australia, have a carefully structured and monitored programme of training and accreditation for those specialising in the field. The rapid development of such allied areas as prenatal diagnosis, screening and early therapy, together with the delineation of numerous clinically recognisable syndromes, has added to the importance of a medical training, even though much of the underlying research responsible for these advances has been made by non-medical scientists.

The author believes strongly that clinical genetic assessments need to be undertaken by people who are medically trained, and that those who undertake these assessments should be able to integrate this with the associated genetic counselling. In other words, clinical geneticists should be capable genetic counsellors too. Indeed, it is often quite impossible to separate the actual 'counselling' from the associated aspects of clinical diagnosis. On numerous occasions, what is referred to as an apparently straightforward problem of risk estimation and counselling produces a completely unexpected diagnostic problem, which a non-medical person would not only be unable to solve but might well fail to recognise. Thus, in planning for the future, the author is in no doubt that training in both medicine and genetics is desirable for those intending to devote all or much of their time to the clinical aspects of genetic disease. It may be argued that to train such individuals is expensive; this is true, but it is preferable to have a relatively small number of well-trained people and for them to be used selectively. This view returns to one of the underlying themes of this book, that most discussion with patients and families affected by genetic disorders about their condition is, and will continue to be, performed by regular clinicians (not specialists in medical genetics) as a part of the overall management of patients under their care, while the medical geneticist is principally involved in those families where the situation is less simple, and in educating clinical colleagues.

Alongside the medical doctors trained in clinical geneticists, we also need a body of well-trained genetic counsellors. Any well-developed clinical genetics service needs to rely heavily on members of its team who are non-medical, and this trend is increasing. Provided that training of such staff is thorough, that their remit is clear and that links and support within the team are satisfactory, this mixed structure of a clinical genetics service should add to its quality and effectiveness, as has been the experience in many other fields of medicine. Indeed, many referrals to clinical genetics services can be handled most effectively by genetic counsellors without the direct involvement of a medically trained clinical geneticist as long as access to a clinical geneticist for discussion is readily available, should questions arise. It has been interesting to see how these changes have evolved over the past three decades or more and that, in the United Kingdom at least, this has occurred harmoniously and (usually) with mutual respect between those involved.

At present, non-medical co-workers in genetic counselling tend to follow two main streams. The first, most common in America, is the 'genetic counsellor' model, with extensive graduate training in basic genetics and in the psychological and social aspects of living with genetic disease and genetic risk. This stream has grown substantially in the United Kingdom too, with two established graduate programmes operating that have both changed from face-to-face programmes into distance-learning programmes that will further expand capacity. In the second approach, the 'genetics nurse specialist', the training in genetics and genetic counselling follows a more general nursing background. In both cases there are important roles that can complement that of the medically trained clinical geneticist. In the United Kingdom there has been rapid development of specific training programmes, career structures and professional bodies, which have united both models. In some parts of continental Europe, the genetic counsellor model has developed, while by contrast, in other areas, especially in the German-speaking countries, a medical qualification remains essential for recognition as an independent professional.

GENETIC COUNSELLING: INITIAL ASSESSMENT AND BEYOND

When a patient is referred to the Medical Genetics service, the referral has to be logged and then allocated to a member of staff for their attention. In our practice, most referrals will be allocated to a genetic counsellor who then speaks with the patient (or their parents). This may be by phone, in the genetic counsellor's clinic or in the family's home (at a home visit).

The purpose of this initial contact is to enable the flow of information in two directions. The genetic counsellor wants to gather background information about the patient and their family, their understanding of the referral and their expectations. They also wish to impart information to the patient (or their parents) about the genetics service and what it can offer. While the genetic counsellor takes down information about the family tree, they will also be alert to the social aspects of relationships within the family (who is, or is not, talking to whom?) and to the family's underlying hopes, fears and expectations. This is invaluable in shaping the service that can be provided to the family. It is unrealistic to expect many families to have a clear idea as to what they want from the service in advance, as genetics services are still so unfamiliar to most people. They hear about genetics as the science of the marvellous but have little idea about what a medical genetics service might do for them. Genetics receives a lot of attention in the media and expectations can be unrealistically high. Patients might hope for gene therapies to cure a fatal disease, or parents might hope for their child's chromosome disorder to be 'corrected'. Equally, those referred may be puzzled or put off by the term 'genetic counselling', thinking that they do not need 'to be counselled'. It is therefore immensely useful for the genetic counsellor to provide information to the patient or parents about what a referral entails and what it is (and is not) feasible for the service to provide or achieve. This allows the patient or family to (re)set their expectations in a more realistic frame.

While some referrals have a very specific focus and do not raise deeply emotional issues, there are others where the referral does touch on something deep. This initial contact with the genetic counsellor often sets the emotional register for the referral, and it is important that these emotional aspects are not closed down by a hurried professional manner or by the interactional distance of a telephone call, when a more relaxed meeting, face-to-face, could have allowed them to surface. It would be ideal if we could conduct the initial contact sessions through home visits, as often used to happen in Wales and many other parts of the United Kingdom. Such home visits give the best chance of developing a rapport between the patient and the genetic counsellor and make it more likely that the family members present will feel able to speak their mind openly. A home visit will usually dispel any fears or misunderstandings the family has and will often also identify sensitive issues that might have been difficult to raise for the first time in a hospital setting or that might have resulted in non-attendance. Likewise, such a visit may uncover the family's true needs and concerns, which may not be those stated in the referral letter.

As there has been a continuous increase in the numbers of referrals over the last two decades without a corresponding increase in staffing, home visits have become very infrequent and often need specific approval. This is an aspect of the quality of the service, and its accessibility to families in poverty or with complex needs, that has (most unfortunately) failed to keep pace with developments in the science of genetics.

One valuable role of a home visit (though this can also often be achieved by an unhurried phone call) is to determine which medical records or family details are needed before a clinic appointment is scheduled. Advance preparation of this kind can avoid much wasted time subsequently. Construction of a pedigree is often also done at this time, although it is then important to ensure that the genetic counsellor who does this is part of the ongoing clinical process. So much informal knowledge of the family can be gathered in this way, and the relationship between the family and the service can develop so effectively during this process, that much may be lost by breaking the continuity of the relationship between the family and the genetic counsellor. Taking the family details gives a valuable opportunity to 'break the ice' and form a relationship with a family being seen for the first time. Much can be learned about their fears and worries, their general attitude to the disorder in the family, how well they are likely to understand risk figures, and whether there are disagreements and tensions within the family. The family's adjustment to the genetic disorder in question may be gauged along with their overall ability to cope. Liaison with other local services may be helpful if a family is seen to be struggling with complex disabilities, financial worries or other problems. On several occasions, it has become clear during this preliminary process that someone coming primarily for counselling is affected by the disorder. Huntington's disease is an example of such a condition, where a period of quiet observation during history-taking may give much more information than a formal examination.

Non-medical staff have further valuable roles to play in the genetic counselling clinic. A trained genetics nurse or counsellor, involved with the family from the point of first referral, will often be able to detect problems that family members have not spoken about, and ensure that they have actually understood what the person providing the information thinks they have; the two often prove surprisingly different. In a tense discussion, with difficult scenarios being considered, it can be most helpful to have two genetics professionals in the room. Such co-counselling, often best provided by a complementary pairing of one medical and one non-medical genetic counsellor, should not be seen as a luxury but may be key to meeting the needs of the family. In many instances, practical support may also need to be arranged; this may prove as valuable as the genetic counselling itself.

The help of such non-medical genetic counsellors is also invaluable in contacting the extended family at home, arranging samples or taking consent from relatives, and obtaining additional information left incomplete at the time of a clinic visit. It is difficult to provide more than a very limited genetic counselling service without the availability of such non-medical personnel, and the authors have been fortunate in having many excellent such colleagues working with them over the years.

Following the initial assessment, whether or not that has occurred at a home visit, the responsible genetic counsellor will need to decide what further contact would be most appropriate for the family. Should this be a diagnostic assessment with a medically qualified colleague? Or another appointment with the genetic counsellor? How does this relate to any question of genetic testing?

It must be remembered that, sometimes, no further contact is needed, especially if the family's questions are straightforward and have already been answered or if the family had no questions but were feeling 'sent' to genetics by another professional. Or perhaps the referral can be managed without another appointment by the interpretation of family history risk information. This may be concluded by a team discussion and then a letter to the family. If the risk level is low or moderate, this may be all that is required, with perhaps the offer of additional contact if future events suggest that a risk reassessment would be appropriate (e.g. if another family member develops a relevant health problem).

It may also be helpful to reiterate here that some referrals may be best handled by a joint approach in liaison with another specialty. This has certainly been the case in relation to inherited cardiac disorders, where multidisciplinary team meetings can discuss referrals and make decisions about the most appropriate route for clinical assessment and also about the most appropriate strategy for genetic testing in the particular circumstances of the family as a whole (e.g. to which member[s] of the family would it be most helpful to offer what type of genetic investigation?).

COUNSELLING AFTER STILLBIRTH AND TERMINATION OF PREGNANCY

The need for parental support and for the natural process of grieving to occur after neonatal death or stillbirth is well recognised, although all too often still ignored by doctors. The need is perhaps particularly great after a malformed infant has been born, and insensitive or inadequate management at this stage can seriously affect the parents' attitude to subsequent pregnancies and to genetic counselling. Frequently, a mother may not have seen her baby and may have exaggerated ideas about the abnormalities; paediatricians now feel that she should see and hold the baby in most circumstances and be offered photographs.

With the increasing use of prenatal diagnosis and termination for genetic disorders, it is becoming clear that parents need corresponding help in dealing with the combination of grief and guilt that is inevitable in this situation. The best way to achieve this will vary from family to family, but a sensitive counsellor, not necessarily a genetic counsellor, will probably be able to help most couples to express and to come to terms with their feelings. It seems likely that this more open approach is preferable to attempting to minimise the entire episode. In the past, this activity has often been left to staff of a medical genetics unit because no-one else recognised the need. Fortunately, obstetric departments are increasingly prepared to take on this role themselves, which is appropriate unless there are specifically genetic aspects involved.

INFORMATION SOURCES: GENETICS AND THE INTERNET

The revolution in information technology has been both a blessing and a problem for the field of genetic counselling. Professionals in medical genetics were among the earliest to develop and use computerised databases, not just in terms of genetic registers (see later in this chapter) but also such information resources as OMIM (the online version of McKusick's Mendelian Inheritance in Man), syndrome databases used in dysmorphology (such as the Winter-Baraitser Dysmorphology Database and POSSUM, see Appendix 1) and computer-based pedigree drawing and risk estimation programmes. Most of these are interactive in nature and are thus of most value to those who are already broadly familiar with the field and have a clear idea as to what information they want.

A further category of useful information for professionals is represented by a rapidly increasing number of databases on the internet, including data on human disease mutations, both general and locus-specific; databases of population genetic variation; directories of laboratory genetic services (e.g. European Directory of Genetics Laboratories); and more general information about genes and genetic disease (e.g. OMIM, GeneReviews). These systems are especially valuable for small or isolated units and those in less-developed countries. In theory, they should make books like this redundant. They can also create a problem of having too much information; digesting and assessing it can be as much work now as obtaining it was in the past. Appendix 1 provides a list of helpful internet-based and other electronic information resources.

The greatest change in the past few years has been in the amount of information available directly to patients and families. There have always been determined individuals who have consulted textbooks and founded lay societies. Now many of these societies publish valuable information for both families and professionals, while most also have websites, allowing direct access by those affected and at risk, or those who are merely interested. More informal groups of patients and others are also developing and can form a valuable link for those who do not wish to become involved personally with specific genetic disease societies.

This rapid development, while undoubtedly beneficial on the whole, can have its drawbacks, apart from the embarrassment of the professional faced with a sheaf of internet information when first meeting a new family. Some of the information encountered may be inappropriate or distressing; for example, a couple searching for information because of a relatively distant history of neural tube defects were immediately confronted with a colour photograph of an anencephalic fetus. Others may be confused or misled by detailed information that would have been better presented as part of a professional consultation. The international nature of the internet, while extremely helpful for those living or working in remote areas or less-developed countries, can often mean that recommendations cannot be implemented or may be unsuitable. Finally, it must be remembered that there is no data privacy on the internet; professionals and patients alike should avoid giving identifying details of other family members, while no computer with internet access should be used for storing confidential patient-related information unless there is an effective firewall.

Whatever one's views, though, those involved in genetic counselling, whether as specialists in medical genetics or in their own disease field, now have to adapt to dealing with a far more informed and articulate clientele than used to be the case.

BACKUP TO GENETIC COUNSELLING

Genetic counselling does not take place in a vacuum. The topics of carrier detection and prenatal diagnosis have already been discussed, but there are a number of other practical aspects that arise in connection with genetic counselling, and these are dealt with here.

Contraception

Ready access to a family planning clinic is essential for any clinician involved in genetic counselling, and it is always wise to enquire tactfully about contraception at an early stage, particularly if the results of investigations are going to take some weeks or months before definitive counselling can be given. It is surprising how often couples aware of the genetic risk and not intending to have children nevertheless take no active measures to prevent pregnancy. We have more than once had the unhappy experience of seeing such a couple on a follow-up visit, to inform them of a high risk of a serious disorder, only to find that the woman had become pregnant in the meantime. Such an event may not always be as accidental as it seems. Although some religious bodies still restrict or prohibit contraception, many of their adherents decide differently, so it is a topic that should not be avoided just because of the family's religious affiliation.

Sterilisation

Sterilisation is often preferable to long-term contraception where a couple has made a definite decision not to have more children. This may apply even to young couples. Before sterilisation is undertaken, however, careful consideration must be given to the following points:

- What is the precise genetic risk to offspring? It is not uncommon for sterilisation to be requested 'on genetic grounds' when the risks of transmitting a disorder are minimal (e.g. sibs of a patient with an autosomal recessive disorder).
- Is there an alternative, such as carrier detection or prenatal diagnosis, that could reduce or avoid the risk?
- Is it likely that advances in knowledge will change the situation in the next few years?
- Do the couple really agree that sterilisation is the best course, and which partner should undergo it?

In general, it is logical to sterilise the affected or at-risk individual in the case of a dominant disease; for autosomal recessive disorders there is no genetic preference. Many couples choose vasectomy on the grounds of simplicity and lower risk. In some instances, the unaffected member of a couple insists on being sterilised; the motivation in such circumstances can be complex. In the case of a fatal disorder, the possibility that the healthy spouse may remarry and wish to have children must be faced. Divorce and remarriage, frequent in many communities, are also relevant for recessive disorders where the genetic risks in a new marriage will often be very low.

Sterilisation of the mentally handicapped patient is a difficult and emotive issue. Genetic risks to offspring are often confused with more general questions concerning whether a child could be safely and satisfactorily reared by parents with physical and/or cognitive impairments. While individuals with disability can be supported to have close, personal relationships, the interests of any child they have will need to be considered and protected. This may entail providing support for the disabled individual in their role as parent. It may also entail discussing the question of sterilisation with them and their partner, parents, carers, and/or advocate. Sterilisation may be a reasonable course, all things considered, if the individual would be unable to take on parental responsibility because of their cognitive impairment, the chance of a child being affected is high and the risk of pregnancy is considerable. However, raising a topic for discussion is far from suggesting it should be compulsory or even that it would be the preferred course of action. Furthermore, this question – of how a couple would cope with pregnancy and with rearing an infant who will become a child – is often raised by the couple themselves or by their close relatives, who may be eager to support them but be anxious about practicalities.

In addition, it must not be forgotten that the disabled adult may need protection from sexual exploitation and sexually transmitted disease, while their right to seek intimacy in relationships is maintained. As with most ethical problems, the right course will often be clear, provided that each case is considered on its own merits and the situation is not allowed to degenerate into general polemics. Often the biggest obstacle to a satisfactory resolution of a problem is the failure to raise it for discussion at all, or the failure to raise it in a supportive and non-judgemental manner.

GAMETE DONATION AND *IN VITRO* FERTILISATION

This is now technically possible for either sperm or egg, although the latter requires the use of *in vitro* fertilisation (see the next section). Sperm donation (artificial insemination by donor [AID]) is simpler. The main genetic indications are as follows:

- Autosomal dominant disorders where one partner is affected or at risk of becoming so (e.g. Huntington's disease).
- Rare autosomal recessive disorders, in particular where prenatal diagnosis is not feasible or termination of pregnancy is not acceptable to the couple. Here a mutated gene must be contributed by each parent, and an unrelated donor is most unlikely to carry the same mutation.

One should not lose sight of the fact that there may also be implications for the donor. If a child is born with a recessively inherited disorder, this will imply that the donor is a gene carrier, while if donor screening tests are undertaken for such common recessive disorders as cystic fibrosis, there will be comparable implications. It is not always clear what information is given on such aspects to donors in advance, nor what support is provided if such a result is obtained.

In vitro fertilisation

In vitro fertilisation (IVF) is now well established as an option for some forms of infertility. It offers the prospect of using an ovum from an unrelated donor to avoid serious autosomal dominant disorders in the female line and X-linked recessive conditions such as Duchenne muscular dystrophy. Because (in contrast to AID) potential ovum donors may be sisters or other relatives, great care will be needed to avoid using individuals who might be gene carriers. It is perhaps surprising that this approach has not been more frequently used by couples with a genetic problem. This may reflect the increasing feasibility and acceptability of first-trimester prenatal diagnosis, as well as the expense, uncertainty and low success rate, that still limit IVF. The topic of pre-implantation genetic diagnosis is discussed in Chapter 9.

ADOPTION

The question of adoption in relation to genetic counselling arises in two main situations:

- Adoption is being considered as one of the options open to a couple at risk of transmitting a genetic disorder.
- A child being placed for adoption has a family history of a genetic disorder and the adoption agency wishes to know how great the risk is before finalising the placement.

In the past it was possible to recommend adoption as a possible course of action for couples not wishing to take the risk of having a natural child with a genetic disorder. With increasing use of abortion for social indications and with most single mothers retaining their children, the number of available children is now small, and couples with a family history of genetic disease will find themselves competing with many healthy but infertile couples for a few children. In these circumstances, couples are often discouraged even from considering adoption, but the author feels that this is wrong and that, if a couple want to adopt, they should attempt to do so. They should realise that considerable determination is needed, since a large amount of 'red tape' and bureaucratic inertia may be encountered that will discourage the faint-hearted. The following advice may help:

- Apply early, since a long wait may be inevitable.
- If one agency states that their list is closed try others, in another region if necessary. There may not be good communication between agencies and areas.
- Be prepared to be inspected and questioned, and to fill out a large number of forms.
- If barriers of religion are raised, work through a local authority or other non-denominational agency.
- Be persistent (without being aggressive) if delays occur.
- Consider the adoption of an older child, or one for whom some other reason has made adoption difficult.

One group of people who may have particular difficulty in adopting are those where one partner is at high risk of actually developing a serious genetic disorder, such as Huntington's disease. Here a decision must be made in each case based on a careful evaluation of the size of the risk, the chance that the disease will develop while the child is being brought up, and the nature of the disorder. For a condition with such serious consequences as Huntington's disease, few adoption agencies will feel able to accept a couple at high risk, except perhaps for placing an older child who would be likely to be grown up in the event of the disorder developing in the adoptive parent.

Adoption and the child at risk

Advice is commonly sought from adoption agencies when a child to be placed for adoption has a family history of a serious disorder. Sadly, this advice is rarely sought before the birth of the child, with the result that unnecessary delay may occur, with resulting uncertainty and harm to the infant, natural mother and adoptive parents. The estimation of risks is no different from that in other genetic counselling situations, although unavailability of (or uncertainty about) the father may cause difficulty. A more difficult problem is where the child results from an incestuous mating (see Chapter 10), where the risks are high for a variety of recessively inherited disorders, not all of which are detectable in infancy. In this situation it may be wise to defer placement for a few months until the major part of the risk can be excluded.

Perhaps the most frequent genetic counselling circumstances to arise in relation to adoption is for a child with developmental difficulties, who is being assessed diagnostically by a paediatrician or clinical geneticist, to be taken into care as a looked-after child and for adoption to be considered. Chromosome studies (usually a chromosomal microarray, CMA) will have been requested and, all too often, a copy number variant (CNV) of uncertain significance or a neurosusceptibility CNV of uncertain penetrance will have been found. This introduces uncertainty into the prognosis for the child. Prospective adopters will often be willing to adopt a child with developmental difficulties, and the CMA result may shed no extra light on this but, nevertheless, it is often experienced as unsettling. Experience suggests that a child, where this additional sense of uncertainty has been introduced, is less likely to be adopted.

The author emphasises to the social workers and community paediatricians involved that he is willing to meet the prospective adoptive parents in such situations, as that can be helpful to put the chromosome results in context. Colleagues have carried out educational liaison for the adoption teams in Wales – for the social workers as well as the paediatricians – to help them understand the relevance of family history information and genetic investigations in the adoption process. This has been welcomed and has proved most helpful.

Where a high risk of a late-onset disorder does exist, many infants are excluded from adoption. This is unfortunate because, from the child's viewpoint, a family would be likely to deal with problems that arise better than an institution would. It is also often overlooked that there are many highly motivated couples who are prepared to adopt or foster children with even very severe disabilities, provided they are fully in the picture as to what they are taking on; Down syndrome is a good example. Very few children should be considered 'unsuitable for adoption'.

The development of presymptomatic tests for late-onset genetic disorders has led to occasional requests for children being placed for adoption to be tested (e.g. for Huntington's disease). This raises serious ethical issues (see Chapter 35), and it seems unjustified to undertake such testing unless there are clear medical reasons for doing so in childhood.

GENETIC REGISTERS

The keeping of accurate and complete records is an essential (although often neglected) part of all branches of clinical medicine, but the long-term and preventive nature of medical genetics makes this an especially important aspect. Much of the information given in genetic counselling may only be fully used many years later. The sister of a boy with Duchenne muscular dystrophy or the child of a patient with familial polyposis coli may have been too young to be given any information at the time of the initial family study; unless careful records are kept, investigations may have to be repeated. Likewise, it is of great help to know that a person with vague neurological symptoms and a family history of possible Huntington's disease is in fact a member of a kindred in which the diagnosis has been fully established.

A genetic register is something more than an accurate records system. The term 'register' implies that the approach is systematic and at least aiming at completeness, and that the information is actively maintained and updated. Genetic registers may be of several types and vary in complexity, although they will now generally be computer based. Most are specific to a particular disorder or group of disorders.

Management-related registers

These are likely to be of greatest interest to the practising clinician with a special interest in a particular group of inherited disorders, and the registers often involve both a clinician and a clinical geneticist. The involvement of disease support groups is also a possibility: they certainly play a most helpful role in some disease-specific specialist clinics. In these clinics, the genetic aspects are only part of the objective, and a register may be of considerable help in overall management and surveillance, as well as in genetic counselling. The familial cancers, notably familial adenomatous polyposis coli and von Hippel-Lindau disease, provide excellent examples of the value of such a register, especially since the advent of molecular testing now means that many individuals can be effectively excluded from risk at an early age. Such registers are also valuable in audit and applied research, although this is not their primary aim.

Contact and genetic counselling registers

Here the specific aim is to allow genetic counselling and associated measures such as carrier detection to be offered in inherited disorders where there may be numerous family members at risk who might be unaware of the risks. The most suitable disorders for such a register (Box 11.1)

BOX 11.1: Disorders worth considering for a genetic register

X-linked recessive
Duchenne muscular dystrophy
Becker muscular dystrophy
Haemophilia (A and B)
Fragile X and other forms of X-linked mental retardation
Other serious rare X-linked disorders

Autosomal dominant
Polyposis coli (and other inherited bowel cancer syndromes)
von Hippel-Lindau disease
Multiple endocrine neoplasia disorders
Polycystic kidney disease
Huntington's disease
Retinitis pigmentosa (also X-linked form)
Myotonic dystrophy
Marfan syndrome

Chromosomal
Translocation Down syndrome (and other chromosomal translocations)

are the late-onset dominant disorders such as Huntington's disease, or X-linked disorders such as Duchenne and Becker muscular dystrophies and fragile X syndrome. Here an accurate knowledge of affected and at-risk individuals in a region is likely to be of considerable help in ensuring that genetic counselling is provided early rather than when an affected or potentially affected child has already been born. In addition, new information that becomes available about carrier females, including information about their risk of physical complications, can be disseminated and/or investigated efficiently, and new policies implemented, through a register system. In contrast, such registers are not suitable for autosomal recessive disorders, the common polygenic conditions and chromosomal abnormalities (apart from translocations) because the risks are either low or confined to immediate family members, who are likely to be aware of them already.

Particular issues with genetic registers

HOW CAN THE REGISTER BE KEPT SPECIFIC AND LIMITED?

It is all too easy for the scope of a register to expand until it is out of control. It is better to confine the register to a small number of well-defined conditions and to deal with them thoroughly.

HOW CAN THE QUALITY OF THE INFORMATION BE MAINTAINED?

An inaccurate or out-of-date register is worse than useless. Accepting data at face value from outside sources is dangerous, and the only person likely to have sufficient sustained enthusiasm to check the information thoroughly is the person actually responsible for maintaining the register. It must also be recognised that updating a register entails a great deal of work and that the expense in time is thus significant.

CONSENT AND CONFIDENTIALITY

Consent for inclusion in a disease register is important. While the legal situation is no more difficult than for other health-related contexts, which are given a privileged position under the European Union's (2018) General Data Protection Regulation (GDPR), explicit consent for inclusion of any such sensitive information is vital. Signing up to the register means that the families are willing to be contacted from time to time and offered updates about their condition and to give updated information about the family to the clinical team. When it might be relevant, they can also be offered clinic appointments. Maintaining a register requires resources, and few UK Regional Genetics Centres are still able to operate these except for some management-oriented registers for selected familial cancers and myotonic dystrophy. In Wales, we are (unfortunately) no longer able to operate a register system for Huntington's disease, the Xp21 muscular dystrophies or the fragile X syndrome.

The protection of confidentiality must be important in any register for a genetic disorder but is of the highest priority for conditions such as Huntington's disease. It is essential that no information be given out without the permission of the individuals concerned, that the register is kept securely, and that no identifying details are put on any computerised system that involves transfer of information outside the genetics unit.

Experience indicates that most individuals in families affected by these conditions are happy to participate provided that they can have a personal relationship with those running the register. If it is under bureaucratic control or any information is divulged without permission, this cooperation would almost certainly be lost.

12

Treatments and trials for genetic disease

TREATMENT FOR GENETIC DISEASES

In comparison with other types of disease, such as major infections, nutritional deficiencies or even cancers, most genetic disorders have been relatively unresponsive to treatment or to primary preventive measures. As these other disease categories have become less common, so the relative contribution of genetic disorders has increased. It is this, rather than any absolute increase, that has resulted in their increasing prominence in chronic disorders of childhood and of later life. It would be wrong, however, to give the impression that treatment is not an area of importance to those working with genetic disorders, or that those affected can be offered little of value. The wide range of increasingly effective approaches is summarised in Table 12.1. Most of the established treatments are now provided by regular medical services and not through medical genetics services. This arrangement will often continue as the new, rational treatments are introduced, although genetics services will have a role in the development of therapies and in decisions about which therapy will be most appropriate when the site or the category of mutation is critical. Genetics services may also continue their historical pattern of involvement in treatment or surveillance for complications of certain conditions, especially when these are complex disorders that involve multiple organs.

The avoidance of serious morbidity or death by the early detection of those at risk is now of major importance in many genetic disorders; the wide range of familial cancers provides many examples, as does the group of inherited neuromuscular disorders, especially myotonic dystrophy.

The importance of supportive measures, even when not curative, has already been stressed in this chapter and in Chapter 1. For many structural conditions, corrective surgical and physical procedures may be valuable secondary measures. Increasingly, though, possibilities are developing for specific therapies for disorders where, until recently, there has been no real prospect of altering the course of the disease. In numerous genetic disorders, large-scale clinical

Table 12.1 Approaches to therapy of constitutional genetic diseases (the order of the table reflects closeness to the primary defect, not degree of proven effectiveness)

Approach	Examples
Replacement of defective gene ('gene therapy')	Inherited immune deficiencies
Replacement of deficient protein product	
For example enzymes	Gaucher disease
Replacement of developmental signal	Ectodysplasin (modified)
Other gene product replacement	Type 1 diabetes mellitus (insulin), haemophilias (factors VIII and IX)
Drug treatment based on molecular defect	Mutation-specific therapies in cystic fibrosis
	Tuberous sclerosis (mTor inhibitors)
Dietary modification	Phenylketonuria
	Galactosaemia
Other medical therapy	Hyperuricaemias (allopurinol)
	Wilson disease (penicillamine)
Organ transplantation	Familial amyloidosis (liver transplant)
	Polycystic kidney disease (renal transplant)
Corrective surgical approaches	Arthrogryposes, limb defects, scoliosis, etc. (numerous orthopaedic conditions)
Prophylactic, risk-reducing surgery (e.g. for intestinal polyposis coli [FAP] or for hereditary breast and ovarian cancer)	Carriers of pathogenic variants in the genes APC, BRCA1 or BRCA2, etc.)
Early detection and surveillance for avoidable complications	Cardiac arrhythmias in myotonic dystrophy

trials are now being organised, based on a new understanding of the underlying pathology. Many patients welcome participation in these, even though they give no promise of benefit, and the treatment may turn out to be at best burdensome and possibly harmful. However, the actual process of involvement in a therapeutic trial may itself be therapeutic, and participation – even as a control – means that the patient should receive at least the best available supportive care. At the same time, patients must be warned against false hope often raised by the media, or by the combination of information with exhortation circulating informally through lay groups. Apart from a few examples of different approaches, we make no attempt to give details of these new advances. The field is moving too rapidly for that to be appropriate.

Clearly, the possibility of effective treatment will be of critical importance in genetic counselling, since it will determine the attitude of family members to the disease, as well as whether they are likely to take up options such as prenatal diagnosis, as already mentioned for phenylketonuria. Remember that treatments can be both a blessing and a burden: the physician's concept of 'successful treatment' may not be the same as that of the patient or family member, especially if painful, stressful and prolonged or even lifelong therapeutic measures are involved. A current of optimism within the disease community may make patients more willing to have potentially affected children. The perception of disease burden and how it may change in light of anticipated but not yet established treatments may influence families' decisions either way, that is, to accept more or less risk on behalf of the next generation.

Treatment may also change from generation to generation; for example, many patients with adult polycystic kidney disease in past generations died from renal failure, coronary artery disease or stroke. Now, in contrast, a combination of dialysis and transplantation with improved cardiovascular disease prevention and management offers a greatly improved outlook. In other conditions, and even within a single sibship, prognosis may alter as a result of early detection and treatment; for example, in congenital adrenal hyperplasia, the first affected sib may die undetected or suffer from serious metabolic problems, while these can be largely anticipated and prevented in subsequent sibs.

Gene therapy deserves a mention, especially in view of the widespread media publicity. It is now possible, when the gene responsible for an inherited disorder has been isolated, to insert a normal copy of it into the DNA of the genetically abnormal cell, and for it to function normally under certain conditions in experimental animals. Clearly there are major practical problems in such an approach, including the insertion of the 'correct' copy of the gene into the correct nuclear site and within the relevant cell types, ensuring that it functions adequately (but not excessively), and being as certain as possible that any virus vector used in the process does not itself cause harmful effects (immediate or long term). Success in treating the animal model of a human disease does not always readily translate into the successful treatment of human patients.

Interest in gene therapy has had a resurgence after a period of lower profile that followed the deaths of participants in trials and in safety studies. There has also been an explosion of interest in the development of other rational treatments that are based upon a knowledge of gene structure and function and the molecular mechanisms of disease although they do not employ gene replacement. Some real successes have been achieved, as in spinal muscular atrophy, and very promising preliminary results have emerged in other conditions, such as Huntington's disease.

Another technology that must be mentioned at this point is gene editing, using bacterial antivirus defences that have been co-opted to modify DNA sequences in cells *ex vivo* or even, once the safety of such methods has been studied and developed further, *in vivo*. The enzyme system best known in this role at present is the CRISPR/Cas9 system, but other enzyme systems with different properties are also being studied. The principal applications of these techniques at present are in research, either to correct a mutation or to introduce mutations into animal models of disease or into human cells, including differentiated cells derived from iPS cell lines.

The slow deterioration and variability of many genetic conditions will often make it very difficult to evaluate the success or otherwise of any therapeutic approach. Long-term safety issues remain a major concern, especially with gene editing that might either cause immediate problems such as cancers from 'off-target' effects or that might affect the germ line and, thereby, impose a mutational load on future generations.

It is likely that gene therapy, gene editing and the new rational, gene-based therapies will enter clinical practice for serious *somatic* disorders (e.g. various cancers) as personalised (i.e. stratified) medicine sooner and more widely than for constitutional genetic disease. It is unfortunate that some workers in the field have promoted the view that the new gene-based treatments are already almost commonplace in the treatment of inherited diseases in real patients (as opposed to the laboratory mouse).

A final point that should be noted in relation to gene therapy and gene editing is that these methods as now envisaged will only affect somatic cells and not the germ line, so that there should be no implications for future generations. There is a consensus that any measures to alter the germ line would, in the present state of our knowledge, be unethical. However, there are enthusiasts who would evade such a consensus, and vigilance will be needed to limit the scope of such potentially hazardous activities until the extent of off-target effects is better understood and controlled.

DESIGNING TREATMENTS FOR GENETIC DISORDERS

The principal message to be conveyed here is that there are multiple levels at which potential treatments may be targeted. We illustrate the broad range of potential therapeutic strategies. Which of the multiple possibilities will be the best one to pursue? That will be a question of judgement that is essentially pragmatic and very specific to the circumstances of each disease and each gene. Indeed, the best approach to pursue is liable to change over time, as our knowledge and the technologies and cost factors are all likely to change. These judgements will have to take account of practicalities that may work out very differently even for closely related disorders affecting the same tissue. Rules of thumb will be difficult to establish until the field has stabilised, and that may take many years. For now, it is a question of how to exploit the opportunities presented by nature, by our knowledge of each specific disease process and the available or affordable technologies. This will be a progress through many small, incremental steps.

When a strategy is not immediately obvious, it may be that knowledge of the disease mechanism(s) needs further development, usually involving a model organism as well as studies of the natural history of the disorder. In genetic diseases, the model organism will usually be a rodent, most likely the mouse.

It is possible that aiming at a single treatment to 'cure' the disease may be too ambitious. Perhaps, a few different strategies may be required to treat different aspects or manage different symptoms of the condition. One condition where there are good grounds for hoping that effective treatments will be possible is Rett syndrome, although there may be numerous obstacles to be overcome before this is achieved (Clarke and Abdala, 2018). It is also salutary to consider what an effective treatment would achieve for an adolescent affected by such a severe neurodevelopmental disorder. How would it feel to have been affected by mutation in the *MECP2* gene and then for this to be reversed abruptly by gene editing *in vivo*? Assuming that the immediate effects on the autonomic system and the somewhat slower effects on intracranial pressure (from enlargement of cells in the brain, as in the mouse model) could be managed satisfactorily, such a girl would not suddenly become an age-appropriate teenager. How would she *feel*? How would those around her cope with the changes, and help her to do the same? Might she be confused and distressed by the changes happening to her? How would she *behave* in response?

STRATEGIES

We list some strategies, working from the purely symptomatic level towards the gene. Note that some therapies may be effective for virtually all forms of the particular disease, whereas others could only be effective for specific mutations or for certain categories of mutation.

1. Symptomatic treatments will always be important and may be all that we can offer, including not only medication (e.g. for seizures, pain, chest infection, cardiac dysrhythmia, growth hormone deficiency) but also physiotherapy and occupational therapy. Even making our cities more accessible to those with motor disabilities, such as those who need to use wheelchairs, counts as a collective, societal 'treatment' provided to reduce these practical difficulties, whatever their cause (whether genetic or otherwise).

2. A focus on nutrition may be effective, as in phenylketonuria, galactosaemia and some other metabolic disorders. A ketogenic diet may be helpful for some children with epilepsy. Not only what is eaten but also when and how it is consumed may be important. Thus, parents

must ensure that their child affected by medium-chain acyl-CoA dehydrogenase deficiency (MCADD) does not become ketotic and hypoglycaemic.

3. Correction of a disturbed physiological state may be the most appropriate therapy. Phosphate supplements are effective in X-linked hypophosphataemic rickets and rehydration, with attention to electrolyte intake, in chloride-losing diarrhoea. The viscous airway mucus in cystic fibrosis can be made less viscous by DNAase treatment, and the arterial wall damage that progressively accumulates in Marfan syndrome may be reduced and delayed by β-blockers and losartan. Hypercholesterolaemia can often be managed by the prescription of statin drugs.

4. Replacing the gene product may be effective. This is already routine with the use of coagulation factors VIII and IX to treat the haemophilias, the use of human insulin to treat some forms of diabetes mellitus and of growth hormone to treat both growth hormone deficiency and some other categories of delayed growth.

   Enzyme replacement therapy is now in use as a standard treatment for a number of 'inborn errors of metabolism', especially some of the mucopolysaccharidoses (including Fabry disease and Gaucher disease). However, these treatments are enormously expensive and will only be generally available in wealthy countries.

   A novel form of 'gene product replacement' for a disorder of development involves the administration of a signalling molecule at the critical period(s) of development, that would not need to be lifelong. This approach has been established as effective in a mouse model of X-linked hypohidrotic ectodermal dysplasia (Gaïde and Schneider, 2003) and has since been used in early clinical trials. In the human disorder, it is likely to be most effective when given *in utero* in pregnancies already known to be at risk of the condition and with an affected male foetus diagnosed by ultrasound scan and/or non-invasive prenatal testing (Schneider et al., 2018). See Appendix 1, 'Treatments for Specific Genetic Disorders'.

5. Genetic testing is being used for therapeutic guidance by selecting the most appropriate therapy, for both genetic disorders and for sporadic or non-genetic conditions. This is what is usually meant by 'personalised treatment' or, perhaps more accurately 'stratified treatment', used now quite widely in oncology. It may involve testing the patient's general genetic constitution or the tumour itself. It may identify specific susceptibilities of the tumour that would indicate the most effective treatment for that malignancy, it may indicate that the usual treatments are unlikely to be effective, or it may identify the potential for an unacceptable degree of toxicity of a drug that might otherwise have been used.

   A good example is the use of PARP inhibitors as an additional treatment in breast or ovarian cancer that has arisen in a patient carrying a *BRCA* gene mutation. PARP inhibitors block the repair of single-strand breaks in DNA, which will then become double-stranded breaks after replication in a dividing cell. The *BRCA* genes are required for the most accurate form of repair for double-stranded breaks (by homologous recombination) and will be unavailable in the cancer cells of a patient who is a carrier for a *BRCA* gene mutation, as the cancer will usually have arisen through Knudson's 'second-hit' mutation at the originally intact *BRCA* gene (as well as other steps in the pathway to malignancy). These malignant cells are then vulnerable to DNA damage and are likely to undergo apoptosis, because they will carry out repair of double-strand breaks using less accurate, less safe, methods.

6. If a disease is usually caused by mutations that disinhibit an intracellular signalling pathway, it may be possible to use drugs to re-establish control over the disinhibited pathway. This approach has been developed for use in tuberous sclerosis, in which the

Ras cell proliferation pathway is disinhibited and inhibitors of mTOR (e.g. sirolimus) can reassert control over proliferation in the resulting tumours, including the renal and pulmonary angiomyolipomas (and the related lymphangioleiomyomatosis).

7. Small molecules may be selected or designed to compensate for a functionally impaired gene product. A good example of this has proved very effective in treating cystic fibrosis where one of the two pathogenic variants is p.Gly551Asp (formerly G551D). Ivacaftor enables this variant of the CFTR protein to locate correctly in the mucosal cell, thereby largely restoring its function.

8. The body's immune system may be utilised by stimulating an immune response to novel targets associated with disease. One potential application for this arises in Lynch syndrome, with people at risk of colon cancer. The mismatch repair-deficient tumours often produce a specific set of novel peptides that can generate an immune response. It has been suggested by Matthias Kloor that immunisation against these peptides may prevent the development of the early stage tumours into carcinomas.

9. The processing of RNA transcripts may be targeted to yield a modified mRNA molecule as a way to make the protein product more effective. This has been the basis of work on the dystrophin gene over many years, working to convert the pathology of Duchenne muscular dystrophy (DMD) (with effectively zero dystrophin) to that of Becker muscular dystrophy (with suboptimal but still useful levels of a functional form of dystrophin) and has been taken to the point of clinical trials. This approach uses DNA oligos to induce exon skipping. Deletion of one or more exons is the most common class of mutation causing DMD, and inducing the skipping of another exon, adjacent to the deleted exon, may be used to restore the downstream reading frame. This may be said to extend the deletion (functionally) and thereby restore production of the C-terminus of the protein. This approach could also be used to skip the exon that includes a stop codon point mutation, as long as the number of bases in that exon is a multiple of three.

   A comparable strategy is to use RNA interference to suppress transcription from the disease-causing allele of a gene that leads to a dominant-negative disease mechanism. This relies on sequence variants that distinguish the pathogenic from the normal allele, so that only the normal allele is transcribed. This approach is currently being assessed in a therapeutic trial for Huntington's disease.

10. The effect of point mutations that convert a coding triplet to a stop codon could be minimised by reading through ('ignoring') the stop codon, although this may lead (in effect) to a missense mutation at the altered triplet. This suppression of nonsense mutations occurs in treatment with the aminoglycoside antibiotics, but these are too toxic to be used as a continuing, lifelong treatment in individuals who might benefit from some read-through. Less toxic derivatives are being developed: the best known (ataluren, PTC124) has been studied in small trials with patients affected by cystic fibrosis and DMD resulting from nonsense mutations.

11. Cell-based therapies have been proposed over the years and are now entering clinical practice. They often employ stem cells with the capacity to repair a tissue that has lost the capacity to heal itself. While full of great promise, however, I should advise caution. This field has been plagued by hyper-enthusiasts who are willing to proceed well beyond what is warranted by the evidence. Despite these difficulties, work has developed on the heart, using stem cells to repair areas damaged by myocardial infarction. Stem cells are also being used

in research programmes to repair injury to the central nervous system – e.g. in the spinal cord – and to replace cells lost through inherited neurodegeneration, as in Huntington's disease. The source of cells is sometimes from embryonic material, but efforts are being made to derive the stem cells from the patient herself, such as iPS cells derived from skin fibroblasts. These cells will then be subject to gene editing techniques (mentioned later) to correct the mutation *ex vivo* and then differentiated into a relevant cell type. Such cells, that have been 'corrected' *in vitro*, should (it is anticipated) be much safer than performing gene editing *in vivo*, as the *in vitro*–corrected cells can be subject to whole genome sequencing to identify iatrogenic off-target mutations before being introduced into the patient.

12. Replacing the gene, or at least a section of the gene, has been attempted with varying degrees of success by inserting the gene in a vector. This is 'gene therapy' in the full sense, and the challenge is either to correct the mutation – by homologous recombination between the inserted vector and the faulty copy of the gene – or to insert the correct version of the gene into the relevant cells but not necessarily into the host's (patient's) chromosome, if the problem can be corrected simply by adding an intact copy of the gene.

    A full understanding of the disease mechanism is needed to plan such interventions, including recognition of whether the disease is dominant or recessive and, if dominant, whether the mechanism is through haploinsufficiency or through a dominant-negative effect, such as through some mechanism of toxicity. In other words, will the insertion of one copy of the intact gene into each relevant cell correct the problem, or will it be essential to remove or inactivate the mutant copy of the gene? (See the discussion of 'dominance' in Chapter 5.)

    If the gene therapy 'construct' has to be inserted not merely into the cell or nucleus but into the host chromosome, then the precision of its site of insertion will be crucial, to avoid insertional mutagenesis.

    The number of copies of the therapeutic construct may also be of great importance. In Rett syndrome, for example, we know that *MECP2* deficiency causes the condition but that there is a different, but also potentially severe, set of problems caused by *MECP2* duplication, so that the window of therapeutic dosage may be narrow.

    The choice of vector, usually a modified virus, is important. A retrovirus will be used if the construct needs to be inserted into the host chromosome, while other viruses may be used if that is not required. A retrovirus was used to infect autologous bone marrow cells of boys affected by an X-linked immune deficiency with an intact copy of the *SCID-X1* gene, *in vitro*, allowing the patients to generate a normal immune system once the treated cells were returned to them. Earlier attempts to achieve this had led to deaths from leukaemia after aberrant insertion of constructs into the host chromosomes.

    Targeting the vector to the tissue of relevance may be another challenge, especially with diseases affecting the brain, although encouraging progress has been made with the intrathecal administration of treatments for spinal muscular atrophy using an AAV vector. Targeting other tissues presents other challenges. Thus, targeting cells in the respiratory epithelium in order to treat cystic fibrosis has to be repeated at regular intervals and this led to an unhelpful immune response against the AAV vector.

13. We can hope that gene editing will, one day, be the 'ultimate' form of gene-based therapy. Gene editing is sometimes termed 'genome editing', although the editing really should be restricted in any one case to just a single site. (If the whole genome was to be edited, then it would be far from therapeutic.) This is well established as a technique in laboratory research but not yet as a directly therapeutic approach in the clinic, administered directly to the

body of the patient: the risk of 'off-target' mutagenesis is substantial and could so easily lead to malignancies in patients who would otherwise have been 'cured'. This area remains contentious and a topic of active policy development, with enthusiasts always keen to push forward into uncharted territory, while the more timid advise caution. Perhaps it is true that 'fools rush in where angels fear to tread'.

The most contentious applications of gene editing are their use in human reproduction, as in the notorious case of twin girls in China in whom gene editing has made them less vulnerable to HIV infection. This breaking of the appropriately cautious moratorium on interference in the human germ line was highly irresponsible, with very few if any circumstances in which one can see an ethical justification for taking such risks with the future of the resulting children, and of their children. This concern is amplified by the subsequent recognition (through research on the UK Biobank cohort) that people with homozygous deletion of CCR5 are at increased risk of several diseases and have a shorter than average lifespan.

Let us hope that we do not see patient deaths from off-target effects as the price to be paid for progress. Let us hope that the community of gene editing researchers can develop a consensus and exercise an appropriate degree of restraint, so that progress can be achieved but not at the cost of patient safety.

TRIALS

Given the range of potential therapies being developed for genetic disorders, and the potential for hazardous complications from some of these treatments, it is vital that trials are set up to assess efficacy and safety and allow comparisons between different approaches.

There are pressures that oppose the requirement for such trials, including the hyperenthusiasm of some who hold strong beliefs that a particular approach will work, as well as commercial and professional interests that stand to gain from such uncritical enthusiasm. There have been too many treatments that 'work well' in the mouse model of a human disease but fail to bring benefit to the human patient; no-one can justify the uncritical acceptance of a new treatment on the grounds that it 'must' work in the human because the rationale for the treatment, and the response to treatment in the mouse, are both so promising.

While clinical trials for rare diseases cannot be structured in the same way as more conventional trials of treatments for common disorders, it is vital that effective trials are mounted to protect patients and their families from both iatrogenic hazards and commercial scams.

It is more difficult to mount clinical trials for rare genetic disorders than for common diseases for a number of reasons that include the following:

1. The number of potential participants is much smaller, so that trials will often need to involve multiple centres, perhaps dispersed across several jurisdictions, which makes a trial more difficult and expensive to mount.
2. The number of potential patients to be treated, once a treatment has been shown to be both safe and effective, is much smaller, so the motivation for commercial enterprises to invest in the development of new treatments for these conditions is much less.
3. The experience of participation in a trial may be difficult for a patient and/or their family, especially if attendance at a distant site is required or if the patient's disease is unstable, so that its current, carefully attained management – already a balancing act – might be disrupted by the trial.

4. The patients of a physician who has a strong interest in a rare disease may feel pressure, or even coercion, to participate in a trial, without any such intention on the part of the physician. The patients may feel reliant – even dependent – on the physician-researcher and his or her clinical team, so that they are unable to decline the 'invitation', even if participation would be difficult and perhaps disruptive for the family and even if it carried a degree of risk.
5. The family may belong to a disease support group that strongly supports the trial in question, and in which refusal to participate might not be seen as an option. In other words, pressure from within the support group may be as powerful as pressure from a clinician.
6. For some patients or families, the question of personal identity might be at stake. When a person's identity is heavily entwined with the condition, then a really effective treatment might undermine their sense of who they are.

COSTS OF TREATMENT

A final topic to consider here is the question of the affordability of a new and expensive treatment for a rare disease. If it becomes possible to treat a rare disorder effectively and safely with gene editing soon after diagnosis, with a single expensive treatment that 'cures' the condition so that continued treatment is not required, then this may be seen as affordable by a social, collective healthcare system (such as the UK's National Health Service). While it requires heavy investment up front, it is likely to save resources in the longer term. But if the cost is high but sustained, as with enzyme replacement treatments for a few inborn errors of metabolism, then the conclusion drawn may be different.

Arguably, such treatments are only affordable, even in relatively wealthy countries, because the diseases being treated are both rare and small in number. While there are many thousands of rare diseases, rational and effective treatments have been devised for only a very few. If the number of rare disorders for which expensive therapies were required lifelong was much greater – say 600, as opposed to 6 – then even wealthy countries may baulk at making these treatments available.

A comparable situation in low-income countries would be treatment for β-thalassaemia. In countries in which the carrier state is fairly common – say 1 in 20 to 1 in 30 – this will affect 1 in 1,600 to 1 in 3,600 live-born children. Once a country has succeeded in controlling the mortality from infectious and nutritional causes in early childhood, those affected by thalassaemia will become a *relatively* common cause of serious morbidity and mortality in childhood. To introduce treatment for the children recently born with the condition may at first be affordable but, in a poor country, the numbers requiring expensive treatments will increase year on year as the survivors will continue to need treatment throughout their lives with blood transfusion and iron chelation.

The two approaches that could transform the situation, with either potentially able to make the treatment sustainable, are (1) the provision of a less costly, once-off therapy (by bone marrow transplant, gene therapy, or gene editing), or (2) the introduction of population carrier screening and/or antenatal screening, linked to the termination of affected pregnancies. Without some such way of limiting the need for lifelong therapy, the treatment of those affected would consume a progressively increasing fraction of the nation's healthcare resources and would rapidly become unsustainable. So, is it reasonable and acceptable for β-thalassaemia carrier screening in such countries to be promoted so heavily that, in effect, it becomes mandatory?

And that the termination of affected pregnancies is also, in effect, 'required'? Or is this justified by the fact that the high uptake of testing (and of selective termination) makes it feasible for those now affected by the condition to survive at all?

Once there are many rare diseases, for which expensive treatments have been developed and which are made readily available, will programmes of non-invasive prenatal testing become (effectively) obligatory? Might families cease to be supported in the care of their second affected child if they have failed to prevent a second case in the family, when this could easily have been achieved? And what if they have failed to participate in population screening or have failed to accept the 'offer' of a termination of the pregnancy? Might the offer of carrier screening and the termination of affected pregnancies become difficult to resist in wealthy, Western countries too, as well as in poor countries? How might this impact on the all-important ethos of genetic counselling?

My position is that it would be understandable and even acceptable for a country to promote population screening for recessive disease, if this enabled it to provide treatment for those affected, and on the condition that it remained voluntary not only in principle, rhetorically, but also in everyday practice.

PART 2

Genetic counselling: Specific organ systems

13

Neuromuscular disorders

MUSCULAR DYSTROPHIES

Many, indeed most, neuromuscular disorders have a Mendelian basis. Partly for this reason, and partly because of the severe chronic disability produced by many of them, they represent a major category of genetic counselling requests and referrals. The muscular dystrophies, a large group of progressive, primary muscle disorders, form a particularly important problem, made more complex by their heterogeneity. On account of the prominence of the X-linked Duchenne muscular dystrophy, though, many laypeople (and some doctors) still have the impression that all muscular dystrophy affects boys but is carried by girls. The first task in genetic counselling is thus to establish the precise diagnosis beyond all reasonable doubt, something that is now normally possible using a combination of clinical and molecular approaches.

There are muscular dystrophies that follow each of the Mendelian modes of inheritance. Table 13.1 lists the major categories and their inheritance. In many types, DNA analysis of blood is the primary confirmatory test, while it is still sometimes necessary to be guided by histopathology and immunohistochemical studies of specific muscle proteins, utilising a muscle biopsy. Appendix 1 points towards sources for more detailed information on the genetic and molecular aspects of the specific conditions, knowledge of which has been entirely transformed since the cloning of the dystrophin gene more than three decades ago.

Clinical management issues (especially respiratory and cardiac complications) are important and complex in the muscular dystrophies. It is still sometimes the case that families seen for genetic counselling have had no expert clinical support, so ensuring that this is provided is an essential part of any consultation.

Table 13.1 Major progressive muscular dystrophies

	Type	Molecular basis
X-linked	Duchenne	Dystrophin (usually absent)
	Becker	Dystrophin (usually present but altered and/or reduced in quantity)
	Emery-Dreifuss	Emerin
Autosomal recessive	Limb girdle muscular dystrophies – with a wide spectrum of severity	Very heterogeneous (different sarcoglycans; dystroglycans, calpain 3; see Straub et al., 2017)
	Congenital muscular dystrophy	Merosin/laminin alpha-2 chain and others
Autosomal dominant	Facioscapulohumeral	*DUX4* on distal 4q
	Distal	Heterogeneous (titin, dysferlin)
	Emery-Dreifuss	Lamin A/C (*LMNA*)
	Oculopharyngeal	*PABPN1* (polyalanine – GCG – trinucleotide repeat mutation)
	Adult-onset limb girdle	Several types (see Straub et al., 2017)
	Myotonic dystrophy type 1	*DMPK* (expanded trinucleotide repeat)
	Myotonic dystrophy type 2 (PROMM)	*ZNF9* (also an expanded repeat)

Xp21 MUSCULAR DYSTROPHY

Duchenne muscular dystrophy

Duchenne muscular dystrophy (DMD) (early-onset Xp21 muscular dystrophy) is one of the major problems in genetic counselling for paediatricians and neurologists, as well as for clinical geneticists. Its X-linked recessive mode of inheritance means that numerous female relatives may be at risk of being carriers, even with only a single affected individual in the family. It is essential that they be advised accurately and that all available information is used correctly in determining carrier status. Molecular genetic approaches to diagnosis and the identification of carriers have minimised the former problems with inadequate information or – worse – the misinformation that used to arise from inaccurate risk assessments. There are now very few families where satisfactory information cannot be given after appropriate molecular studies although, in healthcare settings where these are not available, the older methods of risk estimation may still have some application. These approaches should not yet be entirely forgotten, as disastrous results may otherwise arise for the families concerned.

This condition has seen important progress over recent years and has served as a prototype for other genetic disorders. The gene, located at Xp21 on the short arm of the X chromosome, was isolated by positional cloning. It is the largest human gene (more than two million base pairs, including the non-coding elements) although its protein is not the largest (which prize goes to another muscle protein, titin). The size and composition of the gene make recombination within it frequent, so that even DNA markers within the gene can have a significant rate of recombination with a family's mutation. However, a high proportion of cases (around two-thirds) result from large deletions including one or more exons, and a smaller number result from exonic duplications. Methods of quantifying the copy numbers of exons in the gene can therefore recognise the underlying cause of the disorder in 70% of cases and also identify female carriers in the family. Sequencing approaches can identify the mutation in almost all other families (usually a nonsense mutation), so that linkage analyses are rarely needed (except for single-cell testing in pre-implantation genetic diagnosis: see Chapter 9).

The protein product of the DMD locus, dystrophin, was entirely unknown before isolation of the gene. It is largely muscle-specific, but with smaller alternative forms present in the cerebellum and elsewhere in the brain. It is usually absent in typical cases of DMD, in contrast to the allelic disorder Becker muscular dystrophy (BMD, see later in this chapter), where it is present but altered in structure and/or reduced in quantity, and other dystrophies where it is generally normal. If a young boy presents with typical features of DMD and has a grossly raised serum creatine kinase (CK), molecular testing of leucocyte DNA will often be sufficient to establish the diagnosis, thereby completely avoiding the need for a muscle biopsy. However, immunocytochemical assays on muscle biopsy sections can contribute to the investigation of a limb girdle muscular dystrophy if DMD or BMD cannot be confirmed rapidly by molecular genetic testing. This requires properly stored frozen muscle.

Prenatal diagnosis of DMD by first-trimester DNA analysis is now feasible in the great majority of cases. Every effort should be made to establish the precise molecular defect or genotype of an affected family member in advance of prenatal diagnosis being required, along with the risk that the mother is indeed a carrier. Multiplex ligation-dependent probe amplification (MLPA; a multiplex, dosage-sensitive, PCR-based approach: see Chapter 5) allows prenatal detection of most cases with large (comprising at least one exon) deletions or duplications. Most other cases are now detected by DNA sequencing although in the past they sometimes required more difficult forms of DNA or RNA analysis. However, once the mutation has been identified in the index case, the prenatal diagnosis should be possible using standard types of DNA sequencing. Haplotypes of linked markers may still be required in a few non-deletion cases, especially in pre-implantation genetic diagnosis or non-invasive prenatal genetic testing.

It remains important to retain competence in the pre-molecular methods for those cases where the mutation has not been identified, in settings where the laboratory methods available are limited or where modern methods are too expensive for the family. This requires starting from basic principles of pedigree analysis and using all available information in risk estimation, including biochemical tests of creatine kinase activity, rather than relying on DNA results in isolation. This particularly applies to relatives of an apparently isolated case, where a specific mutation has not been identified.

Even when a mother is shown not to be a carrier of her son's DMD-causing mutation, there is a substantial risk of recurrence (20% or sometimes more) if she transmits the 'same' X chromosome (as defined by linkage haplotype using intragenic and flanking single nucleotide polymorphisms) to another male foetus. This reflects the high level of maternal germ-line mosaicism in this condition.

The general problems of calculating risks for a lethal X-linked disorder are discussed in Chapters 2 and 7. A woman with an affected son and another affected close male relative (e.g. brother or maternal uncle) is an obligate carrier, with a 50% risk of further sons being affected and of daughters being carriers. A woman with two affected sons should be given similar advice, although she may be mosaic rather than a full constitutional carrier of the condition. Detailed examples of risk estimation in DMD can be found in Chapter 2 and in the books of Young and Emery (see Appendix 1).

POPULATION SCREENING

The exceptionally high levels of serum creatine kinase seen in presymptomatic cases of DMD leave no doubt that the large majority of affected males (not carriers) can be detected soon after birth (nearly 90%). Cord blood values are too variable for this, but population screening of males can be undertaken using the newborn samples collected on filter paper for phenylketonuria (PKU) testing at 4–5 days or even earlier. There is still debate as to whether this approach is justified as a service at present, for a number of reasons. The justification would be to avoid the often long diagnostic odyssey from clinical presentation to diagnosis and to give parents the opportunity to access genetic counselling and perhaps prenatal diagnosis in future pregnancies, if they wish to avoid a recurrence. However, some families would much prefer not to know about this lethal disorder at such an early stage if immediate treatment is not going to make a major difference. Whether the distress likely to be caused in these families (and in the families whose tests prove to be false positives) is outweighed by the resulting benefits must be considered. The simplest solution to this is to ensure that the offer of screening is provided within an ethos of real choice, so that families can decide whether they would (not) wish to know if their son had DMD.

This is only feasible if the offer of screening for DMD is clearly marked as very different from the offer of screening for other disorders where early intervention is known to make a major difference and ensures the healthy development of an affected child (e.g. screening for congenital hypothyroidism). In effect, two tiers of newborn screening would be needed, with different approaches to parental consent (see discussion in Chapter 34).

As the prospects for effective, rational treatments improve, the benefits of screening may become more substantial and apply to the individual child as well as to the family. Screening for DMD could then be recommended unequivocally, as for PKU and hypothyroidism, although this does not seem to be imminent. It should also be remembered that, while diagnostic odysseys could be avoided, newborn screening could not (even in principle) prevent the births of most affected infants, as around two-thirds of cases are the first in their family.

Becker muscular dystrophy

While we now know that Becker muscular dystrophy (later-onset Xp21 muscular dystrophy) is determined by mutations at the same locus as DMD, it is valuable to consider this form separately, because the clinical and genetic problems are somewhat different. Onset and course vary greatly from family to family, and asymptomatic males must be checked carefully, even in adult life, before being pronounced unaffected. (I have met one affected man who used to work as a coal miner and was able to walk until 80 years; he had a very large deletion within the dystrophin gene.) Isolated male cases can be distinguished from other muscular dystrophies by the use of DNA analysis on blood and dystrophin analysis of muscle.

Many patients with BMD develop symptoms in adolescence and remain ambulant into adult life, though with increasing disability. This creates a totally different genetic counselling situation to DMD, since many patients will reproduce, and all their daughters will be obligatory carriers. Since no offspring will be affected, the genetic risks may well be forgotten or ignored by the time grandchildren at risk are born. Levels of CK in carriers are more frequently normal than in DMD; even obligatory carriers (obligatory through their position in the family tree) may be erroneously reassured on the basis of such inappropriate testing.

OTHER PROGRESSIVE MUSCULAR DYSTROPHIES

The main forms are listed in Table 13.1. The approach to investigation – to establish a precise molecular diagnosis – is changing. In the past, muscle biopsy to permit analysis by immunohistochemistry was key to distinguishing the different types. Analysis of the biopsy would then guide the selection of the appropriate molecular genetic investigations. With the advent of next-generation sequencing, however, the simultaneous sequencing of many genes has become feasible, so that the need for muscle biopsy to guide the choice of genes to be analysed is becoming much less relevant. Muscle biopsy may still be required in some circumstances but will be needed progressively less often.

Emery-Dreifuss muscular dystrophy

This is often X-linked, determined by a specific gene for the protein 'emerin', allowing specific mutation testing in some families. Affected males and some carrier females are at risk of serious cardiac conduction defects, even though weakness is often mild. Some clinically similar families follow autosomal dominant inheritance, and the disorder is due to defects in the gene *LMNA*, encoding the muscle proteins lamin A and lamin C. This is an unusual gene in which mutations can cause a very wide range of different phenotypes including lipodystrophy and progeria as well as muscular dystrophy.

Facioscapulohumeral dystrophy

This is a variable autosomal dominant disorder that is often mild but is seriously disabling in 15% of cases. Although the gene is 95% penetrant by early adult life, careful examination to exclude minimal signs is essential in counselling asymptomatic family members. Serum CK levels are often normal in mild or presymptomatic cases.

The cause of the disease is inappropriate expression of *DUX4*, a gene on 4q that is usually repressed in muscle by subtelomeric repeats on 4q but which is transcribed inappropriately if deletion reduces the number of these repeats (FSHD1). Homology with subtelomeric repeats on 10q made the recognition of this pattern difficult to achieve and can make it more difficult to achieve accurate diagnostic results. In a small minority of patients (with FSHD2), the disease mechanism is mutation in a separate chromatin structural protein gene (*SMCHD1*) that is needed to regulate *DUX4* in combination with a PAS (polyadenylation signal) on chromosome 4q. Inheritance is therefore digenic in FSHD2. Although complex, molecular tests are usually able to confirm the diagnosis and to enable prenatal diagnosis, although this is requested by only a minority of families.

Autosomal limb girdle muscular dystrophies

Molecular studies have greatly helped to resolve this confusing and heterogeneous group. Most are recessively inherited and due to defects in molecular components of the muscle membrane and contractile complex. The severe and extremely rare (except in North Africa) autosomal recessive dystrophy clinically resembling DMD should be considered, along with X-chromosome abnormalities, in any apparent case of DMD in a girl. More common are the later childhood-onset types of autosomal recessive limb girdle dystrophy, although in most populations this group is considerably less common than Becker dystrophy. It is essential to avoid confusion between female cases of an autosomal limb girdle muscular dystrophy (LGMD) and manifesting female carriers of the Xp21 dystrophies.

Occasional families with LGMD, often following a more benign course with adult onset, show autosomal dominant inheritance. Finally, we mention oculopharyngeal muscular dystrophy. This is a rare, usually autosomal dominant, muscular dystrophy that involves particularly the head and neck region but can also cause a proximal limb girdle muscle weakness. This is associated with an unstable triplet repeat in the *PABPN1* gene.

CONGENITAL MYOPATHIES

Unless the pattern of inheritance within a particular family is clear-cut, genetic counselling for the heterogeneous group of congenital myopathies (Table 13.2) should not be undertaken

Table 13.2 Congenital myopathies

Type	Inheritance	Gene location or defect
Nemaline myopathy	Autosomal recessive (severe congenital)	Nebulin and *ACTA1* (among others)
	Autosomal dominant (milder type)	α-Tropomyosin and *ACTA1* (among others)
Centronuclear (myotubular) myopathy	X-linked recessive neonatal type, often lethal (see text); rarely autosomal dominant or autosomal recessive	Myotubularin (X-linked)
Central core disease	Autosomal dominant	Ryanodine receptor *RYR1*
Bethlem myopathy	Autosomal dominant or recessive	Collagen VI-related
Congenital fibre type disproportion	Uncertain (probably not a single distinct entity)	–
Congenital muscular dystrophy	Autosomal recessive (heterogeneous)	Merosin, fukutin (and others)
Congenital myotonic dystrophy	Autosomal dominant (maternally transmitted)	*DMPK* at 19q (see text)

without a clear molecular diagnosis. This may require a muscle biopsy rather more often than is now true for the muscular dystrophies, although accurate molecular diagnoses can increasingly be made on the basis of DNA-based diagnostics. There can be some overlap of clinical features with the (more progressive) muscular dystrophies (e.g. in Bethlem myopathy). Discussion with colleagues at an appropriate expert centre may be very helpful.

Variation in severity within families may be marked, and both autosomal dominant and recessive inheritance have been recorded for the main types. The X-linked form of lethal centronuclear (myotubular) myopathy is more common than previously thought as a cause of neonatal death and is easily confused with congenital myotonic dystrophy; molecular analysis can distinguish the two. The term 'congenital muscular dystrophy' should be reserved for those specific forms that are progressive, as well as having congenital onset; they may also show central nervous system (CNS) (and sometimes oculomotor) involvement.

METABOLIC MYOPATHIES

Specific metabolic defects are being found for an increasing number of myopathies, as shown in Table 13.3. This emphasises the need for full biochemical and ultrastructural investigation of any obscure case of muscle disease before genetic counselling is given. The relevant individual chapters of the textbooks given in Appendix 1 provide details on the different forms.

Mitochondrial myopathies, which may present as muscle disorders or as CNS degenerations with wider system involvement, may be determined by nuclear genes (such as *POLG*) and follow Mendelian inheritance, or may be maternally transmitted following the general principles of mitochondrial (cytoplasmic) inheritance (see Chapter 2).

MYOTONIC DYSTROPHY

Myotonic dystrophy is an autosomal dominant disorder, for long a special interest of the original author. It ranks second only to Duchenne muscular dystrophy as a major genetic counselling

Table 13.3 Metabolic myopathies

Type	Inheritance
Mitochondrial myopathies (heterogeneous)	
Infantile cytochrome oxidase deficiency	Autosomal recessive
Late onset with ophthalmoplegia (chronic progressive external ophthalmoplegia, CPEO)	Autosomal dominant (some families) or mitochondrial (e.g. deletion of part of the mitochondrial genome)
Very rare hypermetabolic type (Luft type)	Sporadic or mitochondrial
With retinal, cardiac and other changes (Kearns-Sayre type)	May be caused by (heteroplasmic) deletion of part of the mitochondrial genome; often sporadic
Carnitine palmityl transferase deficiency	Autosomal recessive
McArdle syndrome (glycogenosis type V)	Autosomal recessive
Other glycogenoses (except type VIII)	Autosomal recessive

problem in inherited muscle disease and is the most common muscular dystrophy of adult life. Its extreme clinical variability adds special difficulty.

Definitely affected individuals have a 50% risk of offspring being affected. Affected women, even if mildly affected, have a considerable risk (Table 13.4) that an affected child will have the severe congenital form of the disease, which may result in neonatal death or severe respiratory problems after birth and severe physical and mental handicap in survivors. The risk is especially high where a woman has already had such an affected child and very low when she shows no neuromuscular abnormalities. The risk of this form in the offspring of affected males is very low, although childhood onset may occur.

Both genetic counselling and our general understanding of myotonic dystrophy have been entirely transformed as a result of the identification of the specific mutation in the gene on chromosome 19. An unstable trinucleotide repeat sequence is involved, with expansion in a specific CTG repeat found in virtually all cases so far studied. The expansion correlates broadly with severity of phenotype, and tends to increase from generation to generation, thus explaining the progressively earlier onset and greater severity (anticipation) characteristic of this disorder. The gene itself codes for a previously unknown protein, which shows protein kinase activity. Unlike DMD, there does not appear to be absence of the protein in patients – the mutation is in an untranslated part of the gene and its effects are related to its size. An effect on the function of other genes at the RNA level is involved, and the cell biology of the disorder is complex.

Table 13.4 Risks (approximate) of a congenitally or severely affected child with myotonic dystrophy in relation to clinical status of the mother (known to be heterozygous for a pathogenic expansion in *DMPK*)[a]

Maternal status	Risk (%)
Established neuromuscular disease	10–30
Neuromuscular disease minimal or absent	<5
Risk after the birth of a previous, congenitally affected child	40

[a] All groups have the same chance (50%) of a child being genetically unaffected.

Individuals carrying a minimal change in the gene usually show little or no muscle disease, but they may develop cataract at an unusually early age. All patients may have originated from a few ancestral mutations, which may have been relatively stable for many generations, progressive instability resulting once expansion had passed a critical point. As with Huntington's disease and other trinucleotide repeat disorders, asymptomatic individuals with borderline expansions form a reservoir of gene carriers who may transmit clinically significant disease to their offspring.

Although these molecular advances should not become an excuse for omitting a careful clinical assessment, asymptomatic relatives at risk can now be confirmed or excluded as having the mutation by specific molecular analysis, while this is also useful in situations of uncertain diagnosis. Electromyography and eye examination for lens opacities are used to assess clinical status but are no longer needed to establish the diagnosis in apparently healthy relatives. Prenatal diagnosis is also feasible by molecular analysis. Testing of samples from extended relatives in the older generation or from children should not be performed without careful consideration of the implications, since the relation between mutation and phenotype is variable and the risk for instability in family branches where overt disease has not occurred is not clear. The reason why congenitally affected cases are (virtually) exclusively maternally transmitted appears to be that expansions over a certain size cannot be transmitted by sperm. The varying risks of severe disease according to the clinical status of the mother (see Table 13.4) can now be explained, at least in part, by the size of the mother's DNA expansion and its likelihood for further progression in the child.

Presymptomatic testing should be made available with full genetic counselling, as for other disorders, and should be avoided in healthy children in whom clinical examination is normal. Because the disorder is largely penetrant by adult life, the risk of an abnormal result in a clinically normal individual with an affected parent is only around 10%.

Surveillance for complications is important in those with any degree of symptoms, monitoring especially for cardiac conduction defects, nocturnal hypoventilation and diabetes (among many other complications). Affected females and their obstetric or midwifery attendants need to be aware of the dangers in this group of anaesthetic problems and post-partum haemorrhage.

Type 2 myotonic dystrophy

A small number of myotonic dystrophy patients (around 1% in the United Kingdom but considerably higher in Germany) fail to show the expected chromosome 19 mutation, and it is now known that a separate gene (on chromosome 3) is involved, also with an unstable (CCTG) repeat mutation causing the disease. This type 2 myotonic dystrophy is the same as the disorder previously known as proximal myotonic myopathy (PROMM) and shows more proximal weakness, no childhood form, but some similar systemic features to the classical 'type 1' form. Inheritance is autosomal dominant.

OTHER MYOTONIC SYNDROMES

Other myotonic syndromes are rare in comparison with myotonic dystrophy, which must be carefully excluded (Table 13.5). Myotonia congenita (Thomsen disease) is heterogeneous and at least half the cases are recessively inherited, despite the prominence of some large dominantly inherited families. The two types show clinical as well as genetic differences. Because new mutations for this benign condition are likely to be rare, it is wise to give a one in four risk for further children born to healthy parents of an isolated case, until a molecular diagnosis has

Table 13.5 The myotonic disorders

Syndrome	Inheritance	Mutation or gene involved
Myotonic dystrophy (type 1)	Autosomal dominant	Expanded CTG repeat (in 3' UTR)
Progressive myotonic myopathy (PROMM, type 2 myotonic dystrophy)	Autosomal dominant	Expanded CCTG repeat (intronic)
Myotonia congenita		
Thomsen disease	Autosomal dominant	Skeletal muscle Cl⁻ channel
Recessive type	Autosomal recessive	Skeletal muscle Cl⁻ channel
Paramyotonia congenita	Autosomal dominant	Skeletal muscle Na⁺ channel
Periodic paralysis		
Normo/hyperkalaemic (adynamia episodica)	Autosomal dominant	Na⁺ channel
Hypokalaemic	Autosomal dominant	Ca⁺⁺ channel
Chondrodystrophic myotonia (Schwartz-Jampel syndrome)	Autosomal recessive	Perlecan (*HSPG2*)

been achieved. Correspondingly, the risk of such an isolated case transmitting the condition is, in the absence of a molecular diagnosis, small. Careful neurophysiological tests by an expert are important in distinguishing the different disorders in this group.

The molecular advances in myotonic dystrophy have been equalled by corresponding progress in the non-progressive myotonias, but instead of a previously unknown gene and protein, the defects have proved to be those predicted by physiological and pharmacological studies. Following cloning of the adult muscle sodium and chloride channel genes, the former (on chromosome 17) has been shown to be responsible for both paramyotonia and myotonic periodic paralysis, while different mutations in the chloride channel gene on chromosome 7 occur in the dominant and recessive forms of myotonia congenita. It should be remembered that the periodic paralytic disorders do not, unfortunately, quite live up to their name: while there are acute episodes of severe weakness, there can also be an underlying, slowly progressive decline in muscle strength that can show as incomplete recovery from the acute exacerbations.

MALIGNANT HYPERTHERMIA (HYPERPYREXIC MYOPATHY)

Malignant hyperthermia (hyperpyrexic myopathy) is a particularly important dominantly inherited disorder to recognise in those at risk. It gives a subclinical myopathy (often with muscle hypertrophy and raised CK levels), and also profound contracture with hyperthermia following anaesthesia with specific agents, especially the volatile anaesthetics such as halothane, which can be catastrophic if not promptly recognised. Detection of carriers at risk remains unsatisfactory. The previously used *in vitro* contractural test on muscle biopsy is invasive, has proved unreliable, and should be abandoned as the basis for clinical decisions about individuals' risk status. In a majority of families, the condition is due to defects in the ryanodine receptor gene (*RYR1*), in which mutations can also be associated with central core disease (a congenital myopathy). However, the condition is heterogeneous, and this currently limits the applicability of molecular diagnosis.

MYASTHENIA GRAVIS

In the usual adult form of myasthenia gravis associated with antibodies to the acetylcholine receptor, genetic risks are extremely low. In one series of over 400 patients, one pair of affected sibs was the only familial case. A risk of around 1% for myasthenia gravis is appropriate for first-degree relatives, along with an increase in autoimmune thyroid disease. An association has been found between myasthenia gravis and the antigens HLA-DRw3 and HLA-B8. This is a good illustration of the fact that such associations do not necessarily imply high risks to family members. Transient congenital myasthenia gravis is seen in about 20% of the offspring of affected mothers, but, unlike the corresponding situation in myotonic dystrophy, rarely has permanent effects.

The congenital myasthenic syndromes comprise a group of rare and heterogeneous genetic disorders with onset in the perinatal period or infancy. The most frequent cause is acetyl choline receptor deficiency. Most of these conditions are autosomal recessive; anti-AChR antibodies are absent.

SPINAL MUSCULAR ATROPHIES

Proximal spinal muscular atrophy

The spinal muscular atrophies are a group of anterior horn cell disorders that are distinct from the primary myopathies on clinical, electromyographic, histological and molecular grounds. The great majority of all childhood proximal types follow autosomal recessive inheritance, so that sporadic cases should be counselled as such in terms of risk for sibs, even if it is difficult to assign them to a particular type. More than 95% of cases are allelic, caused by deletions in a specific gene on chromosome 5q (*SMN1*). Molecular testing can be used for diagnosis (including prenatal diagnosis) and (by dosage) to determine carrier status. The differences in severity arise largely from differences in the number of copies of the neighbouring (and highly homologous) *SMN2* gene, of which there is a varying number of copies arranged in *cis*.

The congenital type, type 0, is characterised by prenatal onset and short survival (less than 6 months).

In the most common type, type I, known as severe infantile spinal muscular atrophy (Werdnig-Hoffmann disease), onset is at or shortly after birth, with death – in the absence of treatment – invariably before 2 years and usually before 18 months. Severity in other affected sibs is closely correlated, so that the chance of a subsequent affected infant surviving in the long term is very small, as is the chance of an infant who is clinically normal at 6 months going on to develop the disease. This can be confirmed by molecular analysis. DNA analysis or banking on the first affected child is vital to allow subsequent prenatal diagnosis. There have been some promising results in trials of gene therapy for this disease.

Type II, or intermediate spinal muscular atrophy, includes cases with childhood onset but survival beyond 2 years. The majority are severely disabled during childhood, and this may occur in sibs of mild cases. Variability between sibs is greater than for the infantile type, but apparently healthy sibs will have passed through 90% of their risk by the age of 12 years. The same molecular analysis can be used in prediction as for type I.

In type III, or benign spinal muscular atrophy (Kugelberg-Welander disease), most cases follow autosomal recessive inheritance, and are determined by the same 5q locus as types I and II. A few isolated cases may be non-genetic or represent new dominant mutations. The offspring of affected individuals will usually be normal, but where an isolated case is of adult onset and the mutation is unknown, the possibility of dominant inheritance gives a risk to offspring of around 1 in 20.

Other types of spinal muscular atrophy

Distal spinal muscular atrophy is more likely to be confused clinically with Charcot-Marie-Tooth disease (see later in this chapter) than with the types described earlier, which are proximal in distribution. Inheritance is usually autosomal dominant, even in childhood-onset cases; the course is often very slow. It is important to explain to families the very different prognosis and inheritance from the proximal spinal muscular atrophies. A number of cases are difficult to categorise, and since isolated cases may rarely be new dominant mutations, a risk for offspring of around 5% should be given for such atypical spinal muscular atrophies until they are better understood.

There are numerous rare types of SMA, whose genetic basis is becoming clearer. An example is the autosomal dominant distal spinal muscular atrophy with vocal cord involvement (HMN7A).

Some forms of lethal arthrogryposis are due to spinal muscular atrophies with onset *in utero* (SMA0). Some are due to defects in *SMN1*, but one type is X-linked.

MOTOR NEURONE DISEASE (AMYOTROPHIC LATERAL SCLEROSIS)

Motor neurone disease is generally sporadic. Risks to first-degree relatives in two unselected series were under 1%, although these studies need to be extended in light of molecular advances. About 10% of cases are said to be familial, and more than half of these cases now have their mutational basis identified. By far the most important genetic factor identified is the *C9orf72* locus, in which expansion of an unstable hexanucleotide repeat is associated with either amyotrophic lateral sclerosis (ALS) or frontotemporal dementia (FTD). This expansion is found in some 40% of cases of familial ALS and rather less than 30% of familial FTD. Factors influencing the penetrance and the mode of disease presentation (as either motor neurone disease or dementia) are uncertain. There is an intermediate range of repeat expansion where the risk of disease is unclear. These uncertainties make the counselling for predictive genetic testing difficult, as the natural history is still only incompletely understood.

The finding that a modest but appreciable proportion (perhaps 7%) of apparently sporadic cases of ALS is associated with expansion in *C9orf72* is important. When a family history of ALS is taken, it is important also to ask about dementia, as the relevant family history may relate to a different phenotype. The implications for the close relatives of a sporadic case of ALS associated with this molecular pathology have not yet been fully assessed.

Other, much less common familial types have been recorded that follow autosomal dominant inheritance and are due to mutations in the superoxide dismutase gene (*SOD1*) on chromosome 21 and several other genes. Familial clustering also occurs in specific geographical areas (e.g. Guam). Kennedy disease, or X-linked bulbospinal atrophy, is more common than previously recognised and usually follows a more prolonged course. This disorder is due to a mutational defect (a CAG repeat) in the androgen receptor gene, which can be recognised in the isolated case by mutation analysis and clinically by features of mild androgen deficiency; this must also be distinguished.

CHARCOT-MARIE-TOOTH DISEASE

The majority of cases of Charcot-Marie-Tooth disease (also termed peroneal muscular atrophy and hereditary motor-sensory neuropathy) are autosomal dominant. Cases in families previously thought to be recessive probably mostly result from parental germ-line mosaicism. Nerve conduction studies allow two main groups to be distinguished, although there is overlap phenotypically. The nomenclature and classification still remain fluid but are becoming clearer as the different specific molecular defects are identified.

Type 1 (delayed nerve conduction)

In this group, usually dominantly inherited, demyelination is the underlying problem. A specific and unusual molecular defect has been found in many families with type I, with duplication of a small region of chromosome 17p detectable by molecular methods, although not usually visible microscopically, so that affected individuals have three functioning copies of the segment. This is known as CMT1A.

In most families with apparently normal parents but multiple affected children, the disease can now be shown to result from mosaicism in a parent. The specific gene involved is that for peripheral myelin protein (PMP22). This defect provides a specific diagnostic and presymptomatic test, applicable even to isolated cases. A few families show no abnormality of, or linkage to, chromosome 17, and some severe cases are due to changes in a separate myelin gene (P0); interestingly, deletions of the PMP22 gene produce a similar but distinct clinical disorder, 'hereditary liability to pressure palsies'.

The X-linked form of Charcot-Marie-Tooth disease must be borne in mind when considering an isolated male case or a pedigree suggestive of X-linkage. Molecular defects in connexin 32 have been found in this type. Nerve conduction is often variable in this form, and usually normal in heterozygous females, who may be variably affected clinically. Friedreich ataxia (autosomal recessive, see Chapter 14) may also show prominent neuropathic features.

Type 2 (normal nerve conduction)

Type 2 disease, with an underlying pathology of axonal degeneration, is clinically similar to type 1, though often milder. This group is also very similar to the distal spinal muscular atrophies. Indeed, the distinction between these two groups of conditions is unclear and may be 'academic', in that the categories (defined clinically and by electrophysiology) may blur and merge together. Asymptomatic relatives need careful examination to exclude minimal features before they can be given a low risk. In most families with multiple affected sibs but normal parents, inheritance is probably still autosomal dominant but with either mosaicism or undetected parental disease.

Molecular studies show considerable heterogeneity, so predictive or prenatal DNA testing in CMT2 is feasible at present only in those families where a specific defect has been identified. Testing of large gene panels, which will often include the genes responsible for atypical types of SMA, can be helpful in reaching the diagnosis when CMT is not caused by the gene duplication of CMT1A, and especially in CMT type 2.

Other hereditary neuropathies

Now that specific molecular tests are becoming available, it is increasingly possible to distinguish other hereditary neuropathies with greater confidence, and to identify isolated cases with a specific genetic basis. The group of autosomal dominant familial amyloidoses (often characterised by central nervous system, cardiac and other systemic involvement as well as neuropathy) have been shown to result mainly from defects in transthyretin or gelsolin, with different mutations resulting in different phenotypes, and often showing marked geographical variation. Recent evidence suggests that liver transplantation and some drug treatments may reverse or at least prevent progression of the disorder. It should be noted that most cases of primary amyloidosis are not familial, but no clear figure exists to put the proportion that is heritable into perspective.

Familial dysautonomia (autosomal recessive) has highly specific features and is most frequent in those of Ashkenazi Jewish origin, while neuropathy may form an important feature of such metabolic disorders as Refsum disease and the porphyrias (see Chapter 26).

Rare forms of pure hereditary sensory neuropathy (usually autosomal recessive) may result in disabling trophic changes.

The diagnosis of Möbius (or Moebius) syndrome of multiple cranial nerve palsies is frequently misapplied to children with other myopathies (e.g. myotonic and facioscapulohumeral [FSH] dystrophies) or anterior horn cell disorders presenting with facial and ocular palsies. If these can be excluded, the recurrence risk is probably low (1%–2%).

14

Central nervous system: Paediatric and neurodevelopmental disorders

INTRODUCTION

Disorders of the nervous system make up a remarkably high proportion of genetic counselling referrals. This partly reflects the large number of neurological conditions that follow Mendelian inheritance but is also likely to be due to the severe burden resulting from many neurological and developmental disorders and the consequent concern of relatives to avoid recurrence, if possible. We consider childhood-onset disorders of the central nervous system (CNS) in this chapter and CNS disorders of adult onset in Chapter 15. We already considered disorders of the neuromuscular system and the peripheral nervous system in Chapter 13.

The distinction between disorders of early (i.e. childhood) or later (i.e. adult) onset is far from 'tidy'. Indeed, it is rather artificial but is nevertheless helpful in organising the material to be discussed. Diseases do not respect our division of medicine into specialties on the basis of either age or organ; furthermore, affected children will often become affected adults, who then need care from 'adult' neurologists and others. And some disorders have a variable age of onset, sometimes first manifesting in childhood and sometimes not until adult life.

One reason for the early progress in identifying genes responsible for neurodevelopmental disorders, and the dysmorphic syndromes that may also be associated with cognitive impairment, is that clinical geneticists would often be involved in the diagnostic assessment of such patients. As a group, clinical geneticists had early access to the laboratory facilities required to locate the genes through linkage studies or molecular cytogenetics. The resulting progress, and the improved understanding of these disorders, is now informing the development of rational approaches to treatment. The identification of the relevant gene has often been a first essential step to the identification of the protein implicated in the mechanism of disease; this has then enabled the development of possible therapeutic strategies.

The widespread availability of molecular analysis allows both accurate diagnosis and prediction. Neurologists of child and adult patients now employ molecular methods in the first line of diagnostic investigations for many clinical presentations. The ready availability of tests that can be used for prediction makes it particularly important that families in which an inherited neurological disorder has occurred have access to accurate, careful and sensitive genetic counselling. While the neurologist may focus on diagnosis and disease management, clinical genetics services are more concerned with the extended family and with complex situations such as the presymptomatic, predictive testing of individuals who are at risk but have (so far) been healthy.

COGNITIVE IMPAIRMENT (INTELLECTUAL DISABILITY, LEARNING DIFFICULTIES, MENTAL RETARDATION)

Cognitive impairment has been known by a variety of terms, which usually fall out of favour after some years as they are adopted, outside professional circles, as terms of abuse. Outside medical textbooks, 'mental retardation' has been largely left behind for that reason, but the term 'learning difficulty', while very applicable to the problems faced by many children with milder problem or very specific learning impairments, fails to convey the devastating impact that cognitive impairments can have if they are severe or profound. These difficulties have traditionally been divided into two principal categories:

- Mild (intelligence quotient [IQ] 50–70): Prevalence about 3% or 30 per 1,000
- Moderate or severe (IQ 50 or less): Prevalence about 3 per 1,000

All IQ levels above 70 are considered as part of the normal range by definition, with IQ established as a Gaussian distribution with mean 100 and standard deviation of 15. The importance of this division above and below $IQ = 70$ stems from the fact that mild cognitive impairment behaves genetically as the lower end of a normal distribution, so that the IQ levels in sibs or offspring are closely influenced by those of the parents (see later in this chapter). By contrast, in severe cognitive impairment, parental intelligence is usually normal and a sharp discontinuity is seen between family members who are affected and those who are not, with little increase in (mild) learning difficulties in between. It is also in severe cognitive impairment that specific causes are most likely to be found, whose accurate recognition is essential for genetic counselling.

In this book, addressed to health professionals, we still retain the terms 'mental retardation' in addition to intellectual disability and, when it is mild, 'learning difficulty'. No offence or disrespect is intended by any of these terms. When writing for less medical audiences, and also in this volume, we sometimes also use the phrase 'cognitive impairment' as its meaning is clear and it has not (yet) become a term of abuse in popular speech.

Specific causes of cognitive impairment (learning disability)

The number of specific recognised disorders of which cognitive impairment is an integral or major component is exceedingly large and is growing steadily, a fact that makes it important to reassess individuals who have been seen in the past but have no diagnosis or who have not recently had a thorough diagnostic assessment. Some of these disorders have been found to have a definite aetiological basis, which may be biochemical, chromosomal, Mendelian or environmental; in many cases the underlying cause remains unknown, but the occurrence of accompanying physical abnormalities may allow the delineation of a dysmorphic syndrome. The border between 'physical abnormalities' and 'unusual features' may, of course, be difficult to decide upon clinically, to justify scientifically and also, importantly, to negotiate socially.

One major group of specific disorders needing to be recognised is that following Mendelian inheritance, for it is here that the risks of recurrence in sibs are highest, particularly the autosomal recessive and X-linked recessive disorders. Box 14.1 lists some of the major causes; many are considered in more detail in other chapters.

BOX 14.1: Some Mendelian disorders causing or frequently associated with mental retardation

Autosomal dominant, often inherited

Apert syndrome

Myotonic dystrophy (particularly early-onset and congenital cases)

Neurofibromatosis type I (mild learning difficulties are common, more severe cognitive impairment is unusual)

Noonan syndrome and related RASopathies (very variable effects: often cognitively normal but may have learning difficulties)

Tuberous sclerosis

Autosomal dominant, usually arising de novo

This group is too large to specify individual conditions except to mention a few as examples (e.g. Coffin-Siris syndrome including *ARID1B, FOXG1*, Pitt-Hopkins syndrome *TCF4, MEF2C*, Rubinstein-Taybi syndrome *CREBBP* and other genes, Mowat-Wilson *ZEB2, SATB2, SYNGAP1, ANKRD11, SCN1A, DYRK1A, STXBP1, MED13L*). The contribution of this group to developmental disorders has been recognised much more fully through the Deciphering Developmental Disorders (DDD) project in the United Kingdom.

Autosomal recessive

Aicardi-Goutières syndrome (with intracranial calcification)

Ataxia telangiectasia

Bardet-Biedl syndrome

Canavan disease (spongy degeneration of white matter)

Carpenter acrocephalopolysyndactyly

Galactosaemia

Homocystinuria

Marinesco-Sjögren syndrome

Microcephaly (some forms)

Mucopolysaccharidoses (types I, III)

Neurolipidoses (including Tay-Sachs, Gaucher, metachromatic leucodystrophy and numerous others)

Phenylketonuria

Seckel syndrome

Sjögren-Larsson syndrome

Xeroderma pigmentosum (some forms)

X-linked

α-Thalassaemia X-linked mental retardation syndrome (*ATRX*)

Adrenoleucodystrophy

ARX-related disorders (infantile spasms; agenesis corpus callosum)

Börjesson-Forssman-Lehman syndrome (*PHF6*)

Coffin-Lowry syndrome

Duchenne muscular dystrophy (not constant)

Fragile X syndrome

Hunter syndrome (MPS II)

Lesch-Nyhan syndrome (HGPRT deficiency)

Lowe (oculocerebrorenal) syndrome

Menkes syndrome

Norrie disease

Opitz G/BBB syndrome

Orofaciodigital syndrome type I (male-lethal, X-linked dominant) some cases

Pelizaeus-Merzbacher disease (*PLP1*) One of the leucoencephalopathies

Renpenning syndrome (cognitive impairment with microcephaly)

Rett syndrome (X-linked dominant, usually *de novo* and therefore sporadic)

Simpson-Golabi-Behmel syndrome (*GCP3*)

X-linked aqueduct stenosis with associated anomalies, MASA syndrome (*L1CAM*)

Among the non-Mendelian causes of cognitive impairment (Box 14.2), chromosomal disorders are particularly important to recognise (see Chapter 4). Almost all unbalanced autosomal disorders detectable on karyotype are associated with mental retardation; in older patients said previously to have been chromosomally normal, it is worth investigating further with the more sensitive array-based molecular techniques. Imprinting defects (e.g. Angelman syndrome) may need to be considered and may also provide a high-risk subgroup if there is a silent parental defect. This area is a good example of the value of 'targeted' molecular and cytogenetic investigation, where array comparative genomic hybridisation (aCGH) will detect many cases but will fail to detect others, so that more specific testing (tests of methylation or sequencing of *UBE3A*, in the context of suspected Angelman syndrome) will need to be triggered by an experienced clinician, at least until whole genome sequencing (WGS), incorporating tests of the epigenome, becomes a first-line test for developmental problems. Unless a parent also has a chromosomal rearrangement, the recurrence risk for such a disorder will be low.

BOX 14.2: Non-Mendelian and chromosomal syndromes associated with mental retardation

Major chromosomal abnormalities (see Chapter 4)

Down syndrome

Other autosomal abnormalities including especially copy number variants (CNVs) (numerous)

Multiple X syndromes, including XXXY syndrome (The XXX and XXY syndromes are discussed in Chapter 4 and are not usually associated with substantial cognitive impairment)

Mosaicism for cytogenetic abnormalities (sometimes associated with streaky differences in skin pigmentation, when the term 'Hypomelanosis of Ito' used to be applied)

Chromosome microdeletions (not in all cases) (see Chapter 4)

Angelman and Prader-Willi syndromes (15q11 deletions)

Langer-Giedion syndrome

Rubinstein-Taybi syndrome (molecular deletions of locus on chromosome 16p)

Williams (infantile hypercalcaemia) syndrome with deletion encompassing the elastin gene on 7q

Environmental factors (see Chapter 28)

Congenital infections (rubella, cytomegalovirus, *Toxoplasma*, Zika, herpes simplex)

Teratogens (alcohol, phenytoin, sodium valproate)

Hypoxic-ischaemic encephalopathy and cerebral damage (often associated with prematurity)

Intrauterine growth retardation (heterogeneous)

Maternal phenylketonuria

Congenital hypothyroidism (heterogeneous)

Trauma (non-accidental)

Lead poisoning

Structural abnormalities of the central nervous system (see text)

Hydrocephalus and hydranencephalus (heterogeneous and highly variable)

Encephalocoele (sometimes associated with autosomal trisomies or other specific conditions including Meckel syndrome – AR)

Cortical malformation (neuronal migration defects and polymicrogyria: sometimes Mendelian)

Sturge-Weber syndrome (can be caused by somatic mutation in the *GNAQ* gene)

Many previously undiagnosed cases are found, with the newer technologies, to be affected by *de novo* mutations, either CNVs or autosomal dominant disorders. The recurrence risk is then usually small, equivalent to the chance of parental mosaicism.

Where a family history and/or a result on array-based CGH indicates the possibility of a chromosome rearrangement, such as a translocation or inversion, then it is important to perform a karyotype.

The common sex chromosome anomalies are not usually associated with cognitive impairment/mental retardation, although some children with XXX and XXY have a degree of learning difficulty and benefit from educational support; some also show behaviour problems. In the much less common, higher-order X-chromosome syndromes (with four or five X chromosomes), the degree of cognitive impairment can be more significant.

If an environmental cause can be identified, recurrence is unlikely, provided that the harmful agent is not still operating. Care must be taken not to attribute mental retardation falsely to perinatal anoxia or other such factors when that may be the result of the underlying disorder rather than its cause.

The less constant association of cognitive impairment with a large number of specific physical disorders is of great importance in genetic counselling, since many couples who would accept the risk of physical handicap in an affected child are unwilling to accept the additional risk of mental handicap. Unfortunately, bias of ascertainment or reporting often makes the frequency of cognitive impairment in genetic disorders difficult to assess. Duchenne and myotonic dystrophies are examples where there is a true association with learning difficulties and sometimes with more severe cognitive impairment, while in other situations where the association has been suggested (e.g. histidinaemia, X-linked hypohidrotic ectodermal dysplasia), it is no longer considered to be relevant.

Severe non-specific cognitive impairment (learning disability)

Despite the most careful study, including aCGH and exome sequencing, many children with severe cognitive impairment have no clear underlying causative factor or associated syndrome, and there is often no relevant pedigree information. Here one is forced to use the older general empiric recurrence risks (see *Genetics and Neurology* by Bundey, listed in Appendix 1, for details), even though many such cases are likely to prove in the future to have their own specific basis. Fortunately, a number of studies have been carried out with broadly similar results; the overall recurrence risk to sibs appears to be a little under 3% (i.e. about 10 times the population risk). The somewhat higher risk to male sibs in some series probably results from a generally greater susceptibility of males to developmental problems as well as from inclusion of families showing X-linked inheritance (see later in chapter).

As the proportion of cases of severe cognitive impairment in which the cause is known increases, the empiric risks for undiagnosed mental retardation determined decades ago become less applicable. However, fresh population studies would be very difficult to perform as the currently rapid rate of progress in clarifying the aetiology means that the field of study resembles a moving target. One must therefore be cautious in applying such historic studies and remain mindful of diagnostic categories where the risks are likely to differ from these general figures. Once WGS has become the standard genetic investigation for severe neurodevelopmental problems, it will become feasible to follow the families of affected children with and without a genetic diagnosis and thereby determine a new, more contemporary, risk of recurrence of unexplained cognitive impairment.

Table 14.1 gives approximate risks suitable for counselling. These figures assume that a careful search has been made for possible Mendelian causes, including fragile X syndrome (FRAXA). Exclusion of this disorder is essential, even in an isolated case of either sex, in view of its high frequency. Additional family information may modify the risk estimate. Thus, consanguinity in the parents increases the likelihood of autosomal recessive inheritance, giving an empiric risk of one in seven for sibs of such cases.

Where there are two affected sibs, a risk of close to one in four to future sibs is appropriate, regardless of sex, unless a pattern suggesting X linkage is present in previous generations.

Risks to offspring of affected individuals are not a significant problem in severe mental retardation; no estimate of risk can usually be deduced from the rare examples of reproduction

Table 14.1 Genetic risks in severe 'non-specific' mental retardation (IQ 50 or less)

Affected	Individual at risk	Risk
Isolated case, male or female	Sib (both sexes)	1 in 35
	Male sib	1 in 25
	Female sib	1 in 50
Two sibs, regardless of sex	Sib of either sex	1 in 4
Isolated case, male or female, parents consanguineous	Sib of either sex	1 in 7
Affected male with affected maternal uncle	Male sib	1 in 2 (X-linkage probable)
	Female sib	Low
One affected parent (either sex)	Child of either sex	1 in 10
One affected parent, affected child	Child of either sex	1 in 5
Two affected parents	Child of either sex	1 in 2

in such cases. However, the risk to second-degree relatives – the offspring of healthy individuals who have an affected sib or sibs – is a considerable worry to families. This is especially difficult to resolve where a healthy woman has an affected brother or brothers, a situation in which the possibility of X-linked inheritance must be seriously considered. If a maternally related affected male is also present in a previous generation, this is strong support for X linkage. Where the affected individuals are females, or females and males, an X-linked recessive basis is less likely, and risks for second-degree relatives are small. Third-degree relatives are unlikely to be at significant risk unless the family pattern is clearly X-linked, or unless there is a chromosomal rearrangement carried in balanced form.

Fragile X mental retardation (FRAXA)

Fragile X syndrome (type A) is a frequent cause of inherited mental retardation, with a frequency of around 1 in 4,000 in both males and females (lower than earlier estimates). Its recognition is crucial to genetic counselling and to giving accurate information to families who wish to avoid recurrence in future offspring. The delineation of its clinical and genetic basis and the recognition of the underlying molecular defect as a triplet repeat expansion disorder represent advances of the greatest importance.

At a clinical level, the degree of impairment varies from mild to severe, with males usually more severely affected than those mutation-carrying females who manifest the condition. Accelerated growth, characteristic facies and, in postpubertal males, macro-orchidism, are all valuable clinical signs (the Martin-Bell syndrome phenotype). The cytogenetically visible fragile site consists of a constriction near the end of the long arm of the X chromosome (Xq27), with the appearance of a partial detachment of the distal portion (the result of incomplete condensation of the chromosome in early meiosis, at the site of the repeat expansion).

The defect in this disorder is (in >99% of cases) an expansion in a specific DNA triplet repeat (CGG) in exon 1 of *FMR1*, a gene whose normal function is in mRNA transport within neurons. The size of the expansion relates to the degree of cognitive impairment and is usually progressive from one generation to the next. The CGG repeat is in the 5'UTR, not in the coding portion of the gene: the disease mechanism is quite distinct from the polyglutamine repeat disorders, such as Huntington's disease. There are usually about 30 CGG repeats in *FMR1*, with the normal range extending up to 44. A repeat count of more than ~55 repeats is termed a pre-mutation and more than 200–230 repeats is a full mutation, usually associated with methylation of the *FMR1* gene promoter and suppression of transcription (and hence with impaired synaptic function and cognitive impairment).

Rarely, the mutation is a point mutation or deletion elsewhere in the *FMR1* gene that may be missed by conventional testing. It must also be remembered that individuals may be mosaic for *either* the size of the mutation (e.g. pre-mutations and full mutation), perhaps in a tissue-specific fashion, *or* for methylation of the gene promoter, so that a few males who inherit a full mutation (>200–230 repeats) will retain some gene expression. They may be affected but in a milder and atypical fashion.

A minimal expansion, from 44 or 45 to 54 repeats, is termed an *intermediate allele* that may show instability at meiosis. Larger expansions are more unstable and full expansions are unstable at mitosis too, so that affected individuals often do not have a single size of expanded allele but a smear of fragments detected on Southern blot (too large to be detected reliably on polymerase chain reaction).

Males with a pre-mutation will develop normally but will transmit the mutation to their daughters, who will all be carriers, though again usually clinically unaffected. Their offspring, however, have a high risk of severe cognitive impairment, owing to expansion of the triplet repeats, although some of their daughters will be clinically normal carriers, and some sons will be unaffected carriers of a pre-mutation. Whether or not a female carrier of a full mutation is affected depends largely upon the pattern of X-chromosome inactivation. For those female carriers who have affected brothers, those sons inheriting the mutation (50%) will almost all be affected, as will about a half of those daughters who are heterozygous for the mutation.

This accounts for the unusual shape of the family tree, with the condition being transmitted from 'apparently unaffected' males (i.e. with normal early development), once known as 'normal transmitting males', through their daughters to affect their grandchildren. The connection between two affected branches of a family may therefore be through one or more apparently unaffected males, who on testing will prove to carry a pre-mutation. This situation does not arise in any other X-linked disorder and is the result of the instability of the triplet repeat expansion that is the cause of the disorder.

Genetic testing can now assign each member of the family to a specific category, indicating the risks of being affected or transmitting the condition. It must be remembered, however, that pre-mutation carriers can develop health problems even though their intellectual development in childhood is unaffected. Male carriers of a pre-mutation, although not affected by the fragile X syndrome, are at risk of an adult-onset neurodegeneration known as the fragile X-associated tremor and ataxia syndrome (FXTAS) from ~50 years. The effects can also impact memory and motor executive functions. A majority of pre-mutation-carrying males above 80 years are likely to be affected to some degree. Fewer females are affected, and the effects are usually milder.

Female carriers of a pre-mutation (but not an intermediate allele) are also at risk of premature ovarian failure (with menopause sometimes occurring at less than 30 years) or primary ovarian insufficiency. It can be important and helpful for families to be aware of these potential problems; it is also important not to generate information about a child's pre-mutation status without good reason, as this may indicate a substantial risk of neurodegeneration in adult life and testing for this should be at the request of the mature individual and after appropriate counselling.

The possibility now exists of using the recent advances in DNA sequencing to screen for FRAXA (i.e. *FMR1* gene) expansions in the general population, such as in newborn or antenatal screening programmes. If treatments of established benefit were known, then newborn screening could indeed be helpful but the high frequency of intermediate and pre-mutation alleles has the potential to cause much confusion and distress. Antenatal screening to identify female carriers is also technically possible but, again, has several associated problems: (1) many carriers of small pre-mutations or intermediate alleles may be identified, for whom the health and reproductive implications will be unclear. From 100 repeats upwards, the chance of a pre-mutation expanding to a full mutation in the child is ~100%, but below that size the risk is less and expansion to a full mutation has occurred from alleles of <60 repeats. Intermediate alleles of 44 or 45 will often be stable but have been shown (rarely) to expand to full mutations in just two generational steps. Furthermore, in one antenatal clinic study, the frequency of pre-mutation carriers was >1 in 400 and of intermediate allele carriers was >1 in 150; (2) some 40% or so of female carriers of a full mutation will have some learning difficulties or a more serious cognitive impairment, and it may be difficult to address the issues of understanding and consent for this group; (3) there are as yet no clearly helpful treatments for affected children, so that the desired outcomes of such a programme will be difficult to define and to maximise. The chance of expansion from pre-mutation to full mutation may also be influenced by AGG repeats present within the array of CGG repeats. Until further experience has been obtained, it seems to the author to be preferable to concentrate on the complete identification of affected individuals and the offering of counselling and appropriate testing to their relatives rather than population screening.

It should be remembered that there are other fragile sites nearby on the X chromosome, FRAXE and FRAXF. Their association with mental retardation is much less strong. FRAXE is associated with learning difficulties rather than severe cognitive impairment, and there is doubt as to whether FRAXF causes cognitive impairment at all: it may be completely benign.

Other forms of X-linked mental retardation

Apart from a number of well-defined X-linked syndromes (see Box 14.1), there are numerous forms of non-specific (non-syndromic) X-linked mental retardation (XLMR) that are distinct from the fragile X disorder. Fortunately, molecular studies now allow this distinction to be made with confidence. Collectively, they are likely to account for around a third of the cases of XLMR. Family studies suggest as many as 50 different loci, many of which have been identified. With the complete exome or genome sequence now available as a clinical investigation, it is becoming more readily feasible to offer carrier testing and prenatal diagnosis within specific families. Indeed, this area is progressing rapidly, and many additional X-chromosome loci involved in cognition may be discovered.

Rett syndrome

Rett syndrome is a clinically distinctive, but until recently, poorly understood disorder, almost exclusively affecting females and almost always sporadic in occurrence. It is characterised by an active regression – the loss of acquired skills – after normal development for at least 6 months, often for longer, and usually a period of stagnation before the onset of regression. Affected girls may appear to show some autistic behaviours, especially during the period of regression. After this, they typically regain social contact, although continuing with hand stereotypies, and often develop other problems such as seizures, scoliosis and autonomic (respiratory and cardiac) instability. They often appear to be 'locked-in', wishing for contact but usually unable to communicate by speech or by using their hands. Eye-gaze tracking devices may prove to be very helpful in some girls in promoting communication and the making of decisions and in enabling the assessment of cognitive function.

The condition is determined by an X-linked dominant gene, *MECP2*. The mutation most often arises at spermatogenesis, which accounts for the female preponderance. Mutations that cause Rett syndrome in females will cause a more severe neonatal encephalopathy in the hemizygous state (i.e. in males), but we have no reason to suspect that it is lethal *in utero* for the hemizygous male.

There is some association between the precise mutation and the severity of the disease, but this is not very helpful prognostically as so much variation arises from differences in the pattern of X-chromosome inactivation. However, at the milder end of severity, those girls affected by the Zappella (or 'preserved speech') variant, often have the R133C mutation or a deletion towards the 3′ end of the gene. The name for this variant form is somewhat misleading as ambulation and some hand use are more often preserved than functionally useful speech.

Males may be affected by Rett syndrome if, like most affected females, they are functionally mosaic for *MECP2* expression, that is, if they have Klinefelter's syndrome or if they are mosaic for the mutation (if it has arisen as a post-zygotic event). 'Milder' mutations in *MECP2,* that do not cause Rett syndrome in girls, will sometimes cause XLMR in males, transmitted by female carriers who are usually unaffected. The exceptional females, who carry a Rett-causing mutation in *MECP2* but who are unaffected, usually have marked skewing of X-chromosome inactivation in their leucocytes (as well as, presumably, their CNS). They have preferentially inactivated the chromosome that carries the mutated copy of the gene; they will be at high (50%) risk of having affected children.

The recurrence risk of Rett syndrome, when confirmed by *MECP2* mutation analysis and when the mother is known not to be a carrier, is that of gonadal mosaicism in either of the parents and is estimated to be ∼1%. The chance of recurrence in the children of an unaffected sister is remote.

Other neurodegenerative disorders must be carefully excluded before the diagnosis is made, especially if the diagnosis has not been confirmed through finding a pathogenic *MECP2* mutation. Rett syndrome may be confused clinically with Angelman syndrome, especially if the early history is not available, and some other Rett-like and Angelman-like disorders may also have overlapping clinical features. *CDKL5*-related disease causes a developmental disturbance with microcephaly, autistic behaviours and (often) a severe epileptic disorder. The epilepsy typically has onset within the first 6 months, may cause infantile spasms and, in the long term, is often resistant to treatment. Mutations in *FOXG1*, or deletions of chromosome 9 including or adjacent to the gene and recognised on aCGH, cause 'congenital-onset Rett syndrome'. This misnomer (it really is a contradiction in terms, as the early development of girls with Rett syndrome must, by definition, at least appear to have been normal) has many similarities to Rett syndrome except that there is no period of normal early development and it affects boys and girls equally.

Other distinct groups in 'non-specific' (non-syndromic) intellectual disability (mental retardation)

In addition to families showing X-linked inheritance, there are other groups with sufficient distinguishing features to give risk figures different from those in Table 14.1. A particularly high risk is that of symmetrical spasticity with mental retardation; here the recurrence in sibs seems to be around 10%, and more in the presence of consanguinity. By contrast, the recurrence risk for other forms of cerebral palsy associated with intellectual disability (cognitive impairment) is low, although these figures should preferably be applied only in cases with confirmed evidence of perinatal anoxia/asphyxia (see section on 'Cerebral Palsy').

Another important and mostly low-risk subgroup is that of intractable convulsions in infancy (infantile spasms; see later in this chapter), where many of the genetic causes typically arise as *de novo* dominant disorders. A similarly low risk has been found for mental retardation associated with slight microcephaly. This contrasts with the autosomal recessive inheritance of specific types of severe microcephaly with normal facial structure (see later in this chapter).

Mild cognitive impairment (learning difficulties)

It has already been stated that, in contrast to severe cognitive impairment (intellectual disability), mild cognitive impairment behaves as part of the normal distribution of intelligence, as a polygenic trait. One or both parents will commonly have a history of mild learning difficulties at school, and the intelligence of future children will usually be distributed between the mid-parental and general population mean. Correspondingly, the risk of an intelligent couple who have one child affected by mild cognitive impairment having a further affected child is low.

Nevertheless, a careful search should be made for specific causes that may underlie mild cognitive impairment and which, if found, may radically alter the genetic risks. The heterozygous state for the fragile X syndrome should be considered in females, especially if there is a history of more severely affected male relatives.

Normal intelligence

When faced with an enquiry about the inheritance of normal intelligence, the initial reaction of the physician, daily seeing patients with inherited causes of severe mental and physical handicap, is to tell parents to be content with the fact that their child is normal. Nevertheless, intelligence is undeniably an attribute of the highest importance and is not so completely under the control of the environment as some would wish to believe. The following general comments may be helpful if answering questions about families:

- The mating pattern is highly assortative for intelligence; intelligent people tend to marry each other, as do the less intelligent.
- On average, the intelligence of a child is likely to be intermediate between that of the parents (the mid-parental point) and the general population mean, with a considerable scatter around this.
- It is possible for the intelligence of a child to be outside this range; the greater the deviation, the less likely it will be.
- Too much reliance should not be placed on the results of single IQ tests, especially in early childhood. (One of our patients with Marfan syndrome, initially investigated in infancy for 'mental retardation', later studied astrophysics after winning scholarships to three separate universities.)

Current research attempts to identify specific genes involved in normal IQ do not seem, in our view, to have given proper consideration to the important societal issues involved and should only be pursued with public awareness and support. Perhaps fortunately, results so far support the polygenic model of the inheritance of IQ, and the genetic variants identified seem each to contribute only rather small amounts to the variance. Furthermore, the scope for complex interactions among genetic variants and between these variants and environmental factors is so great and so difficult to study (in humans) that it is most improbable that genetic testing to measure 'potential intelligence' will prove meaningful at an individual level (although that may not deter parental, institutional or commercial pressures from seeking or developing such tests).

BEHAVIOURAL DISORDERS AND SPECIFIC LEARNING DIFFICULTIES

Under the heading of behavioural disorders are grouped various abnormalities that cannot be regarded as diseases, but which may result in considerable functional disability. While long recognised as being frequently familial, studies to localise the genes are in progress, in relation both to the disorders and to normal function.

This, like the genetics of IQ, is a highly sensitive area, something that not all research workers in the field appear to appreciate. The social stigma often involved and the tendency for entrenched attitudes regarding the role of environmental and genetic factors add to the difficulties. At present, genetic counselling is rarely requested, but this could change if genetic tests become feasible, something that will present society, as well as professionals, with difficult issues. Any suggestions that specific genes identified in this group should be used for diagnosis or prediction should be viewed critically and with the greatest caution. There is sometimes too free an assumption of the functional equivalence of genes in the human and the mouse, for example, so that the basis of a human impairment may too readily be attributed to changes in the human homologue of a murine gene without any evidence for this in the human. The need for caution and even scepticism applies also to possible forensic applications (in a predisposition to criminality or violence). Perhaps fortunately, the genetic basis of common behavioural disorders is proving to be much more complex than previously anticipated and no genetic tests seem likely for the immediate future.

A further complexity relevant to genetic counselling is the increasing tendency to 'medicalise' the field by giving diagnostic labels to phenotypes that probably have a largely social basis. This dilutes any core of true medical disorders and makes family analyses more difficult. Some nutritional deficiencies, such as beriberi, used to be considered genetic because they often occurred in families; this should remind us to be cautious about these other, much more complex traits.

Dyslexia (specific reading disability)

The status of dyslexia as a diagnosis is sometimes misused so that, in clinical practice, it may be reduced to 'difficulty learning to read' with parents, schools and even psychologists forgetting that this should only be termed *dyslexia* if the child has very specific problems with reading while coping reasonably well with other aspects of learning. One must suspect that a child has a more general cognitive impairment if he or she is struggling with multiple areas of learning and is perhaps labelled as having a number of specific difficulties, such as dyslexia, dyspraxia, dyscalculia, attention deficit and challenging behaviour.

The alternative is that there is some other specific problem that may not be genetic at all but perhaps a difficult relationship within the family or with a teacher, or some unrecognised problem of physical health, neglect or abuse.

Once confident that a child does truly have dyslexia, this is probably best regarded as a disorder showing complex (multifactorial) inheritance with multiple genetic and environmental factors. Most of the recognised genetic factors associated with dyslexia are autosomal but some are on the X chromosome. Some reports have suggested that, if minor degrees are included, dyslexia may be transmitted as a variable autosomal dominant trait; this may be true in some unusual families, which could be of research interest.

Autism

This puzzling and undoubtedly heterogeneous condition requires considerable care in genetic counselling and should be regarded more as a label for a set of behaviours than as a single, specific diagnosis. Parents may benefit from an explanation that a diagnosis of autism and a diagnosis of a genetic condition can complement each other and do not cut across or conflict with each other: they simply derive from different domains of expertise and are of use in answering different questions or concerns. The genetic diagnosis refers to the underlying trigger of a set of problems that interfere with learning and communication and that, in their child, has resulted in behaviours described by psychologists as 'autism'. This term seems to be used popularly to cover a wide and sometimes poorly defined range of phenotypes, the autistic spectrum. The term *Asperger syndrome* may be used to cover the milder cases, in which there are patches of normal or even above-normal ability in someone who has problems in other areas, typically interpersonal communication and the recognition and expression of emotion.

It is essential to consider (and exclude) specific developmental disorders that may trigger such patterns of behaviour in any particular case, including minor chromosome anomalies, fragile X syndrome, Xp21-related muscular dystrophies and many other specific conditions that impact on neurodevelopment and which can present with 'autistic' features. Even though there is no clear Mendelian pattern, there is commonly a familial component, as judged from twin and family studies, with a significant (around 7%) recurrence risk for sibs of isolated cases. One parent may recognise that they have some behavioural or personality features that resemble those of their affected child; in that case, the chance of recurrence in the family may be higher but the severity may be more variable and often mild. When onset is abrupt, without family history, and when there are no associated dysmorphic features, a higher sib risk has been suggested, especially for males. If there are two affected siblings already, then the chance that another boy will be affected is much higher, perhaps as high as 50%, while the chance of a girl being affected is substantially lower.

The arrival of array-based chromosome studies and then exome analyses has identified *de novo* CNVs and loss-of-function mutations in plausibly relevant genes in perhaps 20%–25% of cases. Inherited, familial factors are also important and are now being identified, most notably the 'neurosusceptibility CNVs'. Research on these genetic factors will enable the better identification of important environmental and early life influences on neurodevelopment. To what extent genetic testing will be useful in the diagnosis or management of individual patients is still unclear, especially as an overlapping set of CNVs is also implicated in cognitive impairment and in schizophrenia. The question often arises as to why *this* child manifests *that* problem while another child with apparently the same CNV is unaffected or shows signs of a different condition. Much remains to be learned; in the long run, we can hope that this new (yet to be gained) knowledge will be useful in the treatment and prevention of these serious problems that can have such an adverse impact on human flourishing.

Tourette syndrome

Tourette syndrome, characterised by a childhood onset of motor and vocal tics, often with behavioural abnormalities, usually runs a fluctuating course and may be determined by a major autosomal dominant gene in some families. Several plausible candidate loci have been proposed in different families, but no likely unifying pathogenetic mechanism has yet emerged. This failure (so far), despite extensive study and some suggestive results, may reflect inadequate definition of the phenotype, over-diagnosis of the condition and a complex biology.

HEREDITARY ATAXIAS

Genetic heterogeneity and a previously confused classification of the hereditary ataxias are now being resolved with molecular advances. Careful family documentation and clinical assessment allow accurate information to be provided in genetic counselling in most cases, even when the diagnosis remains uncertain. The following broad framework is a starting point:

- Hereditary ataxia may form part of a generalised syndrome. Over 50 such syndromes have been identified, many from a single family.
- Classic Friedreich ataxia, with absent reflexes due to demyelinating neuropathy, cardiac involvement and early onset, is autosomal recessive, and the risk for offspring of affected individuals is minimal in the absence of consanguinity. The gene has been isolated and the mutation found to be a trinucleotide repeat expansion, but this is not in the coding region of the gene but is intronic, in contrast to the dominant ataxias. Prenatal diagnosis is now feasible.
- Other ataxias with congenital or childhood onset, a very heterogenous group, are generally autosomal recessive, including congenital cerebellar ataxia with aplasia of the vermis (Joubert syndrome) and ataxia telangiectasia. Metabolic causes must be excluded, and magnetic resonance imaging (MRI) of the cerebellum is important to detect or exclude structural defects.

A small number of patients will fail to fit into any of the previous groups, even after molecular studies. If the particular pattern of inheritance in the family is characteristic, this should be the basis for counselling. For isolated cases, it is wise to assume autosomal dominant inheritance for adult cases unless there is evidence to the contrary.

Other movement disorders are considered in Chapter 15. Of these, *hereditary benign chorea* is usually of early onset, and the dystonias can also present in childhood. This is especially true of *primary torsion dystonia* and *dopamine-responsive dystonia*. Some metabolic disorders will often present in childhood, including Lesch-Nyhan syndrome (X-linked recessive) and also Wilson disease (autosomal recessive).

NEUROFIBROMATOSIS

Several forms of neurofibromatosis can be distinguished, much the most common being type I (von Recklinghausen disease). Inheritance is autosomal dominant, with new mutations representing one-quarter to one-half of all cases. Careful examination of apparently healthy family members is essential before pronouncing them to be unaffected. The presence of six or more pigmented spots over 1.5 cm in diameter and of the characteristic appearance is an indication that the gene is present. Young children frequently show only inconspicuous signs of the disorder, but careful examination can often detect signs by the age of 1 year and, if no signs have developed, exclude it with confidence by the age of 5 years. Lisch nodules (harmless hamartomatous lesions of the iris) are a helpful confirmatory clinical sign, although not always present.

This condition affects 1 in 2,000 to 3,000 with up to half arising *de novo* as new mutations. There is no evidence that particular families with neurofibromatosis are free from serious effects although particular individuals can be more or less severely affected, and some mutations are generally more severe in their effects than others. Most surveys have shown that around one-third of affected individuals have one or more serious medical problems at some stage in life (including benign CNS tumours or extra-CNS malignancies that require active treatment, serious orthopaedic complications, epilepsy, moderate or severe learning disability), while two-thirds are mildly affected; about one-half have mild learning difficulties. The *NF1* gene produces an important protein (neurofibromin) regulating cell division and differentiation. A wide variety of different mutations can occur in this large gene, but the clinical utility of molecular confirmation is limited unless there is persistent doubt about the diagnosis, which in practice is usually made on clinical grounds. Molecular diagnosis is likely to become more important as rational treatments are developed.

One small but important subgroup of NF1 is Watson syndrome, when those affected have a pathogenic variant in NF1 but show features of Noonan syndrome as well as NF1. This emphasises the functional relationship between NF1 and the other 'RASopathies', in which the same cell-signalling pathway is affected.

A more severe phenotype is often found in those whose mutation is a whole gene deletion of NF1. A milder variant is caused by a specific 3 bp deletion and typically causes cafe-au-lait patches but very few tumours. NF1 is also milder when it is segmental, arising by somatic mutation, but any affected children of such a parent will be fully affected. An important differential diagnosis of NF1 is Legius syndrome, caused by mutations in SPRED1, in which skin pigmentation and other features are found but in which Lisch nodules and tumours are unlikely to develop.

Surveillance for the complications of NF1 is very important, especially in childhood and in the more severely affected adults, and patients should know who is coordinating this for them. This should include an assessment every 6 months in childhood, annually in adults, with a check on symptoms, on skin features, on blood pressure and vision, and (in children and adolescents) assessment of the spine. Referral to a specialist NF1 clinic is important in managing unfamiliar problems and severe cases. Women with some (activating) mutations in the *NF1* gene are also at modestly increased risk of breast cancer.

For all those affected, regardless of the severity of the medical aspects of the disorder, the social impact – especially the stigmatisation triggered by the cutaneous neurofibromata, and perhaps a plexiform neurofibroma – can have a major and pervasive impact on their quality of life. This stigmatisation can be exacerbated still further for a child who also has learning disability or any behavioural problems.

NF2 (bilateral acoustic or central) neurofibromatosis is a separate, much rarer dominantly inherited abnormality, which also produces multiple schwannomas and meningiomas, with characteristic lens opacities, but has relatively few skin lesions. The first affected in a family may be mosaic for the condition and will then typically have a milder clinical course. Surveillance for tumours on the VIII nerve by audiology and imaging is important. (See Chapter 32.)

VON HIPPEL-LINDAU SYNDROME

Von Hippel-Lindau syndrome is characterised by haemangiomatous cysts and tumours of the retina, brain (especially the cerebellum), kidney and other viscera. Inheritance is autosomal dominant. Penetrance is age dependent, so apparently unaffected members require periodic medical review from early childhood and cannot be completely reassured until late in adult life. Renal ultrasonography, MRI brain scan and ophthalmological assessment are essential. The need for recurrent assessment of both patients and relatives makes this disorder (like other familial tumour syndromes) especially suitable for a genetic register, which can be used to coordinate the management of those at risk. The gene is located on chromosome 3, and mutations can be found in almost all affected individuals (note that more than 25% of mutations will be missed by simple Sanger sequencing without dosage analysis). This enables the genetic testing of relatives, so that those without the mutation can avoid the need for ongoing surveillance.

TUBEROUS (TUBEROSE) SCLEROSIS

Tuberous sclerosis, or tuberous sclerosis complex (TSC), follows autosomal dominant inheritance but can cause problems in genetic counselling because of its extreme variability. Some of the skin lesions (multiple hypopigmented patches, facial angiofibromas, shagreen patches, peri- and subungual fibromas and fibrous cephalic plaques) may be the only abnormalities present in some patients, while most develop epilepsy, and some have severe intellectual disability. MRI is particularly helpful in showing intracerebral involvement. Many patients have renal angiomyolipomas and/or cysts, and affected females may develop lung involvement with lymphangioleiomyomatosis. Affected infants may have cardiac tumours (rhabdomyomas) that are now detected frequently on antenatal ultrasound scan leading to unexpected prenatal diagnosis in many cases. The birth of a severely affected child to a mildly affected parent cannot be excluded. Mosaicism is one mechanism through which a mildly affected parent may have children who are more severely affected than they are.

About 60% of cases appear to represent new mutations, in which case the risks of recurrence in future children of clinically normal parents will be small, although the possibility of parental (germ-line ± somatic) mosaicism leaves a small residual risk (around 1%–2%). Careful study of parents is warranted for accurate genetic counselling, even when their own genetic blood tests for the causative genetic variant in their affected child prove normal. Examination of the skin under ultraviolet light for hypopigmented patches and, if doubt exists, brain MRI scans and renal ultrasonography or MRI should be considered where future reproductive risks are a concern.

Two TSC-associated tumour suppressor genes on chromosomes 9 and 16, *TSC1* and *TSC2*, have been identified, allowing molecular confirmation in most cases. All manifestations of TSC are more severe, on average, in patients with *TSC2*, although a small number of specific *TSC2* variants are associated with a consistently mild phenotype. Some *TSC2* patients may also have involvement of the adjacent polycystic kidney disease gene (*PKD1*) in a contiguous gene deletion syndrome (see Chapter 24), and these patients usually have serious polycystic renal disease.

Understanding the intracellular mechanisms of TSC has enabled the development of a rational, targeted approach to treatment using inhibitors of mammalian or mechanistic target of rapamycin, mTOR. These agents are now recommended by international guidelines and licensed in several countries for treatment of renal and brain tumours, lung involvement and epilepsy in TSC.

Glioma

Although the conditions previously described and others may be associated with the development of gliomas, the risk to relatives of a sporadic and non-syndromic case is minimal, whether occurring in adult life or in childhood.

EPILEPSY

About one person in 20 has an epileptic attack at some time, while the prevalence of recurrent epileptic attacks is around 1% in North America and is probably similar in the United Kingdom. The chance that the child or sibling of someone with epilepsy, all types considered together, will also have or develop epilepsy is of the order of 2%–5%.

Seizures may be secondary to a variety of environmental or hereditary disorders, in which case the primary cause is the determining factor for genetic risks. In neonates, the major cause of seizures is hypoxic-ischaemic encephalopathy, although that explanation should never be accepted without interrogation of the circumstances, and metabolic causes are also of major importance. Later, head injury and infection may precipitate seizures.

Some forms of primary epilepsy have a major genetic contribution but only about 1% of epilepsy is Mendelian. Specific genes have not been recognised as strongly causal in common primary, generalised, 'idiopathic' epilepsy, which appears to have a complex causation to which the genetic contribution is usually oligogenic rather than monogenic. In contrast, many of the relevant genes have now been identified for some of the less common Mendelian types that are proving to be due to mutation in genes encoding ion-channel components, including *SCN1A* in Dravet syndrome. A wide range of autosomal dominant, usually *de novo,* gene mutations has been identified in the infantile epileptic encephalopathies, that overlap with the genes implicated in other severe neurodevelopmental disorders and with the cortical malformations (including neuronal migration disorders). A number of CNVs apparent on chromosome microarray studies – the neurosusceptibility loci, including deletions at 15q11.2, 15q13.3 and 16p13.11 – are associated with seizures, in addition to their association with cognitive problems, autistic spectrum disorders and schizophrenia.

The focus of research on the channelopathies has drawn attention to the pathogenetic parallels among the excitable tissues. Very similar mutations in very similar genes can affect neurons in the CNS, neurons in the peripheral nervous system and muscle, including the heart. The possibility of syncope as a cause of 'seizures' must often be considered and, usually, excluded. Mutations in the sodium channel genes and GABA-receptor genes are known to account for many of the Mendelian epilepsy disorders. It is interesting that the genotype-phenotype relationships are proving complex, with different mutations in one gene resulting in clinically distinct disorders. There is no neat correspondence between clinical phenotype and locus. Fortunately, the advent of gene panels has been most helpful in permitting diagnoses to be made effectively, while minimising the number of variants of uncertain significance results and incidental findings.

Simple absence epilepsy

When accompanied by the typical 'spike and wave' electroencephalographic (EEG) pattern, this type of epilepsy is often caused by mutation in a major gene following autosomal dominant inheritance. Close to 50% of first-degree relatives show the EEG defect when studied in adolescence, but penetrance is much reduced in both early childhood and adult life. A number of loci have been implicated in this type of epilepsy. Not all those with an abnormal EEG have clinical attacks; the empirical risk for sibs is around 6%.

Febrile convulsions

These are extremely common in the general population (2%–7% in various studies). The risk to sibs is increased threefold (8%–29%), the highest figures coming from Japan. Febrile seizures can be a feature of some Mendelian epilepsy syndromes, including mutations in SCN1A, but this is rare.

Benign neonatal convulsions

Although most cases are sporadic, a clear autosomal dominant form is relatively frequent, with the two principal genes coding for potassium channel components. Convulsions cease after infancy in around 90% of patients, and development is usually normal.

Infantile epileptic encephalopathy and infantile spasms

Infantile spasms may occur with or without encephalopathy, at times with devastating outcome, but are rarely familial (recurrence risk for sibs around 2%), provided that underlying conditions such as tuberous sclerosis or metabolic disorders have been ruled out. This is a group that requires expert diagnosis and management. MRI and EEG are especially important, in showing features that may be characteristic of an environmental cause or one of the rare genetic causes. A few very rare types respond to specific treatment (e.g. biotinidase deficiency, pyridoxine sensitive seizures and folinic-acid responsive seizures; all being autosomal recessive).

A persisting and severe epileptic encephalopathy may have many different causes. Among those with an underlying genetic basis, there is a wide range of genes that can be involved. There are two X-chromosome genes to mention, *ARX* and *CDKL5*, and three autosomal dominant genes, *SCN1A*, *STXBP1* and *GRIN2A*, to single out as especially important. The phenotypes associated with *SCN1A* constitute a wide range of clinical disorders, from 'benign' febrile seizures in young children, often familial, to Dravet syndrome, that often begins with severe febrile seizures at ~6 months and then leads into a severe lifelong epilepsy disorder that changes in character, is difficult to treat and is not usually passed to children because patients are unlikely to reproduce. Also difficult to treat is the lifelong epileptic disorder that can result from mutations in *CDKL5*, most often affecting girls and often also causing microcephaly, autism and spasticity and sharing some behavioural features with Rett syndrome. *ARX* mutations will often cause infantile spasms, like *CDKL5* mutations, and are also known as a cause of lissencephaly. Pathogenic variants in *STXBP1* are an important cause of the Ohtahara syndrome. Different mutations in *GRIN2A* may have different effects on the function of the NMDA receptor and may respond best to different treatments. The potential for such a rational approach to therapeutics is one of the eagerly anticipated benefits of molecular precision diagnostics in the channelopathies. However, this will not be as straightforward as 'one drug for (seizures caused by) one gene'.

Myoclonic epilepsy

Rare progressive cases may form part of general neurodegenerative disorders, usually autosomal recessive and sometimes showing tonic-clonic seizures as well as myoclonus with and without seizures. Numerous genes involved in this heterogeneous group of disorders have been identified, and myoclonus may be a feature of a range of other disorders including storage disorders (e.g. sialidosis, Gaucher disease, Niemann-Pick disease) as well as mitochondrial disease (MERRF) and juvenile Huntington's disease.

Juvenile myoclonic epilepsy often has onset in the second decade and is usually benign; a variety of genes is recognised as contributing.

Partial benign epilepsy of childhood

Partial benign epilepsy of childhood is a variable disorder that may follow an autosomal dominant pattern. The prognosis is good with appropriate treatment.

Table 14.2 Genetic risks in idiopathic epilepsy

Individual affected	Cumulative risk of clinical epilepsy up to age 20 years (febrile convulsions excluded) (%)
Monozygotic twin	60 (approximately)
Dizygotic twin	10 (approximately)
Sib	
Onset <10 years	6
Onset <25 years	1–2
Overall	2.5
Parent	4
Parent and sib	10 (approximately)
Both parents	15 (approximately)
General population (variable)	1

Primary idiopathic generalised epilepsy

Numerous surveys of primary idiopathic epilepsy have been carried out, with diverging results, probably depending on the severity of disease in the patients studied and on the social attitudes at the time. Most of the studies were done more than two decades ago and, although they included massive numbers, the earlier ones did not have the benefit of EEG classification or molecular diagnostics.

More recent studies have shown both higher population frequencies and higher risks to relatives, partly as a result of using the cumulative incidence of epilepsy rather than the prevalence.

The risks given in Table 14.2 reflect these higher estimates for both relatives and controls and represent the cumulative risk of epilepsy up to the age of 20 years. The relationship between risk to sibs and age at onset in the proband should be noted. In giving the risks for offspring, the possible teratogenic effects of antiepileptic drugs must be remembered. These are likely to be as important as, or more important than, the risks of genetic transmission (see Chapter 28). It is possible that current pharmacogenetic research may prove helpful in improving control by antiepileptic drugs and in minimising side effects.

CEREBRAL PALSY

A diagnosis of cerebral palsy should be mistrusted. All too often it merely camouflages ignorance of a variety of neurological disorders, some of which are genetic. The question to be asked first is whether sufficient evidence of perinatal anoxia, prematurity or other factors exists to explain the observed clinical problems, which may require access to the mother's maternity notes and the neonatal intensive care unit records:

- If the answer is 'yes', then genetic risks are likely to be small, although it must be remembered that an underlying genetic disorder could compromise neonatal respiratory function and predispose to asphyxia.
- If the answer is 'no', then one should ask whether sufficient investigation has been done to identify any specific primary neurological disorder, such as familial spastic paraplegia (see Chapter 15).

The problem lies less with newly diagnosed patients, carefully studied in a good centre, than with those families in which a relative in a previous generation has been labelled as having 'cerebral palsy' with little or no investigation. It may be necessary to reassess the original patient if accurate genetic counselling is to be given.

One early but thorough British study showed an overall recurrence risk of only 1%, but as environmental factors have been greatly reduced with good perinatal care, it is likely that genetic risks for more recent cases have increased. Several subgroups have been noted to have a higher risk, notably congenital ataxia and symmetrical tetraplegia occurring without definite external cause. In both of these conditions, the recurrence risk is about 10%–12% for sibs, which includes a number of recessive disorders such as Joubert syndrome (see earlier) and disequilibrium syndrome. The athetoid type, formerly associated strongly with kernicterus due to Rhesus haemolytic disease, may also have a largely genetic basis when no external factors exist, in which case a similar recurrence risk is appropriate. We do not have adequate figures for offspring risk in any of the groups, except where a specific genetic diagnosis has been established.

NEURAL TUBE DEFECTS

Despite much work and many hypotheses, the aetiology of neural tube defects remains incompletely understood. Their incidence varies greatly even within restricted geographical areas, and it is recognised that a high proportion of affected foetuses are lost as spontaneous abortions. Nutritional factors, notably folic acid deficiency, form an important environmental component; genetic factors may prove to involve folate metabolism (e.g. the gene *MTHFR*) in addition to other factors. Segmental developmental genes (see Chapter 6) do not seem to play a major role outside specific syndromes, and no clearly Mendelian subset has been defined.

Neural tube defects may occur as part of chromosomal and other severe malformation syndromes, including the recessively inherited Meckel syndrome (see later in this chapter). There is an increased frequency in association with congenital heart disease, diaphragmatic aplasia and oesophageal atresia.

All studies agree that anencephaly and spina bifida are closely related genetically and in pathogenesis. It is essential that this is indicated to families seen for genetic counselling, because a high risk of recurrence of the invariably fatal anencephaly is acceptable to some, whereas a surviving but handicapped child with spina bifida might not be. In general, the recurrence risk is equally distributed for anencephaly and spina bifida, regardless of which condition the index case had. The possibility that low sacral lesions form a separate group is still debatable.

The recurrence risks for neural tube defects are summarised in Table 14.3. The sex of the index case or individual at risk does not appear to alter the risks greatly. A detectable increase in risk is not seen for a relationship more distant than first cousins. The 5% risk for sibs given in early editions of this book is probably now an overestimate in light of the marked fall in incidence in recent years. Where accurate recent incidence data are available, a risk of 10 times the incidence is a reasonable one. In a previously high-incidence area such as Wales, where neural tube defects (anencephaly plus spina bifida) used to affect 1% of live births but have affected only 13.5 per 10,000 total births over the past two decades (or 15.6 per 10,000 total births, if including encephalocoele; data from the Congenital Anomaly Register and Information Service, CARIS), one could suggest the risk of recurrence after one affected foetus or infant of less than 2%, in the absence of syndromic features or chromosomal anomaly.

Table 14.3 Anencephaly and spina bifida: Approximate recurrence risks (percent) in relation to population incidence

Individual affected	Population incidence		
	1/200	1/500	1/1,000
One sib	5	3	2
Two sibs	12	10	10
One second-degree relative (uncle/aunt or half-sib)	2	1	1
One third-degree relative	1	0.5–1	0.5
One parent	4	4	4

The situation for families at risk has been completely changed by both screening and prevention. The widespread use of prenatal diagnosis was originally based on amniotic fluid α-fetoprotein (AFP) and acetylcholinesterase assessments and has now been largely superseded by high-resolution ultrasound scan (see Chapter 9). These will detect virtually all subsequent cases of anencephaly and at least 90% of cases of spina bifida, those undetected being covered defects or small open ones. Thus, the risk of an undetected, serious neural tube defect in the offspring of a couple with an affected child is extremely low. Prevention of recurrence by high-dose folic acid (5 mg/day) from before conception and up to the 12th week of gestation is very helpful in reducing the risk of recurrence in this group. (A lower dose is recommended to other women planning a pregnancy.)

The use of maternal serum AFP assay as a screening test for all pregnancies in the detection of neural tube defects was adopted in many areas of high incidence, and this led to its use also in screening for Down syndrome, while high-resolution ultrasonography is now comparably sensitive in detecting open neural tube defects, provided that the operator is experienced (not always the case) and has adequate time to conduct the scan. As discussed in Chapter 9, it is now possible to detect almost all cases of anencephaly and over 90% of cases of open spina bifida in this way, although the organisational and social aspects of such a screening approach are considerable (see Chapter 34).

Data are now available for the offspring of patients affected with spina bifida and show a risk of around 3%–4% regardless of which parent is affected. Amniocentesis and careful ultrasound screening should be offered for such pregnancies. No increase in other abnormalities has been noted.

The primary prevention of neural tube defects has been greatly helped by the finding that preconceptional folic acid supplementation reduces the recurrence risk for women with one affected child to a maximum of 1%. General population supplementation of flour and other foodstuffs is now widespread. It seems likely that reduction of population incidence as a result of such measures is greatest in areas of high incidence, where defective nutrition has been particularly marked, but uptake of preconception folic acid supplements by those planning a pregnancy in the general population has been disappointing.

Spina bifida occulta

Spina bifida occulta is a term applied both to individuals with spinal dysraphism, showing a significant spinal defect, usually lumbosacral and often associated with a pigmented or hairy patch of skin, and to individuals with radiological absence of one or two vertebral arches, without a visible lesion, usually discovered incidentally following radiography for backache or other unrelated symptoms (sometimes termed 'uncomplicated spina bifida'). The first group shows an increased incidence of overt neural tube defects in their offspring and sibs, with a risk similar to that for overt spina bifida, and it is reasonable to suggest they take higher-dose folic acid and offer them careful ultrasound scanning. The second group, amounting to around 5% of the general population, shows no evidence of any increased risk, and it is unfortunate that the term 'spina bifida' is used at all here, as women aware that they have this variant may be seriously alarmed at the possibility of clinical spina bifida occurring in their children. Fortunately, ultrasound scans can offer an effective test to all women who wish to have this possibility investigated.

HYDROCEPHALUS

Hydrocephalus frequently accompanies spina bifida, and a careful check should be made before assuming that hydrocephalus is an isolated and primary phenomenon. The great majority of families do not follow a Mendelian pattern; an X-linked type with aqueduct stenosis exists but is extremely rare, and counselling as for an X-linked trait should only be given if the pedigree pattern is clearly X-linked or if the other characteristic features of this type are present. Mutations have been shown in this form in the *L1CAM* gene, involving a neural cell adhesion protein. The general recurrence risk for sibs of an isolated case of hydrocephalus is 1%–2%, 4%–5% for male sibs of an isolated male case, and around 8% where two sibs are affected. Where an isolated male case is due to aqueduct stenosis, the risk to male sibs has been shown to be somewhat higher, possibly 5%–10%, although this figure may be an overestimate.

Ultrasound scanning is now able to detect some cases of hydrocephalus in early pregnancy, especially early developing types accompanying spina bifida, and the severe hydranencephaly, for which the recurrence risk is similar to hydrocephalus, unless syndromal. In other cases, though, hydrocephalus may not develop until later in pregnancy. The Walker-Warburg syndrome, with associated retinal changes, is a rare autosomal recessive cause of hydrocephalus, as is the hydrolethalus syndrome. The combination of enlarged fourth ventricle (sometimes with more general hydrocephalus) with aplasia or hypoplasia of the cerebellar vermis (Dandy-Walker complex) may be part of several more general disorders, but otherwise recurrence risks are similar to those in isolated hydrocephalus.

OTHER STRUCTURAL MALFORMATIONS OF THE CNS

Encephalocele

Encephalocele should probably be regarded as part of the anencephaly–spina bifida complex and risks given as such. An important association to recognise is the autosomal recessive Meckel syndrome, in which encephalocele and hypoplasia of the olfactory lobes are accompanied by a variety of other malformations, notably cleft lip or palate, polydactyly, renal cystic disease and eye defects (coloboma, cataract, microphthalmos).

Microcephaly

This diagnosis is best restricted to individuals whose head circumference is more than two standard deviations below the mean. The obvious but poorly resolved heterogeneity present in microcephaly, together with its severe consequences and high overall recurrence risk, makes this a particularly difficult area for genetic counselling. The book by Baraitser listed in Appendix 1 (see especially pp. 17–18), although now rather dated, provides some valuable cautionary notes. Fortunately, the identification of specific genes for some of the recessive types of microcephaly is helping to unravel this complexity.

Microcephaly may result from a variety of intrauterine factors. Congenital infections include TORCH (an acronym for toxoplasma, rubella, cytomegalovirus, herpes and other, now including the Zika virus), and there are chemical teratogens to enquire about and maternal phenylketonuria to consider. It may also be part of many genetic malformation syndromes, including the more severe autosomal trisomies and deletions, and is a striking feature of the autosomal recessive Seckel syndrome. Another important diagnosis to be considered is the very variable autosomal recessive Smith-Lemli-Opitz syndrome. Occasional mild forms of microcephaly inherited as a dominant trait have been recorded. Isolated severe microcephaly with a normal facial structure is often inherited as an autosomal recessive; the overall recurrence risk has been 10%–20% in different studies. Numerous specific genes have now been identified. Where no specific cause can be found, a recurrence risk of 10%–15% is appropriate, but a risk of close to 25% should be used if consanguinity is present.

Ultrasound monitoring can be offered in a pregnancy at risk for the severe forms, but recognition is not always possible until late in pregnancy.

Macrocephaly

Macrocephaly (to be distinguished from hydrocephalus) may be part of a neurological disorder (e.g. neurofibromatosis, various cerebral degenerations), or part of a more general growth disorder (e.g. Sotos syndrome and the *PTEN*/Cowden syndrome, with some risk of malignancy, and others), or an isolated feature usually not associated with serious consequences, and commonly autosomal dominant. It may sometimes be associated with autism. Fragile X syndrome should also be considered as a possible cause in the presence of intellectual disability.

Holoprosencephaly

In holoprosencephaly there is a variable failure of development of the forebrain with associated facial features. It is usually lethal, especially the extreme forms of cebocephaly and cyclopia. More minor forms may occur though; an external indicator may be the presence of fused central incisor teeth (the 'single central incisor'). The condition may be isolated, or it may be part of trisomy 13. Apart from Meckel syndrome (see earlier), other cases of autosomal recessive inheritance have been reported, as well as occasional dominant inheritance with a very mildly affected parent, so caution, chromosome analysis and thorough pathology after death are needed. The frequency is considerably increased in maternal diabetes. The recurrence risk after an isolated non-syndromal case is relatively low (4%–5%). The human counterpart of a specific *Drosophila* developmental gene (*SHH* on chromosome 7q) shows mutations in some dominantly inherited cases.

Lissencephaly and related neuronal migration defects

This group contains various disorders affecting cerebral gyral development, including microdeletions of chromosome 17p (Miller-Dieker syndrome), classical 'type 1' lissencephaly involving specific genes in the same 17p region, and an important X-linked type, with female 'carriers' of mutations in the filamin A gene often showing subcortical band heterotopia and some having mild intellectual problems and epilepsy. It is important to base a specific diagnosis on a combination of neuroradiological, molecular and clinical criteria. The Walker-Warburg syndrome and the related muscle-eye-brain disease include lissencephaly and cerebellar hypoplasia along with a congenital muscular dystrophy and eye anomalies.

Sib recurrence risk is around 7% when specific causes have been carefully excluded. Older diagnoses in this heterogenous group should be reassessed, as a more specific and accurate diagnosis with molecular confirmation may well affect genetic counselling. The use of gene panels and/or exome studies leads to a much-improved chance of identifying the underlying cause of such cortical malformations.

Agenesis of the corpus callosum

This may occur as part of a more general cerebral maldevelopment, or it may be isolated. Most isolated cases have been sporadic, although occasional families following an apparently X-linked recessive pattern have been recorded. Aicardi syndrome is an X-linked dominant

Table 14.4 Degenerative metabolic disorders of the central nervous system (see also Chapter 26)

Disorder	Enzyme or molecular defect	Inheritance
Leucodystrophies		
Metachromatic leucodystrophy	Arylsulphatase A	AR
Adrenoleucodystrophy	Long-chain fatty acid defect	XR
Pelizaeus-Merzbacher disease	β-myelin protein	XR
Krabbe disease	β-Galactosidase	AR
Neuronal storage disease		
Gangliosidoses (including Tay-Sachs, Sandhoff diseases)	See Chapter 26	All AR
Infantile neuronal ceroid lipofuscinosis (including Batten disease)	Heterogeneous: several genes are known	AR
Juvenile and adult-onset lipofuscinosis	Heterogeneous: some genes are known; adult form can present with psychiatric symptoms and lead to cerebellar ataxia and dementia	Often AR, some AD
Canavan disease	Aspartoacylase	AR
Others		
Menkes disease	Copper metabolism	XR
Neuroaxonal dystrophy (previously known as Hallervorden-Spatz disease)	Pantothenate kinase (PANK2)	AR
Leigh encephalopathy (heterogeneous)	Pyruvate metabolism (some cases)	AR, also mitochondrial

Abbreviations: AD, autosomal dominant; AR, autosomal recessive; XR, X-linked recessive.

disorder associated with infantile spasms and patches of retinal pathology or a failure to develop (retinal lacunae). Its genetic basis remains uncertain, but it is almost always sporadic and affects females. It may be lethal to males *in utero* or, like Rett syndrome, it may result from mutations at spermatogenesis. Several syndromes with limb defects (acrocallosal, Neu-Laxova) are autosomal recessive.

Septo-optic dysplasia, with variable optic nerve and pituitary involvement, is generally sporadic.

SYRINGOMYELIA

Recurrence of syringomyelia in a family is unusual.

DEGENERATIVE METABOLIC DISORDERS OF THE CNS

Where degenerative metabolic disorders of the central nervous system are part of systemic metabolic conditions, these are considered in Chapter 26. An important group of disorders is largely confined to the nervous system (Table 14.4). Most are Mendelian, so that the recognition of a specific biochemical and/or molecular genetic diagnosis is of great importance for genetic counselling. Frozen tissue or stored cultured cells are often crucial where the only affected individuals are dead. The recognition of some genes, when the corresponding metabolic defect had been unknown until then, has proved especially fruitful both for genetic counselling (as with the recognition of mutation in CLN3 being the cause of Batten disease) and in efforts to work towards rational therapies.

15

Central nervous system: Adult-onset and psychiatric disorders

INTRODUCTION

The central nervous system (CNS) disorders of adult life considered here fall into two main groups: the neurodegenerative disorders and dementias, and another group, of the psychiatric disorders of adult life, that has intriguingly close aetiological links with neurodevelopmental disorders although these links remain ill defined.

The first category has provided much of the work of the genetic counselling clinic and the genetic diagnostic laboratory for many years, with both predictive and diagnostic testing for Huntington's disease (HD), for example, having been well established for nearly 30 years. Our ability to diagnose some of the other degenerative disorders is not so good, with the major problem of genetic heterogeneity only now being resolved as exome and genome sequencing identifies more of the responsible gene loci.

The second category – of psychiatric disease, especially schizophrenia – is different. These conditions are not, by and large, Mendelian disorders caused by single mutations in genes of major effect. However, schizophrenia often shares many underlying genetic factors with autism spectrum disorders and the non-Mendelian disorders of neurodevelopment. It is not always clear why one person develops autism, whereas someone else with at least some genetic factors in common develops schizophrenia or remains unaffected ('neurotypical'). As discussed in

Chapter 14, this topic is being addressed very actively. Identifying the genetic variants that influence risk of autism and schizophrenia, for example, provides an opportunity to dissect the environmental, early life and lifestyle factors that influence how the individual's genetic susceptibilities work out over the course of their life.

This convergence between psychiatric genetics research and clinical genetics stems from two principal factors: the genomic turn in genetic investigations and the development of rigorous diagnostic criteria for psychiatric disease that can help in the analysis of family data.

While predictive genetic testing for HD provides a steady flow of work in genetics services, the demand for genetic counselling in relation to psychiatric disease has been much less and generally remains small in relation to the burden of disease. A discussion of the range of factors involved in the causation of psychiatric disease – genetic, environmental and early life (including prenatal) experiences – may be helpful for families in its own right, even without the possibility of disease prediction, and referrals to clinical genetics to discuss psychiatric disorders may have been too few in the past so that the needs of families for understanding were neglected. However, as the factors influencing the onset and course of these diseases are clarified, this situation may change. There has already developed a prominent strand of genetic counselling research that focuses on psychiatric disease and attends to the polygenic model of inheritance and disease causation. As clinical practice builds on this model, especially to the extent that it begins to incorporate the results of genetic testing, we may see a move away from the vagueness of a 'purely polygenic' model to one in which risk-modifying variants in specific genes and *de novo* chromosome rearrangements (especially copy number variants [CNVs]) are relevant. Greater interest may then develop in genetic counselling and perhaps genetic testing for psychiatric disease. However, we must remember the great potential for harm from self-fulfilling prophecies.

My own perspective would be to encourage the *counselling* for risk of psychiatric disease, but I would recommend that we should all be wary of the *testing* for three principal reasons: (1) there will be pressure to over-interpret research findings as they emerge and to race ahead of what is warranted by the evidence; (2) those given test results still tend to understand them in a binary fashion – Yes or No – as they did when Abby Lippman conducted her research in the 1970s, but these results will require subtlety to interpret them appropriately. I doubt if human nature has changed much in the (almost) half-century since then, and there is a real danger that patients will suffer from an overly deterministic understanding of psychiatric disease that may arise from within them or that may be imposed on them by overly deterministic professionals; and (3) unlike HD, where a test result often is truly predictive but does not influence the onset of disease, genetic testing 'for' schizophrenia could plausibly be the reverse: it could fail to be really predictive but it could add to the stress or distress of a vulnerable individual so that it could play a part in triggering the onset or provoking further manifestations of the disease. Genetic testing might, in this context, become oracular (in the tradition of Delphi) and result in self-fulfilling prophecies.

HUNTINGTON'S DISEASE

HD, due to an expanded and unstable trinucleotide (CAG) repeat, represents one of the most difficult genetic counselling problems among the Mendelian disorders of adult life. The severe burden imposed on families both by the disease itself and the fear of it, the present inadequacy of preventive and therapeutic measures, and the very real possibility that hasty or insensitive genetic counselling or inappropriate testing may do more harm than good, all add to the difficulties. The advent of accurate molecular presymptomatic testing has provided a particular challenge in ensuring appropriate genetic counselling and support, and HD has become a model for presymptomatic testing in serious late-onset disorders overall. This is discussed further in Chapter 8.

Of course, the situation may change dramatically as soon as effective treatments become available, and current clinical trials as well as research on transgenic animals and cell implantation give good reason for (somewhat cautious) optimism 'in the long run'; we just do not know quite how long the run will prove to be.

HD, although regularly autosomal dominant in its inheritance, is variable in age of onset and in its presentation and clinical course; many of the difficulties in genetic counselling for HD arise from this. To advise affected individuals or their spouses that children have a 50% risk is arithmetically simple, but most individuals requiring advice are the healthy offspring themselves.

While molecular testing can now resolve whether a relative at risk carries the mutation, most people (~80%) decide against testing in advance of disease onset. In any event, it is vital that decisions regarding testing and other aspects are made in the context of an accurate general risk estimate. Fortunately, the careful use of all available genetic information and knowledge of the distribution of ages at onset can be of considerable help in this, as shown in Table 15.1. Although drawn up for a particular population, this table is of general application.

Figure 15.1 shows the more general risk curves for first-degree relatives, corresponding to the data shown in Table 15.1. Tabular data for second-degree relatives are summarised in Table 15.2. This information is especially valuable where a parent at risk has died relatively young but apparently healthy. Risk estimates for limited periods at different ages are also available (using Table 15.2) and may be useful in situations relating to employment or fostering and adoption. Figure 15.2 gives a practical example of how the use of age-modified risks can alter the situation for a second-degree relative.

A difficult question, not confined to HD, is to what extent ages at onset are correlated within families. The variation within a family and our understanding of the unstable nature of the mutation are such that, unless information is available from many members of one family, it is better to rely on the overall, population-derived curve. However, sibs of juvenile cases have passed through about half their risk by the age of 25 years and virtually all of it by the age of 40 years.

Juvenile HD is rare, but often unrecognised in its early stages. It is almost always paternally transmitted (the opposite to myotonic dystrophy) and results from large expansions (with allele size commonly of 60–100 repeats) in the HD gene. It often presents atypically, with general neurodegeneration and rigidity rather than chorea. Familial chorea occurring in childhood is unlikely to be due to HD, and other conditions such as benign hereditary chorea or one of the dystonias should be considered. Molecular testing must be handled with great caution if juvenile HD is suspected, and other possible causes ruled out first; otherwise presymptomatic detection of a mutation unrelated to the symptoms may inadvertently result. Thus, if a mutation with 80 or 90 repeats were found, that might well account for the child's symptoms, the early features of juvenile HD. If, however, the mutation had 42 repeats, for example, then it would not account for problems in a 9-year-old child and would amount to an unsought predictive test in a child already affected by a different neuropsychiatric disorder.

Isolated cases

Most isolated cases of HD prove, on careful investigation of living family members and records of previous generations, not to be isolated at all. In some cases, early death of parents and lack

Table 15.1 Risk for a healthy subject at 50% prior risk of Huntington's disease (HD) carrying the HD gene at different ages

Age (years)	Risk (%)
20.0	49.6
22.5	49.3
25.0	49.0
27.5	48.4
30.0	47.6
32.5	46.6
35.0	45.5
37.5	44.2
40.0	42.5
42.5	40.3
45.0	37.8
47.5	34.8
50.0	31.5
52.5	27.8
55.0	24.8
57.5	22.1
60.0	18.7
62.5	15.2
65.0	12.8
67.5	10.8
70.0	6.2
72.5	4.6

Source: From Harper PS, Newcombe RG. 1992. *J Med Genet* 29, 239–242.

of records make it impossible to exclude transmission of the disease, or paternity may be in doubt; but often a parent (usually the father) may have had a gene expansion in the borderline range giving no symptoms, but expanding in the next generation to give full HD. Most cases of progressive adult-onset chorea prove to be HD, and onset after the age of 60 years has proved to be more common than previously thought. Diagnostic molecular testing can now resolve the situation for most atypical or isolated cases, although autopsy should also be performed on such individuals to confirm the diagnosis, as well as on apparently unaffected relatives dying of other causes in order to exclude it. It is possible, however, for early clinically evident HD to show no neuropathological changes at all unless specialist neuropathology is sought, including techniques of cell counting.

Associated aspects

Calculating the risk of disease transmission is perhaps the least difficult task in the genetic counselling of families with HD. It is the range of more general problems that provides the challenge.

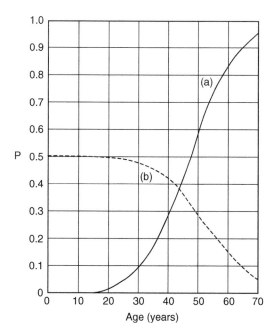

Figure 15.1 Probabilities (a) that an individual possessing the gene for Huntington's disease will have developed the disorder by a certain age, and (b) that the healthy child of an affected parent has the Huntington's disease gene at a particular age. (Based on Harper PS et al. 1979. *Lancet* ii: 346–349; with additional data provided by Dr Robert Newcombe.)

Table 15.2 Risk estimates (percentages) for second-degree relatives of a patient with Huntington's disease (HD): the residual risk of a healthy second-degree relative carrying the HD gene at various combinations of age for the individual and the intervening parent

Age of second-degree relative (years)	Age of parent (years)										
	20–	25–	30–	35–	40–	45–	50–	55–	60–	65–	70–
70–	1.6	1.5	1.5	1.4	1.2	1.0	0.8	0.6	0.4	0.3	0.1
65–	3.8	3.7	3.5	3.3	3.0	2.5	1.9	1.5	1.0	0.7	0.3
60–	5.6	5.4	5.2	4.9	4.3	3.7	2.8	2.2	1.5	1.0	0.4
55–	8.5	8.3	7.9	7.4	6.7	5.6	4.4	3.4	2.3	1.6	0.7
50–	11.2	10.9	10.5	9.8	8.9	7.5	5.8	4.6	3.1	2.1	0.9
45–	14.9	14.6	14.0	13.2	11.9	10.1	7.9	6.2	4.2	2.9	1.3
40–	18.1	17.8	17.0	16.1	14.6	12.5	9.8	7.7	5.3	3.7	1.6
35–	20.6	20.2	19.4	18.4	16.7	14.3	11.3	9.0	6.1	4.3	1.8
30–	22.2	21.8	20.9	19.9	18.1	15.5	12.3	9.8	6.7	4.7	2.0
25–	23.5	23.1	22.2	21.0	19.2	16.5	13.1	10.4	7.2	5.1	2.2
20–	24.2	23.7	22.8	21.7	19.7	17.0	13.6	10.8	7.4	5.2	2.3

Source: From Harper PS, Newcombe RG. 1992. *J Med Genet* 29, 239–242.
Note: Where the individual at risk has an affected grandparent, but the intervening parent is healthy, the risk can be found in the table from the age of the individual and the age of the parent at risk.

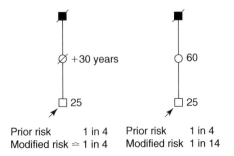

Figure 15.2 Use of age-modified risks for a second-degree relative in Huntington's disease.

In the past, ignorance of the genetic nature of the disorder was a major problem in relation to genetic counselling of those at risk for HD and, while there is no specific legal or professional duty to inform the wider family, the author believes that all adults at high risk have a right to know that they are at risk, preferably before having children. Some parents 'protect' their children from the knowledge well into adult life, with long-term consequences that are often disastrous for them, resulting in deep family discord. An increasingly open attitude to the disease, partly due to active lay groups, seems to be decreasing this problem, but increasing mobility of the population may be having an opposite effect in decreasing awareness of the family background.

Legal action is pushing in both directions: towards preserving genetic privacy and towards recognising the 'right' of family members to be given important information that may be relevant to their healthcare or reproduction. It is difficult to know how these contrary pressures will work out in different jurisdictions. While in the UK there is no specific legal or professional duty to inform the wider family, such an obligation does exist in France and, in the UK, legal developments (the 'ABC' case) may alter medical practice towards ensuring that important information is passed to family members. It would be most unhelpful if the obligation to pass confidential information to family members became primarily a legal obligation imposed on professionals rather than being seen as an ethical obligation that rested essentially on the families.

When the information should be given will vary from family to family, but the best time for the subject to be raised is probably by the early to mid-teens, or before this if the HD is clearly evident in family members or the child asks questions or matures early. It is possible – perhaps ideal – to begin a process of drip-feeding information earlier so that the child has an awareness that there is something to be discussed further when they are older. In this way, a more detailed discussion can arise 'naturally', when relationships and family are being planned, without this coming as a disruptive shock at this time.

It cannot be too strongly stressed that individuals at high risk for HD need support to help them cope with the information that they have been given. This is particularly the case when the disease is newly diagnosed in a family, or when the individuals concerned are being seen as part of an extended family investigation rather than having actively sought advice themselves. Wherever possible, the initial information should come from a responsible family member or sympathetic family doctor, with the genetics clinic providing the opportunity for a fuller and more independent discussion. Where this is not feasible (all too often), the clinician giving advice, whether neurologist or geneticist, must ensure that support is provided. There is no substitute for an experienced genetic counsellor or comparable professional in this respect, although support groups can also be most helpful. In the United Kingdom, the HD associations employ support workers and have established excellent support schemes specifically for teenagers and young persons at risk.

The confidentiality of records and registers, while important for all disorders, is a special problem in HD, as the information may be exceedingly damaging to prospects for careers or insurance. Such information must be severely restricted to clinicians directly involved with the family; access by others should not be allowed without the specific written consent of the individual concerned. This need for consent should include enquiries from other centres about living relatives, although it may be simpler to confirm that the individual seen at another centre is indeed at risk of HD without specifying who in the family is affected unless consent to share information with other family members had been obtained previously.

Reproductive options have increased since prenatal exclusion testing and specific prenatal diagnosis have become feasible (see later in this chapter), although these are used only by a minority of couples. For those who decide not to reproduce, it is important to find alternatives. Adoption is usually ruled out by the severity of the disorder, although adoption or fostering of an older child may be possible, based on a low risk of the disorder developing before such a child has become independent. Gamete donation (see Chapter 11) could potentially be a valuable option but has not been widely used so far. Pre-implantation diagnosis is also proving useful but is not a solution that will suit everyone.

Genetic testing for HD

Although genetic testing using linked markers was possible for almost a decade before the HD gene itself was isolated, the discovery of its specific molecular basis has greatly affected the practical aspects of testing, as well as increasing our understanding of the disease and its possible treatment.

HD results from the expansion of a trinucleotide repeat sequence in a specific gene. Most normal individuals have fewer than 27 repeats, while HD is associated with at least 36 repeats, and usually more than 40 repeats. Age at onset correlates (though only approximately) with repeat length, juvenile cases having the largest repeats (often 60–100) while late-onset cases may be close to the borderline. Those who inherit an allele of at least 40 repeats and live long enough will develop the disease, unless they die early for some other reason. For those who inherit 36–39 repeats, the disease will often develop, but it may be of late onset, and in some cases the individual may never develop the condition (these are reduced penetrance alleles). The estimates of penetrance of these alleles of 36–39 repeats have had to be revised downwards as the population frequencies of these reduced penetrance alleles have been found to be higher than anticipated from the disease incidence in several studies.

Those with an intermediate number of repeats, 27–35, will not develop the disease but the repeat number of that allele may be unstable at meiosis, so that it increases into the possibly or definitely affected range in succeeding generations. The instability of the expanded repeat gives a tendency for the mutation to increase and the disease onset to become earlier in successive generations (anticipation), especially when transmitted by males, although the expansion will sometimes shrink rather than expanding still further. When an intermediate allele is transmitted by a male, the risks of expansion into a disease-associated allele (a reduced penetrance or full penetrance allele) are about 10% when the allele has 35 repeats, about 1% for an allele of 34 repeats and otherwise well below 1%.

The repeat sequence (CAG) appears as polyglutamine in the protein (huntingtin) produced by the *HTT* gene associated with HD, and it is now clear that this has a direct effect on cellular pathology, which can be reproduced in transgenic mice and which is similar to that of other CAG repeat disorders such as the spinocerebellar ataxias. These major advances in understanding should lead to therapeutic possibilities, and active clinical trials are under way. Approaches to treatment include cell-based treatments, gene therapy or editing, and the selective suppression of the expanded allele.

The practical genetic consequences of these major advances are as follows:

- Essentially all cases of HD show the same mutational basis, so both diagnostic and presymptomatic testing can be performed with the same test, regardless of geographical origin or family structure.
- The presence of the mutation correlates very closely with neuropathology of HD. It is wise to ensure that either the mutation or typical neuropathology is present in an affected family member, although testing no longer depends on this.
- The number of repeats is too variable to be of any real use in predicting age of onset in an individual (except if it indicates that onset is likely to be in the juvenile range). Despite that, most laboratories report repeat size, and patients sometimes wish to know this. While ensuring that the significance of the repeat count is kept in perspective (i.e. downplayed), it may be difficult to avoid discussing these details. Table 15.3 sets out some relevant information that can be helpful in these discussions. It makes it very clear how wide the 95% confidence intervals are around the mean age of onset for most repeat counts.

Table 15.3 Extrapolated and approximate ages of onset of Huntington's disease related to the CAG trinucleotide (i.e. polyglutamine) repeat count, based on Langbehn et al. (2004) and subsequent publications

Repeat count	Remarks about penetrance at >65 years	Mean and standard deviation (SD) of age of onset (in years)	95% confidence interval of the age of onset (mean ±2 SD)
27–35	Non-penetrant but unstable transmission (especially from males) (see text)	N.A.	
36	Reduced penetrance (6%)	>70	
37	Reduced penetrance (10%)	>70	
38	Reduced penetrance	77 (approximately 20% penetrance)	
39	Reduced penetrance	69	
40	Almost fully penetrant	62 (12)	38–86
41	Fully penetrant	57 (11)	35–79
42	Fully penetrant	52 (10)	32–72
43	Fully penetrant	48 (9)	30–64
44	Fully penetrant	44 (8)	28–60
46	Fully penetrant	40 (8)	24–56
48	Fully penetrant	36 (8)	20–52
50	Fully penetrant	32 (7)	18–46
52	Fully penetrant	29 (7)	15–43
54	Fully penetrant	27 (6)	15–39
56	Fully penetrant	25 (5)	15–35
60+	Fully penetrant and usually juvenile onset		

- Data on the mean age of onset of HD, and its standard deviation, have been collected by Langbehn et al. (2004). The correct interpretation of that most helpful paper requires careful attention and time spent becoming familiar with how it lays out the information.
- Prenatal testing is feasible (though not commonly requested). This usually employs direct mutation testing although, if the at-risk parent has not already had predictive testing, an adverse result is a double blow.
- Pre-implantation genetic diagnosis is available in some centres (see Chapter 9). This is usually performed by linkage analysis to determine which grandparental haplotype has been transmitted because direct mutation detection can give misleading results from the analysis of only one or two single cells ('allele drop-out'). A variation on this enables prenatal exclusion testing. This is used to identify the grandparental origin of the chromosome inherited through the at-risk parent but without determining whether it is that grandparent's affected or unaffected chromosomal haplotype. See Figure 15.3. If the at-risk parent later has a negative predictive test, then they will realise that a pregnancy terminated as at high risk would have been unaffected. Conversely, if a high-risk pregnancy is continued and the parent develops HD, it becomes clear that their child will also carry the affected HD allele.

Specific mutation testing rapidly replaced indirect testing by linked markers, except in prenatal exclusion and pre-implantation testing, and there has now been extensive experience

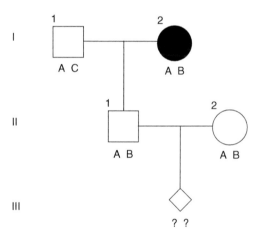

Figure 15.3 The use of haplotypes, each being a collection of single-nucleotide polymorphisms (SNPs) across the *HTT* gene summarised as a single letter. The at-risk parent has clearly inherited haplotype 'B' from the affected grandparent and haplotype 'A' from the healthy grandparent. This figure is being used to make two points: (i) Such testing can demonstrate which haplotype the foetus has inherited from the at-risk parent: the one from the at-risk grandparent or the healthy grandparent. Thus, if the foetus carries two 'B' haplotypes, it must have inherited the at-risk parent's high-risk copy of the *HTT* gene, the one from the affected grandparent (putting the fetus, like the parent, at a 50% risk of HD). If the parent proceeds to develop HD, then the child would be destined to do so too. Conversely, if the fetus has inherited two 'A' haplotypes, then the foetus will be at low risk, whether or not the parent develops the disease. (ii) If the fetus inherits one 'A' and one 'B' haplotype, it will not be possible to draw any conclusion. The situation is said to be uninformative. This does not happen often with haplotypes constructed from a large panel of many SNPs, but it could occasionally arise, especially if only a few SNPs are used.

with predictive testing by direct detection of the mutation (over 10,000 presymptomatic tests in the United Kingdom since 1993). Following are some of the main points:

- Presymptomatic testing for HD should only be performed within a framework of adequate preparation, information and support. Almost all centres use (at least) two separate interviews before giving results.
- Important information needing to be given, and to be considered with care, includes the implications of an abnormal test result (on the individuals tested and other members of their families, for relationships and for insurance, employment, etc.); information on the disorder itself (not all those being tested will have had personal experience of HD); sources of support; and approaches to coping with an abnormal result (see Chapter 8 for further discussion).
- Serious adverse reactions have so far been few and seem to reflect the nature of the individual rather than whether the result was abnormal or normal. This is probably because testing has been done cautiously, with ample opportunity for those who wish to change their mind before testing is done, rather than only realising the consequences afterwards.
- The reasons for requesting testing vary, but commonly involve the wish to resolve uncertainty and to remove risk from children, whether already born or planned for the future.
- It is generally agreed that presymptomatic testing of young children, requested by parents or occasionally by social workers or others, should not be carried out. The consensus view is that individuals have the right to decide for themselves, as adults. Requests from adolescents are few, and these need sensitive discussion before any decision is made.

It has become generally accepted that presymptomatic testing for HD is something that should be performed by the clinical genetics service, by clinical geneticists and/or genetic counsellors, in contrast to diagnostic testing of symptomatic individuals, which is becoming part of the practice of neurologists, psychiatrists and other involved clinicians. It is important that the difference between these two categories of genetic testing be fully appreciated (see Chapter 8, and also Chapter 5), as there are major practical considerations involved.

One issue in presymptomatic testing that has arisen since specific mutation analysis became possible is the testing of those at 25% risk; that is, individuals whose parent is at risk but healthy. If the mutation is detected in the younger generation, then this will imply that the parent also carries it and will probably be much closer to onset of the disease. How should one respond to such a request if the parent does not wish to be tested themselves, or does not know about their offspring's request? Fortunately, data from the United Kingdom and elsewhere show that such difficult scenarios are rare, probably because the situation is usually resolved by sensitive genetic counselling and the facilitation of family communication. In this area, and many others, HD not only highlights an issue that is relevant to presymptomatic testing in general, but also shows how important it is that presymptomatic testing is not isolated from the general genetic counselling process or regarded as an activity purely for the laboratory.

The points noted are equally relevant to the increasing number of other late-onset dominantly inherited neurological disorders where presymptomatic testing has become feasible. See Chapter 8 for further discussion.

PARKINSON'S DISEASE

Parkinsonian features (tremor, rigidity and bradykinesia) may occur in more general brain degenerations, such as frontotemporal and Lewy body dementias, prion disease, spinocerebellar ataxias, Wilson disease and others, including non-genetic disorders (post-encephalitic or drug-induced) and weakly genetic disorders (e.g. progressive supranuclear palsy).

Most cases of Parkinson's disease (PD) are primary rather than secondary to arteriosclerosis or encephalitis, and a prevalence of around 1 in 10,000 is seen in most European countries. PD onset is age related, affecting ~1% of those at least 60 years old and becoming more prevalent with increasing age. Most cases are sporadic, or at least non-Mendelian, but a few large, early-onset (<50 years) dominant families have been recorded, and some of these have shown mutations in the gene encoding α-synuclein on chromosome 4q (*SNCA*). A less rare dominant form is caused by mutations in *LRRK2*, and several rare autosomal recessive genes have now also been implicated.

It should be remembered, however, that Mendelian PD remains rare. A single case of PD increases the risk in first-degree relatives about threefold, overall, to 3%–7%. Even the presence of two affected relatives (an affected parent and grandparent or parent and sibling) does not establish that the disorder is Mendelian in that family and the risks could be exaggerated. One study has demonstrated a risk to sibs that varies with age at onset in the proband, being around 1 in 12 when age of onset is under 45 years; 1 in 20 when it is 45–55 years; and less than 1 in 50 when it is over 65 years. It would seem reasonable to use these figures in the absence of other affected family members, but they may be an overestimate since another study has shown no difference between sibs and controls, while two twin studies have shown low concordance in both monozygotic and dizygotic twins, although the rate is higher if new functional imaging studies are used. The very rare juvenile Parkinson's disease, in which molecular defects have been identified in a gene termed 'parkin' (and some other genes), is usually autosomal recessive in inheritance.

THE DEMENTIAS

It is now recognised that most of the major dementias have a significant familial and genetic component (Table 15.4). At present, dementias following strict Mendelian inheritance are few (HD has already been considered), but susceptibility loci are being identified in some of the non-Mendelian forms through genetic association studies.

Alzheimer's disease

Alzheimer's disease is the most common dementia of old age, and increased survival makes it a major problem for society as well as for individual families. Certain diagnosis is only possible at autopsy and rests upon the demonstration of large numbers of senile plaques and neurofibrillary tangles in the brains of those affected. A specific locus on chromosome 21 was suggested by the occurrence of Alzheimer's disease in older Down syndrome patients, and by the location of the gene encoding β-amyloid precursor protein (the major constituent of the senile plaques) on this chromosome. Specific mutations have now been identified in this gene in a few families showing dominant inheritance of early-onset Alzheimer's disease, while some others show duplications of *APP*, but in more families the disease is determined by mutations in the *presenilin* genes (*PSEN1* and *PSEN2*, on chromosomes 14 and 1, respectively).

Families where the disease shows clear autosomal dominant inheritance are rare (less than 1% of all cases) and onset is usually early (below 65 years). For these rare Mendelian families, a small minority even of early-onset cases, presymptomatic testing may be feasible if a specific mutation can be identified in an affected individual. The issues involved in such testing and the type of protocol involved are closely comparable to those for Huntington's disease (see Chapter 8).

Table 15.4 Major dementias with a significant genetic component

Disorder	Inheritance	Gene or chromosome involved
Huntington's disease	AD	Unstable CAG repeat (*HTT* gene on 4p)
Alzheimer's disease		
Rare dominant early-onset (<65 years) form	AD	β-Amyloid precursor protein (APP), on chromosome 21, and the two presenilin loci account for a subset of cases
Later-onset cases	Unclear, often AD with reduced penetrance	Apolipoprotein E susceptibility locus (see text)
Frontotemporal dementia, sometimes with parkinsonism and sometimes associated in the family with ALS (motor neurone disease)	Usually AD	Heterogeneous; tau protein (occasional families) and *C19orf72* are important
Cerebral amyloid angiopathy	AD	Heterogeneous, and overlap with effects of APP and prion diseases
Familial multi-infarct dementia (CADASIL)	AD (rarely an AR form)	Human homologue of *Drosophila* 'Notch' gene
Creutzfeldt-Jakob disease (and related spongiform encephalopathies)	AD (when Mendelian)	Prion mutations (chromosome 20) in some familial cases
Mitochondrial encephalopathies	Mitochondrial or sporadic	Various mitochondrial DNA mutations

Abbreviations: AD, autosomal dominant; ALS, amyotrophic lateral sclerosis.

For the great majority of Alzheimer cases not showing Mendelian inheritance, which includes almost all those of late onset, genetic risks to relatives are not greatly increased (Table 15.5). They are strongly age dependent, as also shown in a Canadian series including all non-Mendelian cases, which found a risk to first-degree relatives of 2% at age 75 years, rising to 4% by age 80 years. Put in a different way, the chance of such a relative not having Alzheimer's disease (if they live to this age) is around 95%.

Table 15.5 Genetic risks in Alzheimer's disease

	Risk of dementia before age 75 years (%)
Sib affected (onset, >65 years)	2
Sib affected (onset, <65 years)	4–12
Sib and parent affected (onset, >65 years)	4–5
Sib and parent affected (onset, <65 years)	16–22

Source: Based on Bundey S. 1992. *Genetics and Neurology.* Edinburgh: Churchill Livingstone.

The term *Lewy body dementia* is now often used to separate a subgroup of patients with Alzheimer's disease with somewhat different clinical features (e.g. a fluctuating course) and particular brain changes. The synuclein genes α-synuclein (*SNCA*) and β-synuclein (*SNCB*) are implicated. The clinical features can overlap with either Parkinson's disease or Alzheimer's disease.

The accidental finding that common normal variants of the lipoprotein gene *ApoE* showed an association with Alzheimer's disease led to suggestions that this marker might be used in prediction. Further evidence shows that the association is less strong than first thought – a two- to threefold increase for those with one *ApoE* 4 allele and a 10-fold increase for the uncommon homozygotes for this. A series of consensus meetings in both the United States and the United Kingdom has firmly concluded that this should not be used in either prediction or diagnosis. The need for caution is further strengthened by the finding that the association may actually be reversed in some populations, among whom the E4 allele could actually be protective.

The whole *ApoE* story shows how complex such interactions are likely to be in multifactorial disorders (see Chapter 3) and how unwise it is to rush into using genetic susceptibility factors in prediction. This is especially true as the proportion of the heritability for such traits that can be accounted for by specific genetic variants is small, however strong the statistical association implicating some single-nucleotide polymorphisms (SNPs). Furthermore, the elucidation of gene-gene and gene-environment interactions has scarcely begun. Unfortunately, this has not deterred the promotion of such use by some commercial ventures.

Other familial dementias

While all of these are rare, they represent an important group because of the Mendelian inheritance (usually dominant) and high risks to relatives. Increasingly, the ability to detect specific molecular defects allows presymptomatic testing, which should follow a procedure comparable to that for HD (see Chapter 8).

FAMILIAL MULTI-INFARCT DEMENTIA ('CADASIL')

This rare, but probably under-recognised dominantly inherited disorder is due to mutations in a specific gene on chromosome 19q, homologous to the *Drosophila* gene known as 'Notch'. As with Alzheimer's disease, it represents only a very small fraction of all vascular dementia cases. The association with migraine, often from an early age, is strong and will sometimes give an indication as to who is more likely to inherit the disorder in a family. There is a rarer autosomal recessive form at a different locus.

FRONTOTEMPORAL DEMENTIA (PICK'S DISEASE)

This is much less clearly defined and understood in both clinical and pathological terms than is Alzheimer's disease, and genetic risks are poorly defined. *Frontotemporal dementia* is the term now more generally used. As with Alzheimer's disease, only a small subset is likely to follow Mendelian dominant inheritance but, in some of these cases, mutations have been recognised in the *tau* gene on chromosome 17.

The *C09ORF72* locus has also been implicated in familial (and apparently sporadic) frontotemporal dementia, but some who inherit the repeat expansion in this gene develop this dementia rather than the amyotrophic lateral sclerosis (motor neurone disease) that was the phenotype initially associated with the variant.

PRION DEMENTIAS AND CREUTZFELDT-JAKOB DISEASE

The group of disorders comprising the prion dementias and Creutzfeldt-Jakob disease (CJD) is now recognised to be more common and to have a broader and more variable phenotype than as first thought. The late-onset but rapidly progressive dementia known as CJD is familial in around 15% of cases, showing clear autosomal dominant inheritance in a small proportion of these. Mutations in the prion protein gene on chromosome 20 have been shown to be present in most of these rare families, as well as in some families in which cerebellar involvement predominates with a more protracted course (Gerstmann-Sträussler-Scheinker syndrome). An unusual phenotype known as *fatal familial insomnia* has also proved to be due to a specific prion mutation. Other cases may be of a particular susceptible genotype, but no significant increase in risk to relatives of an isolated case exists unless a prion mutation is present.

Analogy with scrapie in sheep (and human kuru) had suggested that human CJD might be mostly dietary in origin, a matter of considerable concern in relation to the UK epidemic of bovine spongiform encephalopathy (BSE) that began in 1986–1987. There is now clear evidence for this being responsible for the small number of 'new variant' CJD cases, but it seems unlikely that there is any dietary basis for CJD overall.

Testing for prion mutations is clearly important in the context of an unexplained familial dementia but may have serious consequences. Widespread testing of all dementias for these mutations, as with those for Alzheimer's disease, would identify high genetic risks for families of some cases not thought to be familial, while testing of samples from relatives should be done only if specifically requested, and only then within a counselling framework comparable to that developed for HD. Testing of healthy children is clearly unethical, and relatives at risk should not be tested as part of a research study without the most careful consideration and specific consent. However, those who know they carry the disease, are affected or at risk, should inform their doctors and dentists to ensure that appropriate care is taken when invasive procedures are performed as medical instruments may convey the infection to other patients.

DISORDERS OF MOVEMENT

Spinocerebellar ataxias

Late-onset ataxia accompanied by upper motor neurone signs (spinocerebellar ataxia) is a heterogenous group and has been found to result from trinucleotide repeat (CAG) expansions in specific genes. The repeat appears in the protein as polyglutamine (as in HD) and is probably directly responsible for the disease pathology. The group is now classified by its specific numbered genetic types, all autosomal dominant, and this largely replaces the previous names (e.g. type III for Machado-Joseph disease). The phenotype of the different forms overlaps extensively; all show a relationship between clinical phenotype and size of repeat expansion, with anticipation present in most. In addition to molecular diagnosis, presymptomatic testing is now increasingly feasible, and a comparable protocol to that used for HD is advisable.

X-linked cerebellar ataxia is very rare but well-documented. Cases are too infrequent to affect counselling for isolated male cases of ataxia. However, it has recently been recognised that a proportion of males carrying the fragile X pre-mutation may develop FXTAS, a progressive, late-onset neurodegeneration with ataxia, something that has wide implications for genetic counselling in fragile X syndrome (see Chapter 14). Females may also be affected, but this is less common.

Hereditary spastic paraplegia

Hereditary spastic paraplegia is often very benign in its course. Autosomal dominant inheritance is usual, but X-linked and, rarely, autosomal recessive inheritance has occurred in several families. Numerous different loci have been identified for the dominant types, with one specific gene ('spastin') on chromosome 2 particularly involved. It is impossible to exclude a high risk for offspring of an isolated case, unless a molecular defect has been found in affected relatives, and parents should always be examined carefully because manifestations can be very mild, especially in females. Fortunately, molecular diagnostics examining a large panel of relevant genes will often identify the underlying cause in a particular case or family. However, confusion with anoxic cerebral palsy and the dystonias can still occur. A magnetic resonance imaging scan of the brain and the spine is essential if there is any doubt about the diagnosis of a patient with signs of spasticity.

Other involuntary movement disorders

Essential tremor is a common and benign disorder, inherited as a late-onset autosomal dominant condition, and is important mainly as a condition to be distinguished from other movement disorders, particularly Parkinson's disease. At the other extreme of life, there are several benign and dominantly inherited tremors of head and chin beginning in infancy.

Primary torsion dystonia follows autosomal dominant inheritance in most cases, though with incomplete penetrance in some gene carriers and minimal expression in others; the disorder is more common in Ashkenazi Jews. A single mutation in a specific gene on chromosome 9 has been found to be responsible for almost all typical cases, Jewish and non-Jewish, including most sporadic early-onset cases. Late-onset dystonia is poorly understood, and most cases may not be genetic. Dystonia may also form part of other more general degenerative brain disorders. Dopamine-responsive dystonia, due to a specific molecular defect, is an important, treatable form to recognise, even though it is very rare.

Hereditary benign chorea is characterised by non-progressive chorea present from infancy, without mental retardation. Inheritance is autosomal dominant, with reduced penetrance in females. It is most important not to confuse this benign condition with HD. It is usually caused by a specific mutation in *NKX2-1* and represents the mildest of the wide range of phenotypes associated with mutations in this gene (that can also affect the thyroid gland and the lung).

Familial paroxysmal choreoathetosis shows intermittent symptoms, as its name implies. It is autosomal dominant.

Chorea-acanthocytosis (neuroacanthocytosis), described mainly from Japan, is autosomal recessive and can be distinguished by the red blood cell changes.

DRPLA (dentato rubral-pallido luysian atrophy) shows a variable combination of chorea, myoclonus and ataxia and is due, like Huntington's disease, to a specific expanded CAG repeat. It is the autosomal dominant movement disorder whose phenotype most closely resembles that of HD. It also is relatively common in Japan but does occur in the United Kingdom.

A variety of other hereditary movement disorders exist, including a number of rare striatonigral degenerations (mostly dominant), while metabolic disorders such as Wilson disease (autosomal recessive) and Lesch-Nyhan syndrome (X-linked recessive) must be considered in the differential diagnosis.

MULTIPLE SCLEROSIS

Familial occurrence in multiple sclerosis is well documented but uncommon. The risk to first-degree relatives is low (around 2%–3% from birth and only around 1% by age 30); even monozygotic twin pairs are usually discordant (risk around 30%). In the rare families in which two first-degree relatives (usually parent and child) are affected, risks are higher (around 10% for subsequent children). It is likely that the major aetiological factors will prove to be immunological, but that a specific genotype may be required for susceptibility. An association with specific HLA antigens exists but is too weak to be used in genetic counselling. The same applies to the other susceptibility loci detected by genome-wide association studies (GWAS). For familial cases presenting with optic neuropathy, care must be taken to exclude Leber optic atrophy and related mitochondrial disorders.

CEREBRAL ANEURYSMS AND STROKE

Occasional family clusters of cerebral aneurysm suggestive of autosomal dominant inheritance have been recorded, but in general these aneurysms are only rarely familial (except when they are associated with polycystic kidney disease). The same is true for most cerebral angiomas (provided that von Hippel-Lindau syndrome has been excluded). The possibility of a connective tissue disorder (e.g. Ehlers-Danlos syndrome type IV) should be considered. Autosomal dominant microaneurysms with cerebral haemorrhage have also been associated with mutations in the β-amyloid precursor protein (APP) gene; they may also present as dementia (see Chapter 14). Haemorrhagic stroke can also arise in another dominant disorder, hereditary haemorrhagic telangiectasia, from the associated AV malformations.

Table 15.6 lists some of the more important Mendelian causes of stroke; all are rare and make up only 1% of all stroke cases. The genetic susceptibility for the great majority of stroke cases is likely, as with most common diseases, to involve numerous genes, each of small individual effect.

Table 15.6 Single-gene causes of stroke and related vascular disorders

Cause	Inheritance
Connective tissue disorders	
Pseudoxanthoma elasticum	AR or AD
Ehlers-Danlos syndrome, vascular type (type IV)	AD
Marfan syndrome	AD
Metabolic disorders	
Sickle cell disease	AR
Homocystinuria	AR
Fabry disease	XR
Thrombotic factor disorders	Various (see Chapter 27)
Others	
Hereditary haemorrhagic telangiectasia	AD
CADASIL	AD
Moyamoya disease	Mostly sporadic but some families are known with variants at specific loci

Source: Based on Markus H. 2003. *J Neurol, Neurosurg & Psychiatr* 75(9): 1229–1231.
Abbreviations: AD, autosomal dominant; AR, autosomal recessive; XR, X-linked recessive.

NARCOLEPSY

Individuals with narcolepsy show a marked excess of the HLA haplotype DR2 and a pattern of other HLA alleles that suggests an association between narcolepsy and dysfunction of the immune system. Some families show a pattern suggestive of autosomal dominant inheritance, but a study of unselected patients has shown only 1% of first-degree relatives of an isolated case to be affected, much less than the figure of 14% for offspring found in a previous study–providing a good example of the limitations of genetic susceptibility testing. Somnolence may be confused with epileptic absences and can also result from other genetic disorders (e.g. myotonic dystrophy).

MIGRAINE

This exceedingly common condition is frequently familial, but specific genes have only been identified in rare Mendelian forms, especially the autosomal dominant familial hemiplegic migraine (associated with mutations in several channelopathy genes, and often also showing intermittent ataxia) and not in common migraine. Migraine is also a prominent symptom in some CADASIL families, with symptoms starting long before the appearance of strokes or dementia (see earlier).

ALCOHOLISM

Distinguishing environmental and genetic components of the familial tendency to alcoholism is particularly difficult. There is no consensus as to whether a separate genetic subtype exists or whether inherited biochemical variation in alcohol metabolism is relevant. The susceptibility to cirrhosis given hepatic injury from alcohol has, we imagine, a separate genetic basis from the behavioural susceptibility to consume alcohol or become addicted. This distinction is important to maintain when interpreting GWAS of alcohol-related problems.

MAJOR PSYCHIATRIC ILLNESS

Two disorders, schizophrenia and affective disorder (which includes both manic-depressive illness or bipolar affective disorder and unipolar disorder with episodes of depression only), account for a considerable proportion of all serious mental illness. They are not only extremely disabling and distressing conditions, often occurring in young people, but also result in a major burden for the community in terms of long-term care. A considerable body of genetic research has been developed over several decades, utilising carefully planned twin and adoption studies as well as family data. Diagnostic criteria have been standardised to overcome inevitable difficulties of interpretation, while quantitative genetic analysis has been developed to circumvent the lack of any clear Mendelian inheritance pattern.

The result of this painstaking research is that, for both schizophrenia and bipolar disease, a strong familial and genetic basis is clear, but a Mendelian basis is not. Biochemical and neurophysiological studies have not provided any clear primary factors either, so it is not surprising that psychiatric geneticists turned to DNA markers as a way of finding specific genetic loci. Unfortunately, early claims of success for both disorders needed to be withdrawn, a salutary lesson for all concerned that molecular methods are no panacea and should be approached (like other new technologies) critically and with scepticism. Large collaborative studies have identified genomic regions for which CNVs can predispose to psychiatric disease, especially autism and schizophrenia, and also functional variants in specific single genes, where the variant may also predispose to disease. Some of the genes implicated in these studies are related to each other in functional pathways; variants in some predispose to a range of psychiatric disorders, including autism, schizophrenia and bipolar disease.

A model of psychiatric disease is emerging that includes some genetic variants that destabilise 'normal' (or 'neurotypical') mental development and others that predispose towards a specific mental disorder, depending upon the presence or absence of other genetic factors, pre- and perinatal exposures and postnatal experiences. The overlap of CNVs that underlie both schizophrenia and autism has been important in generating this model, as has the finding that many of the genetic factors predisposing to schizophrenia also predispose to bipolar disease and major depressive disorder.

For now, the evidence suggests a considerable number of small genetic effects, rather than a few major genes, making it unlikely that the old empirical risks will be superseded by molecular approaches in the foreseeable future. Referrals for genetic counselling, however, may increase in frequency as genetic factors predisposing to mental illness come to be recognised. This is likely to happen both within families with mental illness and in families without recognised mental illness but in which a child with developmental problems is found to have a CNV known to be associated with mental illness and/or autism. It will be important for those supporting such families to be familiar with the latest evidence and to avoid suggestions of an inappropriately deterministic nature.

Schizophrenia

When strict diagnostic criteria are used, the risk of anyone developing schizophrenia during their lifetime is close to 1%.

The seriousness of the disease and its high prevalence make schizophrenia a major problem, although requests for genetic counselling are uncommon. Numerous surveys have been performed in the past on the risks to relatives, and Table 15.7 gives approximate risk figures. It can be seen that the risks are considerable for all first-degree relatives. Several additional points need to be considered in counselling:

- Much of the genetic risk for schizophrenia is for the earlier part of life, so the remaining risk for older, and so far unaffected, relatives is considerably less than the figures given here.
- In addition to the occurrence of classic schizophrenia in relatives, there is an increased frequency of less florid psychiatric states of doubtful classification (so-called *schizophrenia-spectrum disorders*).
- Some genetic factors that predispose to schizophrenia are also associated with developmental problems such as intellectual disability and autism.
- Some genetic factors that predispose to schizophrenia seem also to predispose to other types of mental illness, such as bipolar disease and major depressive disorder. However, other studies have suggested that the increased risk of mental illness in the relatives of those with schizophrenia is especially for schizophrenia.
- Care must be taken to exclude other primary disorders that may present with features suggestive of schizophrenia and that may follow Mendelian inheritance, such as HD.

Adoption studies in a number of countries have shown an incidence in adoptive children close to that predicted from their natural parents rather than their adoptive parents. This not only suggests that the familial nature of the disorder is predominantly genetic in origin, but

Table 15.7 Genetic risks (approximate) in schizophrenia and bipolar disease (manic-depressive disorder)

Affected relative	Risk (%)	
	Schizophrenia	Bipolar disease
No close family history (general population risk)	1	2–3
Sib	9	13
Parent	13	15
Sib and one parent	15	20
Both parents	45	50
Second-degree relative	3	5
Monozygotic twin	40	70
Dizygotic twin	10	20
First cousin	1–2	2–3

it is also of direct importance in advising potential adoptive parents. Of particular interest is the observation that, where a monozygotic co-twin is unaffected, the risk for offspring is as high as in offspring of the affected twin, whereas this is not the case for offspring of unaffected dizygotic co-twins.

Affective psychoses

Affective psychoses, like schizophrenia, represent a major problem in the community. The expectation of developing a major manic-depressive psychosis in a person's lifetime is around 1%, but if milder depressive states are included, the figure may be as high as 5%. There seems to be a genetic distinction among affective disorders between those that are *unipolar* (characterised by recurrent episodes of depression only) and those that are *bipolar* (characterised by alternating mania and depression – manic-depressive disorder – or more rarely by hypomania and mania alone). The risk to relatives also appears to be higher where the proband has early onset of disease than when the onset is later (over 40 years).

Table 15.7 summarises the main risk categories. It should be stressed that different surveys have given a wide range of estimates. Where age at onset in the proband is known, the risk to first-degree relatives should probably be increased to 20% when onset was under 40 years and reduced to 10% when onset was over 40 years.

Adoption studies, as in schizophrenia, have shown risks for adoptive children corresponding to their natural parents rather than their adoptive parents.

No specific major genes have yet been isolated, but GWAS have indicated some possible susceptibility loci.

16

Disorders of bone and connective tissue

PRIMARY BONE DYSPLASIAS

Genetic counselling in the confusing group of primary bone dysplasias requires special care. Full radiographic and clinical assessments are essential for a firm diagnosis to be reached; even so, some cases remain undiagnosed. In such a situation, one must be guided by the pedigree pattern of the individual family. Most types follow Mendelian inheritance, but for an isolated case it is often impossible to distinguish between a new dominant mutation and autosomal recessive inheritance on clinical (and radiological) features. Few clinicians see many cases of bone dysplasia, so it is unreasonable to expect familiarity with every type. Pooling experience is of great help; bone dysplasia groups in different centres, and those that cooperate on a national or supranational basis, can be of great value; they involve radiologists, orthopaedic surgeons and paediatricians, as well as geneticists. Within the United Kingdom the Skeletal Dysplasia Group fulfils this purpose. The discussion of problem cases at such meetings allows accurate diagnosis and genetic counselling that would not be possible otherwise.

A special effort should be made to obtain photographic and X-ray evidence on all skeletal dysplasias, particularly stillbirths. It is both surprising and frustrating how often such vital diagnostic information is not obtained or, in the case of radiographs, has been destroyed by hospitals. Computerised imaging techniques should help to preserve them. Even old family photographs can be of great value in the case of members no longer living. New X-ray investigations should be requested sparingly and selectively, with appropriate gonadal shielding to minimise the mutational load involved. Geneticists have a special responsibility to set an example in this.

Individuals with different (or even the same) forms of dwarfism commonly marry each other, with confusing results in the offspring. Interaction of the genes is to be expected only if the disorders are allelic. The birth of a child of normal stature to such a couple may be unexpected and even pose a difficult problem for them. Many such couples are anxious to adopt children who are also of short stature, and this should be facilitated. Obstetric difficulties in women owing to a small pelvis must not be forgotten.

Ultrasonographic prenatal diagnosis is feasible for a number of the severe neonatal bone dysplasias, especially those with limb shortening, although it can be misleading if used in situations of low prior risk. Specific genes have now been identified for many of the major forms of bone dysplasia, notably those due to mutations in the collagen genes and the fibroblast growth factor receptor genes, but also mutations in important developmental genes.

Box 16.1 summarises the inheritance of some of the major types of bone dysplasia and indicates specific gene defects where these have been recognised. More information is available online and in several atlases that show the radiological and clinical features. Some specific disorders are mentioned as follows.

BOX 16.1: Inheritance of major bone dysplasias (see also Table 16.1)

Autosomal dominant
Achondroplasia *FGFR3*
Hypochondroplasia *FGFR3*
Pseudoachondroplasia *COMP5*
Dyschondrosteosis *SHOX*
Osteopoikilosis (*LEMD3* and other loci)
Spondyloepiphyseal dysplasia congenita *COL2A1*
Multiple epiphyseal dysplasia *COL9A2, COMP5*
Metaphyseal dysplasia, Schmid type *COL10A1*
Congenital bowing (Blount disease, infantile)
Craniometaphyseal dyslasia *ANKH* (also AR)
Freeman-Sheldon syndrome (craniocarpotarsal dysplasia) *DA2A*
Cleidocranial dysplasia *CBFA1*
Diaphyseal aclasis (multiple hereditary exostoses) *EXT 1,2,3*
Progressive diaphyseal dysplasia (also AR)
Nail-patella syndrome *LMX1*
Fibrodysplasia ossificans progressiva (myositis ossificans) *ACVR1*
Trichorhinophalangeal dysplasia *TRPS1*
Kniest syndrome *COL2A1*
Familial expansile osteolysis *RANK (TNFRSF11A)*

Autosomal recessive
Diastrophic dwarfism *DTST* (sulphate transporter) *SLC26A2*
Metatropic dysplasia *TRPV4*
Sclerosteosis *SOST* and *LRP4* (but some cases dominant)
Pycnodysostosis (cathepsin C)
Van Buchem disease *SOST* (most families)

Cartilage-hair hypoplasia *RMLP*
Chondroectodermal dysplasia (Ellis-van Creveld) *EVC*
Ollier osteochondromatosis (heterogeneous)
Jeune thoracic dysplasia (heterogeneous)
Hypophosphatasia (infantile) *ALPL*
Mucopolysaccharidoses (except type II) (see text)
Weill-Marchesani syndrome *ADAMTS10* (dominant form *FBN1*)

X-linked
Spondyloepiphyseal dysplasia tarda (recessive) *TRAPPC2*
Orofaciodigital dysplasia, type I (dominant, lethal in male) *OFD1*
Vitamin D-resistant rickets (X-linked 'dominant') *PEX*
Mucopolysaccharidosis II (Hunter syndrome) (recessive) *IDS*
Otopalatodigital syndrome (phenotype varies with precise mutation in *FLNA*)
Chondrodysplasia punctata (separate X-linked dominant and X-linked recessive types;
    an autosomal recessive form with rhizomelic shortening)

Variable or uncertain
Russell-Silver syndrome (mostly sporadic) – including imprinting disorder on
    chromosomes 7 and 11; some cases due to uniparental disomy
De Lange syndrome (risk to sibs around 2%) (dominant or sex-linked: see text)
Caffey infantile cortical hyperostosis *COL1A1*
McCune-Albright polyostotic fibrous dysplasia (sporadic: post-zygotic mutations in
    GNAS)
Paget disease (heterogeneous; autosomal dominant with incomplete penetrance;
    environmental factors may be involved)
Melorheostosis (usually sporadic from post-zygotic mutation)

Achondroplasia

A diagnosis of achondroplasia should never be accepted without checking. True achondroplasia can be recognised at birth but rarely causes problems in neonatal life, except in the rare homozygous form; most fatal cases of 'achondroplasia' are other dysplasias. Inheritance is invariably autosomal dominant, but around 80% of cases are new mutations, with minimal recurrence risk for future sibs (around 1 in 500 in one study), probably due to gonadal mosaicism. Homozygous achondroplasia occurs in one in four of the children of two parents with achondroplasia and is lethal soon after birth. Another one in four of the children of such couples are normal.

There are a number of important management issues in achondroplasia, both in childhood and adult life, especially those relating to anaesthesia, spinal instability and spinal stenosis, that need to be understood by families and by professionals.

The milder disorder, *hypochondroplasia*, is allelic to achondroplasia; 'compound heterozygotes' have been recorded when one parent has achondroplasia and the other hypochondroplasia. Although most patients with hypochondroplasia have few physical problems and are mentally normal, a small number of cases with mental retardation have been reported. Also allelic to both conditions is the severe thanatophoric dysplasia. All three conditions are caused by (distinct) variants in one of the fibroblast growth factor receptor genes (*FGFR3*).

Pseudoachondroplasia

Most cases of pseudoachondroplasia are autosomal dominant. The face and skull are normal. Multiple affected sibs with normal parents may more often be the result of mosaicism than of recessive inheritance. For an isolated case with typical features and no consanguinity, the risk to offspring is close to 50%, while the risk to sibs is low (around 3%). Molecular defects are recognised in the collagen-associated protein *COMP5*. The condition is allelic with one form of multiple epiphyseal dysplasia (MED), and early hip arthritis is likely.

Spondyloepiphyseal and spondylometaphyseal dysplasias

The group of spondyloepiphyseal and spondylometaphyseal dysplasias is particularly variable clinically. Most are autosomal dominant, and isolated cases should be considered as dominant since cases of affected sibs with normal parents, previously thought to be recessive, have transmitted the disorder, probably representing gonadal mosaicism. Defects in type II collagen have been found in some families. The X-linked 'tarda' form should be clearly recognisable, even in an isolated case, by the characteristic radiographic appearance of the spine, with a central 'hump' of bone and relatively normal distal limb bones.

The severe spondyloepiphyseal dysplasia congenita is frequently confused with Morquio syndrome (mucopolysaccharidosis IV) and usually follows autosomal dominant inheritance. Retinal detachment is an important complication.

Dyschondrosteosis and Madelung deformity

Most cases of Madelung deformity of the wrist are part of the mild but generalised dysplasia, *dyschondrosteosis*, following autosomal dominant inheritance, and due to mutation in (or deletion of) a specific developmental gene in the pseudoautosomal region of distal Xp (*SHOX* and its functional homologue on the Y chromosome). A more severe dysplasia, with more marked short stature, may result from homozygosity (or compound heterozygosity) in the children of two affected parents.

Multiple epiphyseal dysplasia

Mildly affected individuals may have only moderately reduced stature, and the pattern of autosomal dominant inheritance characteristic of most families may be missed as a result. This disorder must be considered as a possible explanation for the diagnosis of bilateral Perthes disease (do not accept that diagnosis unless MED has been considered and excluded). There are multiple loci implicated in this, with mutations at some loci giving additional phenotypic features. The principal loci include those for collagen type 9 and the glycoprotein *COMP5*.

Chondrodysplasia punctata (Conradi syndrome)

Stippled bone epiphyses may be seen in early life on bone X-rays in a variety of conditions, so care must be taken before accepting the specific diagnosis of Conradi syndrome. In this, cataract, mental retardation and ichthyosis may all occur. Both autosomal dominant and recessive forms exist (the latter more severe and due to a peroxisomal defect); X-linked inheritance, both dominant and recessive, occurs occasionally. A phenocopy is also produced by maternal warfarin ingestion in early pregnancy and must be excluded before a genetic basis is assumed.

Lethal newborn dysplasias

The major causes of lethal newborn dysplasia are listed in Table 16.1. Some are invariably fatal, others not so. Sensitive ultrasound scanning is now of real help in prenatal diagnosis for this group; serial measurements are of particular value. Radiographs should always be taken of a stillbirth suspected of falling in this group because this may greatly assist the making of a specific diagnosis. Osteogenesis imperfecta congenita can be easily mistaken for a lethal newborn dysplasia. Although a number of disorders in this group follow autosomal recessive inheritance, the most common, thanatophoric dwarfism, is usually sporadic and shows *de novo* mutations in the fibroblast growth factor gene *FGFR3* (in which other mutations cause achondroplasia and hypochondroplasia). Heterogeneity or mosaicism may well be responsible for the few recurrent cases that have occurred.

OSTEOPETROSIS

A number of conditions are characterised by increased bone density, including pycnodysostosis, sclerosteosis and van Buchem disease, but true osteopetrosis exists in two principal forms, albeit with heterogeneity:

- A mild form, often asymptomatic, following autosomal dominant inheritance.
- A severe childhood form with bone marrow involvement, which is autosomal recessive. A number of loci can be involved.

Table 16.1 Frequently lethal newborn bone dysplasias

Type	Inheritance
Thanatophoric dwarfism	Usually sporadic; new dominant mutations in *FGFR3*
Achondrogenesis	
Type 1	Autosomal recessive; defects in *DTST*
Type 2	New dominant mutation in type II collagen
Ellis-van Creveld syndrome	Autosomal recessive
Thoracic dysplasia (Jeune)	Autosomal recessive
Majewski and other short-rib polydactyly syndromes	Autosomal recessive
Chondrodysplasia punctata	Usually autosomal recessive when severe (but can be X-linked or autosomal dominant)
Metatropic dwarfism	Autosomal recessive
Hypophosphatasia (severe type)	Autosomal recessive
Osteogenesis imperfecta congenita	Usually autosomal dominant but see text on Osteogenesis imperfecta type II
Campomelic dysplasia	Mostly new dominant mutations of *SOX9* but chromosome analysis may be needed (some females are XY).
Spondylothoracic dysplasia (Jarcho-Levin)	Autosomal recessive, but heterogeneous; mutations in *DLL3*

Anaemia and hepatosplenomegaly can occur, as can bone fragility. Cranial nerve compression can complicate several types, impacting on hearing and vision.

MULTIPLE EXOSTOSES (DIAPHYSEAL ACLASIS)

The inheritance of multiple exostoses follows a classical autosomal dominant pattern, although some individuals have only a few lesions that may not be symptomatic. It may form part of the Langer-Giedion syndrome (microdeletion of chromosome 8q), with mental retardation and features of trichorhinophalangeal dysplasia. Specific genes on chromosomes 8 and 11 have now been isolated. By contrast, enchondromatosis (Ollier disease) is rarely transmitted to children. When accompanied by haemangiomas, it is termed Maffucci syndrome. There is a risk of sarcomatous malignant change in the enchondromata.

LIMB DEFECTS

It is impossible to deal with all the different types here, so reference should be made to appropriate textbooks and journals for details. A high proportion of bilateral abnormalities follow Mendelian inheritance; many form a part of more general syndromes, some of which are summarised in Table 16.2. Unilateral defects, by contrast, are usually non-genetic. Where the recurrence risk is high, sensitive ultrasonography allows prenatal diagnosis of the more severe defects (see Chapter 9).

Limb defects have been much studied and substantial progress has been made in describing the molecular pathways of the relevant developmental genes, especially in the mouse, with numerous murine models of human disorders now available.

Polydactyly

Isolated postaxial polydactyly is a harmless but common (especially in African populations) autosomal dominant condition, showing incomplete penetrance. Preaxial polydactyly is more frequently associated with wider syndromes. Important conditions with polydactyly include trisomy 13 and a number of autosomal recessive conditions including Meckel and Ellis-van Creveld syndromes and the Jeune and Bardet-Biedl ciliopathies.

Syndactyly

The Poland anomaly, of unilateral syndactyly and pectoral muscle aplasia, is an important form to recognise because it appears to be non-genetic in the great majority of cases, probably vascular in aetiology. Bilateral isolated syndactyly of hands and/or feet has several forms, all autosomal dominant. Important syndromes include the orofaciodigital syndrome type I (X-linked dominant, lethal in the male) and the acrocephalosyndactylies (see Chapter 17). Greig syndrome, cephalo poly syndactyly (autosomal dominant), combines syndactyly with polydactyly and skull abnormalities. The extreme fusion defect of the lower limbs, sirenomelia, is sporadic.

Brachydactyly

Various distinct types of isolated brachydactyly exist, with clinical types now increasingly able to be correlated with specific mutational defects. Inheritance is generally autosomal dominant. Syndrome associations include Albright hereditary osteodystrophy (pseudo- or

Table 16.2 Syndromes involving limb defects

Syndrome	Inheritance
Polydactyly	
Trisomy 13	Usually sporadic
Ellis-van Creveld syndrome	AR
Jeune thoracic dystrophy	AR
Bardet-Biedl syndrome	AR
Meckel syndrome	AR
Carpenter syndrome	AR
Greig syndrome	AD
Acrocallosal syndrome	AR
Syndactyly	
Poland anomaly	Usually sporadic
Apert syndrome	AD (see Chapter 17)
Other craniosynostosis syndromes	Mostly AD
Orofaciodigital syndrome	XD (male lethal) most common (see Chapter 17)
Brachydactyly	
Albright hereditary osteodystrophy	AD
Turner syndrome	Usually sporadic
Limb reduction defects	
Thalidomide embryopathy	Non-genetic
Roberts syndrome	AR
Thrombocytopenia–absent radius syndrome	AR
Fanconi pancytopenia	AR
Amniotic bands	Usually sporadic
Holt-Oram syndrome	AD
VATER syndrome	Uncertain
Ectrodactyly	
EEC syndrome	AD

Abbreviations: AD, autosomal dominant; AR, autosomal recessive; EEC, ectrodactyly, ectodermal dysplasia, clefting; VATER, vertebrae, anus, trachea, oesophagus, renal; XD, X-linked dominant.

pseudo-pseudo-hypoparathyroidism), a variable autosomal dominant with endocrine features influenced by genetic imprinting, and Turner syndrome.

Ectrodactyly (split hand or lobster-claw defect)

Most isolated bilateral cases of ectrodactyly follow autosomal dominant inheritance. A number of families exist in which multiple affected sibs born to healthy parents have gone on to have affected children themselves. Autosomal recessive inheritance and lack of penetrance seem unsatisfactory explanations, and it is likely that germinal mosaicism is operating (see Chapter 2).

This means that affected individuals have a high risk of producing affected children, even if the family pattern appears to be autosomal recessive. An important syndrome to recognise is the EEC (ectrodactyly, ectodermal dysplasia, cleft lip and palate) syndrome, also autosomal dominant. Cytogenetic anomalies of chromosome 7q are sometimes associated with ectrodactyly.

Limb reduction defects

Limb reduction defects may be extremely difficult to distinguish from each other. Some, in particular asymmetrical amputation defects associated with 'amniotic constriction bands', are likely to be non-genetic. Other asymmetrical defects may be associated with oesophageal, anal, cardiac, renal and vertebral abnormalities (the VATER or VACTERL association); again, the recurrence risk is low. Thalidomide was previously a major cause, but no other definite drug-induced defects of this type are known. The severe symmetrical limb reduction disorder Roberts syndrome, which shows a characteristic abnormality of chromosomal division, is autosomal recessive. Limb changes in Holt-Oram syndrome (autosomal dominant mutations in *TBX5*) can be very similar to those caused by thalidomide and may occur without accompanying cardiac defect.

Fanconi pancytopenia and the syndrome of thrombocytopenia with absent radius (TAR) – both autosomal recessive – are important generalised syndromes to recognise and to distinguish from each other. Fanconi anaemia can be accompanied by growth retardation, microcephaly, learning disability and other congenital anomalies and can leading to aplastic anaemia and/or a variety of malignancies. The thumb is usually involved in the former but preserved in the latter.

Limb asymmetry and hypertrophy

Asymmetry is often found in the Russell-Silver syndrome (with dwarfing), sometimes due to genetic imprinting on chromosome 7 or 11, and in the Beckwith-Wiedemann syndrome (with overgrowth). The asymmetry is hypotrophic in Russell-Silver and hypertrophic in the Beckwith-Wiedemann syndrome. Both of these conditions can be associated with a disturbance of imprinting on chromosome 11p, leading to an increased activity of *IGF2* and decreased activity of *H19* in Beckwith-Wiedemann, the converse in Russell-Silver. The latter condition can also be caused by an imprinting disturbance on chromosome 7 and by other, less clear, mechanisms. Asymmetric hypertrophy can result from various other vascular and lymphatic disorders (see Chapter 18). Recurrence is generally rare in these cases, as they are mostly of somatic (post-zygotic) origin.

CONNECTIVE TISSUE DISORDERS

Collagen has always been recognised as fundamental to inherited connective tissue disorders, but it is only recently, with identification of the numerous and often tissue-specific forms of collagen and their genes, that individual diseases can be matched up with particular collagen defects (Table 16.3).

Osteogenesis imperfecta

Many cases of osteogenesis imperfecta are now recognised as defects in type I collagen, whose helix is determined by two separate genetic loci. Although there may be some correlation

Table 16.3 Molecular basis of bone dysplasias and connective tissue disorders

Molecule	Principal site	Disorders
Collagen I (A1 and 2)	Bone	Osteogenesis imperfecta (various types)
		Ehlers-Danlos syndrome (some types)
Collagen II (A1)	Cartilage	Spondyloepiphyseal dysplasias
		Stickler syndrome
		Kniest dysplasia
		Premature osteoarthrosis
		Achondrogenesis type 2
Collagen III	Vascular	Ehlers-Danlos syndrome, arteriopathic type (IV)
		Familial aneurysms(?)
Collagen IV	Basement membrane	Alport syndrome (see Chapter 24)
Collagen VII	Skin (see Chapter 18)	Epidermolysis bullosa (one dystrophic form)
Collagen IX		Multiple epiphyseal dysplasia (some families); pseudoachondroplasia (some families)
Fibrillin	Vascular; eye	Marfan syndrome
COMP5 glycoprotein	Cartilage	Multiple epiphyseal dysplasia (some families); pseudoachondroplasia (some families)

between phenotype and the type and site of mutation, this is not always clear-cut. Molecular diagnostic testing is now available; this took many years to develop because of the multiple repeat domains in these genes, the wide range of mutations and the difficulty of interpreting some genetic variants. Clinical and radiological assessment remains of central importance. The fact that medication can now influence the prognosis by boosting bone mineral content is changing the outlook for those affected.

TYPE I (PREVIOUSLY 'TARDA')

The great majority of 'classic' non-lethal cases are type I, which varies greatly within and between families and follows autosomal dominant inheritance. Sclerae are usually blue, and deafness and osteoporosis may occur in later life, while the number of fractures is extremely variable. Mutations may be found in either of the two type I collagen loci, but molecular analysis is not normally needed for accurate genetic counselling. The occasional occurrence of germinal mosaicism means that there is a small risk (around 1%) for sibs of an apparently new mutation case.

TYPE II

Although the terms 'perinatal lethal' and 'congenita' have been applied to this group, they are not fully accurate. Several subtypes can be distinguished by careful radiological examination:

- *Type IIa.* This causes stillbirth or is lethal in the neonatal period, with limb shortening and multiple intrauterine fractures; X-ray shows beaded ribs. Recurrence risk is very low (under 2%) and most cases are due to new dominant mutations in type I collagen, some of which can be recognised by molecular studies.
- *Types IIb.* Similar to IIa but less beading of the ribs.
- *Type IIc.* Neither long bones nor ribs are thickened while the ribs show beading.

Although mostly due to new dominant mutations, these groups contain recessively inherited forms and the empirical recurrence risks are higher (probably around 10%, but up to 25% if consanguinity is present). Careful discussion with an expert radiologist is needed.

Where no X-ray evidence is available in a perinatally lethal case, the empirical recurrence risk in a thorough survey was found to be around 4%. Recessive forms are definitely a minority in all subgroups; molecular evidence shows that some recurring cases are the result of germinal mosaicism.

TYPE III (SEVERE DEFORMING TYPE)

Type III is milder than type II but may be difficult to separate from type II in the newborn period, and the distinction may prove artificial. The empirical recurrence risk is around 7%.

TYPE IV

The term 'type IV' is sometimes applied to severe dominantly inherited forms, but it is doubtful whether this is really separate from type I.

Other types are recognised in expansions to the original Sillence classification.

Marfan syndrome

Marfan syndrome is an important disorder now known to be due to deficiency of the connective tissue protein fibrillin, determined by a gene on chromosome 15 (*FBN1*). This disorder tends to be overdiagnosed in tall individuals of slender habitus but with no cardinal signs, especially rapidly growing adolescents. There is rarely doubt, however, when the presence or absence of the various major features is considered as a whole.

Inheritance is autosomal dominant; the occurrence of major aortic complications is unpredictable, and many patients live a relatively normal life until aortic surgery is needed or a sudden demise occurs, although others may have severe early orthopaedic and cardiac problems. Around 15% of all patients appear to be affected by a new mutation. Penetrance is probably full, but apparently healthy family members should be carefully checked (including slit-lamp examination for minor degree of lens dislocation).

The isolation of the gene, and recognition of specific mutations in many cases, now gives the possibility of definitive molecular exclusion or confirmation in families where the causal mutation has been identified, as well as prenatal diagnosis if requested. The primary diagnosis remains largely clinical and, if a composite scoring system is used, most cases can be clearly confirmed or excluded. However, molecular approaches are assuming a greater role in diagnosis, and this is recognised in the 2010 revision of the Ghent diagnostic criteria. Recent striking advances in both surgery and medical treatment make early diagnosis and expert management of particular importance.

Other disorders to be distinguished include homocystinuria (autosomal recessive), patients with isolated lens dislocation due to spherophakia, who by chance are tall and thin, and neuromuscular disorders giving a 'marfanoid' habitus. A separate dominant syndrome of arachnodactyly with contractures but no internal complications (Beals syndrome) has also been described and is due to deficiency of fibrillin 2 (*FBN2*). The Loeys-Dietz syndrome, in which aneurysms are prominent, results from defects in the allied *TGFR-β* genes. The pathophysiology as well as the phenotype of the Marfan syndrome and of the Loeys-Dietz syndrome are closely related through activation of the TGF pathway, which is open to therapeutic intervention.

Ehlers-Danlos syndrome

The Ehlers-Danlos group of disorders is extremely heterogeneous. The main features are hypermobility of skin and joints, skin fragility and bruising, and rarer vascular, visceral and ocular complications. It is important not to confuse the group with the much more common and essentially harmless benign familial joint hypermobility (also often dominantly inherited); it is sometimes associated with pain and limitation of mobility out of proportion to the associated physical signs. The classification of the Ehlers-Danlos syndromes has recently been simplified (Table 16.4).

Autosomal dominant inheritance is the most common. Pregnancy may be dangerous in the severe forms. The vascular (type 4) form, although rare, is particularly important to recognise on account of the risks of bowel and arterial rupture and aneurysm formation. It results from defects in type III collagen. Other genetic abnormalities (including other collagen genes) have been identified in different forms.

Cutis laxa

Cutis laxa may follow autosomal recessive or autosomal dominant inheritance and is even X-linked in a few families, so a high risk for offspring of an isolated case cannot be excluded. Elastin mutations have now been found in some cases.

Pseudoxanthoma elasticum

Most cases of pseudoxanthoma elasticum follow autosomal recessive inheritance, but a few apparently dominant families have been described, mostly with milder clinical features. Asymptomatic individuals may be detected by the presence of angioid streaks in the retina. Most cases are caused by homozygous or compound heterozygous mutations in *ABCC6,* leading to calcification of elastic fibres in skin, the arterial wall and the retina; the apparently dominant families mostly represent examples of pseudo-dominant inheritance.

Mucopolysaccharidoses

All types of mucopolysaccharidoses (Table 16.5) follow autosomal recessive inheritance except for the X-linked type II (Hunter syndrome). The enzymatic basis of the major types is well defined and should be established, together with mutation testing where possible, to allow appropriate prenatal diagnosis, which is feasible for all types.

The Hurler and Scheie types are allelic, as are the mild and severe forms of Hunter syndrome. In each case, the two forms run separately in families. Occasional cases intermediate between Hurler and Scheie types represent a 'genetic compound' with one allele of each type. The related

Table 16.4 Principal types of the Ehlers-Danlos syndromes

Type	(Old classification)	Inheritance	Molecular defect
Classical	1 and 2	AD	Collagen 5 A1 and 2
Hypermobile	3	AD	–
Vascular	4	AD	Collagen 3 A1
Kyphoscoliotic	6	AR	Lysyl hydroxylase
Arthrochalasia	7	AD	Collagen 1A1 and 1A2

Table 16.5 The principal mucopolysaccharidoses

Type	Deficient enzyme and inheritance
1(H) *Hurler:* Severe course, corneal clouding, neurodegeneration	α-Iduronidase (autosomal recessive)
I(S) *Scheie:* Milder course, corneal clouding, no neurodegeneration, adult survival	α-Iduronidase (autosomal recessive)
II *Hunter:* (a) Severe: early onset with neurodegeneration; (b) Mild: late onset, no neurodegeneration; skeletal and cardiac problems	Iduronate sulphatase (X-linked recessive)
III *Sanfilippo:* Severe neurodegeneration often with behaviour problems; less severe physical changes; cornea clear; several biochemical types not clinically distinguishable	(a) Heparan sulphate sulphatase (autosomal recessive); (b) *N*-acetylglucosaminidase (autosomal recessive)
IV *Morquio:* Severe spine involvement with dwarfing; no neurodegeneration but risk of cervical spine compression	Galactosamine sulphate sulphatase (most families) (autosomal recessive)
VI *Maroteaux-Lamy:* Severe physical course, corneal clouding; no neurodegeneration	Arylsulphatase (autosomal recessive)
VII *β-glucuronidase deficiency:* Physical and mental changes; variable	β-glucuronidase (autosomal recessive)

mucolipidoses are all autosomal recessive in inheritance. Several other rare autosomal recessive lysosomal storage disorders can cause clinical confusion, including mannosidosis, sialidosis and fucosidosis. A detailed account of the individual disorders in this group is given in the online successor to the volume originally compiled by Charles Scriver, 'The Metabolic and Molecular Bases of Inherited Disease' (https://ommbid.mhmedical.com/).

Risks for offspring of healthy sibs are very small except in the X-linked Hunter syndrome, where identification of female carriers is of great importance. Combined enzyme analysis of serum and hair bulbs was used in the past for this but was not fully accurate. Isolation of the gene and recognition of frequent deletions and specific mutations now make DNA analysis the definitive test. In prenatal diagnosis of the various types, DNA analysis is the preferred method where mutations are known but amniotic fluid mucopolysaccharide analysis can be used as a rapid and accurate test to complement specific enzyme assay.

ARTHRITIS AND ARTHROPATHIES

The common arthritic disorders are mostly non-Mendelian and recurrence risks are relatively low for close relatives, though not well defined. Disorders with an immunological or vasculitic basis often show clear HLA associations, but not of a strength useful in genetic counselling. In some rare forms, abnormalities have been found in type II collagen, which is mainly found in cartilage.

Ankylosing spondylitis

Discovery of the striking association with HLA-B27 has revealed this – or some closely linked gene within the HLA region – to be probably the main genetic determinant in susceptibility, although genetic risks are not high. One family study showed a risk of 5% (7% for males and 2% for females) for clinical disease in first-degree relatives of patients with ankylosing spondylitis. Sixteen per cent showed radiological sacroiliitis. The chance of a B27 child of a B27 patient developing clinical ankylosing spondylitis is 9%, compared with a risk of less than 1% for offspring without this antigen.

The clinical or genetic applications of HLA-B27 testing are actually of very limited value (see Chapter 3 and Appendix 1), since most B27-positive individuals, whether or not there is a family history of ankylosing spondylitis, will not develop clinical features of the disorder, though a B27-negative result will make the diagnosis or future development of the disorder very unlikely. These limitations are a good example of why 'susceptibility testing' for common diseases is generally of little help in genetic counselling.

Rheumatoid arthritis

This common disorder (around 1% in most populations) rarely follows a Mendelian pattern, and the risks of clinical rheumatoid arthritis to relatives are not high; they appear to be around 3%–5% for first-degree relatives, although the incidence of radiological abnormalities is considerably higher. As might be expected with multifactorial inheritance (see Chapter 3), the risk appears to be higher for relatives of very severe cases (as high as 10%) and minimal for relatives of mild seronegative cases. The antigen HLA-DRw4 is found in rheumatoid arthritis patients with twice the normal frequency and is six times more common in familial cases, suggesting that this may be a major genetic determinant in the disorder. The occurrence of positive tests for rheumatoid factor is associated with HLA-DRw3.

A distinct, progressive 'pseudorheumatoid chondrodysplasia' has been recognised which is probably autosomal recessive in inheritance. Generalised contractures and painful swelling can cause confusion with juvenile rheumatoid arthritis. The hand deformities of Freeman-Sheldon syndrome and mucopolysaccharidoses may also be misdiagnosed as arthritis.

Systemic lupus erythematosus

Association has been found with specific HLA haplotypes and several other genes involved in immune function. There is strong concordance between monozygotic twins (25%–75%), but the empirical risk for first-degree relatives (and for dizygotic twins) is around 3% for systemic lupus erythematosus. As with many autoimmune disorders, there appears to be an increased incidence of other autoimmune conditions in relatives, suggesting that a dominantly inherited general predisposition to autoimmunity may be involved.

Systemic lupus may produce important intrauterine effects, with congenital heart block occurring in some infants born to affected mothers, while the 'lupus anticoagulant factor' (not always associated with overt systemic lupus) may be responsible for recurrent abortion in a small proportion of such cases.

Osteoarthritis

Osteoarthritis occurs with twice the general population prevalence in first-degree relatives of those suffering from this condition. When associated with Heberden nodes, the risk is higher, probably threefold. The nodes themselves have been thought to show autosomal dominant inheritance with incomplete penetrance in males, but the fact that they occur more frequently in the relatives of rarer male propositi makes polygenic inheritance likely. No HLA association has been shown.

Table 16.6 Mendelian forms of osteoarthropathy

Type	Inheritance
Interphalangeal osteoarthrosis	Autosomal dominant
Heberden nodes	Autosomal dominant (see text)
Familial digital osteoarthropathy with avascular necrosis	Autosomal dominant
Hereditary arthro-ophthalmopathy (Stickler syndrome)	Autosomal dominant (often a defect in type II collagen)
Osteoarthrosis, platyspondyly and β_2-globulin deficiency	Autosomal recessive (probable)
Multiple epiphyseal dysplasia	Autosomal dominant
Spondyloepiphyseal dysplasia tarda	X-linked recessive
Other spondyloepiphyseal dysplasias	Mainly autosomal dominant (type II collagen defects)
Premature generalised osteoarthrosis	Autosomal dominant (type II collagen defect)
Hereditary osteoarthritis of the hip	Autosomal dominant
Hereditary chondrocalcinosis	Autosomal dominant or autosomal recessive
Pseudoachondroplasia	Autosomal dominant
Alkaptonuria	Autosomal recessive

An unusual concentration of osteoarthritis in a family should arouse suspicion of an underlying bone dysplasia. Dominant inheritance in families with generalised premature osteoarthritis has been reported; some of these cases showed a defect in type II collagen. Table 16.6 summarises some of the major Mendelian causes of osteoarthritis.

Congenital dislocation of the hip

Apart from environmental factors, it is likely that a genetic contribution is provided both by the shape of the acetabulum and by joint laxity. Congenital dislocation of the hip is three times more common in girls, and there is marked social class and ethnic variation. The overall incidence is around 5 per 1,000 births. Recurrence risks have been studied by Wynne-Davies, whose data are shown in Table 16.7. Care must be taken to distinguish transient 'clicking hips' in newborns, and other generalised bone, connective tissue and neuromuscular disorders which commonly present with hip dislocation.

Table 16.7 Recurrence risks for congenital dislocation of the hip

Individual affected	Individual at risk	Risk (%) Overall	Males	Females
One sib	Sibs	6	1	11
One parent	Children	12	6	17
One parent, one child	Children	36		
Second-degree relative	Nephews, nieces	1		

Source: Wynne-Davies R. 1985. *J Med Genet* 2: 227–232.

Perthes disease

True Perthes disease carries a low recurrence risk, under 1% in sibs and around 3% in children of affected patients. The risks do not appear to be higher in the relatives of patients with bilateral hip disease. Risks for second-degree and third-degree relatives are minimal. Familial concentrations and apparent cases of bilateral disease should arouse suspicion that some other disorder, such as MED, may be present.

Arthrogryposis (congenital contractures)

There is so much heterogeneity in the group of arthrogryposes that the possible causes cannot be listed here. Excellent accounts of this group of disorders have been given in successive editions of *Emery and Rimoin's Principles and Practice of Medical Genetics* (Chapter 161: Arthrogryposis, 6th edition, 2013 by Judith Hall of Vancouver). Every effort should be directed towards making a primary diagnosis, with a careful pregnancy history (to exclude environmental factors) and family history (relevant neurological or skeletal disorders). Full examination and investigations to determine whether the contractures are part of a general syndrome, or have a neurogenic or myopathic basis, are also essential. If, after this, no specific cause has been found and the case is isolated, the recurrence risk is likely to be low.

Two forms that appear to be specific are distal arthrogryposis (autosomal dominant, often very mild) and amyoplasia, with symmetrical contractures of all four limbs (usually sporadic). Where a parent is affected, even mildly, autosomal dominant inheritance is likely. It should be noted that the prognosis with treatment is generally good when the condition is a secondary deformity.

Talipes

As with arthrogryposis, there are many primary causes of talipes, in particular neurological defects, which must be excluded. Idiopathic talipes equinovarus occurs in around 1 in 1,000 births in the United Kingdom, with a male predominance of 3:1. The risk for sibs is around 3% overall, around 10 times the population frequency. The risk for sibs of a male patient is lower (2%) than for sibs of a female patient (5%), as expected on the basis of polygenic inheritance. Full data on risks to offspring of patients are not yet available. Wynne-Davies suggested that the risk may be as high as 25% for further offspring of an affected parent with an affected child. Other forms of talipes (calcaneovalgus and metatarsus varus) appear to run separately in families from talipes equinovarus and may carry slightly higher sib recurrence risks (4%–5%).

Idiopathic scoliosis

Idiopathic scoliosis may be infantile or adolescent.

- The incidence of infantile idiopathic scoliosis is around 1.3 per 1,000 births in the United Kingdom, and much lower in North America. Satisfactory risk figures for sibs are not available.
- The incidence of the adolescent form is around 0.3 per 1,000 births in boys and 4 per 1,000 births in girls. The overall risk for first-degree relatives is around 5%–7% for major defects, but data are insufficient to split by sex and type of relatives.

Dupuytren contracture

When no primary cause is apparent, the inheritance of Dupuytren contracture is thought to be autosomal dominant, but if this is so, one would expect severe forms due to homozygosity for such a common condition, which have not been recorded.

Hereditary digital clubbing

Hereditary digital clubbing is a common and harmless autosomal dominant trait, frequently confused by doctors with acquired clubbing of more serious import. Patients usually correctly recognise its hereditary nature.

VARIOUS SKELETAL SYNDROMES

Nail-patella syndrome

Nail-patella syndrome (autosomal dominant) may present with talipes or hip dislocation in addition to the dysplastic nails and absent patellae. Renal involvement may occur in later life. Linkage with the ABO blood group system was the first autosomal linkage to be discovered (on chromosome 9). A specific gene (*LMX1B*) is known.

Freeman-Sheldon ('whistling face' or cranio-carpo-tarsal) syndrome

The hand deformity superficially resembles severe rheumatoid disease, but the lack of X-ray changes and characteristic pinched face should enable recognition of the syndrome. Inheritance is usually autosomal dominant (*MYH3*), but the birth of affected sibs to normal consanguineous parents suggests a recessive form as well, although germ-line mosaicism remains a possibility.

Rubinstein-Taybi syndrome

Broad thumbs and great toes, short stature, moderate to severe mental retardation and characteristic facies are the principal features of Rubinstein-Taybi syndrome. Recurrence in a family is rare, but patients do not usually reproduce. Molecular studies have identified *de novo* mutations in the CREB-binding protein gene on chromosome 16p as the usual cause; it is less commonly associated with mutations at a few other loci.

Larsen syndrome

A combination of multiple joint dislocation with an unusual facies and often with cleft palate, this syndrome is an autosomal dominant disorder associated with mutations in the filamin B gene. A similar autosomal recessive disorder is associated with mutations in the *B3GAT3* gene.

Stickler syndrome (hereditary arthro-ophthalmopathy)

Stickler syndrome is a variable autosomal dominant disorder, with characteristic flattened facies, often with cleft palate, severe myopia with frequent retinal detachment, and early osteoarthritis. It is most often caused by mutations in *COL2A1*, *COL11A1* or *COL11A2*, affecting collagen type II or type X. However, other forms exist, including some rare recessive forms. All forms involve mutations in a collagen gene.

Klippel-Feil syndrome

Many causes of a short neck find their way into this category but Klippel-Feil syndrome remains heterogeneous even after their removal. Key clinical features (not all required) are a short neck, low posterior hairline and restriction of neck movement, and there is usually some fusion of cervical vertebrae on X-ray. Where the case is an isolated one, the risk for sibs is probably low, although minor degrees of cervical vertebral fusion may be more frequent in relatives, and autosomal recessive families have been reported. The risk for children is significant since some cases are dominantly inherited; no precise figure exists. Familial mutations have been recognised in a number of genes (such as *GDF6*) but most cases are sporadic. Congenital heart disease is a common accompaniment in patients. The specific association with severe deafness and Duane anomaly (Wildervanck syndrome) is more common in girls. Cases with urogenital abnormalities may have the müllerian, renal, cervicothoracic somite abnormalities (MURCS) association. Careful clinical assessment and full skeletal survey should allow future delineation of specific entities within this group.

De Lange syndrome

Low birth weight, dwarfism, mental retardation, characteristic facies with synophrys and a variety of (especially upper) limb defects are the principal features of this syndrome. Severe cases are highly characteristic (with 'pencilled' eyebrows, long philtrum, thin lips and crescent mouth), but there is a spectrum of severity and the milder forms are more difficult to recognise clinically. The principal gene involved in more than half of cases is *NIPBL* at chromosome 5p13.2 (some cases have a cytogenetic anomaly). Two other autosomal genes involved are *SMC3* and *RAD21*, and two X-linked loci are *SMC1A* and *HDAC8*. Most cases are sporadic and the risk to sibs is around 2%.

Popliteal pterygium syndrome

The multiple pterygia are associated with cleft lip or palate, cryptorchidism and often syndactyly. Inheritance may be either autosomal dominant or recessive (usually the latter in the severe infantile form).

Sacral agenesis

Almost all cases of sacral agenesis are sporadic, but there seems to be a specific relationship to maternal diabetes mellitus. There does not appear to be an association with neural tube defects (see Chapter 14).

·

17

Oral and craniofacial disorders

INTRODUCTION

For most clinicians, craniofacial abnormality is a confusing area, on the borderline between medicine and dentistry, yet overlapping broadly into other fields. The plastic or maxillofacial surgeon is the person who sees most of the facial disorders, and there is no doubt that genetic counselling is an integral part of the management of these patients. Even minor facial anomalies can cause great distress, and accurate information regarding possible risks to offspring will usually provide considerable relief from worry for such people.

The amount of information available regarding the inheritance of these disorders is considerable. A number of medical geneticists who began their careers as dentists have provided some thorough reviews of the subject (see Appendix 1, especially Hennekam et al., 2010 and other volumes in the section, 'Dysmorphology').

THE TEETH

Hypodontia and anodontia

Hypodontia, or lack of one or a few permanent teeth, is extremely common (5%–10% in most surveys) and is often inherited as a variable autosomal dominant trait. One gene implicated in both syndromic and non-syndromic tooth agenesis is *MSX1*. Hypodontia may be the only significant finding in female heterozygotes for X-linked hypohidrotic ectodermal dysplasia (see Chapter 18), where incisors may also be peg shaped. Oligodontia and complete anodontia are commonly associated with this disorder in males, but can also occur in other ectodermal dysplasia syndromes, in orofaciodigital (OFD) syndrome type 1 (X-linked dominant) and with iris dysplasia in Rieger syndrome (autosomal dominant). A single central incisor tooth may be associated with midline abnormalities such as holoprosencephaly (e.g. in association with *SHH*).

Enamel defects

Enamel defects are seen in a number of generalised genetic disorders; defects occurring in isolation are termed *amelogenesis imperfecta*. Classifications have tended to be based on the apparent phenotype, either hypoplasia (a reduction in thickness of the enamel) or hypomineralisation (a reduction in the degree of calcification of the enamel), the latter often subdivided into hypocalcification and hypomineralisation according to the severity of the defect. In all probability, both hypoplasia and hypomineralisation occur together in the majority of cases.

Autosomal dominant, autosomal recessive and X-linked modes of inheritance are recognised. In the X-linked forms, characterised by vertical bands of normal and abnormal enamel in heterozygous females, there is evidence of genetic heterogeneity. One locus is the gene coding for amelogenin (the main structural protein of enamel) synthesis in the Xp22 region; there may be a second locus on the X-chromosome long arm.

Enamel pits are a characteristic finding in the permanent teeth in tuberous sclerosis.

Dentine defects

The most common of the defects of dentine is dentinogenesis imperfecta. This may occur in isolation, inherited in an autosomal dominant pattern, or in the various forms of osteogenesis imperfecta. The teeth are opalescent with an amber or grey colour. The teeth may be subject to attrition and chipping, most probably due to fractures within the dentine. Dentinogenesis imperfecta occurring alone is determined by the *DSPP* gene on 4q. When associated with osteogenesis imperfecta, there may be more variation in the severity of involvement, with some teeth being clinically normal, although radiographically and histologically they may show abnormalities.

CLEFT LIP AND PALATE

Before genetic counselling is given, a careful examination must be made to exclude the numerous syndromal associations with clefting. In some of these (e.g. chromosomal trisomies), the other defects are obvious, while in others, e.g. the Van der Woude (lip pits) syndrome (*IRF6* at chromosome 1q), they may be inconspicuous and even absent in some family members. Maternal teratogens (notably anticonvulsants) must also be considered. The most important syndromes to recognise are those that follow Mendelian inheritance; Box 17.1 lists some of the major ones. Cleft lip and palate also occur with other malformations in a non-specific manner and are more common than one might expect. If a careful search for a specific syndrome proves negative, one is forced to use the empirical risks for the abnormalities in isolation. Intriguing associations and interactions of oral clefts have been found with numerous gene loci, including genes in the folate and TGF-β pathways, but there has been a dearth of consistency in these results.

Numerous studies have shown that cleft palate alone runs in most families (apart from Van der Woude syndrome) separately from cleft lip with or without cleft palate. Table 17.1 summarises the overall risks. As expected with polygenic inheritance, the presence of other affected family members considerably raises the risks. The population incidence of cleft lip (with or without cleft palate) is 1 in 500–1,000, compared with around 1 in 2,500 for isolated cleft palate. A small number of X-linked families have been documented with cleft palate and ankyloglossia, associated with mutations in *TBX22*. While of great interest for the developmental biology, these families do not affect the overall risk of recurrence.

BOX 17.1: Some major syndromes associated with cleft lip and/or palate

Autosomal dominant
Van der Woude syndrome (lip pits with cleft lip/palate)
EEC syndrome (ectrodactyly, ectodermal dysplasia and clefting)
Hereditary arthro-ophthalmopathy (Stickler syndrome)
Larsen syndrome (originally thought to be recessive)
Retinal detachment, myopia and cleft palate (Marshall syndrome)
Spondyloepiphyseal dysplasia congenita
De Lange syndrome

Autosomal recessive
Chondrodysplasia punctata (Conradi syndrome)
Diastrophic dysplasia
Smith-Lemli-Opitz syndrome
Meckel syndrome
Orofaciodigital syndrome, type II
Fryns syndrome (with diaphragmatic hernia, limb and facial anomalies)
Roberts syndrome

X-linked
Orofaciodigital syndrome, type I (dominant, lethal in male)
Otopalatodigital syndrome
Isolated X-linked cleft palate with ankyloglossia
De Lange syndrome

Chromosomal
Trisomy 13
Trisomy 18
Chromosome 18 deletions
Various other autosomal abnormalities
Velocardiofacial (Shprintzen) syndrome (22q11 deletion)

Non-Mendelian
Pierre Robin sequence
Clefting with congenital heart disease

One point to note from Table 17.1 is that the risk for sibs of a patient with cleft lip with or without cleft palate is lower when it can be definitely established that no other relatives are affected (2.2%) than is the overall risk to sibs (4%) found by surveys, which will include some families with other affected relatives of varying closeness. Therefore, this higher risk should be used when family information is unavailable or unreliable. Some data are now available on the influence of severity (Table 17.2), and as expected, there is a higher risk when the abnormality is bilateral and a lower risk when there is only cleft lip. It is likely that cleft lip and palate are examples of polygenic inheritance; so far, apart from the Mendelian and syndromal forms, no major susceptibility genes have been identified.

Table 17.1 Cleft lip and palate: Genetic risks in the absence of a defined syndrome or Mendelian pattern

Relationship to index case	Cleft lip and palate (%)	Isolated cleft palate (%)
Sibs (overall risk)	4.0	1.8
Sib (no other affected members)	2.2	
Sib (two affected sibs)	10	8
Sib and affected parent	10	
Children	4.3	3
Second-degree relatives	0.6	
Third-degree relatives	0.3	
General population	0.1	0.04

Table 17.2 Genetic risks in cleft lip/palate: Effect of severity

Anomaly	Risk to sibs (%)
Bilateral cleft lip and palate	5.7
Unilateral cleft lip and palate	4.2
Unilateral cleft lip alone	2.5

Median cleft lip should be regarded as genetically separate from the usual types and may have its own specific syndromal associations (e.g. Ellis-van Creveld syndrome). Lateral and oblique cleft lip and mandibular clefting are likewise due to distinct processes.

Pierre Robin sequence (cleft palate with mandibular hypoplasia)

Mandibular hypoplasia, with or without cleft palate and with resulting respiratory obstruction from the tongue, may be part of a variety of skeletal or muscular syndromes, some Mendelian (e.g. Stickler syndrome, congenital myotonic dystrophy), or with 22q11 deletion. It may also arise as a deformation, in association with severe oligohydramnios. In the absence of a clear genetic cause, the risk of recurrence is low. The prognosis for patients will depend upon the underlying cause but, with careful treatment, the prognosis for the cleft itself is generally good for 'isolated' cases.

OTHER ORAL DISORDERS

Recurrent aphthous ulcers of the mouth

Around 20%–25% of the general population suffer from this minor, but tiresome, complaint to some degree, and around 40% of first-degree relatives appear to be affected.

Gingival fibromatosis

Although most commonly seen as a result of phenytoin treatment, gingival fibromatosis may occur as an isolated autosomal dominant trait or with hirsutism, as well as in some more general syndromes.

Hypoglossia-hypodactylia

Recurrence of hypoglossia-hypodactylia in sibs has not been noted, but insufficient patients have reproduced to exclude new dominant mutation as the cause.

Atrophic rhinitis

Although most cases of atrophic rhinitis are sporadic, occasional families following a clear autosomal dominant pattern have been documented.

CRANIOFACIAL DISORDERS

Craniosynostoses

Several specific genetic and clinical types of craniosynostosis exist, which are important to distinguish in genetic counselling. *Gorlin's Syndromes of the Head and Neck* (see Appendix 1) provides a detailed description. The principal types are listed in Table 17.3. Recognition of the different molecular defects (notably in fibroblast growth factor receptor 2) has been of great importance. All forms except Carpenter syndrome are autosomal dominant, with many cases (almost all in Apert syndrome) due to new mutation.

Isolated craniosynostosis

Most cases of isolated craniosynostosis are sporadic, regardless of which sutures are involved, and probably represent secondary deformations. Risks for sibs where parents are normal are around 5% for coronal and 1% for sagittal suture fusion, although these will need reassessment in light of molecular studies. If multiple family members are affected, it is wise to assume that one is dealing with a Mendelian type and to consider DNA analysis. Some such families have shown mutations in *FGFR2* or *HOX8* genes.

Table 17.3 Craniosynostosis syndromes

Disorder	Clinical features	Molecular defect
Apert syndrome	Severe craniosynostosis, glove-like fusion of most digits, frequent mental retardation	*FGFR2*
Saethre-Chotzen syndrome	Milder craniosynostosis; digital fusion, mostly soft tissue and of digits 2–4	*TWIST* (*Drosophila* homologue)
Pfeiffer syndrome	Mild acrocephaly with broad thumbs and great toes and partial digital fusion	*FGFR2*
Greig cephalopolysyndactyly	Broad forehead, characteristic facies and polysyndactyly	*GLI3*
Acrocephalopolysyndactyly (Carpenter syndrome)	Severe and frequently lethal; autosomal recessive	*RAB23*
Crouzon disease	Involvement of the orbits and mid-face, as well as the cranium	*FGFR2*

Mandibulofacial dysostosis (Treacher Collins syndrome)

Severity of the facial abnormality in mandibulofacial dysostosis varies greatly but inheritance is autosomal dominant, with the treacle (*TCOF1*) gene on chromosome 5 being the most important of several genes. Deafness is a common feature in addition to external ear defects; mental retardation is said to occur but is possibly an artefact of ascertainment. Potential parents will tend to be more mildly affected than average and must be warned that an affected child could be considerably more severely affected. High-resolution ultrasonography can detect severe cases. A separate syndrome of mandibulofacial dysostosis with preaxial limb defects (Nager syndrome) usually follows autosomal recessive inheritance.

Nasal defects

The nose may be characteristically involved in a wide range of craniofacial conditions. Nasal hypoplasia is a feature of Binder syndrome (usually sporadic) and Stickler syndrome (see Chapter 16), while trichorhinophalangeal (TRP) syndrome is characterised by a bulbous nose. The very large normal range and ethnic variation in nasal shape must be taken into account.

Other craniofacial syndromes

Some members of this very extensive group are covered in other chapters and listed in the boxes in Chapter 6. A precise diagnosis is often difficult; *Gorlin's Syndromes of the Head and Neck* provides a detailed and comprehensive guide. Only a few of the most important are mentioned here.

HALLERMANN-STREIFF SYNDROME (OCULOMANDIBULOFACIAL SYNDROME; FRANÇOIS DYSCEPHALIC SYNDROME)

Congenital cataracts, short stature, beaked nose with micrognathia and characteristic facies are all features of the Hallermann-Streiff syndrome. Inheritance is probably autosomal dominant, with most patients being new mutations, but few patients have reproduced. The risk of recurrence in sibs is minimal.

OCULOAURICULOVERTEBRAL DYSPLASIA (GOLDENHAR SYNDROME)

Goldenhar syndrome must be distinguished from the superficially similar Treacher Collins syndrome. The external ear defects are more marked, mental retardation is common, and epibulbar dermoid cyst of the eye is characteristic. Most cases are sporadic, and the recurrence risk where parents are normal is low.

HEMIFACIAL MICROSOMIA

Unilateral hypoplasia of most facial structures is the characteristic feature of hemifacial microsomia. Recurrence is exceptional.

STURGE-WEBER SYNDROME

Sturge-Weber syndrome must be distinguished from other angiomatous malformations of the face. The involvement of the ophthalmic trigeminal area and extension to the deep tissue of the skull and meninges is characteristic, as is congenital glaucoma. The condition can be caused by somatic (post-zygotic) mosaic mutation in the *GNAQ* gene.

OROFACIODIGITAL SYNDROMES

Characteristic features of the most common form (type I) are clefting of the jaw and tongue, with digital abnormalities (usually syndactyly) and sometimes mental retardation. Renal cysts may occur and almost all cases are female, suggesting X-linked dominant inheritance lethal in the male (see Chapter 2). Mutation in the *OFD1* gene is responsible, also known as *CXORF5*; this is the same gene as that for the Simpson-Golabi-Behmel syndrome. A risk of 50% for female offspring of an affected individual should be given. An extremely rare form (type 2 or Mohr syndrome) following autosomal recessive inheritance, and which is clinically distinguishable, has been described. There have been at least 11 other clinical entities proposed within the OFD syndromes, but this group of conditions may benefit from a careful reassessment of the current system of classification. There is substantial clinical and molecular heterogeneity, and there are many phenotypic overlaps with another group of 'difficult-to-classify' conditions, the ciliopathies. A consensus approach is likely to emerge as the results of clinical and molecular studies are integrated.

OCULODENTODIGITAL SYNDROME

Narrow alae nasi and small eyes are characteristic of the oculodentodigital syndrome, often combined with mild digital curvature and fusion, and dental enamel hypoplasia. There are sometimes neurological difficulties, including a spastic paraparesis. Inheritance is autosomal dominant (*GJA1*).

DUBOWITZ SYNDROME

The autosomal recessive Dubowitz syndrome combines microcephaly and mental retardation with a small face, shallow supraorbital ridges and severe eczema.

FRONTONASAL DYSPLASIA AND MEDIAN CLEFT FACE SYNDROME

Almost all cases of frontonasal dysplasia and median cleft face syndrome have been sporadic, but affected individuals rarely reproduce.

AARSKOG SYNDROME (FACIOGENITAL DYSPLASIA)

Aarskog syndrome is an X-linked recessive disorder combining hypertelorism with digital and spinal abnormalities and characteristic scrotal shape. The Opitz syndrome of hypertelorism and hypospadias is somewhat similar but follows either autosomal dominant or X-linked inheritance.

18

The skin

INTRODUCTION

A high proportion of disorders affecting the skin and its appendages follow Mendelian inheritance, and because they are readily available for inspection, they are easier than most to document in families. Since skin disorders are rarely fatal and interfere relatively little with reproduction, it is often possible to identify with confidence what mode of inheritance is operating, even if one is ignorant of the precise pathology or underlying aetiology of the condition. It must be remembered, however, that skin lesions may be the external marker for more serious internal or generalised disease. Furthermore, their cosmetic effect – which may amount to stigmatisation – may be of much greater consequence to the patient than the more narrowly medical effects, and much greater than may be appreciated by the physician.

For the small but significant number of lethal or seriously disabling skin disorders of infancy, including the epidermolysis bullosa and congenital ichthyosis groups, prenatal diagnosis is now often available by molecular genetic testing. This has largely replaced fetal skin biopsy as the method of diagnosis as long as the underlying genetic cause of the disorder in the family is known. Invasive tests would often be used (e.g. chorionic villus biopsy from 11 weeks of gestation), but non-invasive prenatal diagnosis is becoming available under some circumstances.

Most of the Mendelian disorders in this chapter are simply tabulated here without any attempt to describe them (Table 18.1) or provide detailed genetic information. Useful sources of information are given in Appendix 1. Most of the genes in which mutations can give rise to the numerous, but rare, genetic skin disorders have been identified. The clinical disorders,

Table 18.1 Skin disorders that may follow Mendelian inheritance

Disorder	Molecular defect or gene localization
Autosomal dominant	
Acanthosis nigricans	
Acrokeratosis verruciformis	
Angioneurotic oedema	C1 esterase inhibitor
Basal cell naevus (Gorlin) syndrome	Often *PTCH1* but some locus heterogeneity
Blue rubber bleb naevus	Some cases *TEK* gene
Cutis laxa (also autosomal recessive)	Locus heterogeneity including elastin gene *ELN* and *FBLN5*
Cylindromatosis (turban tumours)	*CYLD*
Ectodermal dysplasia (ED), hidrotic types	Especially Clouston hidrotic ED, *GJB6* encoding connexin 30
Epidermolysis bullosa (most families)	Keratin and collagen defects, including COL7A1
Epithelioma, multiple self-healing	*TGFBR1*
Erythrokeratodermia variabilis	especially *GJB3* at 1p34 but some locus heterogeneity
Hailey–Hailey disease (benign familial pemphigus)	*ATP 2C2*
Ichthyosis hystrix	*KRT1* but some locus heterogeneity
Ichthyosis vulgaris	especially the Filaggrin gene, *FLG*
Keratosis follicularis (Darier's disease)	*ATP 2A2*
Koilonychia, hereditary	considerable genetic heterogeneity
Mastocytosis, familial	*KIT*
Monilethrix	Specific hair keratin genes
Nail-patella syndrome	*LMX1B*
Neurofibromatosis (von Recklinghausen) type I	*NF1*
Neurofibromatosis type 2	*NF2*
Pachyonychia congenita	Keratin defects
Palmoplantar hyperkeratosis (tylosis)	Various keratin defects. Rare type with oesophageal cancer *RHBDF2*
Porokeratosis of Mibelli	Locus heterogeneity
Porphyria (all types except congenital erythropoietic)	Specific enzyme and gene defects
Steatocystoma multiplex	Specific keratin defects
Hereditary haemorrhagic telangiectasia	Specific vascular growth factors (especially *ENG*, *ACVRL1* and *SMAD4*)
Trichorhinophalangeal syndrome, type 1	*TRPS* (may also be part of microdeletion syndrome)
Tuberous sclerosis	*TSC1* and *TSC2*
Autosomal recessive	
Acrodermatitis enteropathica	*SLC39A4*

(Continued)

Table 18.1 (Continued) Skin disorders that may follow Mendelian inheritance

Disorder	Molecular defect or gene localization
Albinism, oculocutaneous (tyrosinase negative and positive)	*TYR* and *OCA2*
Ataxia telangiectasia	*ATM*
Bloom syndrome	*RECQL3* but mutations at other loci give very similar phenotypes
Chediak-Higashi syndrome	*LYST*
Chondroectodermal dysplasia (Ellis-van Creveld)	*EVC*
Cockayne syndrome	One of the DNA repair defects. Theer is locus heterogeneity and overlaps with xeroderma pigmentosum. Predominant gene is *ERCC6*
Cutis laxa (also autosomal dominant and X-linked)	Locus heterogeneity including *FBLN5* and *ATP6V0A2*
Epidermolysis bullosa (EB) (letalis and some dystrophic forms)	Predominantly caused by various collagen defects (dystrophic form). EB simplex associated with *EXPH5* or *TGM5*
Ichthyosis, congenita and other types	Enormous genetic heterogeneity but all resulting in defects in barrier function. Genes involved include filaggrin (*FLG*) as well as keratin genes and genes of the ceramide pathway
Lipoid proteinosis	*ECM1*
Netherton syndrome	*SPINK5*
Palmoplantar hyperkeratosis (mal de Meleda and Papillon–Lefevre types)	Mal de Meleda *SLURP1* Papillon-Lefevre *CTSC*
Pili torti	Genetically heterogeneous but often autosomal recessive. Also found in the X-linked Menkes disease
Porphyria, congenital erythropoietic	*UROS*
Progeria	Heterogeneous: Hutchinson-Gifford type *LMNA*
Pseudoxanthoma elasticum	Usually *ABCC6*
Rothmund–Thompson syndrome	*RECQL4* DNA repair defect
Seip (or Berardinelli-Seip) generalised lipodystrophy syndrome	Heterogeneous including *BSCL2* and *AGPAT2*
Trichothiodystrophy	*ERCC2* (DNA repair defect)
Werner syndrome	*RECQL2* (a DNA repair defect)
Xeroderma pigmentosum	Various DNA repair defects
X-linked (*recessive unless stated*)	
Dyskeratosis congenita	*DKC1*

(*Continued*)

Table 18.1 (Continued) Skin disorders that may follow Mendelian inheritance

Disorder	Molecular defect or gene localization
Ectodermal dysplasia, hypohidrotic (HED)	*EDA*
Fabry's disease	α-galactosidase (*GLA*)
Focal dermal hypoplasia (Goltz syndrome). X-linked dominant, lethal *in utero* for the hemizygous male	*PORCN*
Chronic granulomatous disease	*CYBB*
Ichthyosis, X-linked	Steroid sulphatase (*STS*)
Incontinentia pigmenti. X-linked dominant, lethal *in utero* for the hemizygous male. Less severe mutations result in a form of hypohidrotic ectoderaml dysplasia with immune deficiency.	*IKBKG* (also known as *NEMO* for NF-κ-B essential modulator).
Keratosis follicularis spinulosa (X-linked dominant)	*MBTPS2*
Menkes syndrome (copper transport)	*ATP7A*
Wiskott–Aldrich syndrome (immune deficiency, often with thrombocytopenia)	*WAS*

however, often show marked locus heterogeneity. Molecular analysis may be sufficient to achieve a full diagnosis, but this is not always so. Dermatology is a specialty where expert histological and protein studies are often available, and these added levels of investigation can be most helpful in providing a clear causal link between a molecular genotype and the associated phenotype.

SKIN PIGMENTATION AND ITS DISORDERS

Inheritance of skin colour is polygenic, with at least five or six gene loci of additive effect and probably considerably more. Advice regarding the physical appearance of the offspring of interracial marriages or adoptions often used to be sought in genetics clinics in the United States (see later in this chapter) although the present author (AC) has never met this question in his UK-based clinical practice. Questions on this subject may merely be the focussing point of considerable stress and ignorance, as well as prejudice, either latent or overt. The attitudes of other family members such as in-laws or grandparents may be frankly hostile, and it may be not so much skin colour as other racial characteristics, such as hair or facial features, that are the main concern.

In general, children are likely to show skin colour intermediate between that of the parents. Where both parents are of mixed heritage, this will still apply, but here the likelihood is greater that a child could be either darker or lighter than both parents as a result of inheriting a particular selection of pigment-determining genes.

Light-skinned individuals of mixed ancestry married to a 'white' person may enquire as to whether a child or subsequent descendant might have extremely dark skin colour or African features – in other words, might be a clearly black person who perhaps would not be accepted in the 'white' community into which he or she is born. This is very unlikely, but again it cannot be excluded that the degree of pigmentation, though probably not of other features, might exceed that of the darker parent, especially if the 'white' partner is relatively dark-skinned. Where the partner is blond and light-skinned, this possibility can be discounted.

Where mixed-race origin is known or is a possibility, caution must be advised in predicting later appearance from features present in early infancy. Skin colour may darken significantly and African-type hair may not be apparent for some months after birth. Reed, in his 1955 book *Counseling in Medical Genetics*, dealt in detail with these various features, and it is of interest that inheritance of skin colour was the most common reason for seeking genetic counselling at his clinic. Although the climate of opinion has significantly altered since that time, and interracial marriages and adoptions are now a routine matter in many countries and communities, frequent and completely unremarkable, it has become clear from political developments within both the United States and Europe that overt racism is far from having been consigned to history. It would be of interest to know whether the racism manifest as interest in skin pigmentation has moved from the genetic counselling clinic to the direct-to-consumer genetic testing website.

Several of the genes involved in skin colour have been identified. The original author suggested that the use of this knowledge for genetic testing of normal traits and characteristics would raise important and difficult societal questions. These tests are now readily available to anyone, without society having had the debate he hoped for.

Albinism

Generalised oculocutaneous albinism is autosomal recessive. Two main types exist:

- A severe form, OCA1A (with an absence of tyrosinase activity). Those with this form have a total lack of pigment throughout life and have two inactivating mutations in the tyrosinase gene (*TYR*).
- A milder tyrosinase-positive form, OCA2, for which the gene is also known (*OCA2*, corresponding to 'pink eye' in the mouse). Some milder cases of *TYR* mutations (with reduced tyrosinase activity) have a similar phenotype but the disorder is known as OCA1B.

In the latter type, the pigmentation of hair and iris gradually increases, and mild cases may easily be missed. Marriages between albinos of different types will result in all normal offspring as long as the disorders really are not allelic (i.e. are between one person with mutations in *TYR* and another with mutations in *OCA2*). A very rare type, associated with a bleeding diathesis (Hermansky-Pudlak syndrome), is also autosomal recessive. Prenatal detection of severe oculocutaneous albinism may be relevant in tropical countries where the morbidity is high. DNA analysis is much simpler (and can be performed much earlier in pregnancy) than the use of fetal skin biopsy, although molecular testing may not be so easy to access in some of the tropical countries where albinism is especially difficult to manage. It also seems likely that some of the more common genetic variants of pigmentation will be relevant to skin cancer susceptibility.

Ocular albinism (see Chapter 19) is X-linked, the gene being mapped to distal Xp. There are other X-linked disorders of the eye that can also lead to nystagmus and reduced pigmentation within the eye, such as Åland Island eye disease, and practitioners should be aware of these distinctions.

Vitiligo

Vitiligo is commonly associated with a variety of autoimmune endocrine disturbances, and like them often follows a variable autosomal dominant pattern.

Piebaldism

Piebaldism commonly follows autosomal dominant inheritance and has been shown to result from specific mutations in the c-KIT oncogene. It may form part of the more generalised Waardenburg syndrome, which is also autosomal dominant in inheritance and determined by the developmental gene *PAX3*. Isolated white forelock may also occur as a dominantly inherited trait.

PSORIASIS

Psoriasis is a common and variable disorder (prevalence around 1%–2%) which is frequently familial. Families apparently following all major types of Mendelian inheritance have been reported, but it is likely that most of these represent extreme examples of a disorder that is polygenically determined. Concordance between monozygotic twins (70%) is several times higher than between dizygotic twins (15%–20%), indicating a substantial genetic contribution to the condition but also an important role for other influences. Susceptibility loci have been identified in the human leucocyte antigen region of chromosome 6 and at least eight other loci, some of which are related to the function of the immune system. As with most complex disorders, genetic testing has little clinical utility, although this may have a role in research (see Chapter 3).

The risk for first-degree relatives of an isolated case is at least 10%, and probably double this where there are two affected first-degree relatives. Where the disorder appears to follow an autosomal dominant pattern, it is probably wise to give a risk approaching 50% for offspring of an affected member, but it is doubtful whether unaffected members of such pedigrees are completely free from the risk of transmitting it.

The children of two psoriatic patients also have a risk of around 50% of being affected, but there does not seem to be an especially severe form in such children, as might have been expected if homozygosity at a single gene locus was operating.

ATOPIC ECZEMA

Atopic eczema is an extremely common problem, often associated with asthma and other allergic phenomena, and seems to be determined by one or more autosomal dominant genes of rather variable expression. The genetics of atopy is discussed in Chapter 22 in relation to asthma and remains confused; several loci have been identified at which variation is associated with atopy in general or eczema in particular. The risk of some allergic problem where one parent is affected approaches 50%, and is somewhat higher where both parents are affected, although it does not appear that homozygosity results in a particularly severe clinical picture.

One important locus is the gene for filaggrin, *FLG*, also implicated in ichthyosis vulgaris (see next section) as well as in eczema. Specific variants in *FLG* lead to the gene acting as a strong susceptibility factor for eczema. Filaggrin has a role in aggregating keratin molecules and is important in determining the barrier properties of the epidermis; hence its involvement in eczema as well as ichthyosis.

ICHTHYOSES

The inherited ichthyoses are listed in Table 18.2. It is usually possible to distinguish different types on clinical and histological grounds as well as genetically, so that, with care, correct

Table 18.2 The inherited ichthyoses

Disorder	Inheritance and/or gene
Ichthyosis without syndromal association	
Congenital ichthyosis	
Lamellar ichthyosis. Markedly heterogeneous. Note phenotypic overlap between lamellar ichthyosis and nonbullous congenital ichthyosiform erythroderma.	Autosomal recessive. Heterogeneous
Harlequin fetus (may be lethal)	Autosomal recessive. Heterogeneous. One important gene is *ABCA12*
Congenital ichthyosiform erythroderma (nonbullous)	Heterogeneous. Can be autosomal dominant or recessive. When AD, often a keratin gene
Ichthyosis hystrix (overlaps with epidermolytic hyperkeratosis)	Autosomal dominant, often *KRT1* or *KRT10*
Ichthyosis vulgaris	Autosomal dominant *FLG*. More severe when homozygous or compound heterozygous. Two common mutations (allele frequency ∼4% in Europeans) are of high penetrance
X-linked ichthyosis (placental steroid sulphatase deficiency)	*STS*
Syndromes associated with ichthyosis	
Refsum syndrome (peroxisomal: phytanic acid oxidase). Features include ichthyosis, cerebellar ataxia, neuropathy and raised phytanic acid.	Autosomal recessive *PHYH*
Ichthyosis with mental retardation and spastic tetraplegia (Sjögren-Larsson syndrome)	Autosomal recessive *ALDH3A2*
Ichthyosis with male hypogonadism, and sometimes other features including mental retardation	X-linked recessive (contiguous gene deletion syndrome including *STS* and Kallmann syndrome gene *KAL1*, sometimes additional loci)
Rhizomelic chondrodysplasia punctata. The X-linked dominant form is sometimes termed the Conradi-Hünermann syndrome (remember the phenocopy from maternal warfarin)	All modes of Mendelian inheritance are known: autosomal recessive (*GNPAT* encodes dihydroxyacetone phosphate acyltransferase; rhizomelic form *PEX7*) or dominant form (tibia-metacarpal type). X-linked dominant (*EBP*) or recessive (*ARSE*)
Keratitis-ichthyosis-deafness (KID) syndrome	Usually autosomal dominant with heterozygous mutations in *GJB2* or *GJB6* (encoding connexin 26 or connexin 30). Some cases of autosomal recessive inheritance

(Continued)

Table 18.2 (Continued) The inherited ichthyoses

Disorder	Inheritance and/or gene
Congenital hemidysplasia with ichthyosiform erythroderma and limb defects (CHILD syndrome)	X-linked dominant (*NSDHL*). Overlap with features of X-linked dominant Conradi-Hünermann (but unilateral) (both genes involved in cholesterol synthesis pathway)
Trichothiodystrophy. A nonbullous ichthyosiform erythroderma with short stature and cognitive impairment. The hair is brittle, showing pili torti and trichorrhexis nodosa	Heterogeneous. Some cases are photosensitive. Not usually predisposed to cancer. One important gene is *ERCC2*; some overlap with xeroderma pigmentosum
Ichthyosis congenita with cataract	Autosomal recessive

genetic counselling can be given even for isolated cases. Thus severe ichthyosis in a neonate, except for the dominant ichthyosiform erythroderma, almost certainly follows autosomal recessive inheritance, while mild ichthyosis in a female is likely to be autosomal dominant. A careful general examination to exclude the various generalised syndromes is important.

Ichthyosis vulgaris may be associated with mutations in the filaggrin gene, which act in a semi-dominant fashion. Deficiency of steroid sulphatase has been shown to be responsible for X-linked ichthyosis, in addition to causing postmaturity through effects on placental function. A remarkably high proportion of cases (over 90%) are found to result from gene deletion, reflecting its localisation near the chiasma-dense junction with the Xp pseudoautosomal region. Several X-linked syndromes with ichthyosis are due to contiguous gene deletion syndromes in this region, analogous to those around the Duchenne locus.

PALMOPLANTAR HYPERKERATOSIS (TYLOSIS)

Most cases of palmoplantar hyperkeratosis (tylosis) follow autosomal dominant inheritance, and isolated cases thus have a high risk of transmitting the disorder. A variety of specific keratin gene defects have been identified (Table 18.3). The rare form known as 'mal de Meleda' is autosomal recessive and can occur outside the Adriatic area. The remarkable families with dominantly inherited oesophageal cancer and tylosis have late childhood onset of the skin

Table 18.3 Hereditary disorders of keratin (incomplete listing)

Disorder	Keratin type
Epidermolysis bullosa simplex	K5, K14
Epidermolytic hyperkeratosis	K1, K10
Acral type (ichthyosis bullosa of Siemens)	K2e
Palmoplantar keratodermia (hyperkeratosis)	
Epidermolytic type	K9
Non-epidermolytic type	K1, K16
Pachyonychia congenita	K6, K16, K17
Steatocystoma multiplex	K17
Monilethrix (hair defect)	Hb1, Hb6 (hair-specific keratins)

disorder, which does not result from a keratin defect but a pathogenic variant in *RHBDF2*. These cases are, however, exceptional, and families with tylosis from early childhood and no history of oesophageal cancer in the family need not be worried about this possibility.

EPIDERMOLYSIS BULLOSA

Epidermolysis bullosa is another exceptionally heterogeneous group of disorders in which genetic differences are supported by the clinical and histological features and where expert clinical and laboratory diagnosis is particularly important. Thus, the neonatal letalis form (now partly treatable by steroids) is autosomal recessive, while the mild simplex types, without scarring, are autosomal dominant; at least one form results from a molecular defect in keratin. The dystrophic forms with scarring may follow either pattern, but most severe cases are autosomal recessive. A defect in type 7 collagen has been found in most families. Junctional forms are due to defects in the basement membrane zone. Prenatal diagnosis of the letalis and dystrophic forms is usually possible by DNA analysis on chorion biopsy, where the molecular defect is known. This has largely superseded the use of fetal skin biopsy.

ECTODERMAL DYSPLASIAS

These comprise a diverse group of more than 150 distinct conditions that affect two or more ectodermal derivatives, including hair, teeth, nails, and glands (especially sweat glands). They can be thought of as falling into several categories: gene defects in specific developmental pathways (notably *EDA, TP63* or *WNT*) or in macromolecular structures (connexins, keratins or nectin). Note that epithelial-mesenchymal interaction may be disturbed quite generally in some of these conditions, not solely ectodermal-mesodermal interaction, so that development of mucous glands in the lungs and the colon may be impaired (as in hypohidrotic ectodermal dysplasia) as well as the truly ectodermal derivatives.

Hypohidrotic (anhidrotic) ectodermal dysplasia

Hypohidrotic ectodermal dysplasia (HED) is the most common of the ectodermal dysplasias. It is usually sex linked, with full expression in males and variable expression in female carriers, who may show dental anomalies as well as a reduced sweat pore count and a patchy distribution of the sweating pattern on starch-iodine testing. There can be a substantial morbidity and mortality in early childhood in affected males. Morbidity in infancy often includes over-heating, recurrent respiratory tract infections, failure to thrive and incoordinate oesophageal motility, but then health improves around 2 years of age. Those affected readily learn to manage their body temperature but also have to manage their appearance and the stigmatisation it may attract.

Isolation and study of the *EDA* gene has made carrier detection and prenatal diagnosis feasible in many families. Exciting progress has been made towards rational treatment with a few doses of a recombinant form of the ectodysplasin-A protein, starting with treatment *in utero*.

A very rare sex-linked form is found with severe immunodeficiency, caused by mutation in the *NEMO* gene.

Autosomal recessive and dominant forms of HED can result from mutation in this gene that encodes the EDA receptor (*EDAR*); an autosomal recessive form results from mutation in *WNT10A*.

Other types

Other types of ectodermal dysplasia are autosomal. Both dominant and recessive types have been described, as well as a number of more generalised syndromes. There is a family of *TP63*-associated ectodermal dysplasia syndromes, including the ectrodactyly-ectodermal dysplasia–cleft lip/palate (EEC) syndrome, the Rapp-Hodgkin syndrome and the ankyloblepharon-ectodermal defects–cleft lip/palate (AEC) syndrome. Clouston hidrotic ectodermal dysplasia results from alterations to the gene *GJB6*, and hence to the protein connexin 30, disrupting cell-cell junctions.

One notable syndromic form of ectodermal dysplasia, affecting a broader range of tissues, is chondroectodermal dysplasia (autosomal recessive).

PIGMENTED NAEVI

When present in a particular site, pigmented naevi commonly follow autosomal dominant inheritance. Multiple pigmented naevi are also a feature of Turner syndrome and some ring chromosome conditions, as well as neurofibromatosis (especially NF1 but also NF2) (see Chapter 14). The café-au-lait skin lesions typical of tuberous sclerosis must be distinguished from those found in NF1, as must lesions overlying a spina bifida. Other conditions to be aware of are Watson syndrome (the NF1-Noonan syndrome overlap disorder with missense mutations in *NF1*) and Legius syndrome, associated with mutations in *SPRED1*, with café-au-lait macules but not the other features of NF1 and without its substantial risk of malignancy.

Other causes of pigmented macules include mutations in *PTEN* and recessive mutations in some of the DNA mismatch repair genes and related conditions that predispose to tumours.

Lentigines are a feature of the dominantly inherited dysmorphic syndrome of multiple naevi with nerve deafness (LEOPARD syndrome), allelic to one form of Noonan syndrome (the *PTPN11* gene) and also affecting the heart and linear growth. Another cause of lentigines in childhood (as well as on mucous membranes) is the Peutz-Jeghers syndrome.

Irregular patches of pigmentation are found in incontinentia pigmenti (IP) and in chromosomal mosaicism conditions (sometimes in a 'lines of Blaschko' distribution), as well as the McCune-Albright syndrome. The pigmentary disturbance in IP is characterised by hyperpigmentation that later fades and leaves streaks of pale, atrophic skin resembling healed scars.

One type of autosomal dominant dysplastic naevus syndrome (also known as susceptibility to cutaneous malignant melanoma) (gene *CDKN2A*) is important to recognise in view of the risk of melanomas developing. Somatic mutation in *NRAS* leads to multiple congenital melanocytic naevi and also gives a high risk of melanoma.

Segmental pigmentary disorders

Several unusual disorders of skin pigmentation have been described that follow a patchy or whorled distribution corresponding to the lines of Blaschko, and which may be accompanied by mental retardation or other systemic features. Hypomelanosis of Ito, incontinentia pigmenti and focal dermal hypoplasia (Goltz syndrome) are the most clearly defined. Chromosomal mosaicism has been found to underlie many cases previously classed as hypomelanosis of Ito and should be sought in blood and skin biopsies or buccal cells. Recurrence risk is low unless a parent shows mosaicism. The two other conditions are caused by mutation in X-linked dominant (male lethal) genes, and the patchy skin distribution reflects the underlying pattern of X-chromosome inactivation. Somatic mutations and the heterozygous state for X-linked genes in a female both lead, functionally, to a state of mosaicism.

Cavernous haemangiomas

Cavernous haemangiomas of the facial region are usually sporadic, as is the trigeminal area flat vascular naevus of Sturge-Weber syndrome, and the limb angiomas associated with hypertrophy (Klippel-Trenaunay-Weber syndrome). Somatic mutations have been confirmed in vascular endothelial growth factors in some types. Haemangiomatous and lymphangiomatous lesions of the limbs may be associated with hypertrophy and are usually sporadic, although familial cases are described. The usual cause of the Proteus syndrome is somatic mutation in the *AKT1* gene. Knowledge of the molecular basis of these disorders is becoming relevant therapeutically and is therefore gaining in clinical importance.

Rare instances of autosomal dominant inheritance in association with Wilms tumour have also been recorded.

Other specific types of naevus following autosomal dominant inheritance are naevus flammeus of the nape of the neck and the 'blue rubber bleb' multiple naevi.

BALDNESS

Severe, early male baldness is probably due to autosomal dominant inheritance, with expression of the gene limited to the male unless it is present in homozygous state. The authors have never received a genetic counselling request for this innocuous condition, but a specific gene has been identified for a form of total alopecia, so it will be interesting to see if this changes the situation. Premature balding is a feature of myotonic dystrophy. Hair loss or scarcity may also result from a variety of ectodermal dysplasias and specific hair disorders (e.g. monilethrix, pili torti). Alopecia areata is often associated with autoimmune endocrine disorders.

Isolation of the gene responsible for red hair colour (usually autosomal recessive) is more relevant to population genetic studies than to genetic counselling but it is beginning to be used in forensic situations. This raises important issues regarding the wider use of genetic approaches in this area.

ACANTHOSIS NIGRICANS

Primary acanthosis nigricans starts early in life and follows autosomal dominant inheritance. Acanthosis nigricans may also accompany a variety of other genetic disorders. Onset in later life is commonly an indication of acquired visceral malignancy. The inherited type has no such association. Much more common as a cause of acanthosis nigricans than any clearly genetic conditions are obesity and insulin resistance (type II diabetes mellitus).

SKIN TUMOURS

A remarkable number of the rare skin-related tumours follow Mendelian inheritance, mostly autosomal dominant, and appear in the lists in Table 18.1 and Table 32.1. The recessively inherited disorders of DNA repair also frequently present with skin manifestations.

Xeroderma pigmentosum

Xeroderma pigmentosum (autosomal recessive) is a repair defect of ultraviolet-induced DNA damage. Since several separate types exist, it is important for the underling mutation(s) to be identified and confirmed as causal in an experienced laboratory before proceeding with prenatal diagnosis. There is still a place for functional studies of DNA repair in cultured fibroblasts in confirming the pathogenicity of possibly causal variants.

Kaposi sarcoma

Kaposi sarcoma (KS) is not inherited and is caused by infection with human herpesvirus 8. However, the risk of developing KS is greatly increased by co-infection with HIV. There is also evidence that some genetic variants increase the chance of KS developing in a person with HIV infection.

Malignant melanoma

Most cases of malignant melanoma appear to be non-genetic and largely related to UV radiation, but autosomal dominant inheritance occurs in a small subset of families. One type is known as familial dysplastic naevus syndrome (see previous discussion). Transplacental passage of malignant cells is also recorded. Several different specific tumour suppressor genes (notably *CDKNZA* and *CDK4*) have been found to be involved in the dominantly inherited families. Genetic testing can be helpful for such families, both in targeting preventive measures (especially in high-exposure countries like Australia) and also in selecting therapeutic approaches tailored to features of the tumour DNA (e.g. mutations in the *BRAF* gene).

Basal cell naevus (Gorlin) syndrome

Basal cell naevus syndrome is a dominantly inherited disorder which may be recognised from skeletal abnormalities, especially jaw cysts, before tumours appear. There may be also an increased risk of cerebral tumours. The gene most often involved (there is some locus heterogeneity) is *PTCH1* on chromosome 9, a homologue of the *Drosophila* gene 'Patched', involved in cell signalling. Although physically close to the locus for the rare and remarkable familial self-healing epithelioma known principally from western Scotland, the latter condition is known to be caused by mutation in a different gene, *TGFBR1*. Isolated basal cell tumours are not known to be familial.

Congenital fibromatosis

Congenital fibromatosis, also known as congenital generalised fibromatosis, is a rare disorder in which multiple spindle-cell fibromatous tumours occur and commonly mature spontaneously. It has several features in common with hyaline fibromatosis syndrome, but the genes implicated are different. The condition may be fatal if gut tumours occur but is usually benign. Although once considered to show autosomal recessive inheritance, autosomal dominant inheritance with incomplete penetrance (especially in older individuals) is now considered much more probable with at least two loci implicated. Careful search for small lesions in apparently unaffected parents is important.

19

The eye

INTRODUCTION

The study of inherited eye disorders formed a major part of early work on the Mendelian basis of genetic disease, largely because their non-lethal nature led to large families with clear inheritance patterns, but also because many generalised genetic disorders have ocular manifestations important in diagnosis. Since the days of genetic linkage studies and gene cloning, there has been a renaissance of ophthalmic genetics. This has led to exciting developments in localised gene therapy for a few of the retinopathies. These rapid developments make it especially important that patients and family members be given accurate and up-to-date genetic information.

Patients with congenital or childhood blindness frequently marry each other, with complex results although, in contrast to congenital deafness, it is usually possible to distinguish clinically the precise genetic type of each parent's disorder. The original author found that a clinic at a school for visually impaired children, run jointly with an ophthalmologist, was of great help to school leavers and their parents. Children with visual impairments are now much less likely to attend such specialist schools, as they are much more likely to be integrated into mainstream schooling. The affected children may therefore be less likely to have ready access to accurate genetic counselling. When seeing families with severe visual impairments as the major inherited problem, it is best if it can be in a clinic held jointly with a specialist ophthalmologist. If that is not possible, an alternative route of access to expert advice for clinical assessment is crucial if accurate prognoses are to be given and erroneous diagnoses avoided.

Since this chapter cannot possibly list, let alone discuss, all the hereditary ophthalmic disorders, a selective approach has been adopted, aiming to help paediatricians and other clinicians who encounter hereditary eye disorders. It is not primarily intended for ophthalmologists, although they may perhaps find some parts helpful. Around 3–4 per 1,000 children in developed countries have some form of severe visual handicap and at least half of these are genetic in origin. Mendelian disorders are also prominent in progressive blindness of later onset, while genetic factors are known to be important in such common problems as glaucoma, cataracts and age-related macular degeneration.

A remarkable number of X-linked disorders affecting the eye are known, and these are listed separately (Table 19.1), because they produce special problems in genetic counselling. The carrier state can be recognised in a number of these, and they provide direct evidence for mosaicism due to X-chromosome inactivation in the female. Patchy morphological changes

Table 19.1 X-linked eye disorders

Disorder	Changes in heterozygote
Ocular albinism	Patchy fundal depigmentation, translucency of iris
Oculocutaneous albinism with deafness	Partial hearing loss
X-linked congenital cataract	Sutural lens opacities
Choroideraemia	Retinal pigmentary changes (sometimes symptomatic) Abnormal electroretinogram
Colour blindness Deutan Protan Incomplete achromatopsia	Minor defects in colour vision
Iris hypoplasia with glaucoma	
X-linked macular dystrophy	
Megalocornea (also rarely dominant)	Corneal diameter increased
Microphthalmos with multiple anomalies (Lenz syndrome)	
Congenital stationary night blindness with myopia	
Norrie disease (pseudoglioma) often with progressive nerve deafness and/or cognitive impairment and mental illness	Some cases due to gene deletion; only rare manifestations in heterozygotes
Hereditary oculomotor nystagmus	Variable; may be fully affected
Oculocerebrorenal (Lowe) syndrome	Minor lens opacities
X-linked retinitis pigmentosa	Patchy retinal pigmentary and electroretinographic changes
Retinoschisis	

can be seen in a number of these carriers, which allow diagnosis of the carrier state without recourse to investigations. However, molecular genetic analysis can now very often provide accurate tests based on the direct detection of mutations, especially for this X-linked group, but also for some autosomal disorders.

CHOROIDORETINAL DEGENERATIONS

A great variety of types exist, characterised by particular features of fundal appearance, differences in severity and progression, and different responses to various types of electrodiagnostic investigation. It is most unwise for someone who is not an ophthalmologist to venture into diagnosis, but a valuable contribution can be made by documenting the pedigree pattern and carefully searching for any associated syndromic features. This information can then be combined with a specific ophthalmic diagnosis to allow accurate genetic counselling. Two broad groups can be distinguished:

- Those mainly affecting peripheral vision (e.g. the retinitis pigmentosa group)
- Those principally involving central vision (e.g. the macular dystrophies)

Retinitis pigmentosa

Retinitis pigmentosa (RP) is the most common of the retinal degenerations. This group of disorders may follow all three main modes of Mendelian inheritance, autosomal recessive forms being the most common (about 50%), with autosomal dominant inheritance accounting for around 25% of families. X-linked cases account for around 15% of the total, but for about 50% of isolated male cases. A few cases arise as a result of digenic inheritance (heterozygosity at two different loci). Marked variation in course occurs in different families, suggesting further heterogeneity. At least 75 loci have been implicated in non-syndromic RP, although most of these are only rare causes. Although there is some variation between geographical areas, variants in *RHO, PRPF31* and *PRPH2* are the most common forms of autosomal dominant RP, and variants in *EYS, USH2A, CRB1* and *CERKL* are the most prevalent forms of autosomal recessive RP. Most cases of X-linked RP result from variants in *RPGR*, with fewer from variants in *RP2*.

Carriers of the X-linked form may often (but not always) show visible pigmentary disturbance and an abnormal electroretinogram, a useful distinguishing point from the other forms of inheritance in an isolated male case. The carriers for autosomal recessive forms do not generally show abnormalities, so distinction from a new dominant mutation is often impossible. Clinical features are too variable to help much, while an additional problem is incomplete penetrance of the gene in around 10% of heterozygotes for the dominant form. The empirical risk for an affected child being born to a parent who is an isolated case is around one in eight. Should a child indeed be affected, the risk to subsequent offspring would be one in two.

Molecular developments in retinitis pigmentosa are now of practical help in many families because next-generation sequencing panels of ~150 loci (including loci associated with syndromic as well as non-syndromic forms) have a high diagnostic yield. If such a panel fails to identify a pathogenic variant, then a clinical reassessment should be considered along with referral for whole exome or genome sequencing.

Choroideraemia is a specific X-linked disorder that may be confused with retinitis pigmentosa, especially in its early stages. It is infrequently associated with more generalised, and often severe, developmental problems as part of a contiguous gene deletion syndrome.

Norrie disease is the severe end of a spectrum associated with mutation in the *NDP* gene, which also causes the milder X-linked familial exudative retinopathy. It is associated with progressive deafness and more generalised developmental difficulties in 30%–50% of those affected. Retinoschisis is yet another X-linked disorder, with retinal degeneration associated with a characteristic splitting of the retina, where specific molecular analysis is possible.

A number of autosomal recessive syndromes exist in which retinitis pigmentosa is one of the features. These include the ciliopathy Bardet-Biedl syndrome (with polydactyly, hypogonadism and mental retardation), Hallgren syndrome (with deafness, ataxia and mental disturbance) and Usher syndrome (three clinical types, one with profound nerve deafness; there may also be vestibular dysfunction).

Gene therapy is under active development, to the point of clinical trials, for several of the retinopathies including choroideraemia.

Macular dystrophies

The macular dystrophies are a heterogeneous group, selectively involving central vision in contrast to the early peripheral involvement in retinitis pigmentosa. This is readily distinguished by an experienced ophthalmologist, but separating the different forms may be very difficult, causing problems in genetic counselling, especially for the isolated case.

Many late-onset macular dystrophies follow an autosomal dominant pattern, as well as the early-onset best macular degeneration (for which the *BEST1* gene on chromosome 11q is the principal locus), while the juvenile Stargardt form is autosomal recessive. Stargardt disease shows locus heterogeneity; one form is associated with mutations in the *ABCA4* ion transport gene on chromosome 1. Another rare but treatable recessive type is gyrate atrophy associated with a metabolic defect in ornithine aminotransferase. Cone dystrophies are a further heterogeneous group, associated with deterioration in colour vision.

Age-related macular degeneration (AMD) becomes progressively more common with age and is an important cause of visual loss. Most cases, however, are not Mendelian, and smoking is an important risk factor. More than 50 loci are associated with risk for this condition, suggesting involvement of several pathways including the complement, inflammatory and extracellular matrix pathways. Zinc and antioxidant supplements may be protective and several treatments are known to be effective, with more under development. Genetic susceptibility testing for AMD has limited power, even when environmental risk factors are included, and the American Academy of Ophthalmology advises against this.

Leber congenital amaurosis

This must not be confused with Leber optic atrophy (see later). Leber congenital amaurosis is a primary retinal disorder that is one of the most common causes of childhood blindness and is autosomal recessive in inheritance. The condition can be detected in early infancy by electroretinogram. Occasional families with associated cerebral and renal degeneration are known but do not overlap with the isolated form. There is extensive locus heterogeneity, with pathogenic variants found in a retinal homeobox gene (*CRX*) and a separate retinal epithelium protein gene (*RPE65*) among others. Gene therapy is being developed for *CRX*.

Congenital stationary (non-progressive) night blindness

This is usually autosomal dominant or X-linked dominant. An X-linked recessive form with myopia also exists.

NYSTAGMUS

A clear primary diagnosis for nystagmus is essential because the causes may be neurological or vestibular as well as ocular. Even when the nystagmus is primary, there are a number of causes. Probably the most important ones to recognise are the various types of albinism, congenital stationary night blindness (see earlier) and the X-linked hereditary oculomotor nystagmus, which shows very variable manifestation in females (see Figure 2.22).

COLOUR VISION

The common forms of colour blindness, whether protan or deutan in type, are uniformly X-linked recessive in inheritance and occur in about 8% of males.

Because of this high frequency, matings of affected males and carrier females are not uncommon, with a 50% risk of children of either sex being affected. Around 0.4% of women have colour blindness. The genes for red and green colour vision have been cloned, allowing the molecular analysis of colour vision defects.

The rare total colour blindness (monochromatism) is autosomal recessive in inheritance, while the even rarer 'blue cone' type is X-linked. All three disorders should be distinguished from the progressive cone dystrophies.

LEBER OPTIC ATROPHY

This must not be confused with Leber congenital amaurosis (see earlier). Leber optic atrophy follows classical mitochondrial inheritance (see Chapter 2), but other genetic and environmental factors modify the primary pattern. The main empirical risks are as follows:

- Males are affected more often than females (85%) in Europe but not in Japan.
- Males never transmit the disease to descendants of either sex, not even to grandchildren or subsequent generations.
- Where a female is affected or has an affected son, the risk to subsequent sons is ~50% (one in two), while all her daughters appear to be either carriers (80%) or affected (20%), unlike in X linkage.

Mitochondrial DNA analysis can now identify specific germ-line mutations and is especially valuable in cases without a clear genetic pattern. However, as discussed in Chapter 2, the identification of mitochondrial inheritance is of the greatest help in confirming the diagnosis and giving the general pattern of risk, but is singularly unhelpful for the female carrier, since it gives no indication as to whether she will herself become affected, or the risk to particular offspring. An exception is for offspring of a woman who is heteroplasmic for the mutation, who has both normal and mutant DNA; if these offspring show no or very low levels of mutant DNA themselves (in leucocytes), their risk of developing the disorder is correspondingly low (although the level of the mutation may differ between tissues and over time). It is hoped that some preventive therapy that enhances or spares mitochondrial function may be developed that will help those at risk. There have been some promising trials; it may be important to start treatment as soon after the first eye becomes affected as possible. It is also important to avoid risk factors such as smoking and excessive alcohol.

Other forms of hereditary optic atrophy

Several forms exist following both autosomal dominant and recessive patterns. Those of adult life are mostly dominant and usually show a slowly progressive course, unlike the subacute onset of Leber optic atrophy. The Wolfram or DIDMOAD syndrome (diabetes insipidus, diabetes mellitus, optic atrophy and deafness) is a disorder of the endoplasmic reticulum that is usually caused by mutation in the *WFS1* gene (occasionally, the *CISD2* gene) that follows autosomal recessive inheritance. Related but milder phenotypes (e.g. deafness *or* diabetes mellitus) may be associated with different, dominant mutations in *WFS1*.

CORNEAL DYSTROPHIES

Numerous types of corneal dystrophy exist. The slit-lamp appearance is often very characteristic (to the expert), and unless a clear pedigree pattern is seen, it is wise to be guided by ophthalmological opinion. Most types are Mendelian. Corneal clouding and opacification may be a helpful diagnostic feature in various generalised diseases, notably the mucopolysaccharidoses (including Fabry disease in females) and mucolipidoses, but also in some lipoprotein disorders, Zellweger syndrome and cystinosis.

Some dominant forms of corneal dystrophy have recently been shown to result from molecular defects in different forms of keratin, such as K3, K12, kerato-epithelin and type 8 collagen (see also Chapter 18).

RETINAL DETACHMENT

Retinal detachment is commonly associated with severe myopia, and a significant risk to relatives is only likely when they also have severe myopia. Occasional dominantly inherited families are documented with retinal detachment unrelated to myopia or other ocular disorders. Several other genetic syndromes may be accompanied by retinal detachment, including type II collagen defects such as severe spondyloepiphyseal dysplasia and Stickler syndrome, as well as the related, but distinct, condition known as Wagner retinopathy, all of which are dominantly inherited.

RETINOBLASTOMA

Retinoblastoma provides an extremely important and difficult area for genetic counselling. All bilateral cases appear to be hereditary, compared with only about 15% of unilateral cases. Further, only 90% of those with the gene develop tumours, and there are instances where the disorder seems to have been suppressed in an entire branch of a kindred. Occasionally, spontaneous disappearance of a tumour may leave a retinal scar as the only feature, so parents of an isolated case should always be examined carefully. Survivors have an increased risk (around 10%) of other neoplasms, notably osteosarcoma, later in life.

Most cases of retinoblastoma are not associated with other malformations, but abnormalities of chromosome 13q may be accompanied by retinoblastoma, a finding that led to localisation of the gene on this chromosome.

Molecular analysis can be used to provide accurate prediction for those at risk. Tumour DNA analysis is important in unilateral cases. Retinoblastoma provided the first full vindication of Knudson's 'two-hit' mutation theory of cancer (see Chapter 29), and tumour DNA analysis shows that the same locus is indeed involved in both germinal and somatic mutations. The lack of penetrance can now be readily explained by absence of the necessary somatic mutation; while the genetic predisposition is dominantly inherited, the developing retinal tissue must be homozygous for loss of protein activity for a tumour to occur. Equally, a germ-line mutation must have been inherited for more than a single tumour to occur in an individual.

Table 19.2 Genetic risks to offspring in retinoblastoma

	Risk (%)
Unilateral	
Affected, with affected parent or sib	45
Unaffected, parent and sib or two sibs affected	5
Affected, no other affected relatives	5, but higher if multifocal
Unaffected, one affected child	1–2
Unaffected, one affected sib	Varies with penetrance
Bilateral	
Affected, other family members affected	45
Affected, no other affected family members	45
Unaffected, one affected child	2
Unaffected, parent affected	5

Note: The risks given here are estimates from composite data that do not include molecular genetic test results. As next-generation sequencing with high read depth is increasing the chance of identifying low-level mosaicism, these figures will be subject to change.

The empirical risk estimates given in Table 19.2 need to be reassessed in light of molecular developments but remain useful where affected relatives are dead or when DNA analysis is not possible. It should be noted that the risks for some categories have been reduced by comparison with earlier editions of this book in light of further evidence.

Norrie disease (pseudoglioma)

In the past, Norrie disease was frequently confused with retinoblastoma because of the appearance of the exudative vitreoretinopathy. The frequent occurrence of mental retardation makes genetic counselling for this X-linked recessive disease of considerable importance. The gene has been identified, and molecular analysis is relevant to carrier identification and prenatal diagnosis. Norrie disease is also mentioned in the section on retinopathies.

Other retinal dysplasias

A number of other conditions may need to be considered when the retinal appearance is unusual. These include retinopathy of prematurity, retinoschisis (see earlier in this chapter), incontinentia pigmenti (see Chapter 18), other familial exudative retinopathies, Coats' disease and the neuronal migration/congenital muscular dystrophy group of disorders including Walker-Warburg syndrome.

CATARACT

In cases of both congenital and adult-onset cataract, the nature and location of the opacities, especially in the early stages, can be of help in distinguishing the specific types.

Congenital cataract

Numerous types of congenital cataract exist, with all forms of inheritance recorded. The incidence is around 1 in 250 births. Environmental causes (e.g. the toxoplasmosis, other [syphilis, varicella-zoster, parvovirus B19], rubella, cytomegalovirus and herpes simplex [TORCH] congenital infections) and metabolic and other primary disorders (e.g. galactosaemia, hypoparathyroidism, peroxisomal disorders) must be excluded, and syndromal associations sought (e.g. Conradi disease, Lowe syndrome, cerebro-oculo-facio-skeletal [COFS], DNA repair defects). Consider the sex-linked Nance-Horan syndrome in severely affected male infants (females tend to be affected more mildly).

Because most genetic forms without a metabolic cause or syndromic features follow dominant inheritance, the risk for offspring of an affected person is not far short of 50%. The risk for sibs of an isolated case is probably 10% or less, but more accurate figures are needed.

A number of specific genes have been identified as sites of pathogenic mutations, some involving lens crystallin proteins.

Cataracts in later life

Primary disorders, both Mendelian (e.g. myotonic dystrophy) and non-Mendelian (e.g. diabetes), must be excluded. Most families showing a clear-cut aggregation appear to follow autosomal dominant inheritance.

Lens dislocation

Lens dislocation is a feature of the Marfan and Weill-Marchesani syndromes and of homocystinuria but may occur as an isolated abnormality due to an abnormally small and spherical lens (spherophakia), usually following autosomal dominant inheritance. The author has seen tall, thin members of one such family persistently misdiagnosed as having Marfan syndrome, with much unnecessary worry caused. In some families at least, the same fibrillin locus on chromosome 15 is involved as in Marfan syndrome.

GLAUCOMA

Glaucoma can be a part of a surprisingly large number of genetic syndromes and should be checked for in any ocular assessment of the patient with syndromes involving the eye since it may be a treatable aspect in an individual without specific ocular complaints. Major advances are occurring in isolation of genes involved with primary glaucoma, although it is not yet clear how these findings will affect genetic risks for those without a clear Mendelian inheritance pattern.

Primary closed-angle glaucoma

Primary closed-angle glaucoma seems to be determined largely by anatomical orbital factors, particularly shallowness of the anterior chamber; 12% of sibs were found to be clinically affected in one study.

Primary open-angle glaucoma

Primary open-angle glaucoma is common in the general population and is found in 1 in 200 elderly people. Studies of sibs have shown between 5% and 16% to be affected; 10% is probably an appropriate risk for clinically significant glaucoma. The risks for children have been lower but extremely variable. Because the children studied were always much younger than the sibs, it seems likely that the lifetime risk will approach the 10% seen for sibs. The proportion of families that has a Mendelian basis is uncertain, but some large families following autosomal dominant inheritance exist, some adult onset, others juvenile, have been mapped to specific chromosomes. Mutations in several different genes, showing variable penetrance, have been shown to occur in some juvenile families.

Congenital glaucoma

Congenital glaucoma may develop secondary to anterior segment malformation (Peters anomaly, Rieger syndrome, aniridia) and other generalised ocular problems (e.g. Sturge-Weber syndrome). When it is primary, a proportion of families appears to follow autosomal recessive inheritance, but isolated cases are much too common for this mode to explain all cases. The risk to sibs after a single affected child is around 10%; after two affected sibs, a 25% risk should be advised. Risks to children of affected individuals are uncertain. Assuming a mixture of recessive and polygenic forms, a risk of 5% seems appropriate until data are available. A specific cytochrome P450 gene on chromosome 2p, CYP1B1, has been shown to be responsible for some recessively inherited families, but other genetic loci also exist.

REFRACTIVE ERRORS

Twin studies show a very close concordance between monozygotic twin pairs, suggesting a high heritability (the factors affecting variation in ocular refraction being predominantly genetic). Individual pedigrees showing all types of Mendelian inheritance have been produced for each of the major types of refractive error but are of little help in deriving general risks for relatives. Studies of unselected families show high correlations for refractive values between both sibs and parents and offspring, suggesting that a polygenic basis is present with genes of additive effect and little dominance or recessivity. The same situation applies to disorders of corneal shape such as astigmatism, keratoconus and cornea plana.

Some regular syndromes of refractive error exist, including myopia and night blindness, which are usually X-linked recessive. Refractive errors may also accompany other primary Mendelian disorders, such as myopia in Marfan syndrome and some skeletal dysplasias, especially Stickler syndrome. In isolated cases of severe myopia, a risk of 4%–5% for similar severe eye problems in the children has been suggested.

HETEROCHROMIA OF THE IRIS

Heterochromia is frequently an isolated and harmless trait, often autosomal dominant in inheritance. The most important cause of heterochromia to recognise is Waardenburg syndrome (see Chapter 20), in which piebaldness and deafness are major features. Variation in expression of this autosomal dominant disorder is considerable.

EYE COLOUR

In the early medical genetics literature, eye colour was given as one of the most common reasons for requesting genetic counselling, but this rarely seems to be the case now. It is possible that such enquiries were really aimed at establishing paternity. In fact, while brown eye colour in general behaves as dominant to light blue eye colour, the genetic control is considerably more complex than this, and exceptions are sufficiently frequent for this trait not to be used as evidence for or against paternity.

STRABISMUS

Strabismus is a frequent feature of many generalised neuromuscular disorders, which may follow Mendelian inheritance (see Chapter 13). Duane syndrome is due to aberrant innervation of ocular muscles; it is generally sporadic, but a few families follow autosomal dominant inheritance. Isolated strabismus, whether classified as convergent or divergent, fits a polygenic pattern. Variation between studies results, in part, from the extent to which minor deviations are classed as abnormal. From the viewpoint of counselling, it seems that where parents are normal and one child is affected, the risk for subsequent children is around 15%. Where one parent is also affected, the risk is around 40%.

HEREDITARY PTOSIS

Hereditary ptosis is usually autosomal dominant and may persist unchanged through life. Care must be taken to distinguish more general neuromuscular causes (see Chapter 13), such as myotonic dystrophy, oculopharyngeal muscular dystrophy, myasthenic syndromes and the mitochondrial myopathies (e.g. chronic progressive external ophthalmoplegia [CPEO]). Ptosis is also a feature of some dysmorphic syndromes, including Noonan syndrome and the blepharophimosis-ptosis-epicanthus inversus syndrome (BPES).

DEVELOPMENTAL EYE DEFECTS

This field provides an excellent example of the value of comparative genetic studies, genes being strongly conserved between different phyla (e.g. between chordates and arthropods, notably mammals and fruit flies) as well as between mammalian orders (e.g. primates and rodents, notably the genera *Homo* and *Mus*), with many alterations in these evolutionarily conserved genes now recognised in human disorders.

Microphthalmos and anophthalmos

Microphthalmos and anophthalmos constitute an extremely heterogeneous group. Unilateral cases are frequently non-genetic but cannot be securely distinguished from genetic forms. Rubella, toxoplasmosis, maternal thalidomide and other drug exposures are possible causes of bilateral disease. Mental retardation is frequently associated, and microphthalmos is a feature of several chromosomal defects as well as Mendelian syndromes. The X-linked Lenz syndrome of microphthalmos with cataract, mental retardation and digital and genitourinary abnormalities must be considered. Microphthalmos with coloboma is usually autosomal dominant (in the absence of known external causes) and is heterogeneous. Complete bilateral anophthalmia can be difficult to distinguish from extreme microphthalmos and may result from environmental factors. Cryptophthalmos, with absent palpebral fissures, may be part of the previously mentioned disorders, or may occur with relatively normal eye development, usually following autosomal recessive inheritance. Some cases are part of the more general Fraser syndrome (autosomal recessive), where renal agenesis and laryngeal atresia may be major features, and where a specific developmental gene defect is known.

Cyclops

Almost all cases of this lethal malformation, an extreme form of holoprosencephaly (see Chapter 14), have been sporadic. Chromosomal abnormalities have been found in some cases.

Coloboma and aniridia

Both bilateral coloboma of the iris and the more severe aniridia usually follow autosomal dominant inheritance; colobomas may form part of more extensive ocular disorders. Because colobomas may vary considerably in extent, a thorough ophthalmic examination of both the parents and the patient is needed. The rare syndrome of ocular coloboma with anal atresia (cat eye syndrome) follows an autosomal dominant pattern but is associated with an extra chromosome 22 fragment. Mutation in the gene *CHD7* is an important cause of coloboma when it is a part of the condition CHARGE (coloboma, heart defects, atresia choanae, growth retardation, genital abnormalities and ear abnormalities) syndrome.

Aniridia may be associated with Wilms tumour, mental retardation and genital defects, as part of the 11p13 deletion syndrome including the developmental gene *PAX6* and known as WAGR. This is often sporadic but WAGR can be transmitted as a dominant trait. Detailed molecular analysis of the region has shown that a series of overlapping deletions is responsible for the various elements of the syndrome, analogous to those seen in other microdeletion syndromes.

Mutations in the gene *PAX6* and some other developmental genes may occur in aniridia and other anterior chamber abnormalities.

Corneal and anterior chamber abnormalities

These are heterogeneous and at times syndromal (e.g. Rieger syndrome with mutation in *PITX2*, or other loci, and Peters plus syndrome with mutation in *B3GALTL*). They are rare and require expert diagnosis, as well as checking of the parents for minor defects. Molecular abnormalities have been found in some cases, though less consistently than in aniridia.

20

Deafness

INTRODUCTION

At least 50% of cases of congenital and childhood deafness may be genetically determined. In the case of non-syndromic deafness, a precise clinical diagnosis may be impossible owing to phenotypic overlap with deafness of environmental origin. Careful attention to family history and detailed audiological evaluation, not just of the proband but also of other family members, may help to resolve the question of aetiology in apparently isolated cases. Close consultation with audiological colleagues and others is needed if errors are to be avoided.

Recognition of the specific genes involved in deafness has had a major impact on our understanding of this field and is also now playing a significant role in diagnosis and genetic counselling. For non-syndromic congenital sensorineural deafness, the loci and mutations involved vary considerably between different populations, and it is important to know the distribution of molecular defects in the particular population, if possible.

Two groups in particular may request genetic counselling: parents of a severely affected child wishing to have further children, and young adults with deafness, who frequently marry partners similarly affected.

Even without access to specialised audiological testing, it is often possible to assess the genetic situation accurately if the following points are borne in mind:

- What does the pattern of inheritance in the particular family suggest?
- Is the hearing loss severe congenital deafness, or some milder form?
- If hearing loss is milder, is it static or progressive?
- Is there an identifiable syndrome involving other systems?

Genetic counselling for the profoundly deaf is a service that requires a radically different approach from that in most other fields. The process of communication will usually require an intermediary, unless one has special experience with sign language or other forms of communication. Attitudes towards deafness within the community of the profoundly Deaf may well be quite different from those of doctors or of normally hearing patients, as they may regard the Deaf as an ill-understood but profoundly rewarding minority culture. Genetic counselling, like cochlear implantation, may be perceived by some as a threat to their community, unless it is sensitively presented when it is sought, or when it is respectfully integrated into the overall educational provision for young adults and adolescents.

SEVERE CONGENITAL SENSORINEURAL DEAFNESS

The incidence has been estimated to be around 1 in 1,000 births. Care must be taken to exclude external factors such as mild congenital rubella or cytomegalovirus infection.

In the absence of clear evidence of environmental aetiology, there is no doubt that a high proportion of cases result from autosomal recessive inheritance. It is difficult to decide exactly what this proportion is, because the different types are clinically indistinguishable, although they are now often being distinguished at the molecular level. However, one often remains dependent on older, though well-founded, data for an appreciation of the overall pattern of inheritance and recurrence. In less-developed countries, the proportion of deafness that is genetic will vary with the frequency of neonatal jaundice, perinatal asphyxia and congenital and neonatal infection, and also with the prevalence of consanguinity.

Most studies have suggested that 40%–50% of cases are autosomal recessive, with around 10% due to autosomal dominant inheritance and most of the rest due to unknown or undetected environmental (or at least non-Mendelian) factors. This would suggest that the risk of deafness in sibs of an isolated case is about 1 in 10, as long as other causes have been excluded as far as possible (e.g. congenital TORCH [toxoplasmosis, other {syphilis, varicella-zoster, parvovirus B19}, rubella, cytomegalovirus and herpes simplex] infection, perinatal asphyxia, neonatal jaundice, meningitis, aminoglycoside antibiotics). Where consanguinity exists, autosomal recessive inheritance is even more likely, and a one-in-four risk should be given. Likewise, should a couple have a second affected child, autosomal recessive inheritance is almost certain. Table 20.1 summarises the various risks.

The risk for offspring of healthy sibs and other family members is often asked about. This is very low (well under 1%) in the absence of consanguinity or of deafness in the family of the other partner.

The risk for offspring of an affected individual who is an isolated case and whose partner is unaffected is small but not negligible (around 5%). This risk probably results from an inclusion of unrecognised new dominant mutations with the much larger number following recessive inheritance, unless there is consanguinity or other factors suggesting that a recessive gene

Table 20.1 Empiric risk of recurrence of profound childhood deafness of unknown cause

Affected relative	Risk
One child only; environmental factors carefully excluded	1 in 10
One child only; consanguinity present	1 in 4
Two affected children	1 in 4
One parent + one child	1 in 2
One parent only	1 in 20
Parent + sib(s) of parent only	1 in 100
Sib(s) of parent; parent unaffected	<1 in 100

may have been transmitted by the healthy parent. Although severe dominantly inherited congenital deafness is rare in comparison to recessive forms, and is more variable in severity, it nevertheless accounts for the majority of two-generation families. In families with two affected sibs and healthy parents with normal audiograms, where recessive inheritance is almost certain, the risk for offspring of the affected individuals is low (around 1%).

X-linked recessive inheritance is well documented as a mode of inheritance in severe congenital deafness but is not frequent enough to affect the risks for isolated male cases or single sibships containing only affected males. Distinctive findings may be present on cochlear computed tomography (CT) scan in one form of X-linked non-syndromic deafness (*POU3F4*) and also in Pendred syndrome.

Marriage between two individuals with severe congenital deafness is common, and the offspring of such marriages provide clear evidence for the existence of several non-allelic recessive genes. If all cases were due to the same gene, or to different alleles at the same locus, one would expect all children to be affected. In fact, deaf children occur in only around 15% of marriages between affected individuals and the risk of a pregnancy resulting in a deaf child is only around 10%; in around 80% all children are unaffected, being heterozygous at each of the two loci involved. Such an outcome may come as a surprise and may be unsettling and cause difficulties for deaf couples who identify as part of the deaf, signing community. In only 5% of marriages are all children affected; in the other 10%, some children, but not all, prove to be affected, probably representing the situation where one of the partners has a dominant form of deafness.

Table 20.1 shows the various possibilities, while Table 20.2 summarises the risks for individual couples. Genetic testing, now increasingly available in a service setting, is proving especially useful for this group.

It is important to recognise that the risk for subsequent children of a couple may well be markedly altered by whether their first child proves to be affected or not (see Table 20.2), but molecular testing to identify the cause of deafness in both members of the couple will often be able to clarify this in advance of the couple having any children. There should not be so many surprises now that molecular diagnostics are readily available, unless a couple has chosen not to seek genetic counselling ahead of a pregnancy. A deaf couple whose first child is also deaf has at least a 50% chance of this recurring in the next pregnancy.

Numerous different genes may cause severe non-syndromic deafness, and a precise molecular diagnosis is particularly helpful for genetic counselling when both parents are deaf. The principal genes responsible for non-syndromic congenital sensorineural deafness are *GJB2* and *GJB6*, which are co-located at DFNB1 and encode connexins 26 and 30. Mutations in

Table 20.2 Risks for children when both parents have profound childhood deafness (risk for next child)

Number of children already born	Nil	One unaffected	One affected	Two affected
Parents related	>1/2	1 in 10	All	All
Parents unrelated but from same minority ethnic group	>1/2	1 in 10	All	All
Parents unrelated, not from same minority ethnic group	1 in 10	1 in 20	>1/2	All

these genes are responsible for around one-quarter of cases, although the proportion and type of mutations vary considerably between populations. A range of other genes, including other 'connexin' genes, may also be involved in some cases; genes causing syndromal types may also be responsible. Mitochondrial mutations are more often involved in less severe or later-onset deafness but should be considered if there is a maternally inherited family pattern, or a history of exposure to aminoglycoside antibiotics.

Diagnostic assessment will include audiograms of parents as well as the child, urinalysis and electrocardiograph (ECG). Imaging can be very helpful in determining the underlying cause, with structural anomalies giving clues as to genetic or non-genetic factors. Dilated vestibular aqueducts are found in Pendred syndrome, the Mondini cochlear dysplasia in branchio-oto-renal syndrome, and a characteristic deformity of the temporal bone in one X-linked type (*POU3F4*). Renal ultrasound scan may also indicate some syndromic associations.

MILD-TO-MODERATE DEAFNESS

Partial nerve deafness includes numerous genetic forms of deafness whose effect is confined to the ear but where hearing loss is not sufficient to present as congenital deaf-mutism. Some forms are present from birth and are static; others are later in onset and progressive, while detailed audiological testing may show loss of particular frequencies. The classification of this group is currently being reorganised to take account of the contributions of molecular genetics to the taxonomy of the condition. Expert advice should be sought if there is any doubt about interpretation of genetic findings or the correlation between genotype and phenotype.

Molecular analysis is now beginning to identify some of the specific genes, notably those on the X chromosome, and is likely to become helpful in resolving the heterogeneity. Several factors are especially relevant to genetic counselling in this group:

- A considerably higher proportion of cases results from autosomal dominant inheritance than occurs with severe congenital deafness.
- Variability within a family can be considerable, so careful testing is required before an individual is pronounced 'normal' (i.e. neither affected nor a 'carrier').
- Isolated cases are extremely difficult to distinguish from non-genetic forms of hearing loss.
- X-linked deafness of various types is especially important to recognise in view of the risks to the extended family.
- It seems likely that mitochondrial mutations may be involved in predisposition in some families, and also in drug-induced deafness.

Otosclerosis

Otosclerosis is the most common disorder in this group and can be recognised by its progressive course and mixed conductive and neural pattern. It follows autosomal dominant inheritance with rather incomplete penetrance (around 40%).

DEAFNESS AS PART OF SYNDROMES

The number of syndromes associated with deafness is exceedingly large. Previous editions of this book listed some of the more common syndromes, but readers are now advised to consult journal reviews, the GeneReviews website or textbooks (see Appendix 1 for details).

Hearing problems are most important to recognise in any syndrome since they may be remediable, as well as cause avoidable educational problems that may be mistaken for mental retardation.

Four syndromic forms of deafness, three autosomal recessive and one autosomal dominant, are of particular importance and are mentioned here since they have serious consequences if overlooked, and some are (relatively) common.

Pendred syndrome (autosomal recessive)

This disorder has probably been considerably underdiagnosed. Variable but generally severe nerve deafness occurs with goitre; early thyroxine monitoring and treatment are important, but many patients are euthyroid. Vestibular imaging may show characteristic changes. The gene responsible is involved in ion transport.

Jervell and Lange-Nielsen syndrome (autosomal recessive)

Severe nerve deafness is accompanied by abnormal cardiac conduction. Sudden death may occur (see Chapter 21 for further details).

Usher syndrome (autosomal recessive)

Nerve deafness and retinitis pigmentosa are the defining features, but several forms, all autosomal recessive, are now recognised. In type I the deafness is severe, with vestibular involvement, while this is absent and the deafness moderate in type II. Molecular defects in myosin VII have been found in type Ib.

Neurofibromatosis type 2 (NF2) (autosomal dominant)

This condition is mentioned because those who have inherited it or are at risk require careful monitoring with audiology and magnetic resonance imaging (MRI), so that any acoustic neuroma (schwannoma) that develops can be detected and given optimal management. Low-level mosaicism in one parent of an affected child has been difficult to detect, so genetic counselling has had to be cautious, but next-generation sequencing methods are improving the recognition of mosaicism. The causal mutation is now detected more frequently than in the past, which helps guide appropriate health monitoring and provides information about reproductive risks.

Those affected can also develop a range of other complications and require a more general assessment of their health. They are at particular risk of cataracts, meningiomas and spinal and peripheral nerve tumours.

EXTERNAL EAR

Several syndromes, both dominantly and recessively inherited, have been described in which deafness (usually conductive) has been associated with abnormal shape of the external ear as the only visible feature.

External ear malformation is also striking in such craniofacial disorders as Goldenhar syndrome and mandibulofacial dysostosis (Treacher Collins syndrome). Environmental causes include rubella and thalidomide embryopathies, and – usually only in fatal cases – the 'Potter facies' resulting from oligohydramnios secondary to renal agenesis or other causes. Lesser degrees of abnormality form part of the characteristic facies of many genetic syndromes. The CHARGE (coloboma, heart defects, atresia choanae, growth retardation, genital abnormalities and ear abnormalities) and Kabuki syndromes often show dysplastic, cupped ears and can be associated with deafness and anomalies of the inner ear.

Isolated external ear abnormalities, particularly when unilateral, carry a low recurrence risk, but a careful examination should be carried out for minor audiological or branchial arch defects on both sides. The frequent associations with renal abnormalities are especially worth considering.

MÉNIÈRE'S DISEASE

A few familial aggregations of Ménière's disease have been recorded, suggesting either autosomal dominant inheritance with reduced penetrance or multifactorial (complex) aetiology. One can safely say that the risks to family members of a single case of this common disorder are low.

21

Cardiac and cardiovascular disorders

Cardiovascular disorders pose a large number of genetic counselling challenges. The conditions associated with congenital heart disease have been fairly well studied, although further information about some more recently recognised microdeletion syndromes remains to be gathered. In relation to the Mendelian disorders of cardiac muscle and rhythm, however, the application of genetic testing to clinical management is less straightforward. There remains some uncertainty about the contribution of specific genetic variants to the cardiomyopathies and disorders of the thoracic aorta and rather more uncertainty about the genetic basis of the inherited dysrhythmias. Given the context of sudden death, or the risk of sudden death, there is a lot at stake for families.

Congenital heart disease is a large group of disorders for which advice is sought, usually regarding the risks for further affected children and the likely impact of the underlying condition on the quality of the child's life and now, increasingly, concerning the risk to offspring of a successfully treated patient. Our knowledge of the genetic basis of congenital heart disease has grown substantially through the study of the genes involved in cardiac development. In addition, new syndromic patterns of phenotypic features have been recognised that include cardiac features. Chromosomal microarrays have allowed several new diagnoses to emerge – the recurrent microdeletion and microduplication syndromes – and the natural history of these conditions is still being clarified. Similar information is also still being collected in relation to newly recognised disorders that have emerged from exome sequencing projects (such as the Deciphering Developmental Disorders project). The very variable phenotypes associated with some of the copy number variants (CNVs) leave the question open as to whether reports of cardiac malformation in children with, for example, the 15q13.3 and 16p11.2 recurrent microdeletion syndromes reflect a genuine cardiac element in the condition or a comorbidity subject to ascertainment bias but that has arisen by chance. There will be much to learn about these disorders in the coming years.

Major advances have occurred in the understanding of many types of cardiomyopathy and of the inherited dysrhythmias, but coronary artery disease of later life is proving a more complex area to resolve. While large-scale genetic epidemiological studies have begun to dissect the different genetic and environmental risk components, these are not yet at the stage of usefully affecting risk estimation and genetic counselling for the individual patient. Nor is it clear that this will change rapidly (see also Chapter 3), since a series of complex interactions seems likely that makes attempts at individual risk prediction very uncertain and probably unhelpful, outside those families with a clear Mendelian pattern, such as familial hypercholesterolaemia.

The inherited cardiac conditions have developed into a field, alongside familial neurological disease and the familial cancers, where clinical specialists in the area are incorporating genetic advances into their regular diagnostic practice. This is mainly because of the rare but numerous Mendelian forms being recognised, for which genetic testing can be clinically helpful. This is not the case for the common polygenic cardiovascular disorders, where genetic testing still has no significant role to play.

CONGENITAL HEART DISEASE

Clinically significant congenital heart disease occurs in around 1 in 200 births (nearer to 1 in 100 if minor cases picked up by investigation are included). Although around 90% of cases are not obviously familial, it seems increasingly likely that important genetic factors are involved in most cases. The risk of recurrence in sibs indicates that genetic and sometimes maternal effects are important, and specific genes and chromosome regions are being identified. Because the clinical features can be so variable, array comparative genomic hybridisation (aCGH) of the child's chromosomes will usually be performed to look for evidence of the 22q11.2 deletion syndrome or another relevant CNV, of which there are many. It is especially important to examine the child's chromosomes if additional, non-cardiac abnormalities are also present. This can allow other possible clinical problems to be anticipated, such as the immunodeficiency of the DiGeorge syndrome phenotype.

Table 21.1 lists some of the more important Mendelian disorders characterised by cardiac involvement that must be distinguished. There are a number of syndromes that do not always follow Mendelian inheritance (Table 21.2). Congenital heart disease is also prominent in chromosomal disorders, particularly the autosomal trisomies and Turner syndrome; around 15% of congenital heart disease is due to chromosomal defects. The greater resolution of aCGH when compared with conventional cytogenetics has demonstrated that small deletions within chromosome 22q11.2, not always apparent cytogenetically, may be associated with cardiac defects.

Among the identified environmental causes, rubella is still the most important globally, but its incidence in developed countries has fallen as a result of the active immunisation of adolescents in school-based programmes. However, congenital heart defects are produced by almost all the less specific teratogens and environmental factors (see Chapter 28), which should be carefully enquired after, even though it may not be possible to prove cause and effect in an individual case. Prenatal exposure to alcohol is increasingly recognised as an important risk factor (e.g. for ventricular septal defects). Lithium is specifically associated with Ebstein anomaly. Other important teratogenic drugs include retinoic acid and the anticonvulsants. The offspring of diabetic women also form a high-risk group, not only for hypoglycaemia from hyperinsulinism in the first few days after birth but also from teratogenesis. Maternal phenylketonuria (PKU) is

Table 21.1 Heart disease in some Mendelian disorders

Disorder	Main extracardiac features	Usual heart defects	Inheritance
Holt-Oram syndrome	Upper limb defects, especially digits and radius	Atrial septal defect	Autosomal dominant
Ellis-van Creveld syndrome	Dwarfism, midline cleft lip, polydactyly	Ventricular septal defect	Autosomal recessive
CHARGE syndrome	Ocular coloboma, choanal atresia, ear and genital defects	Very variable but conotruncal is relatively frequent	Mutations in CHD7 (allelic with an uncommon form of Kallmann syndrome)
Williams syndrome	Facial features, mental handicap	Supravalvular aortic stenosis	Microdeletions around elastin gene; most cases sporadic
Noonan syndrome (more severe problems in the other RASopathies)	Short stature, wide forehead, hypertelorism, pectus excavatum; may have learning difficulties	Pulmonary valve stenosis; hypertrophic cardiomyopathy	Autosomal dominant
Marfan syndrome	Skeletal abnormalities, lens dislocation	Mitral valve prolapse, dilated aortic root	Autosomal dominant (usually missense) mutations in fibrillin gene FBN1
Alagille syndrome	Intrahepatic cholestasis, facies, butterfly vertebrae, tetralogy of Fallot	Peripheral pulmonary artery stenosis, septal defects, anomalous drainage	Autosomal dominant (JAG1 or del 20p)
Tuberous sclerosis	See Chapter 14	Intracardiac tumours	Autosomal dominant
LEOPARD syndrome	Nerve deafness, lentigines	Conduction defects, pulmonary stenosis	Autosomal dominant mutations in PTPN11 and other loci
Kartagener syndrome	Situs inversus	Dextrocardia	Autosomal recessive
Jervell and Lange-Nielsen syndrome	Nerve deafness	Congenital conduction defects	Autosomal recessive channelopathy (with genetic heterogeneity)
Kabuki syndrome	Characteristic facies, feeding problems	Coarctation and septal defects	Usually de novo dominant mutations in KMT2D; can also be X-linked KDM6A
Friedreich ataxia	See Chapter 14	Cardiomyopathy	Autosomal recessive

Table 21.2 Other syndromes with congenital heart disease

Disorder	Non-cardiac features	Cardiac lesion	Inheritance or recurrence risk
Asplenia and polysplenia syndromes	Complex defects of laterality	Dextrocardia and other complex defects	3%–5%; laterality involves a complex developmental pathway and several genes can be involved
VATER (VACTERL) association	Vertebral, anal, tracheo-oesophageal, renal and (radial) limb defects	Variable	Usually low ~1%
Klippel-Feil syndrome	Fusion and reduction of cervical vertebrae	Cardiac involvement is common; hearing, limbs, association with MURCS	Low, but familial forms exist; many cases arise as de novo dominant mutations
DiGeorge syndrome (due to 22q11.2 microdeletions)	Absent thymus and parathyroids	Commonly conotruncal defects	Recurrence risk low for sibs if parents unaffected and microdeletion is de novo
Velocardiofacial or Shprintzen syndrome	Cleft palate, facial anomalies	As for DiGeorge syndrome	As for DiGeorge syndrome
Goldenhar syndrome	Eye, ear and facial abnormalities	Various defects in half	Low: only rarely familial

Abbreviations: MURCS, Müllerian, renal, cervicothoracic somite abnormalities; VACTERL, vertebral defects, anal atresia, cardiac defects, tracheo-oesophageal fistula, renal anomalies, limb abnormalities; VATER, vertebrae, anus, trachea, oesophagus, renal.

a potent but preventable cause of cardiac malformation and should no longer be a cause of such problems. Monozygous twinning is itself a risk factor for congenital heart disease, such twins having a threefold increase in risk (around 1.5%). In contrast to earlier thinking, there seems to be no evidence of a maternal age effect except through its effect on chromosomal disorders.

Genetic advice is most frequently sought for future sibs of an affected child or the children of a surviving affected individual. Risks other than for first-degree relatives are low in the absence of multiple cases or an identified Mendelian basis. Information is now becoming available for the offspring of affected individuals, and there is increasing evidence that risks are higher for offspring of affected females than of males.

Overall risks are summarised in Table 21.3 but, whenever possible, a specific anatomical diagnosis should be used as the basis for risk estimates. Data for a number of the more common defects, excluding syndromes, are given in Table 21.4. The data are given for sib risk only, since the figures for offspring in different studies have given widely divergent results and are based on small numbers when broken down into individual types. A trend can be seen, however, in

Table 21.3 Overall risks in congenital heart disease (for use when details of specific disorder are uncertain or unavailable)

	Risk (%)
Population incidence	0.5
Sib of isolated case	4
Half-sibs or other second-degree relatives	1
Offspring of isolated case	
Father	2–3
Mother	5–6 (may be higher, up to ~15%, for some conditions)
Two affected sibs (or sib and parent)	10
More than two affected first-degree relatives	50 (approximately)

that the recurrence risk in offspring may be higher than in sibs for some categories of defect (up to 10%–16% for some conditions). This may be the result of some cases being the result of new dominant mutations. Where recurrence does occur, the defect is the same as previously in only about half the cases. This is relevant to counselling because it may mean that a sib of a proband with a correctable defect may have a fatal or untreatable lesion, or vice versa.

Table 21.4 Approximate genetic risks for sibs of isolated cases of non-syndromic congenital heart disease

Defect	Risk (%)
Isomerism sequence	5
Situs inversus	3
Aortic stenosis	3
Hypoplastic left heart	3
Ventricular septal defect	3
Atrial septal defect	3
Patent ductus arteriosus	2.5
Tetralogy of Fallot	2.5
Arteriovenous canal defect	2.5
Pulmonary stenosis	2
Coarctation of the aorta	2
Transposition of great vessels	2
Ebstein anomaly and ventricular septal defect	2
Pulmonary atresia	1
Common truncus	1
Tricuspid atresia	1

Source: Based on multiple studies collated by (1) Nora JJ, Berg K, Nora AH 1991 *Cardiovascular Diseases: Genetics, Epidemiology and Prevention.* Oxford: Oxford University Press; (2) Burn J, Goodship J 2007 Congenital Heart Disease, Chapter 52. In: Rimoin DL, Connor JM, Pyeritz RE, Korf BR (Eds.). *Emery & Rimoin's Principles and Practice of Medical Genetics* (5th ed.). London, New York and Edinburgh: Churchill Livingstone, pp. 1083–1159.

The increasing resolution of cardiac ultrasound imaging can now identify many structural defects in the later part of pregnancy, but prenatal diagnosis before 18 weeks of gestation may only be feasible for the more severe defects. Most published data derive from testing in referral centres where many of the pregnancies monitored are already known to be at high risk, so the performance of ultrasonography in cardiac prenatal screening generally is probably less than the best figures seen in these high-risk situations.

Risks to more distant relatives

Data are inadequate but the excess risk for second-degree relatives of an isolated case of (non-syndromic) congenital heart disease is certainly under 1%, and it is doubtful whether third-degree relatives have a significantly raised risk. Families are sometimes encountered where there are several affected members, none of whom is a first-degree relative. The possibility of a variable but dominantly inherited form should be seriously considered here.

Multiple cases

Familial clusters of congenital heart disease are not uncommon. Their occurrence should prompt a careful search for a Mendelian or chromosomal syndrome or teratogenic factor. After two affected children, the risk of congenital heart disease in future sibs is approximately trebled, regardless of whether the affected individuals have the same heart defect or not. This gives risks ranging from 5% for the rare defects to at least 10% for a common abnormality such as ventricular septal defect (VSD). A similar risk would be likely for future children where an affected parent has an affected child, although data to confirm this are not yet available. Numbers are insufficient to give individual estimates for specific defects. The occurrence of more distant affected relatives does not greatly raise the risks given in Table 21.4. In the occasional families with more than two affected first-degree relatives, risks are likely to approach 50% even though the factors underlying such occurrences are not understood.

Atrial septal defect

Occasional families following autosomal dominant inheritance exist, with a number of loci identified, as well as dominant syndromal associations such as the Holt-Oram syndrome and atrial septal defect (ASD) with atrioventricular conduction defects (several forms of this exist, each associated with a specific locus). These families are too rare to affect the general recurrence risks but should be borne in mind when familial clusters of three or more patients are encountered, which should probably be counselled as Mendelian. Minimal hand defects should be checked for in such families, in case they represent examples of Holt-Oram syndrome, for which the gene is the human counterpart of a previously known mouse developmental gene (TBX5).

Ventricular septal defect

The figures given in Table 21.4 apply to severe VSDs, mostly those patients requiring surgery. It is doubtful whether the risks are as high for relatives of patients with asymptomatic or transient defects.

Patent ductus arteriosus

Congenital rubella and preterm delivery must be considered. In their absence, the recurrence risk of patent ductus arteriosus varies considerably between series, but 3% seems a reasonable figure for sibs. The similar overall risk to offspring seems to mask a higher maternal risk of around 4%. A rare, dominantly inherited form exists (Char syndrome) with distinctive facial features.

Conotruncal and aortic arch defects

This is the group where a careful clinical assessment of the family and aCGH of the chromosomes is most likely to show an underlying chromosome 22q11.2 deletion (see later). Few such cases are truly non-syndromal, but the extra cardiac features can be subtle.

Dextrocardia with asplenia

Absence of the spleen, or the presence of multiple spleens, is an important point to note at autopsy in congenital heart disease, because a combination of defects involving left-sided visceral structures is seen with asplenia, and a corresponding series involving right-sided defects with polysplenia. The recurrence risk overall is probably comparable to other types of congenital heart disease, but there is an X-linked form of isomerism for which a gene (*ZIC3*) has been isolated. An important group of developmental defects involving laterality and isomerism has been defined, with the heart prominently involved. Total situs inversus also provides an association with dextrocardia, as in Kartagener syndrome (see Chapter 22).

Endocardial fibroelastosis

Endocardial fibroelastosis may be secondary to acquired myocarditis or may accompany other congenital heart defects; idiopathic fibroelastosis should be accepted as the diagnosis only with autopsy or biopsy evidence. Some cases may result from systemic carnitine deficiency. A thorough study from Toronto found a recurrence risk of 3.8% in sibs, rather higher than expected from the incidence of the disorder. It is possible that a small subgroup follows autosomal recessive inheritance but, if it exists, it cannot at present be distinguished from the majority and may represent an underlying metabolic disorder. Remember that the cardiac phenotype of the X-linked Barth syndrome can manifest as endocardial fibroelastosis, not always as a simple (i.e. typical) cardiomyopathy.

Syndromes with congenital heart disease

These are numerous and not all show a clear inheritance pattern. The following deserve special note.

NOONAN SYNDROME

The characteristic facies with ptosis and low-set ears, as well as a different cardiac defect from that of Turner syndrome (commonly pulmonary stenosis but also sometimes hypertrophic cardiomyopathy), should allow clinical recognition of this relatively common disorder in either sex. Autosomal dominant inheritance occurs, but the risk to sibs of an isolated case with entirely normal parents is low. Mutations in the gene *PTPN11* have been found in about half of those affected. This gene is also involved in the LEOPARD syndrome of lentigines, deafness and pulmonary stenosis. Other genes of the Ras-MAPK pathway can be involved in Noonan syndrome and several disorders caused by mutations in genes in this pathway have overlapping clinical features; they are known collectively as the RASopathies.

22Q11 DELETION SYNDROME

Loss of chromosome material from the proximal part of 22q, involving a number of genes, is now known to be an important syndromal cause of congenital heart disease, particularly conotruncal defects (around 30% of all cases). It combines conditions formerly considered as distinct, such as DiGeorge syndrome (with thymic and parathyroid hypoplasia) and velocardiofacial (Shprintzen) syndrome (with abnormalities of palatal form and/or function). Facial features are characteristic but often subtle, and some family members have no heart defect. The precise combination of features varies, even within family members affected by the identical deletion. Molecular diagnostic testing by fluorescence *in situ* hybridisation (FISH), aCGH, quantitative polymerase chain reaction (qPCR) or next-generation sequencing (NGS) may show a defect when chromosomes appear normal on karyotype. The recurrence risk is small if parental tests are normal, but it is effectively 50% where a parent has the defect.

With the advent of aCGH studies of patients' chromosomes, it has become clear that microdeletions at either end of the large region usually deleted in the 22q11.2 deletion syndrome can result in developmental disorders but they are not associated with the same cardiac defects or dysmorphic phenotypes. There are different possible breakpoints at each end of the large 22q11 deletion region and the smaller microdeletions result from the loss of sequence between two of these potential breakpoints, at one end or the other of the larger region, when that has not been deleted.

WILLIAMS SYNDROME

This combination of supravalvular aortic stenosis with a characteristic facies, mental handicap and variable hypercalcaemia is now known to be a microdeletion syndrome of chromosome 7q, with loss of several genes, including especially that for elastin, which provides a valuable molecular test. Recurrence is rare if parents are clinically normal and show no elastin gene deficiency. Isolated (non-syndromic) dominantly inherited supravalvular aortic stenosis involves the elastin gene in isolation.

CARDIOMYOPATHIES

Cardiomyopathies can occur in childhood or adult life; they may form part of primary Mendelian disorders such as type 2 glycogenosis (acid maltase deficiency, Pompe disease), the Duchenne and Emery-Dreifuss muscular dystrophies, myotonic dystrophy and Friedreich ataxia, as well as specific syndromes and the various mitochondrial myopathies. Much adult cardiomyopathy is secondary to external factors such as alcohol.

Molecular studies have now defined a range of defects in contractile proteins and ion channels, mostly dominant but with significantly reduced penetrance. Molecular testing is available for many of these disease-associated loci, although there is often uncertainty as to whether a novel variant will be pathogenic. In addition, the natural history of each precise type of cardiomyopathy is often unclear and the penetrance of many variants in disease-associated genes may also be unclear. There are grounds for thinking that interaction between variants at more than one locus can substantially influence the phenotype. It will be important to conduct family studies to clarify these points, and to consider when it may be appropriate to examine a panel of other possibly relevant genes even when a pathogenic variant has been found in one gene in a patient, so that the offer of genetic testing for disease management can be better informed.

Hypertrophic cardiomyopathy

Hypertrophic cardiomyopathy (HCM) in older children and young adults is not rare (prevalence around 1 in 500 prevalence) and often appears to be inherited as a variable autosomal dominant trait (in about two-thirds of those affected). Penetrance is often higher if the family is studied by echocardiography but only around 25% if defined by clinical presentation; that is, there is a risk of approximately one in eight for clinical disease in first-degree relatives. Specific mutations at the myosin β-heavy chain locus have been identified in some families, while others result from defects in tropomyosin, troponin and a longer list of less commonly involved genes. Finding a clearly pathogenic mutation in a known gene can be a great help in assessing unaffected family members and in genetic counselling; it may also help the cardiologist to assess the likely prognosis and thereby inform decisions of management. One of the benefits of NGS gene panel testing for these disorders is that their apparently variable penetrance can be seen in some families to result from the involvement of variants at more than one locus. Thus, some cases seem to arise through a form of digenic inheritance.

First-degree and, sometimes, second-degree relatives may be advised to seek screening for HCM. This is especially true in the teenage years, when those at risk should be assessed at least annually, with less frequent surveillance in childhood or from 20 years. If the family's disease-causing mutation is known, then the numbers of those requiring cardiac surveillance can be reduced and the difficulties with obtaining insurance will be minimised. However, variants of uncertain significance (VUSs) can be a major problem in advising these families, with the potential for problems from either over- or under-attributing significance to a variant. A coordinated multidisciplinary approach to the evaluation of patients, family members and their genetic test results is important.

When arranging genetic testing of an affected patient (the proband in a family), it is important to generate the minimum information that will be sufficient. This means selecting the most focussed panel of relevant genes and avoiding a very wide, all-inclusive panel or an exome; this minimises the chance of finding an irrelevant VUS that would simply cause confusion. Equally, it is important to perform the genetic testing as a panel of relevant genes, because the importance of interactions between mutations at more than one locus is becoming recognised. (The laboratory may in fact perform exome sequencing but the bioinformatic analysis and interpretation of findings should be reported in the way it was requested, as a focussed 'virtual' panel.)

It is important to remember the distinction between (1) the level of confidence that a genetic variant is pathogenic (and caused, or contributed to, the disease phenotype) and (2) the penetrance of the variant or mutation: if someone inherits the variant, how likely are they to be affected? These are very different questions but are sometimes confused.

With a child at risk of an inherited HCM, a cardiac echo will usually be appropriate, and a plan of surveillance can be agreed upon. Making a decision about genetic testing may be more difficult. It will be important to discuss the question of exercise restriction in advance of genetic testing and it may be better to continue with surveillance, without genetic testing, if the child or family fear that their response to a positive (adverse) genetic test result may result in excessive anxiety and caution. Some families have regretted testing undertaken without sufficient prior reflection.

Suggestions for the cardiac screening of all athletes seem unwise, although there may be a role for this in professional sport. Caution is urged until the situation becomes clearer: there is difficulty in distinguishing the ECG features of cardiomyopathy from those of physical training and 'being fit', and enormous distress can result from advising healthy young people to stop training for the sport they love. A long QT interval in the absence of other abnormalities may be entirely benign. Even in professional sport, it is difficult to see any justification for genetic (molecular) screening in the absence of a relevant family history or a disease-associated phenotype, as this may be more likely to detect a VUS and cause confusion than to be helpful.

Dilated cardiomyopathy

This is rarer than hypertrophic cardiomyopathy (around 1 in 2,000 births). Most cases of dilated cardiomyopathy (DCM) are not familial but have a toxic (e.g. alcohol or iron overload), infective, inflammatory or endocrine cause. (Note that iron overload may be associated with other genetic causes, such as haemochromatosis or transfusion for thalassaemia.) In familial cases, less than half have a clear genetic cause. Specific autosomal dominant and X-linked forms are recognised. The dominant forms include mutations affecting sarcomeric or cytoskeletal proteins, lamin A/C and some ion channel proteins. The X-linked Barth syndrome also shows skeletal myopathy and general metabolic changes. Dystrophin-related cardiomyopathies (also X-linked) are another rare group. Mitochondrial disease (including mitochondrial encephalopathy with lactic acidosis and stroke-like episodes [MELAS], myoclonic epilepsy with ragged-red fibres [MERRF] and Kearns-Sayre syndrome) can lead to DCM. Childhood cases may be affected by Alström syndrome, or a mitochondrial disorder, or may be part of a more general metabolic disorder. Families with recessive inheritance are unusual.

Arrhythmogenic cardiomyopathy (ACMP), formerly arrhythmogenic (right ventricular) cardiomyopathy (ARVC) or arrhythmogenic (right ventricular) dysplasia (ARVD)

This is now known not to be a purely right ventricular disorder but remains difficult to diagnose even at examination *postmortem*. It is probably less common than DCM, affecting approximately 1 in 3,000–4,000. It usually follows autosomal dominant inheritance.

In ARVC, the cardiac muscle is replaced by fibrosis and fat, in the right ventricle more than the left. The genes implicated are important for the integrity of cell-cell junctions, such as plakophilin-2 (*PKP-2*). The condition is characterised by ECG abnormalities, dysrhythmias and sometimes heart failure. Changes may also be seen on cardiac echo. ARVC may lead to sudden death. Specialist cardiac pathology may be required to identify the disorder at examination *postmortem*. Treatment can be difficult and may require transplantation.

An autosomal recessive disorder, Naxos disease, is caused by mutations in the junctional plakoglobin gene (*JUP*) and causes palmoplantar keratoderma and woolly hair as well as a biventricular cardiomyopathy resembling ACMP.

Other cardiomyopathies

Other, less common forms of cardiomyopathy are recognised. These include endomyocardial fibrosis, restrictive cardiomyopathy and left ventricular non-compaction.

Restrictive cardiomyopathy is often neither genetic nor familial but can be caused by amyloidosis, endomyocardial fibrosis and a number of genetic and non-genetic conditions. The information relevant for genetic counselling will depend upon the underlying diagnosis (when this can be determined), by the geographical region and by the population of origin of the affected individual.

Left ventricular non-compaction is also often sporadic but it can be caused by mutations in lamin A/C, in some of the genes encoding sarcomeric proteins (overlapping with the genes involved in HCM) and some channelopathy genes.

CONGENITAL CARDIAC CONDUCTION DEFECTS AND DISORDERS OF CARDIAC RHYTHM

These are important causes of unexpected sudden death and may also cause symptoms including loss of consciousness (blackouts, syncope), which can be dangerous in its own right. They are often the result of mutation in one of the channelopathy genes, as are some of the epilepsy disorders that can be difficult to distinguish clinically.

Long QT syndrome

A major advance in the long QT syndrome has been the identification of specific sodium or potassium ion-channel defects for the different forms. All the specific types follow autosomal dominant inheritance but penetrance is incomplete, so a normal ECG (in which the QTc is normal) is not a guarantee of being genetically unaffected. Provocative testing may be needed with an adrenergic agent (e.g. ajmaline) in a cardiac physiology laboratory to demonstrate the ECG phenotype.

At least 12 different loci are recognised. The clinical features may differ somewhat, especially the factors that provoke symptomatic episodes (or death), with swimming and sudden, loud noises being hazardous in *LQT1* and *LQT2*, respectively. All affected should avoid competitive sports and drugs that prolong the QT interval. Timothy syndrome also has non-cardiac features including autism, syndactyly and immunodeficiency.

The form with deafness (Jervell and Lange-Nielsen syndrome) is now known to be due to homozygosity for variants in one of two potassium channel genes. Each parent will carry a mutation in the gene; this may result in LQT syndrome but they need not be symptomatic.

Brugada syndrome

This is an underdiagnosed condition affecting 1 in 2,000 and characterised by specific ECG changes that are not always present or may be missed (including elevation and specific conformational changes of the ST segment across the right-sided anterior chest leads). The associated dysrhythmias, potentially triggered by a number of factors (including some drugs such as anti-depressants, β-blockers, cocaine) can cause syncope, palpitations or sudden cardiac death from ventricular fibrillation. It causes more problems in men than women and is more frequent in Southeast Asia. Responsible genes are known for a modest proportion of cases and include several channelopathy genes, especially *SCN5A*.

Diagnosis of those at risk, as in long QT syndrome, may entail pharmacological challenge in the cardiac physiology laboratory. Management of confirmed cases often requires implantation of an implantable cardioverter-defibrillator (ICD) device, and sometimes also medication (including quinidine).

Other disorders of cardiac rhythm

Catecholaminergic polymorphic ventricular tachycardia (CPVT) is triggered in those susceptible, as might be expected, by exercise or stress. This is mostly autosomal dominant (especially *RYR2*) but a recessive form exists.

Familial atrial fibrillation is often inherited as an autosomal dominant trait and is well reported in Chinese populations. The responsible genes include potassium channel components.

Wolff-Parkinson-White (WPW) syndrome is usually sporadic but families demonstrating dominant inheritance have been recorded (with variants in *PRKAG2*).

Familial heart block may rarely occur congenitally and without other features, but important dominantly inherited forms exist with onset in adult life and no early clinical abnormalities. These are now distinguished as inherited sinus node dysfunction and progressive cardiac conduction defect (several genes are known). Heart block may also arise as one part of the wider phenotype of some inherited disorders, most especially myotonic dystrophy and lamin A/C disease (including Emery-Dreifuss muscular dystrophy).

As with HCM, caution should be exercised when considering testing healthy relatives for these conditions, especially children.

CORONARY ARTERY DISEASE

The epidemic increase of coronary artery disease in the mid- and late-twentieth century, now declining in much of North America and Europe, is likely to have environmental causes. However, susceptibility to the disease has a strong genetic basis, particularly when onset is early. Insurance companies have long recognised this, basing their conclusions on extensive actuarial data, but little practical use has yet been made of our knowledge in terms of information to relatives and the application of preventive measures except in relation to familial hypercholesterolaemia.

The risk of death from ischaemic heart disease in relatives of affected patients has been known for many years (Table 21.5) and has not been altered by recent studies. As expected from the higher incidence in males, the increase in risk to relatives is greater where the index patient is female (see Chapter 3), although the absolute risk figure is greater for male relatives than for females. One-third of monozygotic twin pairs show concordance for coronary artery disease.

Two particular genetic influences have been identified:

- The major gene of familial hypercholesterolaemia and other genetic loci affecting lipid levels.
- Other genetic factors independent of lipid status.

Familial hypercholesterolaemia

This should be suspected whenever a familial aggregation of early coronary artery disease occurs. Many patients will show xanthomas or other cholesterol deposits, but vascular disease

Table 21.5 Risks of death from ischaemic heart disease between the ages of 35 and 55 years in first-degree relatives of index patients with ischaemic heart disease (before the advent of statin drugs)

	Male index case	Female index case
Male first-degree relative	1 in 12 (×5)	1 in 10 (×6.5)
Female first-degree relative	1 in 36 (×2.5)	1 in 12 (×7)

Source: From Slack J, Evans KA 1966. *J Med Genet* 3: 239–257.

may be the only clinical feature. It is most important to recognise that the great majority of lipid abnormalities found in patients with vascular disease are secondary to dietary factors or other disorders and that familial hypercholesterolaemia should be diagnosed only when these have been excluded. Even when only primary cases with typical lipoprotein abnormalities are considered, it seems likely that the majority are multifactorial in origin rather than following simple Mendelian inheritance. Classic familial hypercholesterolaemia, accounting for around 10%–20% of early coronary artery disease, is an autosomal dominant disorder, with a heterozygote prevalence estimated to be around 1 in 500, although in some populations (e.g. South Africans of Dutch origin) the prevalence may be as high as 1 in 100. Affected homozygotes with severe childhood disease are well recognised but difficult to treat (often using plasmapheresis and more experimental approaches) and extremely rare.

The risk of offspring of a heterozygous patient inheriting the gene is 50%, but the risk of heart disease, which is the relevant factor, was considerably lower than this, even before the introduction of statin drugs, and particularly in females (Table 21.6). The risk to offspring of an isolated case showing this lipid abnormality is also considerably lower than where an established dominant pattern exists in the family, since a proportion of the non-genetic lipid defects are indistinguishable from it, unless a specific mutation has been demonstrated. Fortunately, therapy with statins results in a major reduction in vascular complications and mortality.

The disorder is best diagnosed in cascade genetic testing if the family's mutation is known, as that gives a clear result while cholesterol levels vary with age and may be difficult to interpret. It is still uncertain to what extent early childhood therapy modifies the course of the disorder, or whether newborn testing would be justified. While childhood testing of those at high genetic risk is important, there is little case for population-level cholesterol screening in childhood.

The basic defect is an LDL receptor deficiency, or in some families an alteration of the receptor. The *LDLR* gene itself, located on chromosome 19, has been fully characterised, and a variety of mutational defects has been found in patients. Alterations in the genes *APOB* and *PCSK9* are responsible for a small minority of affected families.

At a practical level, familial hypercholesterolaemia provides a lamentable example of a neglected opportunity for primary prevention of a common and treatable genetic disorder, despite clear evidence of benefit shown by systematic cascade testing of family members from studies in the Netherlands and the United Kingdom. The diagnosis is often missed, families are rarely studied systematically, and even more rarely given proper information and management, while there is still no systematic genetic register in many areas. This is probably because the disorder is too frequent to be handled at a regional level by clinical geneticists, while other clinicians and those in primary care are not set up for such a process. The disorder should be a

Table 21.6 Risks of heart disease in familial hypercholesterolaemia (before the advent of statin drugs)

Age (years)	Percentage with ischaemic heart disease	
	Males	Females
<30	5	0
30–39	24	0
40–49	51	12
50–59	85	57
60–69	100	74

Table 21.7 Some rare genetic causes of premature vascular disease

Disorder	Inheritance
Pseudoxanthoma elasticum	Autosomal recessive (sometimes autosomal dominant)
Homocystinuria	Autosomal recessive
Progeria	Autosomal recessive
Cockayne syndrome	Autosomal recessive
Werner syndrome	Autosomal recessive
Menkes syndrome	X-linked recessive

useful indicator as to the success (or otherwise) of moving genetics into regular clinical practice. Fortunately, specific programmes of index case mutation analysis and then family-based cascade screening by mutation testing (not whole-population screening) are now addressing the problem in the United Kingdom.

Other genetic influences in coronary heart disease

Apart from familial hypercholesterolaemia, genetic variations exist in a variety of other lipoproteins and their corresponding DNA polymorphisms – for example, apoAI, apoAII, apoB, ApoE, Lp(a) – which show correlations with atherosclerosis at a population level, and which may well be important risk determinants. Unlike familial hypercholesterolaemia, their relevance within individual families is not yet well understood, and there is no proven case for testing asymptomatic relatives. This may change as we learn more about the Mendelian patterns involved and the precise levels of risk. Epigenetic factors may well play a role in the transgenerational influence of maternal (and perhaps grand-paternal) nutrition on an individual's susceptibility to coronary artery disease as well as hypertension, diabetes mellitus and stroke.

When familial aggregations of early coronary artery disease are encountered in clinical practice, and where there is no detectable lipid abnormality or any other primary cause that can be found, there is little advice that can be given except the importance of healthy lifestyle, including the avoidance of smoking and attention to serum cholesterol and blood pressure. Despite extensive genome-wide searches and investigation of possible candidate gene loci (e.g. homocystine and angiotensin-converting enzyme [ACE] pathways), no major risk factors have been conclusively identified and certainly none relevant at present to genetic counselling and testing. Some rare causes of premature vascular disease are listed in Table 21.7. They account for only a small proportion of the total problem but, as their molecular basis is now recognised, this may give important clues as to factors involved in more common vascular degeneration.

Venous thrombosis is considered in Chapter 27.

SUDDEN CARDIAC DEATH

In many developed countries, sudden (unexpected) cardiac deaths are usually investigated by the coroner. Most such deaths are the result of coronary artery disease but careful investigation can identify other causes in an increasing proportion of cases. This should include toxicology, careful histological examination of the heart, and – after discussion with the family, and where they request this but not otherwise – a focussed molecular genetic search for mutations in plausibly relevant genes. This is sometimes described as a 'molecular autopsy', although that may give a misleading impression. For reasons discussed earlier (see 'Hypertrophic Cardiomyopathy'), it is important not to search for mutations in too many, probably irrelevant genes because that is likely to yield VUSs that cause confusion and unhelpful anxiety. However, if a clearly pathogenic mutation is found in a gene that could well account for the clinical events, then this can be helpful as an explanation of what has happened and as a guide to the appropriate investigation of surviving family members.

ANEURYSMS AND RELATED VASCULAR LESIONS

Thoracic aortic aneurysms and dissection are a feature of Marfan syndrome and a group of autosomal dominant disorders known as the thoracic aortopathies (see also Chapter 16), which include Loeys-Dietz syndrome (types 1 and 2). It can also develop in those with bicuspid aortic valve, which can be non-syndromic and arise in association with mutations in *NOTCH1* or *SMAD6*, or it may be part of a more generalised connective tissue disorder.

The genes implicated in causing aneurysms of the thoracic aorta fall into four broad categories (after Pyeritz, 2014; see Appendix 1). The principal recognised genes include the following:

1. Structural components of the extracellular matrix (e.g. *FBN1, COL3A1, COL4A5, EFEMP2*)
2. Components of the TGF or BMP signalling pathways (*TGFBR1, TGFBR2, TGFB2, SMAD3*)
3. Contractile elements of vascular smooth muscle (*ACTA2, MYH11, MYLK, PRKG1, PKG1, FLNA, TSC2*)
4. Components of other signalling pathways (*JAG1, NOTCH1, SLCA10*)

A more generalised tendency to large vessel rupture and other serious vascular incidents is a feature of several of the other primary connective tissue disorders (see Chapter 16), notably those involving type III collagen, such as vascular (type IV) Ehlers-Danlos syndrome and pseudoxanthoma elasticum (PXE). These mostly follow dominant inheritance, although PXE is often recessive.

Abdominal aneurysms have much the same risk factors as for atherosclerosis, especially smoking and hypertension but also alcohol and hypertension. They are also more common in those with the connective tissue disorders considered previously (including Marfan syndrome, PXE, and the vascular type of Ehlers-Danlos syndrome, etc.). They may show a deficiency of type III collagen, although it seems unlikely that this deficiency follows a Mendelian pattern and such tests should not be used as a basis for risk estimation. Population screening by ultrasound of men of 65 years or more is worthwhile, with further monitoring of those in whom an aneurysm is detected.

Cerebral aneurysms and stroke are considered in Chapter 15.

Hereditary haemorrhagic telangiectasia (HHT) (autosomal dominant) may result in telangiectasiae in the skin and mucous membranes, anaemia (from nosebleeds and chronic loss of blood from the gastrointestinal tract) and AV malformations in a number of organs. In the lungs, these cause a right-to-left shunt with the possibility of chronic hypoxaemia, high-output cardiac failure and embolism into the systemic circulation, especially 'paradoxical' septic embolism of the brain. It is important that a physician should monitor patients with HHT for such complications. The best approach to the surveillance for, and management of, venous and AV malformations in the brain remains uncertain.

The usual cause of HHT is heterozygous mutation in either *ENG* or *ALK1* (= *ACVRLK1*), two genes involved in endothelial growth regulation that account for some 85% of cases. Much less commonly, mutation in *SMAD4* causes HHT with juvenile polyposis.

Cavernous haemangiomas are considered in Chapter 18.

Familial glomus tumours (paragangliomas) provide an unusual example of autosomal dominant inheritance modified by genetic imprinting (see Chapter 32). One of the two genes often involved (*SDHD*) results in the disorder being expressed only when transmitted paternally.

HYPERTENSION

With rare exceptions, this behaves as a classical polygenic disorder, with around a threefold risk increase for individuals with two or more affected relatives. Despite early reports of ACE variants being a risk factor, this has not been confirmed as clinically important, nor has any other specific locus of major effect been found to be involved.

Rare, early-onset, dominantly inherited forms of hypertension are seen in the disorders of aldosterone metabolism, Liddle and Gordon syndromes (familial hyperkalaemic hypertension, also known as pseudohypoaldosteronism), that result from mutation in genes for components of the renal sodium channels or other elements involved in the response to thiazide diuretics.

Hypertension is an important complication of several Mendelian disorders, including polycystic kidney disease, neurofibromatosis type 1 and other tumour predisposition syndromes (especially those that result in neuroendocrine tumours, e.g. the catecholamine-secreting phaeochromocytomas found in von Hippel-Lindau syndrome and the MEN2 syndromes as well as NF1).

Primary pulmonary hypertension is a very rare condition, dominantly inherited in some families, and often associated with *BMPR2* mutations (for which treatments look promising). Even more rarely, PPH is associated with hereditary haemorrhagic telangiectasia, and mutations in *ALK1*.

LYMPHATIC DISORDERS

Mild lymphoedema of hands and feet may be seen in both Turner and Noonan syndromes. Prenatal onset of oedema may be responsible for a number of dysmorphic features, including webbing of the neck. The most common and most severe form of lymphoedema, Milroy disease, follows autosomal dominant inheritance and can usually be recognised at birth. It is genetically heterogeneous with at least four loci involved, including the gene for vascular endothelial growth factor (*VEGFR3*).

A milder and later-onset form (Meige disease) is more variable in inheritance. It appears to be a variable but autosomal dominant disorder and is distinct from two syndromic disorders, lymphoedema with distichiasis (with double rows of eyelashes) and lymphoedema with yellow nails.

RHEUMATIC FEVER

The recognition of a streptococcal basis for rheumatic fever and its dramatic decline in Western populations should not obscure the fact that susceptibility is strongly influenced by inheritance. Early studies (Nora et al., 1991, see Appendix 1) showed a risk of around 10% in sibs and ospring of an affected person developing the condition at some later stage of life and double this risk when a parent and a sib were affected. The risks are now likely to represent susceptibility rather than actual disease but may still be of interest in the many parts of the world where the disorder remains common (although the risk figures may differ between populations).

Respiratory disorders

INTRODUCTION

Malformation and inherited diseases of the lungs and airways often also have effects on the gastrointestinal tract, from which the lungs are derived in the course of development. Thus, two of the important and relatively common inherited pulmonary disorders that follow autosomal recessive inheritance, cystic fibrosis and α_1-antitrypsin deficiency (the latter is discussed in Chapter 23), involve other abdominal organs too (pancreas and liver, respectively). There is no convincing evidence that the heterozygotes for either disorder are more prone to diseases of the lung or other organs. Indeed, it seems likely that the high frequency of the carrier state for mutations in the *CFTR* gene is the result of a heterozygote advantage from the protection these variants afford against diarrhoeal disease.

CYSTIC FIBROSIS

Cystic fibrosis is the most common serious autosomal recessive disorder in northern Europe, where the frequency of the disease is around 1 in 2,500 and the carrier frequency is around 1 in 25.

The remarkable recent advances in our understanding of cystic fibrosis (CF) have sprung almost entirely from genetic studies, the gene being the first to be isolated by the positional cloning approach without the help of chromosome rearrangements. Characterisation of the protein (the CF transmembrane conductance regulator, *CFTR*) is leading to therapeutic progress too, but genetic tests are currently based on the gene itself. A single mutation, a deletion of three base-pairs (c.1521_1523delCTT; p.Phe508Del that was formerly known as delta F508), is responsible for 60%–80% of *CFTR* mutations in northern European populations, although it shows a steady decline towards southern Europe and is rare in most non-European populations. Numerous rarer mutations make up the remainder, although some are more common in particular population groups.

Genetic counselling in CF can now be extremely accurate with use of appropriate mutational tests, making it essential to analyse the mutations present in the particular family, especially any affected individual. Where a couple have had an affected child, with a one-in-four risk for future children, early prenatal diagnosis based on DNA analysis can detect or exclude the disorder in almost all cases; closely linked markers may still be needed if specific mutations have not been identified in time.

Carrier detection within families is also now feasible in most cases where the affected individual is available for molecular analysis. Parents and children of a CF patient will be obligatory carriers, but the risk of disease in the offspring of sibs (in the absence of consanguinity) is low at 1 in 150, and even lower in more distant relatives. In fact, for sibs and for parents of a CF child who subsequently marry other partners, it will be the carrier status of the unrelated partner that will be the major determinant of whether there is risk to a child. Testing for this has been unsatisfactory until very recently and is still not without problems, as indicated later.

Mutational testing for a panel of the more common mutations will usually detect at least 90%–95% of carriers, depending on the mutations included in the panel and the population of origin of the person tested. Using a Bayesian approach, this leaves a residual risk of less than 1 in 200 for a person with a normal (negative) result, and so a residual risk of less than 1 in 800 for a child being affected if the other partner is a known carrier. These low levels of risk are usually adequate for genetic counselling of CF families and those married into them.

Most molecular genetics laboratories will have a battery of tests for the most frequent mutations in particular populations, which can be supplemented by testing for rare mutations if required. This now often entails full sequencing of the gene. For population screening, the issues are more complex, as discussed in Chapter 34. In southern Europe, the mutational spectrum is different, as is generally also true of non-European populations, while in Jewish populations some specific mutations are prominent.

The different CF mutations show varying degrees of correlation with severity of lung and gastrointestinal problems. Some with minimal systemic effects are being discovered, including isolated absence of the vas deferens (many CF males are infertile because of this; see Chapter 25). Those affected in this way may not show the typical clinical features of cystic fibrosis, may have borderline sweat electrolytes and may be compound heterozygotes for a fully pathogenic *CFTR* allele and a less pathogenic variant (often p.Arg117His in *cis* with the 'milder', 7T allele of the polyT stretch in intron 8). They may develop CF in adult life rather than infancy. Infants found on newborn screening to have raised serum IRT (trypsin) levels but with only one definitely pathogenic *CFTR* allele, or with two pathogenic alleles but with intermediate sweat chloride levels, raise the problem of an uncertain disease phenotype after newborn screening, with different views about the best approach to the clinical management of this important group of infants. This is a good illustration of how difficult it can be to predict the phenotype from knowledge of an individual's genotype; diagnostic successes in the reverse direction can lead us to believe that our understanding of genetics is greater than is actually the case.

Knowledge of the precise *CFTR* gene mutation causing disease is becoming ever more important as mutation-specific therapies are entering standard clinical practice.

Cystic fibrosis is one of the conditions that has been suspected when a fetus is found on ultrasound scan to have an echogenic bowel. There may be a modest increase in the risk of a fetus being affected by cystic fibrosis in these circumstances, but other associations include poor outcomes from intrauterine growth retardation (IUGR) or subsequent intrauterine death or, in some but not all reports, chromosomal aneuploidy.

CONGENITAL SURFACTANT DYSFUNCTION

Pulmonary surfactant metabolism dysfunction, which causes the pathologic appearance of pulmonary alveolar proteinosis, is a rare autosomal recessive disorder affecting the ability of the lungs to expand after birth. There is locus heterogeneity.

CONGENITAL PULMONARY AIRWAY MALFORMATION

This malformation used to be known as congenital cystic adenomatoid malformation of the lung. It is rare but more common than used to be appreciated as it is sometimes recognised on fetal ultrasound scan but then resolves before birth or, at least, never causes symptoms. It may be best for the lesion to be removed as it can occasionally contain malignant elements.

The cause is unknown but, if genetic, it is probably caused by a somatic mutational event. It is not known to be familial.

KARTAGENER SYNDROME

Kartagener syndrome is characterised by bronchiectasis, recurrent sinusitis, dextrocardia and other isomerism-related heart defects, and often asplenia, and has traditionally been considered an autosomal recessive disorder. Recent work has shown this disorder to be part of a more extensive group of defects of ciliary structure and function, often accompanied by a disturbance of the usual pattern of left-right asymmetry and male infertility. The finding of a recurrence risk in sibs of one in eight but with no transmission to children would fit well with autosomal recessive inheritance and penetrance of 50%. (The 50% penetrance could result from the risk of inappropriate left-right symmetry if lateralisation has become random instead of being coordinated.)

ASTHMA AND ATOPY

The familial tendency for asthma has been recognised for many years, especially in relation to a general atopic sensitivity, including eczema (see Chapter 18). The fact that it is so common makes it difficult to disentangle a clear genetic basis, since relatives from both parental lines are commonly affected, but it is unlikely to follow Mendelian inheritance. The risk of intrinsic asthma, with no atopic tendency, is around 5% for first-degree relatives, but for atopic cases the figures are higher, especially if the risk for any form of atopy is considered. Some studies have shown higher risks if the mother is the affected parent, but this is not sufficiently established to be incorporated into genetic counselling risks.

The identification of specific genes involved in asthma and atopy remains a controversial area, with conflicting results in relation to specific loci. The role of air traffic pollution in the origin of asthma is increasingly recognised, and 'atopy' is now most often taken to be a complex phenotype arising from many genetic and environmental factors, sometimes mediated through epigenetic influences. There are no genetic tests helpful for counselling at present.

EMPHYSEMA AND CHRONIC OBSTRUCTIVE PULMONARY DISEASE

Even when smoking and other environmental variables have been allowed for, and rare genetic causes ruled out, there is a familial aggregation for this, but no specific genes have yet been identified despite extensive genome searches.

Genetic causes include α_1-antitrypsin deficiency but not its heterozygous state (see Chapter 23), CF and ciliary dyskinesia syndromes, discussed separately earlier, as well as connective tissue disorders such as pseudoxanthoma elasticum and cutis laxa.

SARCOIDOSIS

Sarcoidosis is occasionally familial but affected members are usually related through the maternal line. Ethnic differences in susceptibility and types of sarcoidosis have been found, and differences in the risk to family members have been suggested. Subtypes of sarcoidosis have distinct *HLA* associations, but satisfactory risk figures and useful genetic testing do not appear to exist.

LUNG CANCER

Lung cancer has long been recognised to have a genetic predisposition, interacting with environmental factors, which include uranium mining, residential radon and asbestos exposure, chronic obstructive pulmonary disease (COPD), passive smoking and smoking itself. These environmental factors themselves interact. Small-cell lung carcinoma is associated with somatic chromosome changes involving chromosome 3, but this does not seem to be especially involved in genetic susceptibility. No clear Mendelian form has been recognised, possibly because it is submerged by smoking as an environmental factor, but susceptibility loci are being actively sought and may help in understanding the pathogenesis and in guiding therapy. There does seem to be a modestly increased risk of lung cancer for the first-degree relatives of those affected (perhaps twofold), but it is difficult to completely separate genetic from environmental effects. For now, however, it is fair to state that different genomic regions that have been associated with lung cancer in genome-wide studies yield different results according to ethnicity and smoking history. Some of the association of single-nucleotide polymorphisms (SNPs) with lung cancer may relate to behaviour and susceptibility to COPD rather than a direct relationship with carcinogenesis. As usual in complex disorders, the statistical confidence in the associations found can be very strong but the strength of the effects identified tends to be weak (the relative risks are only modest).

CONGENITAL LARYNGEAL AND TRACHEAL DEFECTS

A variety of these have been described, including laryngomalacia, congenital subglottic stenosis, laryngeal atresia and laryngeal clefts. They may be isolated or syndromal, and sometimes in association with other midline defects. Congenital vocal cord paralysis may also be part of a wider neurological disorder. Very little information is available on genetic risks or specific inheritance patterns, but a useful general review and summary table of syndromes is provided in Tewfik and der Kaloustian (see Appendix 1).

Laryngotracheobronchomalacia may predispose to bronchiectasis.

23

The gastrointestinal tract

INTRODUCTION

Relatively few gastrointestinal disorders follow clear Mendelian inheritance, and so genetic counselling is more dependent on empirical risks than is the case for some other systems. Most data of this type have been collected from western European or American populations, so figures must be applied with caution in other areas, particularly where the incidence of the disorder is known to differ significantly. They are also mostly old data, and likely to be altered by changes in disease incidence and by the recognition of Mendelian subsets.

Gastrointestinal disorders of early life have also proved more treatable than most groups, so that individuals with previously fatal disorders now reproduce. Data for risks to offspring of affected individuals are so far available for only a few conditions, such as pyloric stenosis, and in preliminary form for Hirschsprung disease and oesophageal atresia.

Cancers of the gastrointestinal tract are discussed in Chapter 30.

OESOPHAGEAL ATRESIA

Most cases of oesophageal atresia are combined with tracheo-oesophageal fistula, the incidence varying geographically between 1 and 4 per 10,000 live births. As many as 55% of cases have been found to be associated with other malformations, most notably rectal and duodenal atresia, diaphragmatic hernia, hypoplasia of the radius and renal agenesis, thus often forming part of the VATER (vertebrae, anus, trachea, oesophagus, renal) complex. Other relevant conditions include the CHARGE (coloboma, heart defects, atresia choanae, growth retardation, genital abnormalities and ear abnormalities) syndrome, Feingold syndrome and Goldenhar syndrome (oculo-auriculo-vertebral [OAV] dysplasia). These syndromic cases are progressively becoming better defined, originally in clinical and now in molecular terms. Around 10% of cases are associated with chromosome abnormalities. Excluding syndromic and chromosomal cases, the recurrence risk to sibs of those with oesophageal atresia/tracheo-oesophageal malformation is generally very low: In one large series of 345 patients there was only one affected sib and in another study of 108 patients with 410 first-degree relatives there was no recurrence. A higher proportion of sibs may have some associated defects but, except when this is part of a specific syndrome, this should not be grounds for giving a higher risk. Risk figures for offspring of treated patients are now becoming available although numbers remain small: These risks also appear to be low, probably not more than 1%.

DIAPHRAGMATIC HERNIA

The incidence varies between one in 2,000 to 3,000 births. Although a few instances of affected sibs have been reported, most with complete aplasia of the diaphragm, the overall risk is extremely low, probably no greater than 1%, even though half the cases in one study had associated defects, most commonly of the nervous system. Diaphragmatic hypoplasia is seen in some primary myopathies (e.g. congenital myotonic dystrophy), and in some specific malformations (e.g. Pallister-Killian syndrome, tetrasomy 12p and in trisomies 13 and 18).

Hiatus hernia, whether in infancy or adult life, does not seem to show any notable increase in incidence in relatives.

INFANTILE PYLORIC STENOSIS

Pyloric stenosis follows the pattern expected for polygenic inheritance, with risks diminishing rapidly outside first-degree relatives, and with relatives of index patients of the more rarely affected sex (female) having a higher risk (Table 23.1).

The overall population incidence for the United Kingdom is around 3 per 1,000 births (5 per 1,000 male births and 1 per 1,000 female births). Genome-wide association studies are indicating possible disease mechanisms. Data on risks for families with more than one affected individual are not available, but such families are not rare and may provide additional evidence as to mechanisms of causation.

OMPHALOCELE AND GASTROSCHISIS

The Beckwith-Wiedemann syndrome of exomphalos, macroglossia, general somatic overgrowth and hypoglycaemia is an important and treatable cause to exclude. It is important to prevent symptomatic hypoglycaemia in the neonatal period and so prompt recognition is important. Asymmetry with partial hemihypertrophy may be prominent. Abnormal features may diminish during childhood and are often inconspicuous by adult life. There is an increased risk of various embryonal tumours, especially Wilms tumour (for which surveillance is available).

Table 23.1 Risks to relatives of patients with infantile pyloric stenosis

Relative	Male index patients Risk (%)	Increase	Female index patients Risk (%)	Increase
Brothers	3.8	×8	9.2	×18
Sisters	2.7	×27	3.8	×38
Sons	5.5	×11	18.9	×38
Daughters	2.4	×24	7.0	×70
Nephews	2.3	×4.6	4.7	×9.4
Nieces	0.4	×3.6	–	–
Male first cousins	0.9	×1.9	0.7	×1.3
Female first cousins	0.2	×2.3	0.3	×2.6

Autosomal dominant inheritance applies but is modified by genetic imprinting and many cases arise *de novo*. Microduplications on chromosome 11p involving the insulin-like growth factor (IGF)-2 are responsible for some cases. Other cases result from an effective duplication of the paternal copy of distal 11p by uniparental disomy (e.g. by mitotic recombination or by an anomaly of methylation) or point mutations in the gene *CDKN1C* (see section on 'Genomic Imprinting', in Chapter 2).

Isolated omphalocele has a low (under 1%) recurrence risk in sibs, although a few clusters have been reported. It is a cause of raised amniotic fluid α-fetoprotein levels requiring distinction from neural tube defects (see Chapter 9); ultrasonography provides help in this situation. This is most commonly an incidental finding in a pregnancy tested for other reasons. Gastroschisis is generally not associated with an underlying genetic or syndromal disorder, although it may arise in the context of intrauterine growth retardation and premature delivery and appears more likely to be the result of a disruption to development rather than a primary malformation.

It is most important that such cases, detected by α-fetoprotein measurement or fetal ultrasound scanning, are carefully assessed antenatally and postnatally to detect any associated syndrome or chromosome disorder.

BOWEL ATRESIAS AND MALROTATIONS

Most cases are sporadic, possibly resulting from intrauterine vascular occlusions. Familial aggregations are extremely rare – meconium ileus from cystic fibrosis must be distinguished from true atresia. Duodenal atresia occurs with increased frequency in Down syndrome. Bowel duplications and enterogenous cysts are usually sporadic. Some familial cases of jejunal atresia ('apple peel syndrome') have been reported but are uncommon.

'Echogenic bowel' is an ultrasound finding (not in itself an abnormality) that may, in a proportion of cases, indicate cystic fibrosis, unbalanced chromosomal rearrangement or other pathology, although the outcome is normal in the majority.

PEPTIC ULCER

Genetic studies are difficult in a disorder that in the past was common (around 4% of adult males and 2% of adult females in the United Kingdom, though it has declined sharply) and where symptoms are often ill-defined. Most surveys have shown around a threefold increase in risk in both sibs and offspring. Childhood cases more commonly have an affected relative. The empirical risk for first-degree relations is around 10%, possibly higher if adjusted to a lifetime risk.

The disease has been declining in frequency over the past century but more rapidly over the past two decades. The recognition of infective agents (*Helicobacter pylori*) and non-steroidal anti-inflammatory drugs (including aspirin) as important causes, and the availability of drugs that effectively reduce gastric acid production (even when serum pepsinogen levels are increased), have accelerated this trend. Paradoxically, though, these advances have altered the perception of the disorder to being 'less genetic' and genetic counselling requests are now rare.

Numerous associations exist between peptic ulcer and other primary disorders, some of them Mendelian, such as multiple endocrine neoplasia type I. These should be borne in mind, especially when striking familial aggregations are encountered.

ATROPHIC GASTRITIS AND PERNICIOUS ANAEMIA

One-quarter of first-degree relatives of patients with atrophic gastritis have histological evidence of the disorder, and a similar proportion show parietal cell antibodies. It seems likely that an autosomal dominant gene controlling production of autoantibodies is involved. There is extensive overlap with other autoimmune disorders and autoantibodies within families.

COELIAC DISEASE

Coeliac disease affects about 1% of the population and seems to be increasing in prevalence in developed countries. True coeliac disease is an autoimmune disorder with predisposing genetic factors, some of which are shared with those of other autoimmune conditions. It must be diagnosed with care and distinguished from non-coeliac gluten sensitivity and wheat allergy, which may have some overlap with irritable bowel syndrome. The diagnostic process now focuses especially on IgA antibodies (against tissue transglutaminase, tTG) and the role of jejunal biopsy is less central than in the past, at least for children.

Coeliac disease is strongly associated with two specific HLA-DQ haplotypes, which will of course be transmitted in families. Other predisposing genetic factors vary between populations and an appropriate environmental trigger is necessary for disease. Human leucocyte antigen (HLA) testing is of little help in risk prediction for individual relatives.

The risks to relatives depend on the thoroughness with which they are investigated and the criteria for diagnosis, but around 10% would seem the soundest estimate for first-degree relatives based on several series using jejunal biopsy. Risks to second-degree or more distant relatives appear small, not exceeding 1% for overt disease.

GASTROINTESTINAL ENZYME DEFECTS

Gastrointestinal enzyme defects all follow autosomal recessive inheritance and include the following:

- *Disaccharidase deficiencies* (maltase, sucrase, lactase): Partial lactase deficiency after infancy is normal in most Asian and African populations. Indeed, lactose tolerance can be seen as a recent evolutionary adaptation to dairy herding (an alternative strategy to the culture of yoghurt).
- *Pancreatic enzyme deficiencies* (trypsinogen, enterokinase, lipase).
- *Acrodermatitis enteropathica* (due to a defect in zinc metabolism with variants in the gene *SLC39A4*). The disease is rare in Northern Europe, more common around the Mediterranean.
- *Congenital chloride diarrhoea* (due to mutations in an ion-transport gene related and adjacent to that for cystic fibrosis on chromosome 7).

HEREDITARY PANCREATITIS

Inheritance is mostly autosomal dominant but with locus heterogeneity. In the classic form (associated with the cationic trypsinogen gene *PRSS1*), penetrance is high, around 80%. However, there is locus heterogeneity. Another important dominant gene is *SPINK1*, while a missense variant in *CFTR* (especially with the 5T allele in intron 8 adjacent to the TG repeat polymorphism) can be associated with the disease and may modify the penetrance or severity of variants at other loci.

Hereditary pancreatitis is a rare but important cause of recurrent abdominal pain in childhood and young adults and may predispose to later pancreatic cancer. Predictive genetic testing in someone who is well should be used with caution in view of the great variability of the condition and the scope for gene-gene interaction (as well as the involvement of environmental factors). There is some evidence that the risk of cancer is greater with *CFTR*-associated than with *SPINK1*-associated pancreatitis. Type V hyperlipoproteinaemia (autosomal recessive) may also cause recurrent pancreatitis.

CYSTIC FIBROSIS

Cystic fibrosis is discussed in Chapter 22. Newborn screening has now been introduced in many developed countries. The diagnostic use of DNA analysis as well as the sweat test in cases of meconium ileus now allows most of such cases where cystic fibrosis is the cause to be recognised, which is useful as such cases may not have an elevated serum immunoreactive trypsin (IRT) in the newborn period and so may not be detected on newborn screening.

GALLSTONES

These are only simply inherited when secondary to disorders causing excess haemolysis (e.g. hereditary spherocytosis) or disturbed lipid metabolism. There appears to be an excess among young females affected by Rett syndrome.

INTUSSUSCEPTION

A risk of 1 in 40 for sibs of childhood cases has been shown, compared with 1 in 750 for the general population. Cystic fibrosis and the polyposes (e.g. Peutz-Jeghers syndrome) may be underlying causes in addition to the more usual infectious or anatomic causes, sometimes with a malignancy at the lead point (especially with lymphoid tumours in childhood or colonic neoplasia in the adult).

INFLAMMATORY BOWEL DISEASE

Overlap within families has been shown between ulcerative colitis and Crohn's disease. Recurrence risks are low in both disorders, with a risk of around 3% for first-degree relatives (possibly around 5% if adjusted to lifetime risks), but this may change as the incidence of Crohn's disease is increasing. The risks in families of Jewish origin may be somewhat higher.

In addition to many weakly associated loci at which variation predisposes to Crohn's disease or ulcerative colitis (UC) or both, as well as to autoimmune disorders, some interesting Crohn's-specific factors (not associated with UC) have been found. Most prominent is the *NOD2* locus association as well as association with some loci implicated as Mendelian loci for susceptibility to mycobacterial disease (interesting in view of the cellular pathology in Crohn's disease). The prognosis of those heterozygous for disease-associated variants in *NOD2* is less good, with a greater need for surgery, and ileal disease more likely; the prognosis is worse in those who have variants on both alleles of this gene. However, it remains unclear whether testing can be helpful in guiding treatment decisions (e.g. the timing of bowel resection surgery).

A rare, and often lethal, form of enterocolitis in infancy has been described. Early reports suggested autosomal recessive inheritance, but more recently it has been associated with heterozygous pathogenic variants in *NLRC4*. The condition is called autoinflammation with infantile enterocolitis (AIFEC). It presents with failure to thrive, gastrointestinal symptoms and febrile episodes.

FAMILIAL ADENOMATOUS POLYPOSIS AND COLON CANCER

These are discussed in Chapter 30.

HIRSCHSPRUNG DISEASE

The risks depend on the sex of the index patient and relative, and on the length of the aganglionic segment, as is to be expected in multifactorial (complex) inheritance. The male-to-female ratio in patients is around 3:1, and long-segment involvement makes up 13% of all cases. The overall population incidence is about 1 in 5,000 births (0.02%).

Table 23.2 combines the results of three major family studies. Risks for offspring of affected patients with short-segment disease are becoming available and are low, probably not over 2%. Risks for second-degree and third-degree relatives are imprecise but low.

The underlying cause of Hirschsprung disease should be considered. It may be (1) chromosomal, in about 12% of cases, with the most frequent single condition being Down syndrome. Then (2) there are the monogenic, syndromic forms. Hirschsprung disease is a significant complication of Mowat-Wilson syndrome and FG syndrome and is also a feature of Bardet-Biedl syndrome, congenital central hypoventilation, cartilage hair hypoplasia, Goldberg-Shprintzen syndrome and Waardenburg syndrome type 4 (among others). (3) There are the monogenic non-syndromic forms, associated especially with variants of low penetrance in the *RET* proto-oncogene but variants in other genes can be associated (including *EDN3* and *EDNRB*). Pathogenic variants in *RET* act as a Mendelian predisposition to the condition but are not sufficient to cause it. Then, finally (4) there are those cases that are non-syndromic but without a recognised molecular predisposition.

Note that pathogenic variants of *RET* also cause multiple endocrine neoplasia type 2 (MEN2), and that both MEN2 and Hirschsprung disease relate to neural crest tissue.

The risk estimates in Table 23.2 will need to be refined once the results of more systematic, population-based molecular studies have appeared.

ANAL ATRESIA

Anal atresia is seen in various syndromes, notably with ocular coloboma in association with an extra chromosome 22 fragment (cat eye syndrome), with anomalies of the hand and ear in Townes-Brocks syndrome, with dysmorphic facies and hypotonia in Opitz (FG) syndrome, as well as with vertebral and radial limb defects (and other defects) in the VATER/VACTERL (vertebral defects, anal atresia, cardiac defects, tracheo-oesophageal fistula, renal anomalies, limb abnormalities) association. There is no evidence of a high recurrence risk to sibs either in the VATER/VACTERL association or in isolated anal atresia.

Table 23.2 Genetic risks to sibs in Hirschsprung disease

	Brothers (%)	Sisters (%)	Offspring (both sexes)
All lengths of aganglionic segment			
Male index patient	5.3	2.3	2.0
Female index patient	11.3	13.6	2.0
Short aganglionic segment			
Male index patient	4.7	0.6	2.0
Female index patient	8.1	2.9	2.0
Long aganglionic segment			
Male index patient	16.1	11.1	High (about 50%)
Female index patient	18.2	9.1	High (about 50%)

Source: Based on Passarge E 1972. Birth Defects 8, 63–67; also see Amiel and Lyonnet's review 2001. J Med Genet 38, 729–739.

GENETIC LIVER DISEASE

Liver involvement occurs in numerous metabolic disorders, including lipidoses, mucopolysaccharidoses, glycogenoses and galactosaemia. A few require separate mention.

Wilson disease

This autosomal recessive disorder may present to neurologists or to haematologists as well as with liver disease and is treatable if recognised early. Prenatal diagnosis and carrier detection are both possible now that the gene (ATP7B on chromosome 13) is recognised. However, it remains essential to use conventional studies of copper and caeruloplasmin in establishing the diagnosis and making decisions about therapy as the ability to predict the phenotype from a genotype remains limited.

Haemochromatosis

This condition, characterised by excessive iron storage in a variety of organs, including the liver, pancreas and heart, has traditionally been considered to follow autosomal recessive inheritance, but the genetic component should really be considered more as a susceptibility locus than as a true Mendelian disorder; it is perhaps a 'Mendelian (autosomal recessive) predisposition' to iron overload. The overt disease is largely but not totally sex-limited to males as females are protected by the loss of iron at menstruation and during pregnancy. Transmission of the full disease by an affected person is rare, but sibs have a higher risk (clinical onset being delayed and reduced in females). Although earlier studies suggested this might be as high as one in four, this is likely to be a considerable overestimate in light of subsequent research. A close HLA linkage indicating an important and common gene controlling iron storage in this region led to isolation of the gene itself (HFE). As with cystic fibrosis, one particular mutation (p.Cys282Tyr) seems to be particularly common in northern European populations, with 80%–90% of patients homozygous for it.

This knowledge has led to pressure for widespread testing and screening, but this move has been both premature and inappropriate. Particularly relevant is the disparity between the high frequency of homozygosity for the main mutation (around 1 in 150–200) and the frequency of the disease, as measured by clinical and pathological studies (around 1 in 5,000–6,000),

30 times less. Even allowing for underdiagnosis, this can only mean that most homozygotes are, and remain, clinically unaffected, rendering it both unnecessary and unwise for them to be converted into patients and 'treated' by regular venesection.

Thorough studies in Britain, Australia and the United States have confirmed that as few as 1%–2% of homozygotes for the predisposing mutation may develop clinically significant iron overload, although the figure could well be higher for close relatives of patients on account of other shared genes. Recent findings suggest that penetrance over the whole life course may be somewhat higher than the lowest estimates from population cross-sectional studies, so there may be further calls to reassess the question of population screening. One difficulty is that early symptoms can be very non-specific and so the attribution of symptoms to homozygosity for a pathogenic variant can be difficult in the individual case.

Heterozygotes (10% of the population in parts of northern Europe) are at no significant risk and it is most important that they are not falsely worried. Until considerably more is known about the relationship between genotype and disease, in both sexes, genetic testing should be focused on high-risk individuals – sibs, and possibly offspring in particular circumstances. A further complexity is that a considerable proportion of patients with porphyria cutanea tarda are also homozygous for the main haemochromatosis mutation: there is an interaction between these loci so that homozygosity for haemochromatosis acts as a trigger for that other condition, also of rather low penetrance.

Alpha-1-antitrypsin deficiency

This relatively frequent (1 in 2,000–4,000) autosomal recessive disorder is an important cause of neonatal hepatitis and cirrhosis. Some adults develop emphysema, accounting for around 1% of all cases, while others remain healthy. A Swedish newborn screening survey has shown 17% with liver problems as infants, two-thirds of these recovering, the others progressive. This variable prognosis and lack of specific therapy (apart from avoidance of both active and passive smoking, and early treatment of chest infections in childhood and adult life) make the disorder unsuitable for newborn population screening. (Indeed, the Swedish programme was discontinued at least in part because screening was associated with the families of affected infants becoming more likely to smoke.) Families tend to be concordant for mild or severe disease. The disorder is rare in those of African origin and in Asian populations. Heterozygotes are healthy, with no good evidence of increased risk of either lung or liver disease. Unfortunately, they are frequently misinformed and unnecessarily worried as the result of genetic testing, and this may increase with the promotion of DNA-based genotyping as a 'diagnostic' test. Prenatal diagnosis is technically feasible by molecular analysis but has been used only rarely.

Hyperbilirubinaemias

The hyperbilirubinaemias are a heterogeneous group, including the following conditions:

- *Dubin-Johnson syndrome*: A variable autosomal dominant that rarely causes significant symptoms.

   Two related disorders of different severity caused by variants in the same gene encoding the transferase, UDP-glucuronosyltransferase (*UDPGT*):

- *Gilbert's syndrome*: A mild autosomal dominant trait, a harmless condition that is so common (around 5% of the population) it should be considered a normal variant rather than a disease
- *Defective bilirubin conjugation (Crigler-Najjar syndrome)*: A complete absence of the transferase in type 1 (autosomal recessive) and a partial absence in type 2 (autosomal dominant)

There are three conditions caused by different variants in the gene *ATP8B1*:

- *Benign recurrent cholestasis*: Autosomal recessive
- *Intrahepatic cholestasis of pregnancy*
- *Familial progressive cholestasis (Byler disease), often leading to hepatic failure before adulthood*: Autosomal recessive

Biliary atresia

Biliary atresia may occur in chromosomal trisomies or be the result of intrauterine viral hepatitis. Most cases are of unknown cause, and recurrence seems rare in sibs regardless of cause, although no satisfactory figures exist.

Alagille syndrome (arteriohepatic dysplasia)

Alagille syndrome shows a combination of bile duct hypoplasia with facial anomalies, cardiac defects (commonly peripheral pulmonary artery stenosis) and vertebral anomalies (typically, butterfly vertebrae). Microdeletions of chromosome 20 are found in some cases, and this finding led to isolation of a specific gene (*JAG1*) homologous to the *Drosophila* 'Jagged' gene, in which pathogenic variants may also cause the condition. Recurrence risk is low if the defect is present in the child but not in a parent. Parents showing partial expression may transmit the disorder.

Polycystic disease of the liver and congenital hepatic fibrosis

A variety of forms can be recognised pathologically, depending on the predominance of fibrosis or cystic change and the degree of renal involvement (see Chapter 24). Some of these conditions follow autosomal recessive and others autosomal dominant inheritance. The recessive polycystic kidney disease type 4 shows variable liver involvement that can include Caroli disease (of dilated biliary ducts, congenital hepatic fibrosis and portal hypertension). Adult polycystic kidney disease (autosomal dominant) rarely has more than a few hepatic cysts in early life. A separate entity of adult polycystic liver disease without renal involvement may exist but is rare compared with polycystic kidney disease, so offspring of patients may have a risk of renal as well as hepatic involvement.

In addition to the cystic diseases of the liver and/or kidneys, congenital hepatic fibrosis can also arise in association with Leber congenital amaurosis and juvenile nephronophthisis (the heterogeneous Senior-Løken syndrome), or as part of a spectrum of ciliopathies (**c**erebellar vermis aplasia, **o**ligophrenia, congenital **a**taxia, **c**oloboma and **h**epatic fibrosis [COACH] syndrome, with features overlapping with Joubert syndrome and Meckel syndrome). It is also a feature of congenital disorder of glycosylation (CDG) type 1B.

Adult chronic liver disease

In patients with an autoimmune cause for their liver disease, a strong association with other autoimmune disorders and the presence of various autoantibodies suggest the action of at least one dominant gene affecting immune responses. A few striking familial aggregations of cirrhosis and hepatoma have been found to result from the hepatitis virus and to have been maternally transmitted. It is clear that there are numerous genetic factors that influence persistence of the various hepatitis viruses and the progression of the body's responses to them.

24

Renal and urinary tract diseases

POLYCYSTIC KIDNEY DISEASE

Renal cystic disease may occur in a number of generalised syndromes (Box 24.1). It may also be secondary to obstructive anomalies *in utero* and to end-stage renal disease in later life. Thus, the question to be asked in a clinical context is not just whether the case is one of renal cystic disease but also what is the cause.

Once the various other causes have been excluded (not always an easy task), primary polycystic disease most commonly falls into two distinct groups:

- *Adult polycystic kidney disease*: Autosomal dominant
- *Infantile polycystic disease*: Variable but often following autosomal recessive inheritance

Adult polycystic kidney disease

Autosomal dominant polycystic kidney disease (PKD) is one of the most common Mendelian genetic disorders in adulthood (incidence around 1 in 1,000), but it is extremely variable. Occasionally, newborn infants present with massive renal enlargement, while mild cases may be recognised only incidentally at autopsy in old age. Genetic counselling of young, apparently healthy, adult family members presents problems. Such individuals can have molecular genetic testing if the family mutation is known. Otherwise, they should have a careful examination, urinalysis and renal ultrasound scan before being told that they are unlikely to carry the condition.

Apparently isolated cases should not be accepted as new mutations unless both parents are alive and have been shown to be unaffected.

Studies of adult PKD suggest that high-resolution ultrasonography will detect almost all carriers of the principal form (*PKD1*) over 19 years old, the risks of carrying the altered gene being under 5% for those at 50% risk who are normal per these tests. There is a strong case for a genetic register for all families in a region to ensure full ascertainment of those affected, with information and access to testing for relatives at risk. A systematic study from Australia

---

BOX 24.1: Genetic disorders associated with renal cystic disease

Autosomal dominant
Tuberous sclerosis
Von Hippel-Lindau disease
Beckwith-Wiedemann syndrome

Autosomal recessive (N.B. many are ciliopathies)
Meckel (Meckel-Gruber) syndrome
Cerebrohepatorenal (Zellweger) syndrome
Bardet-Biedl syndrome
Joubert syndrome
Short rib-polydactyly syndromes
Fryns syndrome

X-linked
Orofaciodigital syndrome type 1

Chromosomal
Trisomy 13, 18
Turner syndrome
Triploidy

---

has shown that early detection of the disorder in young adults can recognise and often avoid treatable complications, such as those due to hypertension or infection. Intracranial aneurysms are an important cause of mortality but are more difficult to detect and manage. Liver cysts are frequent but not usually of clinical significance.

Both the major genes for adult PKD have been isolated. The gene for the most common and more severe type (*PKD1*) is located on chromosome 16, immediately adjacent to one of the genes for tuberous sclerosis (*TSC2*), and some of the renal cystic disease observed in that disorder is due to both genes being involved, as when a contiguous gene deletion affects both loci. Molecular tests are now feasible for most cases of *PKD1*-related disease, but linked markers have been used until recently and renal ultrasound remains of central importance in family testing for those at risk. The *PKD2* gene, on chromosome 14, is associated with milder disease and later onset, and has probably been underdiagnosed in the past.

The demand for prenatal diagnosis is currently small, but pre-implantation genetic diagnosis (PGD) is available (often using linkage through haplotype analysis). It has been debated whether young children should be tested in the absence of clinical indications, whether by ultrasound scan (which can be regarded as a 'genetic' test in terms of its implications) or molecular genetic methods. The current author considers that there are factors weighing in both directions and, very often, the parents of an at-risk child would choose not to request investigation. Indeed, they may, not infrequently, be slow to pass on information about the risk of disease to their children even once adult. This can be a response to the unfortunate diagnostic experiences of those affected or concern about the impact of the diagnosis on career choice or life insurance and so it is 'understandable'. However, denying teenagers information about their risk of disease makes it more likely for them to run into avoidable or deferrable complications. An early knowledge of being at risk can lead to a child (and then the adult) having an annual health assessment (blood pressure, urinalysis) and a low threshold for more specific investigations (ultrasound scan, genetic testing) in the presence of any indication of renal problems, including urinary infection or haematuria. This ensures that active management can begin early in the course of disease, giving the best outlook for future health and hopefully deferring the onset of renal failure, coronary artery disease and stroke. Ultrasound imaging of the kidneys can be performed in the event of any suggestion of urinary tract problems and may be helpful occasionally even without such signs or symptoms.

It is often best to negotiate a family-specific strategy to monitoring a child at risk of PKD. Careful consideration of the issues as perceived by the parents is important to strike up an arrangement that will both look after the 'medical' welfare of the child and be accepted in practice by the family.

Autosomal recessive (infantile) polycystic kidney disease

Infantile polycystic disease is a disorder of both the kidneys and liver. The renal cysts are a manifestation of collecting duct ectasia and are accompanied by variable degrees of hepatic fibrosis and biliary dysgenesis.

The predominant presentation is in infancy. More recently, however, onset at later ages and survival into adulthood have been recognised. Generally, affected sibs show close concordance of onset and severity.

The histological appearance is distinct from that of adult polycystic disease presenting in infancy. Thus, it is most helpful for an accurate autopsy to be done on probands who die, to avoid confusion with early childhood cases of this form and to distinguish from other conditions, including multicystic dysplastic kidneys. In isolated cases with onset after the neonatal period, ultrasound examination of the liver, spleen and pancreas may be helpful. Increased hepatic echogenicity or dilated biliary ducts are characteristic findings. Although parents are usually clinically normal, both parents should be studied to exclude an asymptomatic case of the dominantly inherited form.

Genetic heterogeneity was originally thought likely, but most cases now appear to be due to a single gene locus on chromosome 6p. Prenatal diagnosis is usually available by mutation detection or, occasionally, with closely linked DNA markers. Prenatal diagnosis is also feasible in the more severe types by ultrasonography, but molecular testing is generally preferred if the molecular basis has been determined as it is available earlier in a pregnancy and is more reliable (false-negative and false-positive results have occurred on ultrasound scanning). In addition, some severe cases result from deletion of the *PKD1* gene, and perhaps of *TSC2* too.

Multicystic dysplastic kidney disease (renal hypo-/dysplasia)

Many genes have now been implicated as causing this highly variable but often early lethal disorder. Genotype-phenotype correlations are emerging but for now, and until a precise molecular aetiology has been identified in any one family, I would be concerned that it might represent a highly variable dominant disorder (although one that can arise *de novo*). It may affect one, both or neither of a person's two kidneys. When it does affect the development of a kidney, it may lead to agenesis, to a non-functioning or poorly functioning cystic renal mass, or to an effectively normal kidney. Thus, a lethally affected fetus may have a parent who is perfectly healthy but who has a single, unilateral kidney; in those circumstances, the risk of recurrence would be substantial although the effects on the next affected pregnancy could vary from lethality *in utero* or soon after birth to the trivial. Very similar appearances may result from urinary obstruction or other problems, and cystic dysplasia may be confused clinically with inherited polycystic disease. While high-resolution ultrasonography is making diagnosis easier, careful histological review by an experienced pathologist is wise if there is any doubt.

This group of conditions can itself be seen as the severe end of an even broader spectrum of congenital abnormalities of the kidney and urinary tract (CAKUT). In many cases, gene panel testing can be used to achieve a fairly rapid diagnosis.

Medullary cystic kidney disease

Medullary cystic kidney disease (MCKD) is an autosomal dominant disorder of usually adult onset that is caused largely (not exclusively) by mutation in one of two genes, either *MUC1* or *UMOD*. The kidneys are small and sonographically echogenic. Despite the emphasis on cysts, they appear to contribute relatively little to the functional renal abnormality.

Juvenile nephronophthisis and renal microcysts

Juvenile nephronophthisis is an autosomal recessive disease that has early onset and will often lead to end-stage renal failure in childhood. It is autosomal recessive in inheritance and is often accompanied by non-renal features, such as features of a more generalised ciliopathy as in Jeune's asphyxiating thoracic dystrophy, Joubert syndrome (with cerebellar hypoplasia), Bardet-Biedl syndrome (with polydactyly and obesity) or Meckel-Gruber syndrome (with malformation of the central nervous system, notably occipital encephalocoele and polydactyly). The ciliopathies comprise a varied group of disorders that share many features but also show great locus heterogeneity. They have been a focus of some very productive research into disease mechanisms in embryogenesis.

Small cortical cysts occur in the rapidly fatal, autosomal recessive Zellweger (cerebrohepatorenal) syndrome in which peroxisomal development is disrupted.

These types of renal maldevelopment, and indeed MCKD as well, should be distinguished from the much more benign medullary sponge kidney, where no clear familial tendency has been shown, although genetic predisposition may play a role as there is some evidence to support familial clustering.

OTHER HEREDITARY NEPHROPATHIES

Congenital nephrosis

Congenital nephrosis comprises a heterogeneous group. In the rare Finnish type (autosomal recessive), prenatal diagnosis has long been feasible from a greatly raised concentration of amniotic fluid α-fetoprotein (AFP, presumably derived from fetal urine). Specific mutation analysis is now available and would usually be preferred.

Idiopathic (minimal-change) childhood nephrotic syndrome

A careful family study has shown a 6% risk to sibs.

IgA nephritis

There is a familial component to IgA nephritis, an immune-mediated disorder that accounts for up to a quarter of primary glomerulonephritis cases in adults. There are some familial clusters of the disease and there is a reported increase in the frequency of HLA-Bw35 or HLA-DR4, or both.

Amyloidosis

Renal involvement may occur in association with some of the primary amyloid neuropathies (due to defects in transthyretin; see Chapter 13) and with familial Mediterranean fever (autosomal recessive).

Alport syndrome (hereditary nephropathy with nerve deafness)

Once other hereditary nephropathies have been excluded, true Alport syndrome is almost always X-linked, with variable expression in females and deafness a variable feature even in affected males. Microscopic haematuria is probably the most accurate clinical detector of heterozygous females. Renal electron microscopic detection of extensive thickening and splitting of the glomerular basement membrane helps to distinguish true Alport syndrome from various other hereditary nephropathies, most of which are dominantly inherited when onset is in adult life. Pathogenic variants in the gene for one of the chains of type IV collagen is now known to be responsible. Specific variants can usually be identified in affected families, so that accurate carrier detection and prenatal diagnosis are possible. Molecular analysis is also helpful in the rare autosomal Alport families, also due to type IV collagen defects but involving different chains; it has largely replaced renal biopsy in the distinction from other nephropathies.

Benign familial haematuria

This type of haematuria, usually recurrent and painless, sometimes gross or microscopic, is not associated with deafness, ocular defect, hypertension or renal impairment. Moderate basement membrane thinning is sometimes found. Transmission is usually consistent with autosomal dominant inheritance when analysis is performed on all available family members. A molecular defect in either of the type IV collagen genes on chromosome 2q (*COL4A4* or *COL4A3*) is often responsible.

Fabry disease

Fabry disease is X-linked with partial manifestation in some females. Cardiac involvement, characteristic skin lesions and painful neuropathy are other predominant features, in addition to nephropathy and also ocular involvement. Diagnosis of the affected hemizygous male can employ enzyme assay (α-galactosidase), but the detection of heterozygous carrier females (whether or not they manifest clinical features of the disorder) is often best achieved by molecular methods. Prenatal diagnosis is also available by molecular diagnostics or by enzyme assay (for a male fetus). Enzyme replacement therapy is available (and useful) for affected males and for females who manifest complications of the condition.

Cystinosis (cystine storage disease)

Progressive renal failure is one of the main features of cystinosis, which is an autosomal recessive disorder. The specific gene *CTNS* encodes a lysosomal membrane protein, cystinosin. The condition must not be confused with the renal transport defect cystinuria (see later).

Urinary tract malformations

Many chromosome abnormalities and other general malformations are associated with structural urinary tract abnormalities, associations that are important to detect in order to avoid preventable obstruction or infection. Ultrasonography is playing an increasing role in the prenatal diagnosis of urinary tract malformations but requires expert interpretation. In the case of some obstructive uropathies, it has been used in conjunction with intrauterine insertion of shunts, although the results have not, so far, been conclusive.

Renal agenesis

The estimates of the recurrence risk in sibs range from 3% to 8% for bilateral renal agenesis, which may have associated congenital abnormalities. There may be some additional risk for unilateral agenesis (often undetected without ultrasound). See the previous section, 'Multicystic Dysplastic Kidney Disease (Renal Hypo-/Dysplasia)'. Whereas that condition is caused by heterozygous variants in any of several genes, 'pure' renal agenesis may sometimes result from homozygous variants at a different locus.

Renal agenesis may also be part of more general syndromes, including the autosomal recessive Fraser (cryptophthalmos) syndrome and several other recessive disorders.

Hydronephrosis

Most bilateral cases of hydronephrosis are secondary to obstruction or other disorders. Unilateral hydronephrosis apparently following autosomal dominant inheritance has been recorded, but most cases are not obviously familial.

Horseshoe kidney

Horseshoe kidney is rarely familial when it arises as an isolated defect. It is frequent in Turner syndrome.

Bladder exstrophy

Recurrence of bladder exstrophy in sibs is very rare (below 1%). Prenatal diagnosis may result from a raised serum AFP level detected by a screening test, as well as from ultrasound scan. With omphalocoele, imperforate anus and spinal defects, it forms one part of the OEIS complex.

Smith-Lemli-Opitz syndrome

This autosomal recessive multisystem disorder is due to a primary defect in cholesterol biosynthesis. Hypospadias, other genital defects and a variety of structural urinary tract abnormalities are prominent features, together with mental retardation, characteristic facies, syndactyly and cardiac involvement.

Prune belly syndrome (abdominal muscle deficiency, megaureter, megacystis, undescended testis)

Almost all cases of prune belly syndrome are male. Recurrence in sibs is rare (below 1%) and several discordant monozygotic twin pairs are known. A substantial body of opinion is of the view that the syndrome is a consequence of early urethral obstruction and that the recurrence risk is dependent on the specific cause of the urethral obstruction.

Urethral valves

Satisfactory risk figures are not available, but the risk is certainly small in sibs.

Hypospadias

Incidence of hypospadias is at least 1 in 1,000 males. The recurrence risk in male sibs is around 10%, and in children of affected males the risk is similar. The risk for offspring of female sibs of patients is uncertain. Care must be taken to distinguish various intersexual states and Mendelian syndromes such as the autosomal recessive Smith-Lemli-Opitz syndrome, the separate Opitz syndrome (autosomal dominant or X-linked), and the X-linked Aarskog syndrome, as well as deletions in the Wilms tumour gene region of chromosome 11. Association with maternal hormone therapy has been suggested, and mutations in the androgen receptor have recently been found to be responsible for some cases.

Cryptorchidism

The recurrence risk in sibs is around 10%. The underlying primary causes must be borne in mind.

Vesicoureteric reflux

A family study of vesicoureteric reflux has shown a risk of around 10% to sibs (about 10 times the population frequency), which is relevant to the early detection and prevention of renal scarring. A similar proportion of parents were affected. In some families, a single dominant gene may be acting, but there is substantial locus heterogeneity. The genetic contribution to reflux is strong, but it may be more reasonable to regard it as multifactorial than autosomal dominant with incomplete penetrance and locus heterogeneity. There may be overlap in causation with urinary tract obstruction and multicystic dysplastic kidney disease/renal hypo-/dysplasia.

Enuresis

This common problem is frequently familial and appears to follow an autosomal dominant pattern in some families, with loci on chromosomes 12q and 13q suggested, and of moderately high penetrance.

RENAL STONES

Most cases of renal stones, whether calcium, urate or associated with infection, are not Mendelian in inheritance. There appears to be an increased risk for close relatives, but no precise figures are available. Numerous rare metabolic causes exist for renal stones; some of those due to renal transport defects are listed in Table 24.1.

Isolated hyperparathyroidism is rarely familial. In most families showing dominant inheritance, renal stones are due to familial hypocalcaemic hypercalciuria or are part of

Table 24.1 Inherited renal transport defects

Disorder	Inheritance
Cystinuria (see Chapter 26)	Autosomal recessive
Xanthinuria	Autosomal recessive
Renal glycosuria	Autosomal recessive
Hartnup disease	Autosomal recessive
Dibasic aminoaciduria	Autosomal recessive
Fanconi syndrome (usually secondary to cystinosis)	Autosomal recessive
Lowe syndrome	X-linked recessive
Familial hypophosphataemia (vitamin D–resistant rickets)	X-linked dominant (often somewhat milder in females)
Nephrogenic diabetes insipidus	X-linked (variable female expression)
Renal tubular acidosis	Several types; most commonly autosomal dominant (when familial); occasionally X-linked
Familial hypocalcaemic hypercalciuria	Autosomal dominant

multiple endocrine neoplasia type 1 (see Chapter 25). Urate stones are frequent in the X-linked Lesch-Nyhan and related hyperuricaemic syndromes.

Cystinuria (see Chapter 26) is autosomal recessive in inheritance, so sibs of affected children deserve careful screening for this relatively common (about 1 in 7,000) and readily treatable disorder.

Renal transport disorders

Table 24.1 lists some of the inherited renal transport disorders. As expected with inborn errors of metabolism, most are autosomal recessive, but the three X-linked conditions are all expressed variably in the heterozygous female. Most carriers of Lowe (oculocerebrorenal) syndrome are detectable by lens opacities, while heterozygotes for familial hypophosphataemia may be short in stature and have low serum phosphate levels. Renal tubular acidosis is heterogeneous; many cases are sporadic, but numerous families with autosomal dominant inheritance exist, as well as rarer autosomal recessive and X-linked forms, so careful classification of the precise tubular defect is important.

RENAL TUMOURS

Wilms tumour and the related syndrome complex are discussed in Chapter 32. An important Mendelian cause of adult renal cell carcinoma is von Hippel-Lindau disease (also see Chapter 32), which is determined by a specific tumour suppressor gene on chromosome 3. Tuberous sclerosis is another cause, although angiomyolipoma is the more usual renal lesion. In the absence of associated disorders, occasional families with renal cell carcinoma following dominant inheritance have been reported, but most cases are sporadic.

25

Endocrine and reproductive disorders

DIABETES MELLITUS

The genetics of diabetes mellitus provides a paradigm for the role of genetic factors in common disorders of complex determination. The following summary is an oversimplification of a difficult subject, but recent reviews are available that give more detail.

Diabetes can be divided broadly into three main groups:

- Type 1 (insulin-dependent or juvenile) diabetes
- Type 2 (non-insulin-dependent or maturity-onset) diabetes
- Diabetes associated with specific primary genetic disorders (Table 25.1)

Neonatal diabetes is extremely rare and usually sporadic. Transient neonatal diabetes is the result of an imprinting defect on chromosome 6.

Type I diabetes

Type I diabetes (T1D) affects around 1 in 300 individuals in most of Europe, and a moderate familial tendency has long been recognised. Approximate risks to different categories of relative are given in Table 25.2.

Table 25.1 Specific genetic disorders frequently associated with diabetes mellitus

Disorder	Type of diabetes	Inheritance
Cystic fibrosis	1	AR (see Chapter 22)
Haemochromatosis	2	AR (see Chapter 23)
Myotonic dystrophy	2	AD (trinucleotide repeat, see Chapter 13)
Seip syndrome (lipoatrophic diabetes)	2	AR
Lipodystrophy (various types, often partial)	2	Usually AD (often *LMNA*)
Alstrom syndrome (with deafness, retinal degeneration)	2	AR (see Chapter 20)
Werner syndrome	2	AR
Prader-Willi syndrome	2	15q microdeletion or imprinting defect
Bardet-Biedl syndrome	2	AR (ciliopathy)
DIDMOAD (Wolfram) syndrome (diabetes insipidus, diabetes mellitus and optic atrophy)	1	Usually AR (also AD or mitochondrial)
Friedreich ataxia	Variable	AR (intronic trinucleotide repeat, see Chapter 14)
Leprechaunism (Donohue syndrome)	2	AR (insulin receptor defect)
Ataxia telangiectasia	2	AR (see Chapter 32)

Abbreviations: AR, autosomal recessive; AD, autosomal dominant.

Autoimmune destruction of the insulin-producing β cells of the pancreas, associated with T-cell dysfunction, results in low or absent insulin production. Viral infection may be an important environmental trigger. In terms of genetic susceptibility, it still seems that the human leucocyte antigen (HLA) region of chromosome 6 is one of the principal determinants. Sibs with an identical HLA haplotype have around double the usual sib risk, while those with a completely different haplotype have only a 1% risk. It is uncertain how useful such modest risk modifications are in genetic counselling. The HLA-DQ region appears to be particularly important, with some alleles giving susceptibility and other alleles conferring protection,

Table 25.2 Approximate genetic risks in diabetes mellitus

Risk category	Type I	Type II
General population	1 in 300	Very variable (commonly 1%–5%)
Sib of isolated case	1 in 14	1 in 10
Sib, no shared HLA haplotype	1 in 100	–
Sib, two or more shared HLA haplotypes	1 in 6	–
Sib and another first-degree relative affected	1 in 6	1 in 5
Offspring of isolated case	1 in 25	1 in 10
Monozygous co-twin affected	1 in 3	1 in 2

the findings applying in a number of population groups. These associations have now been confirmed by studies at the DNA level.

Outside the HLA system, a series of other susceptibility loci have been proposed, including the region of the insulin gene on chromosome 11. Despite much research, no other associations have proved to be sufficiently strong or consistent to alter the empiric estimates in Table 25.2.

Type II diabetes

Type II diabetes (T2D) is an exceptionally common disorder that shows extreme geographical variation but is continuing to increase in prevalence with the trend to higher body mass index (BMI) levels in many populations. A range of genetic, environmental and epigenetic factors are involved, with the epigenetic modifications seeming to mediate the effect of early experiences (*in utero* or in infancy) and perhaps of transgenerational factors too (e.g. grandparental experience of famine or smoking).

T2D is proving to be a major problem in developing countries as they increasingly adopt 'Western' dietary habits and sedentary lifestyles. Attempts have been made to replace Neel's 'thrifty genotype' hypothesis by a 'thrifty phenotype' (Barker's phrase) based on inadequate intrauterine nutrition that marks the body's metabolism so that it is pre-adapted to cope with chronic undernutrition. It has been proposed that this would account for the increase in T2D shown in certain populations, as they are unable to cope well with an unexpectedly generous supply of calories. These ideas of an underlying explanation for such a 'predictive adaptive response' remain suggestive and of interest but their place relative to conventional genetic factors has not yet been firmly established. The chronic stresses of unemployment, marginalisation and racism may also add to the causal factors that contribute to the development of T2D and related disorders. Insulin levels are initially increased in someone developing T2D, and insulin resistance is present but the specific genetic determinants remain even less clear than in T1D. Risks to relatives are high (see Table 25.2), especially for monozygotic twins, but are mainly for the same form of diabetes, not for the more severe type I disease.

With insulin resistance a feature of the disorder, molecular defects in the insulin molecule or its receptor might have been expected, but these have been found only in a few individuals. The rare MODY (maturity-onset diabetes of the young) form with juvenile onset, which appears to follow autosomal dominant inheritance (although with incomplete penetrance), has been linked to the glucokinase locus in some families, with specific mutations found in this gene, and more frequently in the hepatocyte nuclear factor-1-α (*HNF1A*) gene, as well as less commonly in others. MODY appears to make up about 1% of all T2D, although MODY may be more accurately seen as distinct from T2D and, in any case, heterogeneous. Other susceptibility loci have so far proved too inconsistent to use in practice. Variants in the mitochondrial genome have also been found in some families showing maternal transmission.

Diabetes and pregnancy

The risk of a family member developing diabetes is not the only factor to be considered in giving genetic counselling to diabetic families. The offspring of a diabetic mother face special hazards, although these appear to be declining markedly with better diabetic control during pregnancy. Perinatal mortality has been shown to correlate with the severity of maternal diabetes – one large early study gave an overall perinatal mortality rate of 20%, rising to almost 40% in the most severely affected group. Although risks have declined since these data were collected, they remain far from negligible.

There is also an increase in the incidence of congenital malformations in the offspring of the diabetic mother, with a threefold excess over the general population. There is a clear relation to control of the diabetes, with a low risk where this is well controlled. There is no detectable increase in malformations when the mother has preclinical or gestational diabetes.

A number of specific malformations seem to occur particularly in the offspring of diabetic mothers, including sacral agenesis, proximal femoral deficiency and related caudal regression syndromes. However, most of the increased risk is for malformations that are much more common and that do not act as strong indicators of maternal diabetes (such as anencephaly, cardiac defects, bilateral renal aplasia or dysplasia and vertebral anomalies).

PITUITARY GLAND DISORDERS

Although the pituitary gland may be involved in a variety of generalised syndromes, most of the genetic counselling problems arise in relation to specific hormonal deficiencies, many of which follow Mendelian inheritance, as indicated in Table 25.3. Molecular defects in the hormones or their receptors are now known in some of these conditions (e.g. Laron dwarfism), which should help to resolve heterogeneity, as well as provide tests for family members.

Isolated growth hormone deficiency may follow autosomal recessive, autosomal dominant or X-linked inheritance. In the autosomal recessive Laron dwarfism, growth hormone levels are high as the receptor function is deficient and IGF1 levels are low, usually with defects in both copies of the GH receptor gene, *GHR*. In the recessive (and often treatable) dwarfism caused by homozygosity or compound heterozygosity for growth hormone gene defects or deletions, growth hormone levels will of course be low; the dominant negative action of some pathogenic variants can cause a similar effect in the heterozygous state.

Among the posterior pituitary deficiencies, the DIDMOAD (Wolfram) syndrome has been noted in Chapter 19 and is usually autosomal recessive. A severe form of the condition can

Table 25.3 Genetic disorders involving pituitary hormone deficiency

Disorder	Inheritance
Anterior pituitary	
Familial panhypopituitarism	Autosomal recessive or X-linked recessive
Isolated growth hormone deficiency	All types of inheritance (see text)
Laron pituitary dwarfism	Autosomal recessive (human growth hormone [HGH] receptor defect)
Decreased responsiveness to growth hormone in rainforest dwellers (including African pygmy groups)	Polygenic adaptation
Septo-optic dysplasia	Usually sporadic
Holoprosencephaly group	See Chapter 14; mainly sporadic (but heterogeneous)
Posterior pituitary	
Familial diabetes insipidus (vasopressin sensitive)	Autosomal dominant
Familial nephrogenic diabetes insipidus	X-linked semidominant
DIDMOAD (Wolfram) syndrome (diabetes insipidus, diabetes mellitus, optic atrophy)	Autosomal recessive (usually)

result from dominant mutations in the same gene, and similar phenotypes can be associated with disorders of the mitochondrial genome. Isolated vasopressin deficiency causing diabetes insipidus is usually autosomal dominant, whereas most cases of primary nephrogenic diabetes insipidus are X-linked, with variable manifestation in females.

Acromegaly and related disorders of pituitary hypersecretion are mostly sporadic but may form part of the autosomal dominant type 1 multiple endocrine neoplasia (see later).

Primary growth deficiencies

A heterogeneous group of proportionate growth failure, most often from intrauterine life, remains after endocrine causes have been excluded. Most chromosomal disorders impair growth, but specific causes to be considered include Russell-Silver syndrome and Seckel syndrome. Russell-Silver syndrome often shows asymmetry and is usually sporadic, often being the result of a disturbance of imprinting processes. It is often associated with triangular facies and sometimes with problems affecting swallowing and/or speech; in a boy, it is sometimes also associated with hypospadias.

Seckel syndrome (autosomal recessive) is a cause of severe growth failure and microcephaly and is the best recognised of the group of conditions known collectively as 'microcephalic osteodysplastic primordial dwarfism'. Next-generation sequencing (NGS) gene panels are available to help achieve a diagnosis in this group.

Overgrowth syndromes

These are likewise mostly sporadic and include Sotos syndrome (often due to new mutations), Weaver syndrome, Beckwith-Wiedemann syndrome (commonly with macroglossia and omphalocoele), and the *DNMT3A*-related overgrowth syndrome.

Gorlin syndrome, Simpson-Golabi-Behmel syndrome, the *PTEN*-related disorder Cowden syndrome and the fragile X syndrome FRAXA may also be associated with macrocephaly and overgrowth.

Surveillance for tumours needs to be considered in this group of conditions, especially for Wilms tumour during early childhood in Beckwith-Wiedemann syndrome and for breast cancer in adult women with Cowden syndrome. Being alert to the risk of various types of malignancy is important also in Gorlin syndrome (varying with the gene involved).

Developmental difficulties are found in many but not all of these conditions, so that those with Gorlin syndrome and Beckwith-Wiedemann syndrome may have normal cognitive development.

THYROID GLAND DISORDERS

Congenital hypothyroidism

Most cases of congenital hypothyroidism are due to failure of thyroid gland development and are sporadic. Occasional occurrence in sibs may indicate recessively inherited forms that cannot at present be distinguished. Recessively inherited cases of thyroid-stimulating hormone deficiency have also been recorded. Newborn screening is now universal in developed countries and has led to the recognition of hypothyroidism being part of several unusual malformation syndromes. There are no satisfactory data on offspring risks at present, but a knowledge of the underlying genetic aetiology, where it is achieved, can allow families to be given carefully considered advice.

The presence of a goitre in a non-endemic region indicates that an inborn error of thyroxine synthesis is likely. The various types all follow autosomal recessive inheritance, including Pendred syndrome, in which defective iodine organification is associated with nerve deafness (see Chapter 20) and is due to defects in a specific ion transport gene.

Absence of thyroxine-binding globulin may be X-linked recessive or autosomal dominant. It is usually harmless but may be confused with hypothyroidism biochemically.

Autoimmune thyroid disease

Autoimmune thyroid disease may frequently form part of a broader autoimmune disorder, with other endocrine glands and different systems affected (e.g. myasthenia gravis, pernicious anaemia). This possibility must be borne in mind when investigating families. An autosomal dominant susceptibility gene is likely to be involved in many such families.

Both Graves disease and Hashimoto thyroiditis show strong familial aggregation, with both disorders commonly seen in the same family. A common autoimmune basis is now recognised, association with antigens HLA-Dw3 and HLA-B5 being seen in addition to other abnormalities. About 50% of monozygotic twins are concordant (compared with 5% of dizygotic twins). Clinical thyroid disease in other relatives is much less frequent than the incidence of thyroid antibodies. The lifetime risk probably does not exceed 10%, except in a small number of families where a pattern strongly suggestive of autosomal dominant inheritance is seen.

Transient neonatal hyperthyroidism may occur in infants of mothers affected with Graves disease because of long-acting thyroid-stimulating IgG antibodies that cross the placenta and persist in the infant. The joint treatment of a thyrotoxic mother and fetus may be indicated (e.g. with carbimazole) but needs to be managed with great care.

A distinct, recessively inherited, autoimmune polyglandular syndrome (APECED), which involves parathyroid and pancreas as well as thyroid, is due to pathogenic variants in the *AIRE* gene on chromosome 21. There may also be skeletal features and mucocutaneous candidiasis.

PARATHYROID GLAND DISORDERS

Most, but not all, familial cases of hyperparathyroidism are part of multiple endocrine neoplasia type 1 (see later), but the great majority of parathyroid tumours are non-Mendelian, with a low recurrence risk for relatives; the same applies to Cushing syndrome and to pituitary tumours.

A dominantly inherited, benign entity of hypercalcaemia with hypocalciuria has been recognised that can mimic hyperparathyroidism. It is caused by defects of the calcium-sensing mechanism.

Hypoparathyroidism is commonly sporadic, but a rare X-linked recessive type has been recognised, as has an autosomal recessive syndrome with adrenal failure and candidiasis. Absent parathyroid glands are a feature of DiGeorge syndrome, part of the broader microdeletion syndrome involving chromosome 22q (see Chapter 21).

Albright's hereditary osteodystrophy (encompassing pseudohypoparathyroidism and pseudopseudohypoparathyroidism) is now understood in molecular terms as being due to receptor defects in the adenyl cyclase system, the gene *GNAS* encoding the Gs-α protein. Formerly considered to be X-linked, it is now recognised as autosomal dominant but subject to imprinting effects. Most fully expressed cases are maternally transmitted, as the endocrine aspects are much less fully expressed when transmitted through the father.

MULTIPLE ENDOCRINE NEOPLASIA

Multiple endocrine neoplasia comprises two major types, both usually inherited as autosomal dominant disorders:

- *Type 1 (MEN 1)*: Parathyroid, anterior pituitary and pancreatic endocrine tumours are the most frequent.
- *Type 2 (MEN 2)*: Medullary carcinoma of the thyroid may occur alone or coexist with phaeochromocytoma and with mucosal neuromas (type 2B). Some patients may be 'Marfanoid' in appearance. The gene responsible is the *RET* oncogene, with a small number of specific mutations responsible for most cases of both 2A and 2B types.

Both major forms are important examples of high-risk neoplastic disorders, where recognition of the Mendelian inheritance and the existence of a genetic register can prevent fatal disease in relatives, quite apart from the importance of genetic counselling in relation to reproduction (see Chapter 32).

Phaeochromocytoma may form part of other tumour syndromes than MEN2, such as von Hippel-Lindau disease and familial paraganglioma.

OBESITY

A few cases of severe childhood obesity have syndromal associations (e.g. Prader-Willi and Bardet-Biedl syndromes), but most cases are not clearly genetic and arise as a result of excess food intake. Research into the genetics of severe obesity has elucidated important biological mechanisms that relate to metabolism and to satiety; a very few cases of autosomal recessive leptin deficiency have been recorded. The therapeutic applications of such research are perhaps more developed in the management of the lipodystrophies.

CONGENITAL ADRENAL HYPERPLASIA (ADRENOGENITAL SYNDROME)

At least eight types of congenital adrenal hyperplasia (CAH) exist, resulting from different disorders of steroid hormone biosynthesis; all follow autosomal recessive inheritance. The most important type, 21-hydroxylase deficiency, is closely linked (in terms of chromosomal location) to the HLA system. A variety of deletions and other mutations have been identified, correlating with phenotype to some extent and allowing accurate prenatal diagnosis and carrier detection.

Intrauterine treatment with dexamethasone used to be given to women carrying an affected female fetus at risk of virilisation. The safety of this approach for the pregnant woman is being reassessed, and there are reports of adverse effects on the child's cognition. A much more cautious approach may be emerging.

Early diagnosis of affected infants is important, especially in the salt-losing form of CAH where it is critical. Newborn screening is offered in some countries.

Prenatal diagnosis is available and can be helpful to ensure the prompt treatment of an affected infant. Whether termination of an affected pregnancy is chosen may be strongly influenced by the severity of the effects, particularly virilisation of a female, in the first affected child. With the more cautious approach to fetal treatment with dexamethasone, attitudes to the termination of affected pregnancies may change.

HYPOGONADISM AND ALLIED STATES

The molecular basis of sex determination has considerable relevance to the classification and pathogenesis of the different forms of hypogonadism and intersex. The principal points of relevance are as follows:

- A specific gene on the Y chromosome (*SRY*) has been identified that commits the undifferentiated gonad to become a testis. If this is absent or defective, the gonadal phenotype will be female.
- Male phenotype is dependent on the presence of and sensitivity to androgen, which is itself dependent on a differentiated testis.
- Two functioning X chromosomes are needed for formation of a fully developed ovary with viable ova.
- Other hormonal influences (e.g. adrenal steroid precursors) may modify genital development and result in ambiguous genitalia.

Genetic counselling in this area must rest on a well-defined diagnostic assessment that integrates clinical assessment with endocrinological and genetic investigations as appropriate. Recognition of X-linked and autosomal recessive disorders, along with translocations involving X and Y chromosome material, is especially important, as it is in these groups that recurrence within the family is most likely.

The following broad groups are important to distinguish for genetic counselling.

Primary sex chromosome disorders

In particular these include XXY (Klinefelter) and 45,X (Turner) syndromes, which are discussed in Chapter 4. Recurrence in a family is exceptional, except where there is mosaicism.

Disorders where chromosomal and phenotypic sex do not correspond, including XX males and XY females

The complexities of this group have become greatly clarified with isolation of specific genes on the Y and X chromosomes involved with sex determination. A careful endocrine, cytogenetic and molecular assessment is essential before genetic counselling can be given. The main disorders include XX males and XY females:

- *XX males*: These are usually sporadic, resulting from Y chromosome material including the *SRY* gene translocated onto an X chromosome and usually detectable by molecular tests.
- *XY females*: The most frequent cause is the androgen insensitivity syndrome (formerly known as testicular feminisation) where a normal female phenotype is associated with the presence of testes. This diagnosis may not be suspected until failure of menarche or absent pubic and axillary hair is investigated. Partial androgen insensitivity may result in ambiguous genitalia at birth. In XY gonadal dysgenesis, due to molecular defects in the Y-linked sex-determining *SRY* gene, or to corresponding X-linked defects, there may be a normal phenotype or varying degrees of intersex. The dysgenetic gonad is at risk of malignant change and should be removed. Both these disorders may follow X-linked recessive inheritance with phenotypic and chromosomally normal female relatives at risk of having an affected XY daughter.

- *Ambiguous genitalia*: This may result from some of the conditions mentioned previously (e.g. CAH, sex chromosome disorders), from partial androgen insensitivity, from disorders involving the *SRY*, *SOX9* or *WT1* genes, associated with campomelic dysplasia, Wilms tumour, the Denys-Drash syndrome and other genital anomalies). It will require careful endocrine, chromosome and clinical assessment to be sure of the cause.

Genetic counselling in all of these conditions needs to be especially sensitive to the sexual identity of those affected and to link closely with the overall, multidisciplinary management of the condition. In general, it will be the phenotypic and psychological sexual identity that is more relevant than chromosomal sex. Great care must be taken not to confuse or upset affected individuals by inappropriately assuming that sex chromosomal status must necessarily determine actual sexual identity.

The sense of urgency of gender assignment at birth can be very real, but the perceived need for surgical intervention to make this irreversible is perhaps somewhat less marked than in the past. The deferral of irreversible surgery until the affected individual has the capacity for real involvement is to be encouraged to the extent that is practicable.

Hypogonadism due to specific genetic disorders

Here the recurrence risk will be that of the underlying disorder, while the hypogonadism itself may be of gonadal, pituitary or hypothalamic origin (Box 25.1).

BOX 25.1: Some genetic causes of infertility and hypogonadism

Phenotypic male
Sex chromosome anomalies and reversal
Y-chromosome microdeletions
Androgen insensitivity (partial)
Kennedy disease (spinobulbar muscular atrophy)
Kallmann syndrome
Pituitary hormone defects (various)
Dysmorphic syndromes with hypogonadism (e.g. Bardet-Biedel, Prader-Willi)
Myotonic dystrophy
Cystic fibrosis
Primary ciliary dyskinesia

Phenotypic female
Sex chromosome anomalies and reversal
Androgen insensitivity (complete)
Fragile X pre-mutation (premature ovarian failure)
Congenital adrenal hyperplasia (some types)
Pituitary hormone defects (various)
SRY gene defects (Y chromosome)
Galactosaemia (premature ovarian failure)

INFERTILITY

There are two important questions that need to be asked (but frequently are not) by those attempting to investigate, counsel and treat infertility:

- Is the infertility one aspect of a genetic disorder that might be transmitted?
- Will correction of infertility give an increased risk of malformations in the offspring?

The genetic causes of both female and male infertility are numerous and in part overlap with those of hypogonadism already mentioned (see Box 25.1). As with these, it is only X-linked or autosomal recessive disorders that are of practical importance for genetic counselling, because only in these will unaffected people be at risk of having an affected child.

Premature ovarian failure has been shown to result in some cases from X-autosome translocation involving a critical region of the long arm, but it may also be associated with pre-mutations in the fragile X (*FMR1*) gene.

Disorders of sperm production include primary sex chromosome disorders such as XXY (Klinefelter) syndrome, other disorders affecting the testis (e.g. myotonic dystrophy), balanced chromosomal translocations causing abnormalities of chromosome pairing in meiosis, clinical defects affecting sperm motility, and a variety of poorly defined biochemical disorders. Molecular deletions of the Y chromosome involving the azoospermic factor *AZF* are an important cause. Blockage or aplasia of the vas deferens causes infertility in most males affected by cystic fibrosis or carrying the condition in one copy of the *CFTR* gene along with otherwise benign variants in their other copy of the same gene. A mild form of this may be responsible for some apparently primary cases of such obstruction.

The question of increased risk to offspring arises principally in those patients in whom apparent infertility is really a reflection of early unrecognised fetal loss as a result of abnormal gamete production. The most important group to detect is where one parent carries a balanced translocation, where the risk of an unbalanced chromosome abnormality in a pregnancy that goes to term is considerable, especially when the defect is carried by a female (see Chapter 4). This problem is closely related to that of recurrent abortion, considered later.

Artificial insemination by donor (AID) and *in vitro* fertilisation are mentioned in Chapter 11 as increasingly used modes of treating infertility. There has now been sufficient experience with AID to make it clear that there is no increase in abnormalities. The same is probably true of *in vitro* fertilisation from preliminary studies of children conceived in this way, but there are doubts remaining about the safety of intra-cytoplasmic sperm injection (ICSI).

RECURRENT ABORTIONS

Most women with a history of recurrent abortions will be under the care of a gynaecologist, who will have already searched for a gynaecological cause and will have excluded most serious maternal disorders. Rhesus haemolytic disease is now usually prevented as a cause of later pregnancy loss. Factors such as lupus anticoagulant antigen or maternal thrombotic disorders may be relevant in a small proportion, but numerous proposed factors and corresponding remedies have failed to be confirmed and the cause of most recurrent abortions remains unknown.

The main question to be answered is not so much whether another abortion will occur, but what are the chances of having a healthy child, together with the risk that a pregnancy reaching term will result in an abnormality. The question of amniocentesis may also arise: clearly, one does not want to expose a pregnancy to any added risk of abortion unless there is a likelihood of an abnormality detectable by this method.

There will be many women in whom a careful search reveals no genetic or other factors involved, but with care considerable help can be given by the following measures:

- Pathological examination of the abortus, where possible, may identify major structural malformations. Genetic analysis may also be helpful, including a karyotype (although that may not be feasible).
- Cytogenetic study of the parents is especially important where a translocation is a possibility and should always be done. In general, the finding of a chromosome abnormality in the abortus but not in a parent is not likely to be relevant or to affect the genetic risks (see Chapter 4).
- Search for possible lethal Mendelian causes. Consanguinity may be relevant, as it increases the risk of autosomal recessive lethals; X-linked dominant disorders lethal in the male; and myotonic dystrophy, which gives heavy fetal losses in the offspring of mildly affected women.

The most important group to detect are the autosomal translocations, where one parent is a balanced translocation carrier. As stated in Chapter 4, these carry a significant risk of an abnormal live-born offspring, probably around 12% where the carrier is female, but nearer 5% where the male is the carrier, the precise risk depending on the type of translocation. Amniocentesis or chorion biopsy is clearly indicated in any such pregnancy, and there is no evidence that it is accompanied by a greater risk of abortion in such a situation. One study has shown that couples where a parent has a balanced chromosome rearrangement have as high a chance of eventually having a healthy child as a control group.

It is important for couples to realise that spontaneous abortion is an exceedingly common event, occurring in at least one in eight recognised pregnancies. Thus, 1 in 64 women might be expected to have two consecutive abortions on the grounds of chance alone, and unless there are other reasons, it is probably not worth undertaking investigations unless they have had at least three spontaneous abortions, when around 5% of couples will be found to carry a balanced translocation.

OTHER REPRODUCTIVE PROBLEMS

Hydatidiform moles

Hydatidiform moles are masses of trophoblastic tissue that are rarely familial but show unusual chromosomal features. The complete hydatidiform mole has a normal chromosome number that is of entirely paternal origin, while the partial mole is a complete triploid, with two paternal complements. These structures represent perhaps the most extreme examples of genomic imprinting (see Chapter 2). A 1% recurrence risk in future pregnancies is likely for the complete mole and may represent persistence of the original mole with the risk of malignant change; the recurrence risk is probably less than this for the partial form, which is not associated with malignancy.

Sacrococcygeal teratomas are now usually detected by ultrasound and are mostly sporadic.

TOXAEMIA OF PREGNANCY (PRE-ECLAMPSIA)

Toxaemia of pregnancy may be associated with genetic disorders affecting placental development (e.g. trisomy 18), but in the absence of a specific cause it is frequently familial, possibly determined by a common autosomal recessive gene giving toxaemia when both mother and fetus are homozygous for this. However, the causation of pre-eclampsia remains unclear.

Recurrence risks are around 20% for a pregnancy in a woman whose own mother had toxaemia in the pregnancy leading to that woman's birth; and about 15% where a sister has had toxaemia in pregnancy, figures rather less than suggested in earlier studies (the population risk is around 10%).

26

Inborn errors of metabolism

INTRODUCTION

Since most Mendelian disorders eventually prove to be the result of a deficient or defective product of a specific gene, there is no absolute distinction between inborn errors of metabolism and other genetic disorders. Indeed, the concept of 'inborn errors of development' has now become a reality, as discussed in Chapter 6 (and as foreseen by Garrod himself). For this chapter it seems wise to restrict the term to those conditions where some form of metabolic basis, usually enzymatic, has been clearly identified, but each year more diseases are added to the group. In many cases, the discovery of a specific metabolic basis radically changes the concept of a disease. Thus, Tay-Sachs disease is no longer thought of as purely a brain degeneration but as a generalised metabolic disorder, and the interventions of carrier detection and prenatal diagnosis involve laboratory techniques far removed from those traditionally associated with neurology. Xeroderma pigmentosum and allied disorders of DNA repair are further examples of disorders entering the inborn error category. The recognition of genes in which the process of mutation introduces a propensity for disease used to be achieved by positional cloning but now, with the availability of the human genome sequence, it entails parallel processes '*in silico*'. The upshot of this work is that the 'genes for' many important metabolic disorders (such as Batten disease, Menkes syndrome and Lowe syndrome) and the resulting pathogenic processes have been recognised, when the primary protein defect and even the function of the relevant gene were previously unknown.

The development of specific tests for direct identification of pathogenic variants (the term now preferred to the earlier 'gene mutations') (see Chapter 5) is causing rapid changes in our understanding of many inherited metabolic diseases. In particular, heterogeneity in the types of mutation involved is becoming apparent; in some contexts it is becoming possible to predict the form or severity of phenotype from the type of mutation, although it remains much more difficult to make inferences from genotype to phenotype than in the reverse direction.

From the viewpoint of genetic counselling, inborn errors of metabolism have several characteristics that must be taken into account:

- Almost all follow a Mendelian recessive pattern of inheritance, the great majority being autosomal.
- Precise molecular and/or biochemical techniques for early recognition, carrier detection and prenatal diagnosis are often available, although the biochemical methods (such as enzyme assays) may be confined to a very few expert centres. Molecular genetic methods are generally much more robust and so are usually preferred as long as the causal gene variant is known with certainty.
- Genetic heterogeneity in terms of multiple loci is frequent but can usually be resolved with appropriate investigations, if not clinically. Further redefinition of apparently well-defined disorders will undoubtedly continue.

No attempt is made here to describe or even list the large number of inborn errors, mostly very rare, that have been documented. *The Metabolic and Molecular Bases of Inherited Disease*, now in electronic form (see Appendix 1), is a definitive source of information. Some disorders have been covered in the present volume in the specific system chapters. Peroxisomal disorders are mentioned in Chapter 6. For the great majority of disorders where the inheritance is autosomal recessive, this means that a high genetic risk (one in four) is usually confined to sibs of the affected individual. Unless consanguinity exists, or the gene is especially common in a particular population, the risks to the offspring of healthy sibs or more distant relatives are low or extremely low, and carrier detection or prenatal diagnosis is not likely to be required in such situations. Indeed, it may be unwise to embark on tests whose margin of error may be greater than the individual's prior risk of having an affected child (see Chapter 7), unless there are particular reasons in the individual situation. The risk of error used to arise from difficulties in interpreting enzyme assay results, where there could be a clear overlap between healthy 'carriers' and those affected; now, the scope for error or confusion enters when the unrelated partner of a patient's healthy sibling has gene testing ('to provide reassurance', or to 'make sure they don't also carry the same condition') and a variant is identified whose clinical significance is uncertain.

Table 26.1 and Box 26.1 give some important disorders known to follow X-linked or autosomal dominant inheritance. The X-linked group is especially important for carrier detection, because the female carrier will have a 50% risk of transmitting the condition to her sons (see Chapter 7). Prenatal diagnosis is feasible in almost all serious inherited metabolic disorders, although rarity often means that very few centres will have extensive experience with the particular disorder. This is not such a problem as in the past, when enzyme assays were the principal investigations, but can still be a problem, especially if unanticipated results emerge. Further discussion of this area is provided in Chapter 9.

The following notes deal with some of the situations particularly relevant to genetic counselling in individual conditions. Some other inherited metabolic disorders are dealt with in specific chapters.

Table 26.1 X-linked inborn errors of metabolism

Disorder	Protein defect (usually enzymatic)
Barth syndrome (3-methylglutaconic aciduria type II [MGCA2])	Taffazin, TAZ, a mitochondrial transacylase
Chronic granulomatous disease	β-Cytochrome subunit
Fabry disease (angiokeratoma)	α-Galactosidase
Glucose-6-phosphate dehydrogenase deficiency	Glucose-6-phosphate dehydrogenase
Glycogenosis type VIII	Liver phosphorylase kinase
Haemophilia A	Factor VIII (procoagulant subunit)
Haemophilia B	Factor IX
Hyperammonaemia type I	Ornithine carbamoyl transferase
Hypophosphataemic rickets	Renal tubule phosphate transport defect
Ichthyosis, X-linked	Steroid sulphatase
Lesch-Nyhan syndrome	Hypoxanthine-guanidine phosphoribosyl transferase
Lowe syndrome	Inositol phosphate phosphatase
Menkes syndrome	Defective copper transport protein
Mucopolysaccharidosis II (Hunter syndrome)	Iduronate sulphatase

---

BOX 26.1: Inborn errors of metabolism following autosomal dominant inheritance

Porphyrias
  Acute intermittent
  Variegate
  Coproporphyria
  Protoporphyria
Familial hypercholesterolaemia (low-density lipoprotein receptor [LDLR] defects) (rarely homozygous, then much more severe)
Hereditary angioedema

AMINO ACID DISORDERS

Phenylketonuria

With a mean frequency of around 1 in 10,000 births in the United Kingdom (carrier frequency 1 in 50), this is one of the more common inborn errors, although it is geographically variable. Successful dietary treatment and newborn screening (see Chapter 34) have resulted in a generation of young adults who are, in most cases, mentally normal and are living healthy, active lives, although it has become clear that treatment needs to be strictly controlled and prolonged, at least in some degree, into adult life to achieve optimal results.

This undoubted success story has largely transferred the burden of genetic risks onto the adult females who were identified in the newborn period. Here, although the risk of transmitting phenylketonuria is low (around 1%), there is a high risk of brain damage and other malformations in all offspring of affected women due to phenylalanine crossing the placenta. It is now clear that only strict dietary treatment started prior to conception offers the likelihood of a normal child, and that even therapy started as soon as pregnancy is recognised is likely to be associated with microcephaly and severe cognitive impairment.

The possibility of maternal phenylketonuria causing additional teratogenic problems, such as cardiac defects, must also be considered in those countries without newborn screening programmes. There is no evidence that such problems occur among the offspring of asymptomatic individuals with moderately raised blood phenylalanine detected by screening.

Prenatal diagnosis is feasible but rarely requested except for the very rare and usually fatal form of phenylketonuria, due to dihydropteridine reductase deficiency, which does not respond to the usual dietary treatment. In the classic form, due to phenylalanine hydroxylase deficiency, the enzyme is confined to the liver. There is a useful degree of genotype-phenotype correlation, so that the particular pathogenic variants found in an affected individual correlate with the disease severity and the need for dietary control. Carrier detection is feasible by mutation analysis, but prenatal diagnosis is finding significant application only in countries without effective dietary treatment. It should be borne in mind that the great majority of treated phenylketonuria patients are now entirely normal.

Histidinaemia

Most cases of histidinaemia appear to be asymptomatic, and the original association thought to exist with speech problems and mental retardation seems doubtful. There is no evidence of a significant maternal effect in the heterozygous offspring of affected women.

Cystinuria

Renal calculi are the only significant clinical features in cystinuria. Heterozygotes in one of the two main types may excrete small amounts of amino acids in the urine but are symptomless and must not be confused with the affected homozygotes, where large quantities of cystine and other dibasic amino acids are excreted. The disorder is quite distinct from cystinosis (also autosomal recessive), which is a generalised storage disease of cystine, with much more serious clinical effects including renal failure. (See Chapter 24 for other causes of renal calculi.)

BARTTER SYNDROME

This disorder of electrolyte metabolism, causing hypertension and hypokalaemia, is proving to be heterogeneous, with different ion-channel genes responsible in different families.

GALACTOSAEMIA

Recognition of galactosaemia, a rapidly fatal disorder without early treatment, is important not only because effective treatment exists, but also to allow immediate diagnosis from cord blood in a subsequent pregnancy. Distinction of classic galactosaemia must also be made from the form due to galactokinase deficiency in which cataract is the only abnormality, and from harmless enzyme variants that may be picked up by screening programmes.

Prenatal diagnosis is feasible, but decisions about prenatal diagnosis and the termination of affected pregnancies is difficult for some parents in view of the relatively good outcome of treatment for physical health in most cases, although many treated children have a degree of intellectual disability. The various options and their consequences must be fully discussed with the couple concerned before a decision is made. Pituitary-ovarian dysfunction may result in infertility in treated women.

SPHINGOLIPIDOSES

Specific lysosomal enzyme defects have been identified for most disorders in the severe and clinically confusing group of sphingolipidoses, all autosomal recessive, and prenatal diagnosis is feasible in these. Carrier detection is of particular significance for Tay-Sachs disease, where the gene is at high frequency in Ashkenazi Jewish populations. Screening for adult carriers, with prenatal diagnosis offered to couples who both carry pathogenic variants in the gene, has been successfully applied in many Jewish communities in the United Kingdom, Canada, the United States and Australia; the carrier frequency is approximately 1 in 30 in many of these communities. A comparable approach has also been developed in Finland, Quebec and Israel, where the genes for some other specific metabolic neurodegenerations are at high frequency. Carrier screening programmes have started to switch technologies to high-throughput DNA sequencing, which allows a wider range of disorders to be screened for in 'extended carrier screening' programmes that can be applied to entire populations without the need to target the screening according to an individual's ancestry (see Chapter 34).

Other important sphingolipidoses, almost all autosomal recessive in inheritance, include Gaucher disease, Niemann-Pick disease, metachromatic leucodystrophy and generalised gangliosidosis. Batten disease had no specific enzyme defect known until positional cloning identified one form on chromosome 16, with one particularly frequent mutation, allowing, for the first time, prenatal diagnosis for some families with this devastating disorder (see also Chapter 14). The genes involved in the other forms of Batten disease have since been identified.

Fabry disease is X-linked, with minor signs and biochemical changes often detectable in female carriers. However, the effects in some female 'carriers' can be severe, indeed life-threatening in the case of the cardiac effects, so that enzyme replacement treatment can be indicated for them as well as for affected male hemizygotes. The mucopolysaccharidoses are mentioned in Chapter 14.

The importance of obtaining a precise diagnosis in inborn errors of metabolism (based on enzymatic assay and/or molecular genetics) has already been stressed, but it is probably more important in the group of lysosomal enzyme deficiencies than in any other, since clinical differentiation is often extremely difficult and the prognosis is poor, but prenatal diagnosis is feasible if one knows which enzyme is defective (see Chapter 9) and rational treatments are being developed. Bone marrow transplantation is proving effective in some members of this group, while in Gaucher disease and Fabry disease (and some others) direct enzyme replacement therapy is feasible although it remains very expensive.

GLYCOGEN STORAGE DISEASES

All members of the heterogeneous group of glycogen storage diseases are autosomal recessive in inheritance, apart from the exceedingly rare type VIII (X-linked recessive). Type II (Pompe disease), caused by lysosomal acid maltase deficiency, can be diagnosed prenatally and exists in two distinct forms:

- An infantile type with severe cardiomyopathy and cerebral involvement.
- A later neuromuscular type that may mimic a muscular dystrophy.

The classic type I (von Gierke) glucose-6-phosphatase deficiency has the enzyme confined to the liver.

HYPERLIPIDAEMIAS

The classification of the hyperlipidaemias is still in a state of flux but is becoming clearer as specific molecular defects underlying the condition are being recognised. Most hyperlipidaemias, even with multiple affected family members, are likely to be secondary to diet and other external factors. Type I hyperlipidaemia (hyperchylomicronaemia) and type V are autosomal recessive. The relatively common type II (familial hypercholesterolaemia), which affects about 1 in 500 in northern Europe, is especially important because of its association with early coronary artery disease, as discussed in Chapter 21, and because it is often simply but effectively treatable.

THE PORPHYRIAS

The acute porphyrias form the most striking exception to the rule of recessive inheritance for most inborn errors due to enzyme defects. Acute intermittent porphyria, porphyria variegata, hereditary coproporphyria and protoporphyria all follow autosomal dominant inheritance. Careful investigation of urine and faecal porphyrins, enzyme studies and, where possible, molecular analysis are needed to exclude subclinical disease. Now that specific enzyme and gene defects are known, prenatal diagnosis may be possible but is rarely requested. The severe congenital erythropoietic porphyria follows autosomal recessive inheritance. Porphyria cutanea tarda, the most common of the group, is usually sporadic, with low recurrence risk for family members. This can be dominant or recessive. Much the commonest type is a 'dominant' disorder but of low penetrance and that requires adverse environmental factors such as alcoholic liver damage and/or homozygosity (or compound heterozygosity) for iron overload susceptibility variants in the haemochromatosis gene, *HFE*. Its common representation in textbooks as being inherited in a typically autosomal recessive fashion is misleading.

PSEUDOCHOLINESTERASE DEFICIENCY

Pseudocholinesterase deficiency – an important cause of apnoea following muscle relaxants (notably suxamethonium) – follows autosomal recessive inheritance. Sibs are thus the principal relatives at risk, although, because the gene is relatively common, it may also be worth testing the parents. Heterozygotes (4% of the population) are not at significant risk of clinical problems, and in testing relatives, it is most important not to confuse them with affected homozygotes. Since heterozygotes commonly show a moderate reduction in pseudocholinesterase level, the dibucaine number, which measures the degree of inhibition of the enzyme by dibucaine, should be measured. This will be under 25 in affected homozygotes, 50–70 in heterozygotes and over 75 for normal homozygotes. Other rare genetic variants exist; their nomenclature is most confusing, but the subject is clearly discussed by Whittaker (1986) (see Appendix 1).

Molecular analysis is now well established in clinical use alongside biochemical assays. There are circumstances where molecular methods can replace enzyme or other biochemical assays, as when the pathogenic variant(s) in a family is (are) known and molecular testing permits clear discrimination between normal and heterozygote or heterozygote and affected homozygote, which may not be possible with assays of metabolites or enzyme activities because the ranges may overlap. Molecular techniques are often more robust, as in tracking familial hypercholesterolaemia through families ('cascading' the test) or distinguishing affected from carrier fetuses in many recessive metabolic disorders when both pathogenic variants have been identified.

PHARMACOGENETICS

Inherited differences in metabolism of, and response to, drugs has been recognised for over 50 years (e.g. gene loci such as those for cholinesterase, see earlier, and acetylation), but the possibility of finding simple DNA-based tests that will predict the therapeutic response to a drug or, conversely, predict a hazardous reaction to the drug, could bring enormous benefits in treatment outcomes and cost savings. However, it is not clear at present to what extent such inherited variation might also be predictive for disease risk, nor whether it will really lead to individually tailored therapy based on the individual's genetic constitution. Treatment of a malignancy can be usefully informed by genetic testing of the tumour, but it is less clear that the individual's non-tumour genome will often guide the treatment very effectively. There are settings where this does occur, however, as with the use of synthetic lethality through the action of anti-poly-ADP ribose polymerase (anti-PARP) drugs in the treatment of malignancies in women who carry a constitutional, pathogenic variant of a *BRCA* gene (see Chapter 12).

The term 'pharmacogenomics' is now often used for this DNA-based approach to prescribing drugs. Even more misleading is the term 'personalised medicine', which often refers to the stratified targeting of chemotherapy in oncology, guided by the genomic construction of the tumour. Each person is assigned to a group and given the treatment deemed appropriate for that group, rather than being given a unique treatment created for that one person alone. It is rather like testing the sensitivity of a bacterium in order to guide the patient's antibiotic therapy; would it be reasonable to call that the 'personalised prescription' of antibiotics?

Opportunities for pharmacogenetic testing that have attracted most interest include examples such as (1) establishing the appropriate therapeutic dosage of warfarin in a patient and (2) avoiding rare adverse effects, such as the severe cutaneous drug responses to abacavir, carbamazepine and flucloxacillin that are associated with specific human leucocyte antigen subtypes.

As with all common disease genetics, the underlying basis seems likely to require a considerable amount of more basic research before it reaches practical applications, including genetic counselling.

FATTY ACID METABOLIC DEFECTS AND SUDDEN INFANT DEATH

Several previously unrecognised defects in fatty acid and organic acid metabolism (e.g. medium-chain acyl-CoA dehydrogenase [MCAD] deficiency) have been shown to be responsible for some unusual cases (probably around 1%) of unexplained sudden infant death, and for some cases of what was formerly termed Reye syndrome, with rapidly developing hypoglycaemia, acidosis and encephalopathy. There have been disagreements about the applicability of the term 'unexplained sudden infant death' in situations where a child had a minor ailment before going to bed and then died overnight, but we can steer clear of these discussions in this brief mention. The proportion of such cases that are genetic has probably risen since the removal of likely environmental factors such as aspirin in infancy. The forensic implications in this field are exceptionally serious and provide a striking example of how essential it is to use and integrate all available information in a statistically appropriate manner before attempting to estimate the chance that an underlying metabolic defect may be responsible for a particular case.

Since effective therapies appear possible by dietary modification, recognition of a possible metabolic basis in such situations is most important for a future sibling or for a surviving, near-miss case. Autosomal recessive inheritance is usual, and prenatal diagnosis is theoretically possible even if the child has been buried with inadequate investigation, as long as both parents are willing to provide samples for genomic analysis (leading, one hopes, to a presumptive diagnosis with hindsight).

The frequency of most such disorders appears to be very low in the general population. Population newborn screening is now technically feasible using tandem mass spectrometry, but countries differ greatly in how this has been implemented. Some countries offer screening for many (>100) disorders, even when the evidence does not suggest any great benefit to children affected by some of these conditions, while in other countries screening is only introduced for a disease once the likely consequences of doing so have been scrutinised with great care and a decision has been made on the basis of the best available evidence. Unfortunately, pressure groups have led to tandem mass spectrometry screening for a wider range of disorders introduced on a population basis in some countries before the appropriate evidence is available. The difficulties of withdrawing such services once they have been introduced makes it imperative to evaluate such programmes critically in advance wherever possible, because of the potential harms, including the opportunity costs, the impact on biochemically affected infants who would never have come to any clinical harm, and the potential for over-medicalisation (see Chapter 34).

27

Disorders of blood and immune function

DISORDERS OF HAEMOGLOBIN STRUCTURE AND SYNTHESIS

The large group of haemoglobin disorders, of great importance in many parts of the world, contains perhaps the best understood disorders (in molecular terms) that exist. Most are autosomal recessive in inheritance, and only a few points will be mentioned here.

Sickle cell disease

Sickle cell disease, caused by homozygosity for a glutamic acid to valine substitution at amino acid number 6 in β-globin, is exceptionally common in some regions, and the heterozygote frequency reaches and can even exceed 1 in 8 in some parts of Africa. Thus, carrier testing is of great importance, but fortunately it is readily feasible using a sickling test screen on the red cells, with haemoglobin electrophoresis as a confirmatory measure. Only couples who are both carriers will be at risk of having an affected child. Heterozygotes are essentially healthy and have partial protection against malaria in endemic areas. It is important for them not to be given the erroneous impression that they have a mild form of the disease. Severity in homozygotes can vary greatly according to geographical region.

Prenatal diagnosis, originally using fetal blood but now usually based on DNA analysis of chorionic villi or amniotic cells, has been feasible for some years but has not found wide application, in part because of the variation in clinical severity. The early screening programmes for carriers also met with little success, partly because of their hasty and ill-judged introduction, and partly because of the stigmatisation of carriers that resulted. Recent, more sensitively approached programmes are proving more acceptable, as is newborn screening in high-risk groups or, in some instances, whole populations, to allow the early treatment of complications.

Numerous other β-globin chain abnormalities are known, some of which, such as haemoglobin C, may be encountered in combination with haemoglobin S. This may result in complex genetic situations, emphasising the need for expert haematological and molecular diagnosis to be available to those undertaking genetic counselling for haemoglobinopathies.

Thalassaemias

Thalassaemias, characterised by an imbalance or failure of globin chain synthesis owing to a variety of underlying causes, are another disease group that is exceedingly common in some regions of the world, as well as in immigrant populations in Europe and America. All the thalassaemias are recessively inherited, and various compounds with different abnormal alleles may occur.

β-thalassaemia major is an important problem in parts of the Mediterranean, the Middle East and Asia, while in South-East Asia forms of α-thalassaemia make a large contribution to intrauterine and neonatal deaths. Carrier detection of most forms is feasible, and so is prenatal diagnosis, particularly for β-thalassaemia major, with which there is now considerable experience. Molecular techniques had their first diagnostic applications in this group of disorders and identified a wealth of different defects at the DNA level. The advent of first-trimester prenatal diagnosis based on DNA makes it particularly important to establish the precise molecular nature of the disorder.

In planning prenatal diagnosis, it is important to recognise that the great majority of cases in any particular population will result from a few specific mutations and that the programme must be adjusted to this local biological context, as well as to the cultural background of the population involved. Deletions may be frequent in some situations (especially for α-thalassaemias), while DNA polymorphisms, especially when used in combination as a haplotype, may still be used for cases of β-thalassaemia where the specific mutation is unknown. Carrier detection and prenatal diagnosis have been taken up on a large scale by many populations, notably in Mediterranean and Middle Eastern countries. Population and screening aspects are discussed further in Chapter 34.

The uncommon but important α-thalassaemia mental retardation syndromes, due to deletions on chromosome 16 and to mutations in the X-linked *ATRX* gene, are mentioned in Chapter 14.

OTHER RED BLOOD CELL DISORDERS

Hereditary spherocytosis and elliptocytosis

Hereditary spherocytosis is a disorder of the red cell membrane which usually follows autosomal dominant inheritance, but haemolysis is often mild, requiring red cell fragility tests to be sure that an individual is not affected. Numerous other causes of spherocytosis must be excluded before this diagnosis is made. Specific forms of hereditary spherocytosis have been identified as due to defects in several different red cell membrane proteins, including spectrin and ankyrin.

Hereditary elliptocytosis is also autosomal dominant. Several forms exist, due to defects in glycophorin C and other membrane proteins.

Glucose-6-phosphate dehydrogenase deficiency

This important red cell enzyme defect is particularly common in parts of the Middle East, the Mediterranean and South-East Asia and in people of African descent but is not unknown in others. Numerous enzyme variants exist, with varying loss of activity which determines the haemolytic severity of the disease. The disorder is X-linked recessive but alterations in the gene are so common in some areas (e.g. the Arabian Peninsula) that homozygous affected females are frequent. Carrier detection is often feasible, but this depends on the type of abnormality and the techniques being used.

Other red cell enzyme defects

Other red cell enzyme defects are mostly autosomal recessive, with the exception of phosphoglycerate kinase deficiency, which is X-linked. Some are confined to the red cell, others have generalised clinical effects (e.g. triose phosphate isomerase deficiency). Prenatal diagnosis from fetal blood is a possibility for this group but, as the genes have been cloned and sequenced, DNA analysis is generally preferable, being available much earlier in pregnancy.

Sideroblastic anaemia

Most cases, especially in later life, are acquired, but an X-linked recessive form, though rare, is important to recognise.

Pernicious anaemia

Pernicious anaemia has already been mentioned in connection with atrophic gastritis (see Chapter 23). Congenital vitamin B_{12} deficiency is an exceptionally rare disorder caused by intrinsic factor deficiency, following autosomal recessive inheritance.

Rhesus incompatibility

The prevention of haemolytic disease of the newborn due to Rhesus incompatibility has been so successful that there is a danger of overlooking the problem completely. It certainly ranks as one of the major contributions of genetics to medicine, largely thanks to the work of Cyril Clarke and his colleagues in Liverpool.

Although the molecular genetics of the Rhesus system has been established, it is complex and is not presented here. In essence the problem arises when a homozygous Rhesus-negative woman with a Rhesus-positive partner (heterozygous or homozygous) develops antibodies that will react with the red cells of a Rhesus-positive fetus. Sensitisation may be the result of a previous pregnancy (whether successful or aborted), prenatal diagnostic procedures or transfusion, and is now usually prevented by giving anti-RhD antibody at the appropriate time.

Once sensitisation has occurred, any Rhesus-positive fetus will be at risk. This relates to 50% of pregnancies where the father is heterozygous, and 100% where he is homozygous for the RhD antigen.

The management of established Rhesus disease is difficult and hazardous: it is much better prevented. An affected pregnancy has to be monitored to assess fetal haemolytic anaemia and cardiac failure, leading to hydrops fetalis. The fetus may require transfusion or the delivery may be expedited, with the neonate requiring exchange transfusion. Without this, the fetus may not survive, or the neonate may suffer brain damage from kernicterus, or may die.

Hydrops fetalis

The control of Rhesus haemolytic disease means that other causes must now be sought for hydrops. These are often genetic and include various haemoglobinopathies, red cell enzyme defects and congenital heart defects (some associated with Down syndrome and other chromosome abnormalities), as well as non-genetic causes such as fetal infections.

Other blood group systems

In the past, these were relevant to paternity and zygosity testing (see Chapter 9). Most blood group systems do not cause regular clinical problems, although haemolytic disease of the newborn may occur, particularly with the ABO and Kell systems. Most blood group antigens are co-dominant, expressing themselves without interfering with the action of other alleles that may be present.

A variety of disease associations have been described with the ABO blood group system but are too weak to be of use in genetic counselling. The Duffy blood group is associated with malaria susceptibility. Similarly, although blood groups have been useful genetic markers in the study of genetic linkage, it is rare to be able to apply this form of information in risk prediction. DNA markers have superseded blood group typing for such purposes.

WHITE BLOOD CELLS AND PLATELETS

There are a number of rare genetic disorders of white blood cells and platelets and information is summarised in Table 27.1. There is some overlap with the immune deficiency disorders considered in the following section.

A number of syndromal associations with skeletal dysplasias also exist and should be carefully looked for.

Leukaemias are considered in Chapter 32.

IMMUNE DEFICIENCY DISEASE

Numerous forms of immune deficiency exist, mostly Mendelian in inheritance (Table 27.2). The X-linked types, probably involving at least five distinct loci, are particularly important to recognise in view of the high risk to offspring of female carriers. Some carriers can be recognised by lowered immunoglobulin levels in their blood but levels are frequently normal, so molecular analysis is preferable if the specific defect has been defined. Study of the clonal origin of lymphocytes may indicate the carrier state. Fetal blood sampling will often allow prenatal detection of both immune deficiencies and blood cell disorders but has largely been replaced by molecular analysis of chorion villus samples, as the specific genes have been identified. Bone marrow transplantation is proving valuable in some situations, but the scope for gene therapy or gene editing is still uncertain in terms of long-term safety.

The autosomal recessive, severe combined immunodeficiency due to adenosine deaminase deficiency can be recognised prenatally in chorionic villi or cultured amniotic cells. X-linked chronic granulomatous disease is located close to the gene for Duchenne muscular dystrophy at Xp21 and may be associated with it in the very unusual event of a contiguous gene deletion that spans both loci.

Disorders of the complement system form a sequence of recessively inherited defects, some characterised by immune deficiency, others of which are symptomless. An exception is the

Table 27.1 Hereditary disorders of blood cell production

Disorder	Inheritance
Blackfan-Diamond red cell hypoplasia	Autosomal recessive
Fanconi pancytopenia	Autosomal recessive
Infantile hereditary agranulocytosis	Autosomal recessive
Cyclic neutropenia	Autosomal recessive or dominant
Chediak-Higashi syndrome	Autosomal recessive
Chronic granulomatous disease	X-linked recessive (rarely autosomal recessive)
Hereditary isolated thrombocytopenia	X-linked recessive (rarely autosomal recessive or autosomal dominant)
Thrombocytopenia with absent radius (TAR) syndrome	Autosomal recessive
Familial lymphohistiocytosis	Autosomal recessive

Table 27.2 Immunological deficiency disorders

Disorder	Inheritance
Hypogammaglobulinaemia	
Bruton type	X-linked recessive
Swiss type	Autosomal recessive and X-linked recessive
Combined immunodeficiency due to	
Adenosine deaminase deficiency	Autosomal recessive
Nucleoside phosphorylase deficiency	Autosomal recessive
Other types	X-linked and autosomal recessive
Pure thymic dysplasia	Autosomal recessive
Thymic and parathyroid aplasia (DiGeorge syndrome)	Small chromosome 22 deletion; most cases sporadic (see Chapter 19)
Ataxia telangiectasia	Autosomal recessive
Wiskott-Aldrich syndrome	X-linked recessive
Chronic granulomatous disease	X-linked recessive (rarely autosomal recessive)
Complement factor deficiencies (various types)	Autosomal recessive (properdin deficiency is X-linked)
Hereditary angioedema (C1 inhibitor)	Autosomal dominant
Defects of innate immunity in hypohidrotic ectodermal dysplasia (HED) including EDA, EDAR and IKBKG deficiency (HED with immunodeficiency; NEMO)	Most are X-linked recessive (but EDAR is autosomal, either dominant or recessive)
Dyskeratosis congenita (leading to bone marrow failure)	Usually X-linked but can be autosomal dominant or recessive
Phagocyte dysfunction: many types	Mostly autosomal but the sex-linked forms include the X-linked lymphoproliferative syndrome and X-linked neutropenia

dominantly inherited C1 esterase inhibitor deficiency, responsible for hereditary angioedema. In view of the potentially lethal laryngeal problems and the success of preventive and acute therapy, it is important for all close relatives of a patient with this disorder to be carefully checked for the deficiency.

GENETIC ASPECTS OF INFECTIOUS DISEASE

Susceptibility and resistance to major infectious diseases have a strong genetic basis, something that has been recognised for many years, especially when the environmental agent was close to universal (e.g. tuberculosis, rheumatic fever). The underlying genetic basis is beginning to be understood and may involve both rare genetic changes in the immune system as well as more common population variants (e.g. susceptibility to meningitis).

So far, these developments have not impacted on genetic counselling, although this could change. It should be remembered also that, in the past, major infections are likely to have played an important role in the population distribution of a number of common polymorphisms, not just those related to malaria where the relationship can still be seen today. Thus, it is conjectured that the carrier state for cystic fibrosis may be as common as it is in populations today because it conferred resistance to diarrhoeal diseases such as cholera.

HAEMOPHILIA

Haemophilia represents a major genetic counselling problem, particularly since most haemophiliac males now reach adult life with only moderate disability, and frequently reproduce. Both major forms of haemophilia are X-linked; haemophilia A results from a deficiency of factor VIII, while haemophilia B (Christmas disease) results from a deficiency of factor IX. It is now recognised that factor VIII is found in association with its carrier molecule, von Willebrand factor (VWF). Factor VIII is encoded by the X-linked locus that is defective in haemophilia A, while von Willebrand factor is encoded by an autosomal locus, defective in the disorder von Willebrand disease (VWD).

Occasional forms of 'autosomal haemophilia A' occur owing to defects in the factor VIII-binding site of VWF.

Genetic advice for men affected with haemophilia (A or B) is straightforward, although mistakes are often made. As with any X-linked recessive disorder, all sons will be healthy, as will their descendants; all daughters will be carriers. It is unnecessary and often misleading for such daughters to have tests of carrier detection, because whatever results these give, the daughter of an affected male must be a carrier.

A daughter will be fully affected by haemophilia, as if she were an affected male, if she is either homozygous or hemizygous for the condition. She will be homozygous (an exceptionally rare event) if her father is affected, her mother is also a carrier and her mother passes it to her. She will be hemizygous for the condition if there is a sex chromosome abnormality, such as Turner (45,X) syndrome. Otherwise, the severity of manifestation in a woman will depend upon the pattern of X chromosome inactivation (XCI) in the cells that produce the F8 or F9 proteins, which will be both random and highly variable (Lyon's hypothesis). For F8, these cells are found in the liver and in various endothelia.

Risks for the offspring of definite (heterozygote) female carriers are also clear, there being a 50% risk of sons being affected and of daughters being carriers (see Chapter 2). The main problems in genetic counselling lie in determining how great is the chance of women at risk being carriers, and this is of particular importance if decisions are to be made regarding fetal sexing and prenatal diagnosis or the mode of delivery of an affected male.

The risk of being a carrier will depend on:

- The prior genetic risk
- Other genetic information
- The results of carrier detection studies

The general approach to the subject for X-linked diseases is discussed in Chapters 2 and 7. Although specific molecular defects can now identify most carriers, it remains extremely important to identify the genetic risks appropriately from pedigree information if molecular investigations are to be interpreted accurately.

The factor VIII gene, located at Xq28, is a large gene that shows relatively few polymorphisms and is deleted in only 4% of affected males, but an inversion within the gene is responsible for around 40% of severe cases. Point mutations differ widely between families, so prediction is still sometimes dependent on DNA polymorphisms. The polymorphisms at the factor IX gene, located more proximally at Xq26, are more informative. In both disorders, the identification of a mutation in one family member will usually allow much simpler prediction for any relative, so it is important for this information to be recorded and to be available. The concept of a 'mutational register' has been established for both haemophilia A and B.

The shift to first-trimester DNA testing, especially non-invasive prenatal testing (NIPT), makes it imperative for carrier status to be established before a pregnancy occurs. This anticipatory approach is greatly enhanced if there is close communication regarding testing and counselling between the haemophilia and genetics services within a region. NIPT may be used to determine fetal sex and could in principle be used to establish whether a male fetus is affected although that is more technically challenging.

The use of immunological and coagulation assays is now largely ancillary to DNA analysis in carrier testing but should not be ignored. In prenatal diagnosis, DNA analysis from chorion biopsy samples is the approach of choice but, where the family is not informative or presents too late, fetal blood sampling and analysis of the appropriate factor is still a reliable test.

These striking advances in the haemophilias have been overshadowed, in some countries, by the tragic and potentially avoidable catastrophe of HIV infection and AIDS in many families. Not only must HIV infection be especially considered in the handling of samples, but it has to be recognised that this disaster has radically affected attitudes to haemophilia, both within families and in the community at large. Many families now opt for prenatal diagnosis and termination who would not have done so before, and the stigmatisation of families that has occurred gives reason for profound concern in relation to the attitudes of society towards those with presymptomatic tests proving positive for other serious disorders.

OTHER COAGULATION DISORDERS

Von Willebrand disease, determined by the autosomal portion of the factor VIII molecule, is usually mild in heterozygotes, although a very rare, severe homozygous form also exists. Deficiencies of numerous other coagulation factors have been recognised (Table 27.3). All are autosomal recessive. A variety of forms of thrombocytopenia have also been identified, showing various modes of inheritance, but an X-linked recessive form is the best recognised. Prenatal diagnosis from a fetal blood sample or by molecular analysis is possible for most of these disorders.

Table 27.3 Inherited coagulation disorders

Deficiency/disorder	Inheritance
Deficiency resulting mainly in bleeding	
Factor VIII (haemophilia A)	X-linked recessive
Factor IX (haemophilia B)	X-linked recessive
Von Willebrand disease	See text
Other coagulation factor deficiencies (V, VII, X, XI, XII, XIII)	Autosomal recessive
Deficiency resulting mainly in thrombosis	
Antithrombin III deficiency	Autosomal dominant
Protein C deficiency	Autosomal dominant
Protein S deficiency	Autosomal dominant
Factor V (Leiden variant)	See text
Plasminogen deficiency	Autosomal dominant
Dysfibrinogenaemias	Autosomal dominant

An increased risk of venous thrombosis is now known to result in some families from coagulation factor alterations. In some instances (e.g. factor V), deficiency may cause bleeding, whereas other alterations may predispose to thrombosis. Table 27.3 lists some of this group. In general, the thrombotic tendency (which may be very variable) is shown by heterozygotes; that is, the inheritance is autosomal dominant.

The relatively common 'Leiden' population variant of factor V deserves note here since it occurs at a frequency of around 5% in northern European populations. Those carrying it have a two- to threefold increase in thrombotic risk, and higher in relation to oral contraceptive use. This should be regarded as a susceptibility factor that modifies risk, rather than a genetic disorder, and it is not clear that widespread screening or testing of family members is of value, since the risk of venous thrombosis for heterozygotes is less than 0.1% a year.

Unfortunately, because results on patients are reported often as genotypes, inappropriate testing of relatives has become widespread, usually without adequate information, so that genetic counselling referrals are mainly occupied with attempting to reduce problems already created.

28

Environmental hazards

INTRODUCTION

At first sight, the subject of environmental hazards might seem to bear little relation to genetic counselling, but in practice there are several reasons why environmental agents and their risks need consideration:

1. They may come into the differential diagnosis of malformation syndromes. For example, congenital rubella must be considered among the possible causes of congenital cataract, and the recurrence risks will be greatly affected if such an agent can be either confirmed or firmly excluded. Congenital infections share a number of features, including growth retardation, microcephaly and liver involvement, that may easily be confused with a primary developmental or metabolic cause.
2. Many agents causing fetal damage in pregnancy may also cause harmful mutations; radiation is a prime example.
3. Enquiry may be made as to whether cytogenetic or prenatal diagnostic tests may be of help in confirming or excluding fetal damage.

Three groups of agents are briefly discussed here: congenital infections damaging the fetus, drugs believed to be teratogenic, and radiation and other potential mutagenic agents. The role of genetic factors in susceptibility to infectious diseases is also considered briefly.

CONGENITAL INFECTIONS

Table 28.1 lists the major types of congenital infections. Of these, congenital syphilis is rarely seen now in Western populations; overwhelmingly the most important until recently has been congenital rubella. Systematic immunisation is reducing the frequency of this in some populations, including in the United Kingdom, but it remains a major problem worldwide.

The global pattern of infectious diseases is always in flux and can change rapidly. Thus, attention was focused on the rise of congenital infection with the Zika virus in Brazil in 2016

Table 28.1 Congenital infections

Agent	Common defects
Rubella	Cataract, deafness, congenital heart disease
Cytomegalovirus	Microcephaly, chorioretinitis, hepatosplenomegaly, deafness
Varicella	Microcephaly, chorioretinitis, scarring limb defects
Zika and herpes simplex (similar range of pathologies)	Microcephaly, structural brain anomalies including neuronal migration defects and calcification; in the eye: chorioretinopathy, cataract, microphthalmia, strabismus; range of associated features secondary to neurological dysfunction (e.g. clubfoot) and some other anomalies (orofacial clefting)
Other viruses	See text
Toxoplasma	Chorioretinitis, microcephaly, hepatosplenomegaly
Syphilis	Facial and other bony abnormalities, keratitis

and since. The media attention was magnified in part because of the 2016 Football (Soccer) World Cup being held in Brazil. The scientific response has been dramatic and constructive.

Congenital rubella

The principal malformations seen in congenital rubella include cataracts, nerve deafness, congenital heart defects (commonly patent ductus arteriosus) and microcephaly with mental retardation. Since congenital rubella may occur in the absence of overt maternal infection, it is a condition that must be considered seriously in the differential diagnosis of any syndrome where these abnormalities occur.

The risk to a subsequent pregnancy after a child with congenital rubella has been born is negligible. The critical information usually sought is the risk to a current pregnancy in which the mother has developed or has been exposed to the infection. When the mother is already known to have immunity, on the basis of immunisation or previous serological tests, the risk to the fetus is exceedingly low. When this information is not available, it is extremely difficult to obtain rapid direct evidence for fetal infection or lack of it. Tests on amniotic fluid are not reliable, but preliminary evidence suggests that immunoglobulin M (IgM)-specific antibodies on a fetal blood sample may be an accurate indicator of infection. Techniques for detecting viral antigens or nucleic acids are available but of uncertain reliability.

General information that can currently be used to predict risks is that infection in the first month of pregnancy carries an extremely high risk of abnormality (around 60%), which falls to about 25% for infection in the second month and about 8% in the third month. Risks are small for serious abnormality after infection in the second trimester, and negligible after this. Indications for termination of pregnancy are clearly strong in the early stages, but the decision may be difficult around the third month, or if dates are uncertain. More specific tests will be of great help. Careful examination of an apparently normal infant at risk (especially audiometry) is important to exclude minor degrees of damage.

Cytomegalovirus infection

Microcephaly with mental retardation, cerebral palsy, chorioretinitis, deafness, hepatosplenomegaly and purpuric rash are common features of cytomegalovirus (CMV) infection. Magnetic resonance imaging (MRI) brain scan shows helpful distinguishing features, although only around 5% of cases have serious neurological problems. Maternal infection is often asymptomatic, and no preventive measures – apart from avoidance of known or potential sources of infection – are available. Childcare and healthcare workers may be at increased risk of acquiring CMV infection. Good hygiene, particularly washing hands after changing nappies, regular cleaning of toys and surfaces, and care with food preparation, may reduce this risk. Both maternal and neonatal infection with CMV may be more likely in those also infected with HIV.

Varicella zoster virus

Varicella in pregnancy poses a risk to the fetus. If acquired during the first 5 months of pregnancy, maternal varicella can occasionally result in the congenital varicella syndrome. Varicella-induced defects include areas of skin scarring with a clear dermatomal distribution, hypoplasia of the bone and muscle of a limb, microcephaly, mental retardation, cataract, microphthalmia and chorioretinitis.

Parvovirus B19

Infections are common in childhood. Infection in pregnancy, particularly the second trimester, may not be apparent clinically but may present as hydrops fetalis with severe anaemia, congestive heart failure, generalised oedema and fetal death. A prospective study of symptomatic and asymptomatic maternal infection found an overall fetal loss rate of 16%. There is no convincing evidence that B19 is teratogenic. Animal parvoviruses are not known to be transmissible to humans.

HIV infection

Congenital HIV infection is a serious problem among the offspring of women carrying the virus. It seems unlikely that it produces significant dysmorphic features in affected infants, but it may need consideration in the context of immune deficiencies and of unusual infections. Co-infection with CMV or syphilis is also possible. Antiviral drugs are not known to be teratogenic.

Other viral infections

Although there have been many suggested associations, evidence for the teratogenicity of other viruses is not well established. Maternal infection with hepatitis B virus may lead to congenital infection, but this does not seem to be teratogenic; it leads to chronic infection and, in a substantial minority, to chronic hepatitis and adverse sequelae. Maternal transmission of hepatitis C gives a high risk for chronic liver disease, including liver cancer in later life, in susceptible individuals.

Congenital herpes simplex virus infection is unusual but can be very severe, resembling congenital Zika virus infection (see Table 28.1). Both are much more likely to occur when a pregnant woman has her primary episode of infection in the pregnancy, especially during the early stages.

Vertical transmission of herpes simplex from the mother to the infant can occur during delivery or soon afterwards, and this will sometimes lead to a severe set of problems, including encephalitis or disseminated, multi-organ disease with a high mortality. If a pregnant woman has signs of genital herpes simplex infection while pregnant, this should be treated actively (with oral acyclovir), and it may be good practice to treat a pregnant woman known to have genital herpes infection in any case from ~34 weeks or so to make it less likely that she will have genital lesions during delivery.

Influenza virus has been claimed to be responsible for some of the cyclical peaks of malformations such as neural tube defects. Live viral vaccines, while obviously undesirable in pregnancy, have in fact only occasionally produced any evidence of fetal damage.

Toxoplasmosis

Chorioretinitis (which may be progressive and not always apparent at birth), central nervous system involvement with convulsions, hepatosplenomegaly, pneumonia, myocarditis and rash are the main features of *Toxoplasma gondii* infection. The incidence of severe fetal infection falls from 75% associated with first-trimester maternal infection to under 5% when the woman is exposed to *T. gondii* in the third trimester. Children born infected but symptom-free will develop retinal disease in over 85% of cases. Late development of mental retardation and hearing defects can occur. Maternal infection is often asymptomatic and is usually from domestic animals, cats in particular.

DRUGS AND MALFORMATIONS

Since the epidemic of limb defects due to thalidomide, not only has there been stringent testing of new drugs for teratogenicity, but many studies have investigated possible associations. In fact, the number of specific malformation syndromes clearly related to individual drugs is extremely small (Box 28.1). Much more difficult to assess are situations in which a commonly used drug (e.g. an anticonvulsant) appears to be associated with an increased incidence of certain malformations, and where the type of malformation is either variable or commonly seen in the absence of the agent. It is likely that most of the associations still to be discovered are in this latter group, where proof of a causal relationship is exceedingly difficult to obtain.

Despite the small number of firm teratogenic syndromes due to drugs, it is clearly prudent for all drugs that are not strictly essential to be avoided in pregnancy, and indeed avoided by all women who are at risk of conceiving. Avoidance of cigarette smoking and the taking of a nutritious, balanced diet with folate supplementation are additional common-sense factors that are desirable. General advice of this type can often be given as part of more general pre-conception advice because most couples known to be at increased risk for abnormality in the offspring will be anxious to do anything possible to reduce this risk (see Chapter 34).

Thalidomide

A generation of children with thalidomide-induced limb defects and other abnormalities has now grown up, particularly in continental Europe but also in the United Kingdom. Those used to seeing malformations in younger children may not think of thalidomide as a possible cause; a useful clinical review by Smithells and Newman (1992) (see Appendix 1) gives the range of features.

Where the relationship with thalidomide is clear-cut, there should, of course, be no increased risk of abnormalities in the offspring of these patients, but it seems likely that some dominantly inherited limb reduction defects, including Holt-Oram syndrome, may in the past have

---

BOX 28.1: Drugs with teratogenic effects

Definite
Thalidomide
Warfarin
Alcohol
Retinoids
Aminopterin and methotrexate
Anticonvulsants (in particular valproate, phenytoin, trimethadione)

Probable
Lithium
Anaesthetic gases

Possible
Sex hormones
Anti-emetics
Industrial chemicals

---

mistakenly been attributed to thalidomide, in which case affected children may well be born. The recessively inherited pseudothalidomide or Roberts syndrome should not be confused if full radiographs are available.

Warfarin

Warfarin has been clearly associated with a syndrome identical to the severe form of chondrodysplasia punctata, in effect a phenocopy. Although occurring only in a small proportion of exposed pregnancies, there is a high fetal and perinatal loss overall, so it seems clear that warfarin and related anticoagulants are undesirable in women who are pregnant or at risk of becoming so. In one case known to the original author, the pregnancy resulted from stopping oral contraceptives which had produced a venous thrombosis, warfarin then being used for therapy in a double iatrogenic misfortune.

Alcohol

There is no doubt as to the existence of a syndrome of abnormal facies, reduced somatic and brain growth usually apparent at birth and that continues without catch-up afterwards, mental retardation and congenital heart disease in the children of mothers with a high alcohol intake during pregnancy. This fully characteristic 'fetal alcohol syndrome' (FAS), however, is really the tip of a large iceberg of 'fetal alcohol effect' (FAE), where some of the features are apparent but not sufficient for the diagnosis of FAS. Either (FAS or FAE) can be caused by binge drinking or by chronic but lower-level alcohol consumption, and there must be genetic variation in susceptibility to FAS (perhaps related to variability in N-glycosylation activity).

Studies suggest that the consumption of alcohol by pregnant women is an enormous global problem; perhaps 10% consume alcohol and more than 1% of their infants will be affected by FAS itself. This is an entirely preventable disorder, and its prevention has accordingly been given progressively greater priority. There is not known to be any entirely 'safe' level of alcohol consumption, but the risks fall as less is consumed.

There is useful guidance available on FAS and related alcohol effects (see Appendix 1).

Anti-epileptic drugs

Chapter 14 has more information on epilepsy. There is no doubt that there is an overall increase in the incidence of malformations in the offspring of epileptic mothers. This effect varies with the drug(s) being used in treatment. Valproate has the highest risk of malformation of any anti-epileptic drug used in monotherapy (estimates range as high as 10%) while lamotrigine, levetiracetam, and oxcarbazepine carry little if any extra risk above the background 2%–3% risk found in many populations. Other drugs give intermediate risks of malformation. The evidence suggests that these risks are more related to therapy than to the epilepsy per se. The spectrum of defects is broad, including congenital heart disease, orofacial clefting and neural tube defects. The risks appear to be dose-related; experience with valproate suggests that doses above 650 mg/day are more likely to cause malformation but that there is still an effect at lower levels. In addition, there are risks of neurodevelopmental and behavioural problems.

Multiple drug therapy is more likely to be teratogenic than monotherapy, so it is the aim of epilepsy clinics to help women of reproductive age who require treatment towards effective control on one drug alone. It is clearly essential that all epileptic women of childbearing age receiving therapy be told of the potential risks, as well as the parents of young girls who may remain on drugs initially prescribed in childhood. Before embarking on childbearing, there should be a reassessment of the need for therapy and, if possible, a trial period on no drugs or a minimal dose, with careful blood level measurements. Sime neurologists may protest that this is unnecessary, but they do not generally see the resulting problems. This is probably the major avoidable source of teratogenic agents at present, after alcohol.

Specific syndromes related to anti-epileptic drugs exist but are much less common than the overall effects:

- *Phenytoin*: This drug is associated with a moderately specific syndrome of low birth weight, mental retardation, unusual facies with hypertelorism, congenital heart defects and hypoplastic digits, which appear to occur rarely. There is an overall increase in the incidence of cleft lip and palate and the overall malformation rate is doubled in comparison with the general population.
- *Trimethadione*: After trimethadione administration there appears to be an occasional specific combination of congenital heart defects, genitourinary abnormalities, unusual facies with V-shaped configuration of eyebrows and mental retardation, with a considerable increase (possibly as high as 20%) of congenital heart disease in isolation.
- *Valproate*: An increased incidence of neural tube defects is likely with the use of sodium valproate, and a characteristic craniofacial appearance has been suggested as well as learning and behaviour problems. Overall the malformation rate is increased fourfold to ~11%.
- *Lithium*: This is a frequently used agent in affective disorders. It has now been convincingly associated with the occurrence of congenital heart disease, in particular Ebstein anomaly.

Vitamin A analogues

A relatively characteristic pattern of defects with some similarities to DiGeorge syndrome is associated with the administration of vitamin A analogues in early pregnancy, and with vitamin

A excess for other reasons. Agents such as isotretinoin and etretinate are used increasingly for various skin disorders, while an increasing use of high-dose vitamin A supplements in some areas has caused concern.

Sex hormones

The use of female sex hormones in early pregnancy for prevention of threatened abortion and for treatment of infertility is now rare, partly due to concern regarding fetal abnormalities. There is no evidence of teratogenic effects from oral contraceptives. An increased malformation rate has been seen following ovulation-inducing drugs, but it is not known whether this is a direct effect, related to the frequently associated twinning or related to the underlying cause of the infertility.

An important albeit rare example of delayed teratogenicity has been the occurrence of vaginal adenocarcinoma in the daughters of women treated with diethyl-stilboestrol during pregnancy because of threatened abortion.

Immunosuppressive and cytotoxic drugs

Increasing numbers of women are reproducing while taking immunosuppressive or cytotoxic drugs for previously lethal diseases or following renal transplantation. So far, few obvious abnormalities have been found in pregnancies going to term. Aminopterin and its derivative methotrexate have been associated with specific craniofacial and vertebral anomalies, mental retardation, limb reduction defects and growth impairment. Problems in this group are perhaps more likely to arise from their mutagenic properties (see later).

Industrial and other chemicals

Despite widespread and reasonable concern, actual evidence for human teratogenic effects is scanty. Claims for increased abnormalities after deliberate mass spraying or industrial accidents involving the herbicide 2,4,5-T are circumstantial, as is the case for other chemicals such as hair dyes. An effect of anaesthetic gases inhaled by pregnant operating theatre staff and anaesthetists seems more soundly based; an increase in spontaneous abortions and in a variety of common malformations has been seen, rather than any particular malformation or combination. There is also some evidence that healthcare workers exposed to sterilising agents, and perhaps also to radiation, antineoplastic drugs and reproductive hormones, have a higher risk of miscarriage.

GENETIC EFFECTS OF RADIATION

The genetic effects of radiation are of much concern in view of the very real possibility of a localised accident involving a civil or military nuclear installation. While the genetic effects of nuclear conflict would be overshadowed by the scale of the immediate catastrophe, the consequences of an isolated disaster or near-disaster should be anticipated. Although reactions to such an event are likely to be largely based on fear, the Chernobyl disaster, which exposed large parts of Europe to radioactive contamination and which resulted in large numbers of probably unnecessary terminations of pregnancy, has emphasised how ill-prepared are the radiation protection services of most countries.

The great majority of individuals exposed are likely to receive a low or even insignificant dose of irradiation, but it may be difficult to be certain of this at the time. Provided that the dose is approximately known, information on the possible genetic effects can be given with a reasonable degree of confidence, because of the very large amount of work that has been done on the topic.

Much of the biological information available on the effects of radiation relates to population effects (see later), but first the risks for a particular conception or pregnancy must be dealt with. Two separate situations must be considered, which are often confused by those requesting information:

- Mutagenic effects, resulting in damage to germ cells before fertilisation.
- Teratogenesis, i.e. damage to the developing embryo.

Mutagenesis must be considered separately for the two parents, because the method of germ cell formation in each sex is entirely different. In males, animal experiments have shown two major classes of abnormality:

- Major chromosomal abnormalities, occurring mainly in the offspring conceived a few days or weeks after irradiation.
- An increased incidence of point mutations, persisting in offspring conceived long after irradiation has been given.

For the human male, some direct evidence is now available from the study of human sperm chromosomes. The incidence of abnormalities more than doubles after radiotherapy and changes may persist for at least 3 years. One can probably draw the following conclusions regarding risks to offspring:

- Diagnostic and similar low-level irradiation does not significantly increase the risk to an individual offspring.
- Conception in the few months after therapeutic or other high-dose irradiation (especially of the gonads) is unwise. Amniocentesis is advisable should pregnancy occur in order to detect chromosomal defects. The same probably applies when a man is, or has recently been, taking cytotoxic drugs or other known chemical mutagens.
- A variable period of infertility is common after gonadal irradiation (and with cytotoxic drugs) but should not be relied upon.
- Long-term risks for a pregnancy conceived many months or years after irradiation are small, and result mainly from increased dominant mutations, which are unlikely to be detected by amniocentesis. However, the incidence of such abnormalities is low (not more than 1%).

In women the oocyte is especially radiation-sensitive around the time of fertilisation. Outside this period, the risk is likely to be similar to or less than that for males. Diagnostic radiation is unlikely to be a significant risk factor for future children of an individual woman, although unnecessary exposure clearly should be avoided to prevent even a small population increase in point mutations and chromosome defects.

Irradiation during pregnancy is a somewhat different problem and is the most common cause of referral for genetic counselling in relation to radiation. Such irradiation is almost always diagnostic, with a dose of 0.01 Gray (Gy) or less; it is usually inadvertent and given in the earliest weeks of pregnancy before a pregnancy has been recognised. It is not uncommon for such irradiation to be given during the course of investigation for infertility, and the combination of a wanted pregnancy with the feelings of guilt shared by patient and doctor that radiation exposure should have occurred may produce considerable anxiety.

Until recently, termination of pregnancy has frequently been advised in such a situation, but it is likely that the risks to the fetus have been considerably overestimated and are in fact very small for diagnostic levels of radiation. A valuable but older review by Mole (see Appendix 1 under 'Radiation') concludes that after 0.01 Gy (the upper limit for most diagnostic radiation) the total added risk to the fetus is unlikely to exceed 1 in 1,000 – this risk being partly for malformations, partly for mental retardation and possibly childhood cancer. In such circumstances, neither termination nor amniocentesis seems warranted, although it is probably wise to stress the relatively frequent occurrence of abnormalities in the general population, because there is a real danger that any such occurrence will be attributed to the radiation.

Information on the risks of heavy doses of radiation (see UNSCEAR reports in Appendix 1 under 'Radiation') has come mainly from follow-up of Japanese atomic bomb casualties. At levels over 0.6 Gy there is a clear and dose-related increase in mental retardation and microcephaly in such exposed pregnancies (10% at 2 Gy). Because amniocentesis or other prenatal procedures are unlikely to exclude this, there is a strong indication for termination of pregnancy. Such an exposure is rare in peacetime and would probably be associated with severe maternal illness anyway if therapeutic irradiation were involved. No clear increase in the incidence of malformations or other genetic disorders in children conceived after exposure has been shown, despite much concern and publicity.

Leukaemia and other malignancies involving somatic cells currently seem to be a greater short-term hazard, but the hidden load of recessive mutations will take many generations to show itself and may ultimately prove to be the more serious aspect. Neel (1993) provides interesting background information and an assessment of this important study (see Appendix 1 under 'Radiation'). Evidence of mutations from direct studies of DNA is becoming available and so far supports the older studies.

Similarly, there is no clear evidence to support any increase in malformations or genetic disorders in the offspring of military personnel exposed to nuclear test explosions, despite considerable publicity.

More recent data following Chernobyl – with three decades of follow-up data becoming available – indicate the anticipated dose-dependent risk of some adverse health effects, including cancers, especially thyroid cancer in the young, as well as cardiovascular disease and cataracts. Studies on the outcomes of pregnancies exposed to the radiation from Chernobyl and, more recently, from Fukushima have been more difficult to conduct. Indeed, it has been difficult to define the levels of radiation suffered by many of those potentially exposed *in utero* after Chernobyl. There have also been more thorough follow-up studies in some countries with less exposure than in the more heavily contaminated areas. There was an increase in perinatal mortality in heavily contaminated areas of Europe and Japan following the two disasters, although these findings do not establish causality, and there were additional environmental problems in Japan from the tsunami that triggered the nuclear contamination. There has been a sustained increase in neural tube defects, microcephaly and microphthalmia in heavily contaminated regions of Ukraine, that coincides with higher levels of Caesium-137 in pregnant women there. There may have been some effect on the somatic and cranial growth of exposed fetuses in Scandinavia, but the effects have not been large, and uncertainty remains as to their clinical relevance. There has been little evidence of serious neurodevelopmental problems, but it has not been possible to exclude an increase in some specific learning difficulties.

Irradiation and the population

The generally low risks to future offspring and to radiation-exposed individuals themselves have been emphasised here, as most relevant for genetic counselling. The population and long-term effects stand in contrast to this but are difficult to consider because they are so spread out in both space and time. Even a slight increase in background radiation will be likely to cause a significant increase in both point mutations and chromosome disorders, although in the case of recessive mutations, the full effects will not be noticed for many generations. Thus, the exposure of a population of one million to an increased level of radiation of 1 Gy per generation has been estimated as likely to result in an extra 2,000 genetic disorders per million births in the first generation; the eventual total, including the effect on subsequent generations, would be considerably higher. Because these cases are indistinguishable from 'naturally' arising mutations, they tend to be overlooked; were such an occurrence to be concentrated in a single town, it would be considered a disaster.

At present, most gonadal radiation received over the background level comes from medical diagnostic X-rays. Responsibility for this is shared by all physicians, who should help to reduce this load to the minimum necessary. In the author's view, the profession has an equal social duty to help to ensure that this load is not further increased by the avoidable exposure from other sources, notably nuclear weapons or accidents in the future. The widespread nuclear contamination resulting from the disasters at Fukushima and Chernobyl, the earlier nuclear disaster in the Urals region of Russia, and a series of lesser accidents in other countries (including the United Kingdom and the United States) are examples of the potential danger of nuclear energy and have resulted in greatly increased awareness of the problems in the population as a whole. Whether effective action will be taken and continued in the long term is a different matter.

PART 3

Genetic counselling and testing for cancer

ALEX MURRAY AND JULIAN SAMPSON

29

Cancer as a genetic disorder

INTRODUCTION

Cancer genetics forms a major part of genetics services and although the large majority of cases show only weak inherited influences, a small proportion show Mendelian inheritance, often with very high risks.

With the advances in molecular testing technology, the detection of familial cancer syndromes showing Mendelian inheritance has increased, allowing affected individuals and their relatives to be offered surveillance and, in some cases, preventive or targeted treatments.

Nevertheless, it can still be challenging to accurately distinguish those families with a Mendelian cancer syndrome from the great majority for whom risks are low. Careful clinical assessment and review of the pedigree are vital in recognising these rare syndromes, but other pointers towards a high-risk family history can also be helpful, including young age of onset, occurrence of multiple tumours in one individual and, increasingly, particular pathological characteristics of the tumours.

These pointers can be turned into useful clinical guidelines or used to frame healthcare policy, as in the United Kingdom with the development of National Institute for Health and Care Excellence (NICE) guidance on familial breast cancer.

A second challenge, of providing a systematic service to patients and families appropriate to their level of risk, is increasingly being met, at least in those countries with planned rather than consumer-led health services. This requires partnerships between specialist genetics services, the relevant clinical specialities, including oncologists, surgeons and radiologists, as well as close communication with primary care. Genetic counsellors play an important role in the delivery of cancer genetics services, especially in linking with the other health professionals involved and ensuring that extended families are fully informed and counselled.

Genetic counselling in cancer covers several different areas that are considered in the following chapters of this section:

- Common cancers of later life and their genetic subsets
- Colorectal cancers and cancer of the breast and ovary
- Familial tumour syndromes following Mendelian (usually but not always autosomal dominant) inheritance

- Genetic disorders giving a general predisposition to malignancy (commonly autosomal recessive)
- Embryonal and childhood cancer

Before these areas are considered, it is essential to give a brief background to some of the key scientific advances that have so radically affected possibilities for genetic counselling.

MOLECULAR GENETIC BASIS OF CANCER

It has long been recognised that chromosomal changes are seen in many cancers and that, while these are not completely specific in most cases, neither are they random. Molecular analysis has brought added precision to these findings, with the result that a number of tumour types can be associated with somatic changes in specific chromosomal regions. Loss of heterozygosity is the most important finding, as measured by comparing the DNA of the tumour with DNA of blood (i.e. leucocytes) from the same individual.

Genetic linkage studies in rare Mendelian tumour syndromes showed that the same loci (or at least the same chromosome regions) are often involved as in sporadic tumours, indicating a direct relationship between the familial and non-familial forms of the same tumour type.

These findings validated Knudson's 'two-hit hypothesis' for tumour suppressor genes, which proposes that for a tumour to occur, both copies of a cancer predisposition gene must be deactivated. Normally this will be the result of two independent somatic mutations, but if an individual has inherited a mutation in one allele, only a single somatic event will be required to initiate a tumour. This readily explains why, in inherited forms of cancer, the tumours tend to occur earlier and can be multiple. Retinoblastoma and Wilms tumour provided the initial examples of these changes being directly identified. This hypothesis also explains the concept of 'non-penetrance' seen in retinoblastoma and many other Mendelian cancer syndromes, because a 'second hit' may fail to occur. If the second hit fails to happen, or if it occurs but the downstream chain of molecular events required for malignancy fails to occur, then there will be non-penetrance.

The genes involved in this process are *tumour suppressor genes*, which play important roles in growth, development and cell-signalling pathways. Most familial cancer syndromes are due to inherited defects in tumour suppressor genes. The 'second hit' or somatic event is often a more extensive loss of the relevant chromosome region in the cell.

A second category of genes involved in cancer is that of the *oncogenes*, whose activation may predispose to tumour formation. The structure of these oncogenes is homologous to that of particular RNA retroviral sequences. Their normal counterparts, the cellular or *proto-oncogenes*, present in all individuals, are the site of somatic point mutations or chromosomal rearrangements characteristic of a number of tumour types, especially leukaemias and lymphomas. Thus, the 9/22 translocation characteristic of chronic myeloid leukaemia (the 'Philadelphia' chromosome) occurs at the site of the *c-ABL* oncogene locus on chromosome 9 in most cases of chronic myeloid leukaemia (CML). This results in the generation of a new protein, from the fusion of *c-ABL* with the *BCR* gene on chromosome 22, which stimulates unchecked cell division. The elucidation of such mechanisms has opened up important new approaches to the development of rational therapies for particular tumour types, as with the use of tyrosine kinase inhibitors to block the constitutively active BCR-ABL fusion protein in CML.

Numerous oncogene loci are well recognised and are known to represent important growth factors or receptors involved in the regulation of cell division and other cell behaviours. These loci may also be important in early development and many (e.g. the *RET* oncogene) are involved in developmental malformations as well as tumours, linking the two important areas of cancer and developmental genetics.

Genetic variation at many other sites can influence the initiation, progression, metastasis and response to treatment of different tumour types. Such studies are not only of interest in research but are increasingly impacting the management of inherited and sporadic cancers.

30

Colorectal cancer syndromes

COLORECTAL CANCER SYNDROMES FOLLOWING MENDELIAN INHERITANCE

Although individually rare, the number of Mendelian tumour syndromes is considerable (see Table 30.1) and there is little doubt that many cases are missed from lack of careful history-taking in what initially may appear to be an ordinary 'common or garden' variety of non-familial neoplasm. Almost all these conditions follow autosomal dominant inheritance, and the recognition of specific loci for a number of them has been one of the major contributions of molecular genetics. Not only is it now possible to provide practical tests for relatives at risk but, as outlined previously, these loci are also proving to be involved in the somatic mutations producing common non-inherited tumours of the same organs. More than any other group of genetic disorders, the familial cancers are proving the value of systematic genetic register systems. The combination of early ascertainment, molecular diagnosis and effective prevention and therapy provides direct benefits to the health of those who are affected or at risk, and also allows risks to be reduced or excluded for many family members. Familial adenomatous polyposis (FAP) provides an excellent example of this, allowing genetics services to develop a prototype for the delivery of services for the rare, dominantly inherited cancers.

Familial adenomatous polyposis

This is an important autosomal dominant disorder that shows almost complete penetrance for colorectal polyps by early adult life and carries a virtual inevitability of colorectal cancer if left untreated. It is thus a prime candidate for a genetic register, which can facilitate the direct management of those at risk and those affected, as well as genetic counselling. Testing of the *APC* gene allows genetic confirmation of the diagnosis and accurate prediction for almost all families. DNA analysis allows the avoidance of invasive procedures in those shown to be at low risk, while giving extra motivation for these procedures, particularly surveillance colonoscopy from adolescence onwards, where the risk is confirmed to be high. Colorectal disease is managed by a number of different prophylactic surgical procedures to remove the large bowel, undertaken after the development of polyposis but before progression to cancer.

Table 30.1 Familial tumour syndromes following autosomal dominant inheritance

Disorder	Chromosome	Gene
Retinoblastoma (inherited and syndromal)	13q	RB1
Wilms tumour (syndromal form)	11p	WT1
Neurofibromatosis (type 1)	17q	NF1
Neurofibromatosis (type 2)	22q	NF2
Von Hippel-Lindau syndrome	3q	VHL
Gorlin syndrome (basal cell naevus syndrome)	9q	PTCH1
Hereditary paraganglioma phaeochromocytoma syndrome (familial glomus tumours)	5p	SDHA
	11q	SDHAF2
	1p	SDHB
	1q	SDHC
	11q	SDHD
Familial melanoma	9p	CDKN2A
Multiple self-healing keratoacanthoma	9q	TGFBR1
Multiple endocrine neoplasia type 1	11q	MEN1
Multiple endocrine neoplasia type 2A and 2B	10q	RET
Li-Fraumeni syndrome	17p	TP53
Oesophageal cancer with tylosis	17q	RHBDF2
Polyposis coli	5q	APC
Cowden syndrome	10q	PTEN

Manifestations of the disease outside the colorectum are common. Duodenal adenomas and cancer are a major cause of morbidity and mortality in patients who have effective treatment of colorectal disease, and endoscopic surveillance is recommended from 25 years of age. The occurrence of bony and soft tissue desmoid tumours, previously considered to be a separate disorder (Gardner syndrome), is now known to be part of FAP, as is the occasional association with brain tumours (Turcot syndrome); rare manifestations also include thyroid cancer and, in infancy, hepatoblastoma.

The occurrence of eye lesions representing congenital hypertrophy of the retinal pigment epithelium (CHRPE) is a further systemic feature, but it is too inconsistent for use in clinical or presymptomatic detection.

Familial aspects of colorectal cancer without polyposis are considered in Chapter 31.

Other important forms of polyposis

Other forms of polyposis include the following.

- *Peutz-Jeghers syndrome* (autosomal dominant): This is characterised externally by circumoral pigment spots as well as by polyps and neoplasms, which may occur throughout the gastrointestinal tract and also increase risks for extra-intestinal malignancy including breast and testicular cancers. The risk of malignancy is lower than in polyposis coli but is considerable and less preventable owing to the wider distribution of lesions. Most cases are associated with inherited mutations in *LKB1/STK11*.

- *Juvenile polyposis syndrome* (autosomal dominant): This is characterised by occurrence of hamartomatous gastrointestinal polyps and increased colorectal cancer risk. It is caused by pathogenic mutations in *SMAD4* or *BMPR1A*.
- MutYH-*associated polyposis* (MAP) (autosomal recessive): This is associated with attenuated polyposis and colorectal cancer due to defects in the DNA repair gene *MutYH*. This disorder is of considerable significance, since it means that one can no longer assume that all familial colorectal cancers and polyposis are dominantly inherited.

Lynch syndrome

Pathogenic variants affecting the DNA mismatch repair (MMR) genes *MLH1*, *MSH2*, *MSH6* and *PMS2* cause the common autosomal dominant cancer syndrome Lynch syndrome. Although colorectal cancer is a major part of Lynch syndrome, risks for cancers of the endometrium, ovary and other organs are also high. Historically, families with Lynch syndrome were usually identified because of their histories of early onset-cancers and the occurrence of multiple cancers in individual family members. Increasingly, however, cases are being identified by pathology services through the molecular characteristics of tumours that in Lynch syndrome show a form of genetic instability termed *microsatellite instability* (MSI) and loss of expression of MMR protein expression.

Molecular presymptomatic testing for Lynch syndrome is widely available, once a pathogenic variant has been identified in an affected family member. As with FAP, this allows regular clinical surveillance to be specifically targeted at those who are definite gene carriers, rather than all family members potentially at risk.

Pathogenic variants in each of the MMR genes are associated with different cancer risks, with the highest colorectal cancer risks in carriers of variants in *MLH1* and *MSH2*, compared to minimal if any increase in colorectal cancer risk in carriers of *PMS2* variants, and intermediate risks in *MSH6*. Current international management guidelines recommend surveillance colonoscopy every 1–2 years for all genotypes, but these guidelines are likely to be revised soon to stratify patients by gene and gender. Although cancer risks are high in Lynch syndrome, most cancers have significantly better prognoses than their sporadic counterparts, and strong evidence from clinical trials demonstrates effective chemoprevention with aspirin.

In giving genetic risks for non-Mendelian colorectal cancer, one has to rely on the older empirical data, as given in Table 30.2. Computer programs have been developed to individualise risk estimates, as for breast cancer, but it must be remembered that there will be a considerable number of patients with Mendelian cancer whose family history does not suggest this, while the true risks for most patients may be smaller than current data suggest once all Mendelian cases have been recognised and excluded from the calculations.

Table 30.2 Genetic risks in colorectal cancer

Lifetime risks of colorectal cancer for relatives (excluding Lynch syndrome and FAP)	Risk	% (approx.)
Population risk	1 in 20 (males)	4-5
	1 in 25 (females)	
One first-degree relative affected	1 in 17	6
One first- and one second-degree relative affected	1 in 12	8
One first-degree relative with onset under 45 affected	1 in 10	10
Two first-degree relatives affected	1 in 6	15
Clear dominant inheritance pattern; first-degree relative affected	1 in 2	50

Source: Based (loosely) on Houlston RS et al. (1990), *Br Med J* **301**: 366–8 and Butterworth et al. (2006), *Eur J Cancer* 42: 216–27

Note: These risks vary substantially between countries and even between regions. These figures apply to a relatively low-risk area. The overall incidence of CRC in developed countries may be falling slightly but with an increase in incidence in younger adults (<50 years).

31

Breast and ovarian cancer

INTRODUCTION

Breast cancer is the most common cancer affecting women. A woman in the developed world has a lifetime risk of developing breast cancer of as much as 12%. The risk of developing breast cancer for women in the general population increases with age. Other factors known to increase the risk include the use of hormone replacement therapy (HRT), especially combined oestrogen and progesterone preparations, hormonal contraceptives, obesity and alcohol. High parity, young age at first childbirth, breastfeeding, late menarche and early menopause all decrease the risk.

The clustering of breast cancer in families is almost entirely due to genetic variation rather than shared lifestyle or environment. The risk of developing breast cancer is twice as high in women who have an affected first-degree relative (FDR) compared to women in the general population. The majority of the genetic risk is due to low-risk or moderate-risk susceptibility alleles. Some moderate risk loci may be helpful to include in risk stratification assessments (e.g. *CHEK2, ATM, NF1*), but these alleles confer only a very small increased risk and are not used in the routine clinical management of individual patients. Might they be combined with variants of even smaller effect and lower penetrance to help in the context of population screening programmes for disease prevention? That situation would arise if the 'polygenic risk scores', that can be generated by genome-wide tests for risk-modifying single nucleotide polymorphisms (SNPs), turn out in the future to be of some clinical utility, although there is real doubt about the prospects of that being achieved (Wald and Old, 2019, see Appendix 1). Pathogenic mutations in high-penetrance genes such as *BRCA1* and *BRCA2* confer a high risk of breast and ovarian cancer, but these variants are rare and only account for a small percentage of these cancers.

COLLECTING THE FAMILY HISTORY

This is the first step in assessing an individual's risk and determining whether a Mendelian cancer syndrome may be present. It is important to ask about both the maternal and paternal relatives, but each side of the family should be considered separately. Not everyone with a family history of breast and/or ovarian cancer will have an increased risk of developing the disease. Where appropriate, referral can be made to the local regional genetics service for risk assessment, counselling, advice about screening programmes (surveillance for tumours) and sometimes genetic testing. Many regional genetics services have local referral guidelines that help to identify those who should be referred. Although there will be some regional variations, it is reasonable to consider making a referral if a person has any of the following:

- One family member with breast cancer diagnosed before age 40 years
- Two family members with breast cancer diagnosed before age 60 years
- Three or more family members with breast cancer at any age
- A family member with bilateral breast cancer
- A male family member with breast cancer
- A family member with both breast and ovarian cancers
- Two family members with ovarian cancer at any age

If the individual seeking referral is not personally affected by cancer, their affected relatives should be first- or second-degree relatives. Some family history information that modifies risk is given in Table 31.1.

Table 31.1 Genetic risks in breast cancer

		Lifetime risk	Percentage (%) (approximate)	Risk relative to population risk
General population[a]		1 in 8	12	1
One affected first-degree relative (parent RR 1.7; sister RR 1.9; brother RR 2.5)[b]		1 in 4–7	14%–25%	2
Relative risk adjusting for age of diagnosis of the affected female first-degree relative	Diagnosis >55	1 in 6–7	14%–16%	1.6
	Diagnosis 46–55	1 in 5–6	17%–20%	2.8
	Diagnosis <45	1 in 4	25%	3.6
Two affected first-degree relatives[c]		1 in 3–5	20%–30%	2.8
First-degree relative with bilateral[c] breast cancer		1 in 3–5	20%–30%	2.7

Abbreviation: RR, relative risk.

[a] Northern Europe, North America.
[b] It is not valid to multiply lifetime risk by RR as RR varies with age distribution in studied population.
[c] Depends on age of relative(s) at diagnosis.

If the family history is complex and involves other types of cancer, such as prostate cancer, pancreatic cancer, sarcoma, adrenocortical carcinoma, gastric cancer and thyroid cancer, it is best to refer to the local guidelines or contact the regional genetics service directly.

Once the family history has been collected, the reported diagnoses should be confirmed by reviewing medical records, pathology reports and cancer registry records. Although breast cancer is usually reliably reported, there have been instances of patients reporting fictitious family histories, and the reliability of reporting for other cancers, especially ovarian cancer, is certainly not as good. The different gynaecological cancers are often confused, perhaps because they are all treated with the same surgical procedure, which is a good example of why it is so important to confirm reported diagnoses: ovarian cancer can be linked to breast cancer but it can also, less commonly, be associated with colorectal cancer as part of Lynch syndrome (see Chapter 30). The predominant gynaecological cancer risk in Lynch syndrome is for endometrial cancer, while cervical cancer is generally not a genetic cancer but is linked to infection with the human papillomavirus (HPV).

RISK ASSESSMENT

The next step is a formal risk assessment, often facilitated by the use of computer programmes or other algorithms that estimate either the probability of the individual carrying a pathogenic mutation in the *BRCA1* or *BRCA2* genes or the risk of the individual developing cancer. In the United Kingdom, women are usually assigned to one of three risk categories for breast cancer risk: 'near population' or 'average' risk (10-year risk of less than 3% for women aged 40–49 years and a lifetime risk of less than 17%), 'raised' or 'moderate' risk (10-year risk of 3%–8% for women aged 40–49 years or a lifetime risk of >17% but <30%) or 'high' risk (10-year risk of >8% for women aged 40–49 years or a lifetime risk of >30%).

SCREENING (SURVEILLANCE FOR EARLY DIAGNOSIS)

A woman's risk category will determine what breast screening she is offered. Women at average or near population risk will not be offered any screening over and above what is available to women in the general population. In the United Kingdom, screening recommendations for women at different risks are included in the National Institute for Health and Care Excellence (NICE) guidance on familial breast cancer. This is largely done by mammography, but women at particularly high risk should also be offered magnetic resonance imaging (MRI) screening, especially at younger ages when mammography is less sensitive due to greater breast density.

There is no proven screening for ovarian cancer so women who may have an increased risk of this cancer should be counselled about symptom awareness, and if they are at high risk it may be appropriate to consider referring them for risk-reducing bilateral salpingo-oophorectomy.

GENETIC TESTING

When the family history is suggestive of a *BRCA* gene mutation, genetic testing can be undertaken. Ideally, this is performed on DNA extracted from a blood sample from a family member affected by a *BRCA*-related cancer. However, with advances in genetic testing technology, the sensitivity of mutation analysis is now sufficiently good that, even where there is no living or available affected family member, testing can nevertheless be offered to unaffected, at-risk individuals.

Whether to offer genetic testing will depend on the likelihood of an individual carrying a pathogenic variant. As previously discussed, this can be determined by one of the readily available computer software packages or by using a numerical scoring system such as the one developed in Manchester. This assigns a score to each potentially *BRCA*-related cancer, according to the age of diagnosis, and the overall score correlates with the probability of the cancer being associated with a *BRCA1* or *BRCA2* mutation. Many centres in the United Kingdom have set a Manchester score threshold above which testing will be offered. The advantages of this system include its simplicity and versatility, allowing easy re-calculation during a clinic consultation if the patient's family history turns out to be different from what was thought.

Testing strategies vary but must allow for the detection of point mutations and small deletions as well as larger-scale deletions and duplications of one or more whole exons. Traditionally this has required two separate techniques, a sequencing method and a dosage method such as multiplex ligation-dependent probe amplification (MLPA). Most laboratories now use next-generation sequencing (NGS) techniques, which are being refined to allow detection of larger deletions and duplications as well, making separate dosage methods increasingly redundant. Many centres are offering gene panels, which allow for analysis of multiple genes simultaneously. This can be particularly useful if the combination of cancers in the family could be due to more than one familial cancer syndrome. The advantages of being able to test more than one gene at a time need to be balanced against the potential disadvantages, such as identification of variants of uncertain significance and, perhaps more importantly, the incidental finding of variants in genes unrelated to the patient's family history.

If a pathogenic mutation is identified in one of the high-risk genes, at-risk family members can be offered predictive testing to clarify their risks. Predictive (or presymptomatic) testing should only be undertaken in regional genetics centres, with appropriate pre-test and post-test counselling.

MANAGEMENT OF *BRCA* GENE MUTATION CARRIERS

Women found to be carrying a *BRCA* gene mutation should be offered annual breast screening from a young age, initially by MRI and then by both MRI and mammography. However, some women want to be more proactive in managing their risk, in which case they can consider chemoprevention with drugs such as tamoxifen, raloxifene or anastrozole, or risk-reducing surgery. Chemoprevention may reduce a woman's risk of developing breast cancer by up to 40%, although the reduction appears to be confined to oestrogen receptor (ER) positive cancers, and since *BRCA1* gene carriers have a propensity to develop ER negative cancers, the benefits in this group are less clear.

The two surgical options available to these women are bilateral mastectomy and bilateral salpingo-oophorectomy (BSO). Risk-reducing mastectomy in *BRCA* gene carriers reduces the risk of breast cancer by around 95%. Ideally, women considering risk-reducing mastectomy should be seen and assessed by a multidisciplinary team who can assist in the decision-making process. These women need appropriate counselling and sufficient time to weigh up the advantages, namely a reduced risk of breast cancer and the alleviation of anxiety, against the disadvantages, which include the risk of surgical complications and possible psychological problems.

Bilateral salpingo-oophorectomy reduces the risk of ovarian cancer by approximately 90% and may also reduce a woman's risk of developing breast cancer, depending on her age at the time of the procedure. Aside from infertility, the effects of the surgically induced menopause can be alleviated by the use of HRT. The decision to use HRT will depend on a woman's personal circumstances. Although HRT is known to be associated with an increased risk of breast cancer, it appears that the use of HRT does not reverse any reduction in breast cancer risk in these women.

MEDICAL MANAGEMENT OF AFFECTED *BRCA* GENE MUTATION CARRIERS

The *BRCA* status of women affected by cancer is increasingly impacting on how they are treated. Affected female gene carriers have a significantly higher risk of developing a second breast cancer in the contralateral breast (approximately 25% compared to 10% in non-carriers). This raises the question of whether a risk-reducing contralateral mastectomy should be performed, possibly as part of the initial surgical procedure. There is no evidence that *BRCA* gene mutation carriers are more radiosensitive than the general population, in terms of response or toxicity.

There is now considerable evidence that *BRCA*-associated tumours are more sensitive to certain chemotherapeutic drugs, thanks to advances in the understanding of the biological function of the *BRCA1/2* genes and the role of the BRCA1/2 proteins in DNA repair. The poly-ADP ribose polymerase (PARP) proteins also play important roles in DNA repair, and we now know that inhibiting PARP in the presence of BRCA deficiency leads to cell death, while cells with normal BRCA function remain unaffected. This concept, that the mutation or inhibition of two pathways can lead to cell death when mutation or inhibition of either alone would not, is termed *synthetic lethality* (see also Chapter 12).

PARP inhibitors have been tested in clinical trials in patients with *BRCA*-related cancers and, although results in breast cancer patients to date have been mixed, there is clear evidence of benefit for women with high-grade serous ovarian cancer. The first PARP inhibitor has now been licenced and approved for use in the United Kingdom and further clinical trials are in progress.

OTHER GENES

There are other genes in which pathogenic variants can increase the risk of developing breast cancer to varying degrees. However, how to build this information into decisions about appropriate screening, and whether to do so at all with the more moderate risk genes, has not yet been fully resolved. This list of genes includes *PALB2, TP53, PTEN, STK11, CHEK2, ATM* and *NF1*.

32

Rare Mendelian cancer syndromes and other cancers

INTRODUCTION

Previous chapters have considered the Mendelian subsets of the common cancers: colorectal cancer (Chapter 30) and breast and ovarian cancer (Chapter 31). This chapter covers some of the rarer syndromes associated with an increased cancer or tumour risk, although the list is by no means exhaustive. Some of these conditions are characterised by a combination of specific tumour types with associated clinical features, whereas others have a more generalised tendency to malignancy. We also consider the genetic aspects of other 'common' cancers.

RARE MENDELIAN CANCER SYNDROMES

Although individually rare, the number of Mendelian cancer syndromes is considerable. Almost all these conditions follow autosomal dominant inheritance, and genetic testing is readily available for the large majority. Identification of a pathogenic mutation in a known cancer predisposition gene allows family members to request predictive testing to clarify their risk, thus ensuring that surveillance, if available, is offered only to those at risk.

Note that several of these conditions may be encountered by the paediatric geneticist or dysmorphologist, because of the function of these genes in development, before any syndrome-associated tumour has developed.

Li-Fraumeni syndrome

This rare, dominantly inherited multiple tumour syndrome, due to mutations in the tumour suppressor gene *TP53*, primarily gives a high risk of osteosarcoma, soft-tissue sarcoma, breast cancer, adrenocortical cancer, leukaemia and brain tumours including choroid plexus tumours, most with childhood or early adult onset. Other tumours have also been associated with the condition. Apart from breast cancer surveillance by magnetic resonance imaging (MRI) from early adulthood, there is limited evidence for screening for the other cancers found in Li-Fraumeni syndrome (LFS) although the idea that annual whole-body MRI could be beneficial is now gaining traction, and there is increasing pressure from families to provide this.

Due to the lack of evidence of benefit from surveillance, predictive testing for this condition has not routinely been offered to at-risk children. However, some families do request predictive testing for their children, and these requests should be discussed on a case-by-case basis, at all times keeping the best interests of the children at the forefront of the discussion. When testing is not undertaken in childhood, parents can be supported by a local paediatrician with rapid access to a paediatric oncologist as needed, allowing the children to make an independent decision about predictive genetic testing when they are older. Of course, if a screening programme to detect complications is introduced in childhood, it is likely that testing in childhood would then become the norm, since it would not be appropriate to subject a child to intensive screening if they were not, in fact, at risk.

Cowden syndrome

Due to mutations in the *PTEN* tumour suppressor gene and part of the wider *PTEN* hamartoma tumour syndrome, this condition is associated with an increased risk of early-onset breast cancer, thyroid cancer and endometrial cancer. Other characteristic features include macrocephaly, hamartomatous intestinal polyps, mucocutaneous lesions, for example, trichilemmomas, and Lhermitte-Duclos disease (a dysplastic gangliocytoma of the cerebellum, which is thought to be a slow-growing hamartoma). Some individuals will have developmental delay or intellectual disability, although these are seen less commonly than in other *PTEN*-related conditions, for example, Bannayan-Riley-Ruvalcaba syndrome.

The lifetime risk of breast cancer for women with Cowden syndrome is high, probably equivalent to that of *BRCA* gene carriers, so these women should be offered regular breast screening and possibly risk-reducing surgery. The thyroid cancer is usually follicular, rarely papillary but never medullary; annual ultrasound screening is recommended for those at risk. There is no recommended screening for endometrial cancer, but women can be offered risk-reducing surgery if they wish.

Gorlin syndrome

This condition, also known as naevoid basal cell carcinoma syndrome, predisposes to the development of both malignant and non-malignant tumours. The most commonly occurring cancers are basal cell carcinomas, which tend to start developing in adolescence or early adulthood. Other tumours include benign jaw tumours, called keratocystic odontogenic tumours, and cardiac and ovarian fibromas. A small number of individuals with Gorlin syndrome will develop a medulloblastoma during childhood. In addition to tumour formation, individuals with this condition may have palmar and plantar pits, macrocephaly with frontal bossing, calcification of the falx cerebri and skeletal anomalies such as bifid ribs. The condition is caused by mutations in the *PTCH1* gene, and the inheritance is autosomal dominant.

Von Hippel-Lindau disease

Von Hippel-Lindau (VHL) disease is another autosomal dominant condition, caused by mutations in the *VHL* tumour suppressor gene. The characteristic features are cerebellar and spinal haemangioblastomas, retinal angiomas, phaeochromocytomas and renal cell carcinomas. Some individuals with VHL also develop endolymphatic sac tumours of the inner ear, which can cause hearing loss and tinnitus, and pancreatic tumours. Many of the tumours will develop in young adulthood so screening should start during childhood. For this reason, VHL is one of the few conditions where predictive genetic testing for a known familial mutation is indicated in childhood, ensuring that only those who are truly at risk are offered surveillance.

It is also worth noting that, as this disorder affects several different organs, it provides a good example of those conditions where a clinical genetics department can be especially effective at the coordination of surveillance. If surveillance is organised by the relevant specialists for each single organ working independently, the chance of problems arising in practice will be substantially greater.

Tuberous sclerosis

Tuberous sclerosis (TS) is discussed in Chapter 14, as neurodevelopmental problems are so much more common than malignancy among those affected.

Neurofibromatosis type 2

Neurofibromatosis type 2 (NF2) is an autosomal dominant condition caused by mutations in the *NF2* gene. It affects about 1 in 35,000 people, making it much less common than NF1 (see Chapter 14). The hallmark features of NF2 are bilateral vestibular schwannomas, which are benign tumours growing on the vestibular nerves. Other tumours found in NF2 include meningiomas of the brain and spinal cord, spinal schwannomas and cutaneous schwannomas. The vestibular schwannomas almost inevitably cause hearing loss of some degree, and this is commonly one of the first signs of the condition.

About half the individuals with NF2 have not inherited the condition from a parent. Some of these have a milder phenotype, and genetic testing may not identify the causative mutation. Many of these will be mosaic for a mutation in the *NF2* gene, this having arisen as a post-zygotic event. The risk to their offspring appears to be less than 50%, but those children who do inherit the condition may be more severely affected as they will not be mosaic.

Multiple endocrine neoplasia

The main clinical features of multiple endocrine neoplasia type 1 (MEN1) are tumours of the parathyroid glands, pituitary gland and pancreas, which are usually not malignant. The symptoms of the condition tend to arise as a consequence of overproduction of hormones, for example, hyperparathyroidism. Once an index case has been recognised, and the pathogenic variant identified in the *MEN1* gene, family members at risk can be tested to identify those affected. Screening for complications starts in childhood (often between 5 and 7 years) and should be coordinated by a paediatric endocrinologist with seamless transfer later to adult services. Inheritance is autosomal dominant (see also Chapter 25).

Multiple endocrine neoplasia type 2 (MEN2) is due to mutations in the *RET* gene. The main features are medullary thyroid cancer (MTC) and phaeochromocytomas. Annual biochemical screening for phaeochromocytomas is by measurement of 24-hour urinary metanephrines. Due to the high risk of MTC, mutation carriers are advised to have a prophylactic thyroidectomy. There are three subtypes of MEN2, known as MEN2A, MEN2B and familial medullary thyroid cancer (FMTC). Individuals with MEN2B may also have mucosal neuromas of the lips and tongue, ganglioneuromatosis of the gastrointestinal tract, and a 'Marfanoid' body habitus. The MTC in MEN2B typically develops in early childhood so surgery should normally be done in the first year of life. In other cases, thyroidectomy should be performed before age 5 years, unless certain low-risk criteria are met. Before undertaking any surgery in an individual with MEN2, biochemical screening should be arranged to exclude a functioning phaeochromocytoma. As for MEN1, the inheritance of MEN2 is autosomal dominant (see Chapter 25).

Hereditary diffuse gastric cancer

Caused by mutations in the *CDH1* tumour suppressor gene, hereditary diffuse gastric cancer (HDGC) is another autosomal dominant cancer predisposition syndrome. As suggested by the name, the risk is for a specific pathological type of gastric cancer, which is described as 'diffuse' because of the characteristic infiltration of malignant cells beneath the stomach lining without the development of a discrete mass. (This used to be termed 'leather-bottle stomach' or linitis plastica.) This makes detection of the cancer particularly difficult, and prophylactic gastrectomy may be more appropriate than regular gastroscopic surveillance, although this surgery does carry a significant risk of morbidity and even mortality. In addition to the risk of gastric cancer, women with a *CDH1* mutation have an increased risk of lobular breast cancer.

Familial atypical multiple mole melanoma syndrome

This syndrome, which is characterised by multiple melanocytic naevi and melanomas, is caused by mutations in the *CDKN2A* gene. In addition to a high lifetime risk of melanoma, there is a significant risk of pancreatic cancer. Regular follow-up by a dermatologist is recommended to monitor the development of melanomas, but there is no screening of proven worth for the pancreatic cancer risk.

Hereditary paraganglioma-phaeochromocytoma syndrome (familial glomus tumours)

Characterised by the development of mainly non-malignant tumours in paraganglia, this condition is caused by mutations in the succinate dehydrogenase subunit genes *SDHA*, *SDHAF2*, *SDHB*, *SDHC* and *SDHD*. The paragangliomas are mostly found in the head and neck, especially around the carotid bifurcation, or in the adrenal glands, when they are known as phaeochromocytomas. The inheritance is autosomal dominant, but the *SDHD* gene is maternally imprinted, which means that only those individuals who inherit the mutation from their father will manifest the condition.

GENETIC SYNDROMES PREDISPOSING TO MALIGNANCY

In contrast to the dominantly inherited specific tumour syndromes previously discussed, most of the Mendelian disorders showing a generalised tendency to malignancy, especially in early life, follow autosomal recessive inheritance (Table 32.1). Some of these have been shown to be inborn errors of DNA repair, and it is likely that others will prove to have a comparable basis. Others are immune deficiencies (see Chapter 27).

There remains uncertainty about whether heterozygotes for these rare recessive disorders are also at increased risk of developing malignancy. The evidence for this remains largely unclear, but there seems to be a consensus that carriers of ataxia telangiectasia have an increased

Table 32.1 Some Mendelian syndromes predisposing to malignancy

Syndrome	Inheritance	Type of neoplasm
Xeroderma pigmentosum	Autosomal recessive	Various skin tumours
Fanconi anaemia (pancytopaenia)	Autosomal recessive	Leukaemias
Ataxia telangiectasia	Autosomal recessive	Leukaemias and carcinomas
Bloom syndrome	Autosomal recessive	Leukaemias
Chediak-Higashi syndrome	Autosomal recessive	Lymphomas
Werner syndrome	Autosomal recessive	Various
Dyskeratosis congenita	X-linked recessive	Pharyngeal and oesophageal cancer
Wiskott-Aldrich syndrome	X-linked recessive	Leukaemias, lymphomas
Lymphoproliferative disease	X-linked recessive	Lymphomas

risk of breast cancer and should be offered additional breast screening, although standard mammography may be best avoided.

The recessively inherited form of colorectal cancer with polyps has also proved to be a DNA repair defect due to mutations in the *MutYH* gene (see Chapter 30).

EMBRYONAL AND CHILDHOOD CANCER

When known genetic syndromes are excluded, the overall risk of malignancy in childhood is around 1 in 600. The risk of malignancy occurring in sibs is approximately doubled (1 in 300), with most cases concordant for the same neoplasm. The relative increases in risk, divided into the major groups of leukaemias, lymphomas and other malignancies, were calculated by Draper and colleagues some five decades ago (Draper, Heaf and Wilson, 1977). Note that some of these familial factors may prove to be environmental rather than genetic.

It would seem reasonable to use these estimates for the various rare forms of childhood cancer where individual data are not yet available, where no other cases of childhood cancer have occurred in the family and where a clear genetic basis for the neoplasm has not yet been identified. Cytogenetic and molecular analysis of the tumours has become increasingly important in defining, distinguishing and planning the treatment of these disorders. As whole genome sequencing becomes more readily available through diagnostic services, genome sequencing of the affected child and the child's tumour are likely to be among the more fruitful disease categories in terms of clinically helpful diagnostic yield. Retinoblastoma is considered more fully in Chapter 19.

Wilms tumour (nephroblastoma)

The incidence of Wilms tumour is approximately 1 in 10,000. Survival has improved considerably with about 90% of children now surviving 5 years or more. A proportion of cases follow Mendelian dominant inheritance, including most of those with bilateral tumours, but it can be difficult to separate the Mendelian from non-heritable cases in the absence of a significant family history or other features. Empirical risks for relatives of patients with Wilms tumour appear low for the siblings of an isolated case with no syndromic features, even with bilateral tumours (no more than 1%). The risks to the offspring of an affected individual are less clear but probably no more than 5% in the absence of family history, syndromic features

Table 32.2 Risks for relatives in Wilms tumour (without molecular studies)

Affected member	Risk for subsequent children (%)
Parent with bilateral tumours	30
Parent with unilateral tumour; affected relative	30
Parent unaffected: two affected children	30
Parent with unilateral tumour	10
Sib with bilateral tumours	10
Sib with unilateral tumour; no chromosome defect or associated malformations	1

or bilateral tumours. Molecular studies in the affected relative will be crucial in clarifying the situation in each family. (See Table 32.2.)

In addition, Wilms tumour may occur as part of several conditions including WAGR syndrome (Wilms tumour with aniridia, genital defects and mental retardation), Denys-Drash syndrome and Frasier syndrome. All of these are associated with mutations involving the *WT1* gene on chromosome 11, as well as with hemihypertrophy and Beckwith-Wiedemann syndrome. Cases of familial but non-syndromal Wilms tumour have also been described, which may be related to alterations of chromosome 11p15.5 rather than *WT1*. Mutation in *DICER1* can cause complex phenotypes that also include Wilms tumour.

Neuroblastoma

In contrast to Wilms tumour, the great majority of cases of neuroblastoma are sporadic, but poorer survival means that adequate data are not available for the offspring of affected patients. In the few two-generation families known, the parent has usually had spontaneous maturation of the tumour. The risk for further siblings of an isolated case is unlikely to exceed 1% and is probably nearer the 1 in 300 risk found overall for siblings in childhood cancer. Where two siblings, or a parent and child, are affected, the risk for further siblings is much greater, probably that of an incompletely penetrant dominant gene, about 30%. Two genes have been found to be associated with familial neuroblastoma, *ALK* and *PHOX2B*, and research suggests there may be other loci involved, on chromosome 1 and chromosome 11. The case for regular screening of siblings, or for general population screening of infants using urine, has not yet been proved. Neuroblastoma can also arise in the LFS.

LEUKAEMIAS AND RELATED DISORDERS

The great majority of cases of all types of leukaemia do not seem to have a significant hereditary basis, but specific oncogenes and somatic mutations are involved.

Acute leukaemia

Acute leukaemia is most commonly seen in childhood, where it accounts for a major proportion of all malignancies. The risk for siblings is increased, possibly two to four times greater than normal, but the absolute risk remains low. Monozygotic twins appear to carry a risk of around 20%–25% for concordance of childhood leukaemia, a finding that might seem to suggest a strong genetic influence but probably results from shared circulation of precursor cells. Whatever the case, the high risk has important implications for the careful surveillance and early therapy of such twins.

The various chromosomal abnormalities described in blood cells appear to be the result of somatic genetic changes, some involving particular oncogenes. The well-recognised relationship between leukaemias and irradiation has led to concern about the possible epidemiology and association of childhood leukaemia clusters with radiation sources such as nuclear power stations. At one point it was suggested that such cases may be related to occupational exposure of the father, implying that a germ line rather than somatic mutational mechanism might be operating, but there is no evidence to support this hypothesis.

Acute leukaemia may also be a complication of a number of primary genetic disorders, including immune deficiencies, DNA repair defects and Down syndrome. No data are yet available for the offspring of the increasing number of survivors. Risks of leukaemia are likely to be small, but an increase in other abnormalities as a result of therapy cannot be excluded.

Chronic myeloid leukaemia

Chronic myeloid leukaemia carries little risk to relatives, although the 'Philadelphia' chromosome abnormality – a partial deletion of chromosome 22 resulting from translocation of part of it onto chromosome 9 – is a consistent finding in most cases. This is a somatic event, not affecting the germ line, and involves the *ABL1* locus on chromosome 9.

Chronic lymphatic leukaemia

Chronic lymphatic leukaemia rarely recurs in a family, but a small number of multigeneration families makes it possible that a dominantly inherited form exists among the much more common non-genetic cases.

Lymphomas

As with leukaemias, most cases of lymphoma are sporadic; clustering is suggestive of an infective or immunosuppressive agent and may well not be genetic. Burkitt lymphoma shows a characteristic translocation at the site of the immunoglobulin genes on chromosome 14. The same primary genetic diseases as predispose to leukaemias, such as ataxia telangiectasia, may also be responsible for lymphomas, although this does not apply to Down syndrome. The same reservations about the offspring of 'cured' patients apply. Lymphomas may also occur in the X-linked immune deficiencies, notably in X-linked lymphoproliferative disease.

Study of the siblings of childhood lymphoma cases shows a fivefold increase in risk for lymphomas, but the overall risk of childhood malignancy is still only around 1 in 300.

Histiocytosis

Histiocytosis comprises a confused and heterogeneous group including somatic mosaic disorders and several Mendelian disorders that present in childhood. Adult cases appear to be non-genetic (i.e. arising at post-zygotic events). The Mendelian group includes familial erythrophagocytic lymphohistiocytosis (autosomal recessive), which is rapidly progressive and fatal, as well as familial reticuloendotheliosis with eosinophilia (Omenn syndrome, autosomal recessive).

OTHER COMMON CANCERS

After the impressive genetic developments in colorectal and breast cancer, it is not surprising that both clinical and basic research workers have looked closely at other common cancers to see if comparable Mendelian subsets exist. So far, no high-penetrance genes similar to *BRCA1* and *BRCA2* have been identified for other common cancers. It is possible that families with a Mendelian pattern do exist, but these appear to be few and less easy to define. From the viewpoint of clinicians asked about genetic risks, accurate documentation of family history is the most important task. If this looks clearly Mendelian, then it is probably wise to consider the risks high, especially if the affected members show the same specific tumour type, if age at onset is unusually young, or if there are multiple tumour types or tumour sites in a single individual.

Ovarian cancer represents a particular problem, partly because the *BRCA* genes and mismatch repair genes are all known ovarian predisposition genes but also because methods of screening and prevention are of uncertain value. Other gene loci (e.g. *RAD51C* and *RAD51D*) have recently been identified in ovarian cancer families both with and without breast cancer, but relatively little is known about the magnitude of ovarian cancer risk associated with variants in these genes. There is no clear consensus on the appropriate management of women who carry such variants, but it may be reasonable to consider them to have a moderately increased risk, and some gynaecological oncologists are willing to offer them risk-reducing bilateral salpingo-oophorectomy.

Prostate cancer has been a relatively neglected field of research in comparison with breast cancer, although recent studies have made considerable progress. Problems are created by the late age at onset, making recognition of a Mendelian pattern difficult, and by the high proportion of tumours that are not relentlessly aggressive. The most clinically significant genetic loci for prostate cancer are the *BRCA1* and *BRCA2* genes, but specific mutations of the *HOXB13* gene have also recently been shown to confer a significantly increased risk. The prostate cancers associated with the *BRCA2* and *HOXB13* genes tend to have a poorer prognosis. Monitoring for prostate-specific antigen (PSA) levels may be helpful for men with a strong family history although there is no formal screening programme for prostate cancer.

Gastric cancer incidence shows a considerable geographical variation, in which genetic factors may play a part (e.g. in the Welsh and Japanese). Unlike colorectal cancer, clear Mendelian forms are exceptional (see section 'Hereditary Diffuse Gastric Cancer' in this chapter), although there has been an increased risk historically in some families with Lynch syndrome, that appears to have fallen in frequency as with sporadic stomach cancer in the general population (see earlier). A modest two- to fourfold increase has been shown in first-degree relatives of patients with gastric cancer as a whole.

Oesophageal cancer risk is not obviously increased in relatives of affected individuals, at least in western Europe. The situation may be different in areas of high incidence such as central Asia and parts of Africa, where striking familial clusters have been reported. Environmental factors, particularly smoking and dietary factors, are probably responsible for the major differences in incidence. The remarkable, but exceedingly rare, families with oesophageal cancer and tylosis (hyperkeratosis of palms and soles; see also Chapter 18) following autosomal dominant inheritance should be borne in mind if a familial cluster is found in an area of low incidence. The gene, called *RHBDF2*, is on chromosome 17 and somatic mutations at this locus have been identified in sporadic oesophageal cancers.

Pancreatic cancer is a feature of several familial cancer syndromes including Lynch syndrome and Peutz-Jeghers syndrome (see Chapter 30). There is also an increased risk for carriers of mutations in the *BRCA2* (see Chapter 31) and *CDKN2A* genes (see earlier). However, even in the absence of a known familial cancer syndrome, first-degree relatives of affected individuals have an increased risk, particularly if the cancer is diagnosed before age 60 years.

Renal cancer can occur in families with a number of different Mendelian cancer syndromes, for example, von Hippel-Lindau (VHL) (see Chapter 14), Birt-Hogg-Dubé (BHD) and hereditary leiomyomatosis and renal cell cancer, but familial aggregations outside these conditions also occur, and the risk seems to be particularly significant for siblings of affected individuals.

Endometrial cancer is well recognised as part of Lynch syndrome, but there is also an increased risk for women with Cowden syndrome (see earlier). There may be other low-penetrance susceptibility alleles, but these are yet to be identified.

Cervical cancer and *lung cancer* are almost always attributable primarily to external agents. Whereas the predominant risk factor for lung cancer is smoking, for cervical cancer it is the human papillomavirus (HPV).

For those attempting to ensure that an efficient system of service delivery is developed for cancer genetics, it is perhaps fortunate that scientific discoveries in this field have been sequential rather than simultaneous. The evolution of a system such as that outlined for breast cancer, using the combined resources of primary care, cancer clinicians and geneticists, will allow genetic counselling and testing guidelines to be developed and applied across the entire area of common cancers. This will help to avoid wasteful use of resources and needless worry for many patients and their relatives. It should also be useful when future population screening programmes for cancer begin to incorporate genetic approaches, as is beginning to happen in relation to breast cancer.

PART 4

Genetic counselling in context: The broader picture

33

Communication in genetic counselling

COMMUNICATION

What do we want to communicate in genetic counselling?

We want to convey information that will be relevant to patients and answer their questions and their concerns. We also wish to convey to patients our interest in them and our concern for their situation.

To be able to give relevant information in an appropriate manner, however, we first need to acquire some information. We need to know as much as we can about the biological basis of the problem or condition in the family and have some understanding of the way the patient views this and makes sense of it. We may also need to consider how the wider family sees the situation.

For these reasons, as discussed earlier in this volume, we need first to listen – to listen to the patient's questions, to see what the patient (or parent or other relative) already knows about the condition and to gain a sense of their perspective on it. Giving people space to talk aloud about a difficult topic will often lead them to make apparent their underlying concerns, which may go beyond the questions that they put to us explicitly. This requires us to listen intently and make inferences from what has been said – to 'read between the lines'. We also want to find out the extent to which the topic of their concern is discussed within the family, especially if it might be relevant to others not present in the consultation.

Once the patient or parent has had their say, we may then wish to ask questions, to obtain a more detailed description of the patient's symptoms and a more general account of how the patient is affected and how the condition impacts on their life. And we want to find out about how any others in the family are affected, if they are, or if they feel at risk.

At that point, we may need to pursue further investigations or to check family medical records before we can draw conclusions. However, if the diagnosis is apparent and we have enough biological understanding to give a coherent response to their questions, we can begin to give information back to the patient. This may be given very directly or in a much more tentative manner, with frequent checking of their understanding and their emotional state. How this is done will depend upon the patient's prior level of understanding, the level of anxiety we sense, and the relationship we have established.

Once we have been able to impart some information, the next topic to address may be the implications of this new knowledge for the patient. There may need to be a process of personal adjustment to new diagnostic information or risk information for the patient to make. There may be other members of the family who need to be informed, and perhaps offered testing. This will sometimes be very challenging for the patient, especially if they wish to protect their children or parents from distressing or confusing information. We can offer to support them in this or share the task with them. But it will usually be their decision as to how to approach their relatives with such information.

When the patient is weighing up their future course of action, we can help by listening and by talking. The balance for the professional between giving information or helping a patient to weigh up different potential courses of action, will of course vary both within a consultation and over the course of several consultations. The practitioner will want to be flexible and adapt to the present understanding of the patient or family, aiming to contribute either information or 'points for consideration' at a pace that will allow the family to incorporate these ideas in a constructive fashion.

Professionals differ in how they communicate and in their styles of communication. These are partly learned and habitual differences but may also relate to deeper issues of personality. Those who work in frontline, acute medicine with necessarily short consultation times may find it difficult – indeed, disorienting – to have the opportunity to adopt a 'slow' approach to consultations. However, this 'slow' approach is often necessary when the outcome of a consultation is not a prescription or (yet) another investigation but, instead, deals with education and understanding, with adjustment to a difficult reality, or with weighing up personal decisions where the medical facts provide little guidance.

Decisions about relationships, about reproduction, looking into the future or sharing information within the family may all require knowledge of the medical facts, but the facts alone will fail to provide the answers. The professional engaged in genetic counselling (whatever their base speciality) will need to adjust their tone and style to the circumstances. This aspect of communication, the 'tuning' of communicative style to the needs of the patient, can be expressed in terms of content and context, information and reflection, or facts and values.

Another aspect of the practitioner's approach to the patient is the balance between neutrality and guidance, and we address that later in a brief discussion on non-directiveness and counselling. It is important to appreciate that information is not necessarily neutral: whether or not to pass on a particular item of information, and when and how to do so, can convey strong recommendations about future action. We address this later.

COUNSELLING

The word 'counselling' in the phrase 'genetic counselling' carries baggage: It can lead to misapprehensions about what goes on within the genetics consultation. What it should convey is the sense that the practice of genetic counselling addresses both the biology of the condition under discussion and its personal, emotional and family impact, treating people in their full social, relational context. The word 'counselling' here should reassure the patient that they will not be abandoned with a surfeit of indigestible information. Instead, they should be supported to assess its implications and to weigh up the likely outcomes of different possible future courses of action, both in terms of managing disease or the risk of disease and in terms of adjustment, family communication and relationships.

Not all those who perform 'genetic counselling' will be equally competent or experienced in all aspects of this activity. Some of the medically qualified will focus on the diagnostic elements, while those formally trained as genetic counsellors may attend with particular care to the emotional aspects and support for those making important decisions. However, one should remember that medicine is – aspires to be – a holistic profession. Medical professionalism has always (for centuries, millennia) addressed the personal aspects of disease, and it does not sit well with this tradition for genetic medicine to focus only on the pathogenic variant and to ignore the person in whom that variant is found. As well as differences in interest and scope of practice between individual practitioners, remember that there will also be systematic differences in professional roles between countries, depending upon whether genetic counsellors are recognised as a distinct professional group.

The unhelpful expectations that the term 'genetic counselling' can generate vary from a sense of threat (intrusion into the patient's personal space) to a sense of being immune to criticism. Some patients feel that they may have their inner thoughts and feelings exposed for all to see – and for all to judge. This can lead people to feel vulnerable and to decline referral. Others, perhaps familiar with the unconditional positive regard of Carl Rogers's client-centred therapy, may feel that their genetic counsellor could not possibly challenge them or recommend that they change a decision already made. In fact, patients can be reassured that the inner workings of their souls will not be held up to scorn, but some patients may have their plans challenged and a course of action recommended that they find challenging.

In reality, the practitioner – whether a clinical geneticist, a genetic counsellor or a different specialist – will not probe intrusively but will sometimes have to challenge a patient. Yes, they should always respect and support the patient, but they may put forward unwelcome information that the patient should perhaps take into account in reaching important decisions. And they may challenge the patient to consider how a course of action is likely to work out. They may ask the patient to consider the implications of their actions for others as well as her- or himself. Such 'scenario decision counselling' is not to everyone's taste or inclination – and some patients are unable or resolutely unwilling to engage with it – but it can be very helpful to give patients the opportunity to look afresh at how their plan of action may impact upon themselves and others.

VOCABULARY OF CONVERSATION

In thinking through one's general approach to communication, it can be helpful to have a vocabulary for doing so and for discussing particular instances of communication in consultations. A common vocabulary that one shares with colleagues is even more useful. One such verbal framework, that promotes reflection and discussion on the use of particular words in a specific context, is John Heron's Six Category Intervention Analysis. This sets out six categories of intervention that the counsellor can make: six types of practitioner contribution to the verbal communication within the consultation.

Three of these categories are described as 'authoritative' and three as 'facilitative'. The authoritative interventions are prescriptive, informative and confronting. The facilitative interventions are cathartic, catalytic and supportive. These descriptions are neutral, not loaded, and it can be perfectly appropriate to use any of these interventions, depending upon the context. When the intervention has been appropriate, this use can be described as valid. If an intervention is used inappropriately, if it does not 'succeed' or 'work' (if it 'falls flat'), then its use was ill-judged and is described as degenerate. If an intervention is used maliciously, perhaps in a manipulative fashion, then this is described as being perverted.

This set of words – prescriptive, informative and confronting ('authoritative'), cathartic, catalytic and supportive ('facilitative'), along with valid, degenerate and perverted – can help to describe what has happened in an exchange, what one hoped would happen, and what one could have done differently or what one might still be able to do in the future to repair any awkwardness or any lasting difficulty that has resulted.

For such reflection and discussion to occur, genetic counselling professionals need to create opportunities to do so. Consultations that are likely to be difficult – especially in prenatal genetics and when a patient is considering predictive genetic testing for non-medical reasons (e.g. for Huntington's disease, until it becomes readily curable) – should usually involve two practitioners working together, sometimes termed co-counselling. This naturally creates the opportunity to reflect jointly upon a difficult consultation and for two (perhaps slightly different) accounts to be discussed with others, either with a supervisor or in a team or departmental meeting. Such safe spaces for those doing genetic counselling to reflect upon and to discuss their clinical work are of great importance.

AUTHORITATIVE INTERVENTIONS AND NON-DIRECTIVENESS

By its very nature, genetic counselling will often entail the passing of information to the patient or a family member. We usually do this in an appropriate manner, tailored to what the patient needs at that moment and to what the patient is able to absorb. There can be a temptation to give more, and especially more technical, information than is needed for the patient to understand their situation and make their decision, and this is to be guarded against. The history of how an important fact emerged, and the details of the laboratory methods used in carrying out a test, may be of interest to the practitioner but are not usually required by the patient.

Genetic counsellors are often committed to being non-directive, that is, to the principle of supporting patients in making their own decisions and not steering them towards one outcome rather than another. This is a very appropriate ethos for much of genetic counselling practice, but there are decisions for which we will wish to encourage and, frankly, to recommend one outcome rather than another. These are our prescriptive interventions.

Our general aim is to enhance the quality of decisions made by our clients, in the belief that a sound understanding of the relevant biological facts and an opportunity to think through the possible consequences of any course of action for one's self and for others (e.g. as in having a genetic test, seeking a termination of pregnancy, not disclosing important information to a relative) will lead to better long-term outcomes for all parties. There are some areas of practice where we will *not* want to steer patients towards one outcome rather than another, but there are other areas where we may wish to do so.

We will *not* want to steer patients' decisions about prenatal decisions – whether to have prenatal diagnosis, whether to terminate a pregnancy – as that area of life is so intensely personal and so tied up with fundamental values. This is an area that can be intensely challenging for the professionals as well as for the families. Another area in which non-directive practice is of great importance is that of predictive genetic testing for late-onset genetic disorders, when there is no scope for medical intervention to improve the outlook for the patient in advance of the clinical onset of disease. The reason for seeking such a test is because of how it will play out in one's personal and social life, in the family and in relation to future decisions about reproduction.

In contrast, there are several areas where we may wish to be prescriptive, or directive, by making clear recommendations to our patients:

- We will almost always wish to encourage openness within a family about an inherited disorder for which other family members are at risk rather than encouraging secrecy. We see too much family disruption because decisions are made that seem 'easier' in the short term but that store up major problems for later.
- We will recommend that patients at risk of an inherited condition have genetic testing to clarify this, if testing can improve medical decisions about their care. This applies, for example, to genetic testing for a number of familial cancer syndromes, where surveillance has a substantial impact on cancer prevention and/or on survival. Testing for some inherited cardiac conditions can also be recommended.
- We will encourage parents not to seek genetic tests on their young children for conditions known about in the family, whether predictive tests for late-onset disorders (where there is no medical intervention that can help at this time of life) or tests for reproductive purposes ('carrier status'). Such tests are better left until the child can at least take part in the discussion, although it may be very helpful to promote communication about the problem long in advance of testing so that the child can adjust to their situation and take responsibility when older.

Thus, there is a place for making recommendations in genetic counselling practice as well as a place for non-directiveness. Where non-directiveness remains key to good practice, it is important that the professionals involved should absorb that ethos and work with care and determination to ensure that they support but do not steer their clients. 'Steering' can be subtle, and it takes effort and insight to avoid it: this can be worked at, along with one's colleagues.

Finally, among the authoritative interventions, there are the confrontational interventions. We will wish to give more – and perhaps unwelcome – information to those patients who, we fear, may be making poor decisions because they are ill informed. This may require us to confront them with information (including conjecture about what might happen if …) that they would prefer to avoid. Similarly, there are those patients who seem to be choosing the path of least resistance – the easy option – instead of passing information to their families about a disease for which they (and perhaps others in the family) are at risk. There may be many reasons for such decisions, and it can be our task to confront our patients – sensitively – with the likely problems they are causing. If they persist in failing to pass on information, we may even have an ethical – and perhaps a legal – obligation to do so instead.

FACILITATIVE INTERVENTIONS

These interventions are generally simpler and involve us behaving in a way that is both natural and professional at the same time. Furthermore, as is also true with the authoritative interventions, these three types of intervention are not necessarily distinct but can often overlap. Simple, non-specific ways of being supportive – such as listening, encouraging, reassuring – will often facilitate (catalyse) insight and the making of constructive decisions. The habit of being supportive may also trigger tears and sobs in someone who until then has maintained his/her composure in the face of great unhappiness and perhaps concern about others in the family. Such catharsis can be very helpful, although I would not usually set out to 'achieve' it as a deliberate goal.

Sobs and tears will come often enough in those who have been living with genetic disease in themselves or their loved ones, without much need for us to induce it deliberately. We are conducting genetic counselling, and sometimes disease or risk management too. However, we are not usually acting as, or trained as, psychotherapists.

34

Population aspects of genetic counselling and genetic screening

INTRODUCTION

The primary aim of this book is to provide information that will help particular families in which a genetic disorder exists or is at risk of occurring. Throughout the book, the family – at times nuclear, at times extended – has been the unit under consideration. It is hoped that both the general discussions and the more specific information in the various chapters will have helped readers deal with many of the problems they are likely to meet, as well as alerting them to some of the pitfalls and unsolved problems that exist.

Most people, however, will not be fully satisfied dealing with these individual problems in isolation but will wish to place them in the more general context of the disorder overall – and to know how far they can relate these individual instances of genetic counselling to the wider prevention of inherited disorders in the population they serve.

These wider population aspects have so far received very little emphasis in this book, in part because the author's view is that the primary duty of a physician is to individuals and their immediate families, and in part because the general aspects can usually only be approached through study of the specific conditions. However, it would be entirely wrong to suggest, as is sometimes done, that these wider aspects are not the concern of those involved with genetic disorders. In the author's opinion, to take such a view would be as short-sighted as it would have been for the nineteenth-century physician to insist that only the individual case of typhoid fever was his concern, not the broader epidemiology or prevention of the disease.

The increasing application of prenatal and other screening programmes has highlighted the differences in approach and, indeed, the potential for conflict between approaches that focus on the population and those that attend to the individual family; indeed, this has in some instances resulted in considerable disagreement. However, these debates have been helpful in clarifying both the issues and the thoughts of those involved. The authors' principal conclusions are as follows:

- Genetic counselling is an activity whose goals and processes relate to individuals and families and will thus inevitably and appropriately vary according to the nature, attitudes and wishes of different families, as well as the society in which they live.
- Success or failure in genetic counselling (extremely difficult to evaluate) must be gauged by the extent to which it has helped the problems of individual families, not by any effect on the frequency of a genetic disorder or by a particular type of outcome (e.g. termination of affected pregnancies).
- Prevention or avoidance of a genetic disorder in an individual family is a valid goal provided that it is also the goal of the family. For most severe genetic disorders, this will commonly be the case, but with milder or more variable conditions it may well not be so. Whether this is the view of any one person will depend upon many factors including the family's experience so far of the condition (or of other genetic conditions) and wider societal factors.
- It may also be a perfectly valid goal for health services to enable and even encourage the population prevention of serious genetic disorders, provided that it does not conflict with the individual aims of families, and provided that it is clearly recognised as something separate from genetic counselling.
- It is crucial that the care of affected patients remains a high priority even when the health services hope to reduce the incidence of the condition. Efforts to 'prevent' a condition must be accompanied by efforts to treat it, so that treatment and prevention go hand in hand and are not seen as being in opposition.
- It may actually be the case that provision of high-quality treatment is enabled by disease prevention, but the population-level goals must not be allowed to set the ethos of the healthcare or genetic counselling of affected individuals and their relatives. The potential for conflict will depend partly on the nature of the disorder, but also on the degree to which those introducing any population-based programmes are aware of, and sensitive to, the wishes and needs of individual families. Experience with medical care and genetics services for the haemoglobin disorders provides good case studies of how prevention and treatment work well together, however, not if prevention wins out over treatment.

For those responsible for the delivery and development of genetics services to particular regions and populations, it is clearly important to know the extent to which a genetic counselling service is reaching the families that need it, and whether it is having beneficial effects. It is also important to be aware of changes in the overall frequency of the more common disorders. Equally, though, it is essential to resist pressure to establish or extend programmes on 'economic' grounds, where the primary aims could be of a 'public health' or 'eugenic' nature in terms of reducing disease frequency and thereby the costs of health services.

There may be a considerable temptation to use economic arguments when attempting to obtain funding for programmes, but the author's strong view is that any possible short-term benefit from such an approach would be greatly outweighed by longer-term loss of trust and respect for the field of medical genetics by families and professionals alike. The clinical genetics community and other professionals involved in genetic counselling have often been found arguing against population-based programmes that are inappropriate or not fully considered. We must now watch with care, as laboratory genetics services come to be used by a wider range of professionals, to ensure that these lessons are not forgotten and do not need to be learned over again.

The wider population aspects considered in the rest of this chapter fall into two main groups:

- Extensions of 'family-based' services to ensure equity of and full access to services – the wider aspects of genetic counselling
- Population screening for genetic disorders

WIDER ASPECTS OF GENETIC COUNSELLING: WHOM DOES GENETIC COUNSELLING REACH?

Anyone regularly involved in genetic counselling will be under no illusions that their advice is reaching all the individuals who wish for it – or would do so if they were aware of it. In general, one will be seeing a small segment of the community which is both sufficiently informed, motivated and articulate to ask for referral or to ask the type of question that prompts their own doctor to arrange for referral. Inevitably, this means that the less privileged, generally with the greatest need, are less well served. Even in a system like the UK's National Health Service (NHS), where no direct payment is required, the same situation applies, and at present it seems likely that genetic counselling is still only dealing with the 'tip of the iceberg', even in those situations where it could have a profound effect on people's healthcare, their options for dealing with the risk of disease or its complications, and their decisions about family life. It is still all too often the case that healthcare provided to a population is often delivered in an inequitable manner, with more care provided to those groups that need it least. It was a distinguished Welsh general practitioner from within the UK's NHS (Dr Julian Tudor Hart) who formulated this Inverse Care Law (Hart, 1971).

Improved awareness of genetic problems among medical and paramedical staff in both primary care and hospital-based specialities will undoubtedly help and is one of the principal aims of this book. This alone, however, is unlikely to have more than a minor effect unless there is a comparable change in the awareness and motivation of the population as a whole. Genetic counselling given to those who do not wish for it or who are unaware of the underlying problem is often an unrewarding and even futile procedure for professional and patient alike. Indeed, the idea of genetic counselling being imposed as an obligation conveys a strong sense of the ethos of eugenics. 'Compulsory counselling' would, indeed, be a contradiction in terms.

The author's view is that genetic counselling will have its full impact only when an awareness of its importance and availability is built into the general education of young people, especially around school-leaving age, and when the population is rather more scientifically literate in general. At a time when small families are the rule, it seems essential for those having children to be given every opportunity to ensure that their children will be healthy and to avoid known risk factors if they so wish. At present, public awareness of the subject, largely the result of television and increasingly the internet, is often focussed on problems and diagnostic techniques during pregnancy itself – quite the worst time for a considered appreciation of the situation. As a result, there is a real danger at present of increasing the general level of anxiety without any corresponding increase in the overall level of people's knowledge.

Fortunately, a shift of emphasis is occurring from pregnancy to the phase before conception (pre-conceptional rather than pre-conceptual, one hopes) with genetic counselling, or at least genetic screening tests, increasingly being requested prior to reproduction. This should permit a much more balanced and objective approach to the problems involved, but the positive effects can easily be undone if the offer of reproductive genetic testing is made within a for-profit business that glamourises the testing process, provides misinformation or perverts an otherwise decent sense of responsibility towards one's future children. These problems are apparent even within the United Kingdom, where most healthcare is still provided through the NHS, and appear much graver elsewhere. The commercial offer of antenatal screening by non-invasive prenatal testing (NIPT) is especially fraught by such pressures and problems (Nuffield Council Report, 2017).

A logical extension of these ideas is the development of 'preconception clinics' where couples planning a pregnancy or school-leavers considering their future families could receive information on a wide range of subjects relating to the health and well-being of a future child. Genetic aspects could be included along with other factors such as diet (notably folic acid), the avoidance of smoking, alcohol, 'recreational' drugs and medications, and the need for rubella immunisation. Rather than formal genetic counselling being directly associated with such a venture, it should be reserved for the small minority where a clear problem is identified by the taking of a simple family history.

A well-organised and motivated family practice would make an excellent setting for a preconception clinic and could allow contact with the less educated and motivated parts of the population who, as already mentioned, are the least likely to request advice although the most in need. If our health services are indeed to be led from within primary care, this seems an important and appropriate field in which primary care can take the lead. So far, largely due to the pressures of work load in primary care, there are still few signs of this happening on a wide scale, and this remains an unmet challenge for all those involved.

PREVENTION OF GENETIC DISEASE

Even with the most complete ascertainment and cooperation from the population, the prevention of inherited disorders has to rest on the basic facts of the genetic situation. Thus, in such dominantly inherited disorders as the familial cancers, where the proportion of cases due to new mutation is low, the prospect for prevention is ultimately good, in the sense of preventing disease in those genetically at risk although not for reducing the numbers born with the harmful mutation. For many other more severe and earlier-onset conditions, such as those many congenital malformations where almost all cases arise as new mutations, or even in a more common disorder such as achondroplasia (where new mutational events account for 80% of cases), genetic counselling and the application of genetic tests will have little impact on the population incidence of the disorder, since most cases will arise 'out of the blue' into a family that is not known to be at risk.

In earlier editions of this book, Huntington's disease was cited as an example of a dominant disorder with very few new mutations, where a genetic register and systematic genetic counselling might be expected to result in a marked long-term decline in disease prevalence. Recognition of the molecular basis has shown that, for this and other trinucleotide repeat disorders, such a suggestion is an oversimplification. The unstable nature of the mutation means that most apparent new mutations have arisen from a pool of healthy individuals carrying 'intermediate alleles', which can expand and cause overt disease in later generations. This does not in any way invalidate the systematic approach to genetic counselling for such conditions, nor the value of genetic registers, but it reinforces the need for careful consideration of what the goals for such efforts should be and on which diseases they should focus.

The same lack of population effects will apply to most rare autosomal recessive disorders, since the overwhelming majority of the abnormal genes are in healthy heterozygotes, who will not be aware of this unless they marry someone carrying the same harmful gene and have an affected child. Only the small number of second or subsequent cases in a sibship are likely to be preventable unless population screening of heterozygotes is feasible and appropriate, as discussed later.

X-linked disorders seem at first sight to be a suitable area for prevention in the population, and certainly the testing of the extended family for carrier status is probably one of the most valuable parts of genetic counselling. Even here, however, new mutations may account for a considerable proportion of cases, and efforts at prevention have to be seen in perspective. However, the experience of centres that have maintained a genetic register of Duchenne muscular dystrophy (DMD) patients and carriers has shown a progressive decrease in recurrent cases within families, alongside an increase in healthy births to couples at risk, while new mutation cases are still as common as before. Where centres do not maintain a register, to promote active continuing contact with families, experience shows that cascade screening within families rapidly falls away within a family network so that many female carriers do not, in practice, have the opportunity to be identified before they have an affected son. This major potential benefit of genetics services has often not been delivered largely because of a shortage of trained professionals.

For chromosome disorders, the benefits of the 'extended genetic counselling' approach are of great value where a harmful translocation or inversion is identified that could be carried in balanced form by healthy relatives (see Chapter 4). Prevention of the great majority of serious chromosome disorders (including Down syndrome) is only feasible through prenatal screening programmes (see later), implying the acceptance of the termination of affected pregnancies.

PREVENTION OF DISEASE IN THOSE AT RISK

While the reduction of serious genetic disorders by prenatal diagnosis and the selective termination of a pregnancy carrying an affected fetus can be a valid goal for families when treatment is absent or unsatisfactory, there are numerous other situations where the application of genetic approaches may result in the avoidance of serious morbidity or death for those who are at risk or affected, as discussed in Chapter 12. A combination of systematic ascertainment, maintenance of a genetic register and the offer of genetic testing to those at risk forms the basis of many preventive programmes. Examples that have already been discussed include the familial cancers, drug-induced disease (e.g. the porphyrias and malignant hyperthermia) and other chronic diseases such as adult polycystic kidney disease, where control of blood pressure and infection is facilitated by early detection. The most common disorder in this category, familial hypercholesterolaemia, has been relatively ignored until recently (see Chapter 21), reflecting perhaps inadequate awareness of genetic approaches by the clinicians and epidemiologists involved.

Common, 'multifactorial' disorders such as diabetes, hypertension and certain cancers are often raised as examples where the widespread identification of those at increased genetic susceptibility might be of benefit through allowing subsequent prevention of disease (see also Chapter 3). 'Changes in lifestyle' and 'targeted drug therapy' are arguments given in favour of this, but it has to be said that, at present, the evidence of benefit is almost wholly lacking. 'Lifestyles', whether in relation to diet or other aspects, are often remarkably resistant to change unless this involves the entire population and is driven by a systematic government policy. Although the UK's NHS is sometimes criticised for not being very effective at preventing disease, this criticism is really misdirected as major changes in diet, physical activity and air quality are simply not within the scope of action of any Health Service. To be effective at prevention would require interventions in government policy on housing, transport, agriculture and food, and retail law (at a minimum). Another possible approach is the use of genetic information in selecting drug therapies – 'therapeutic guidance' – but this remains a promising area of research rather than soundly established as being of proven benefit, however attractive to pharmaceutical manufacturers.

WILL GENETIC COUNSELLING INCREASE THE LOAD OF DELETERIOUS GENES?

The pessimist predicting harmful effects of genetic advances is likely to be as wrong as the optimist who hopes to eradicate (i.e. 'wipe out') genetic disease, if generalisations are made. We have already seen that genetic counselling may result in a reduction in frequency of serious disease in certain dominantly inherited and sex-linked disorders, but that with other conditions there is little effect. Influences increasing gene frequency are likely to be equally diverse.

Successful treatment of previously fatal or disabling dominant disorders might certainly allow a rapid rise in frequency if accompanied by unrestrained reproduction, although it would be the treatment, rather than genetic counselling, that would tend to produce this. If treatment of a disorder really proves successful, then the problem might be considered to have disappeared anyway unless the cost of treatment is very substantial; that decision will be specific to each particular set of circumstances.

Thus, the treatment of β-thalassaemia is arguably too costly for many of the countries where it is common, in the absence of any carrier screening programme alongside the provision of treatment. The only way for some poorer countries to afford treatment for affected children would be if their numbers were much reduced as a result of carrier screening and then the choice to use prenatal diagnosis (and selective termination) in pregnancies with a one in four chance of an affected child. A similar question might well arise in wealthier countries in the near future. Thus, the costs of enzyme replacement treatments – as for some of the mucopolysaccharidoses – are very high (>£100,000 annually) – and this would be prohibitive if the disorders were more common. However, the costs would also become prohibitive if comparably expensive treatments became available for many more rare diseases: they could not all be treated, even in wealthy countries.

X-linked disorders where fetal sexing used to be employed without a direct prenatal diagnosis might have provided an important example of where genetic measures could increase the population frequency. By allowing female carriers to have daughters (half of whom will themselves carry the gene) without the risk of having an affected son, it is likely that a steady (though ill-defined) increase would be seen. However, the use of this approach occurred during a transient phase of genetic technology. The direct prenatal diagnosis of affected males is now feasible for these conditions. This counters the effect by avoiding the abortion of healthy male fetuses, and so fewer pregnancies are needed to reach the desired family size.

A more important potential source of increase in deleterious genes might be expected to arise with the numerous polygenic malformations which in the past were generally fatal but for which treatment (usually surgical) now allows a near-normal lifespan and fertility. Congenital heart disease, pyloric stenosis, Hirschsprung disease and hydrocephalus are but a few examples. Although the risks for offspring of such individuals are relatively low (usually under 5%), there is no doubt that reproduction of such individuals will produce a slow but eventually appreciable rise in the overall level of genetic liability in the population. Again, it is the provision of treatment rather than genetic counselling that is likely to be the basis for any such change, and any effects are likely to be slow and open to being countered by an improved understanding of disease mechanisms leading to genuine 'primary' prevention.

MARRIAGE BETWEEN AFFECTED INDIVIDUALS

Marriage between affected individuals is common in some groups of disorders, such as congenital deafness, blindness and dwarfism. It may well also be increasing as a result of the social activities of 'disease-specific' lay societies. The genetic risks for couples in particular situations have already been discussed, but worry is sometimes expressed as to the overall effects of such assortative patterns of mating on the population level of the particular condition.

In fact, such effects are negligible in the case of rare Mendelian disorders and usually also for the more common polygenic disorders (e.g. diabetes). The general effect is a redistribution of affected children so that more are likely to be born to affected parents and fewer to unaffected parents. Thus, although genetic counselling is of great importance for these high-risk couples, their reproduction will have little overall effect on the population frequency of the disease or the genes.

The one circumstance where there could be a real effect might be marriage between people with autosomal recessive deafness, where all children will be affected if the deafness in the parents is caused by pathogenic variants in the same gene. However, this will never be common because there are so many different genetic causes of deafness. In any case, those affected usually have a static impairment rather than a progressive disease and may regard themselves as belonging to a minority culture (the Deaf) rather than having a serious disorder. The impact of newborn screening to detect hearing impairment, combined with the use of cochlear implants to ameliorate severe impairments, is relevant to these discussions; they may be experienced as a threat to the future of the minority Deaf culture. Their effects are difficult to predict over the long term.

INBREEDING AND OUTBREEDING

Many inbred populations are characterised by high levels of autosomal recessive disorders and, where this is the case, there is no doubt that outbreeding would greatly reduce the frequency of the disease. Thus, a marked increase in the proportion of marriages between Ashkenazi Jews and gentiles would sharply decrease the incidence of Tay-Sachs disease, especially common in the former. The overall gene frequency would not be decreased, but a greater proportion of the genes would be present in healthy heterozygotes whose partners would be less likely also to be carriers.

Conversely, fragmentation and isolation of populations combined with inbreeding, as seen in some minority migrant populations, are likely to increase the incidence of autosomal recessive disorders, even when the parent population does not have a particularly high frequency of deleterious genes. Again, it is not the gene frequency but the frequency of affected homozygotes that is increased. Prolonged inbreeding over many generations might in theory actually 'breed out' harmful recessive genes by progressively eliminating them as homozygotes. However, this would require much suffering over many generations – longer than the current social arrangements are likely to persist. This would not be a helpful course to recommend prospectively, and there is no evidence that it has actually occurred in inbred populations. While the precise effects on gene and phenotype frequencies are thoroughly analysed in a number of books on population genetics, the moral for the clinician is to be wary of generalisations, and to realise that in the great majority of situations the advice given to individual couples may have a profound effect on them and their offspring but will rarely alter the population structure to a significant extent.

The social aspects of consanguineous marriage are discussed in Chapter 10.

CULTURAL ASPECTS OF GENETIC COUNSELLING

Genetic counselling cannot be carried out in a vacuum, and the way it is practised inevitably reflects and interacts with the attitudes and structure of the society in which one works. In most Western countries, this society is now heterogeneous, containing a variety of ethnic, cultural and religious groups whose views on medicine, genetics and life in general may differ considerably. The authors, trained in a 'Western' milieu like most medical geneticists, have become increasingly aware that the approaches to genetic counselling outlined in this book cannot always be applied easily to families coming from different societies.

A comparable recognition has led to the involvement of workers, including non-medical genetic counsellors, from specific minority groups, especially when population programmes are involved, as with the haemoglobin disorders. The issue of consanguinity, already discussed, is another major area of societal difference, while the importance of using a language familiar to those seeking information is a further obvious, though often overlooked, point.

Some differences are difficult to reconcile with accepted concepts of genetic counselling but need to be recognised and perhaps confronted. The attitude to women in many more traditional societies may result in stigma and even divorce if a particular genetic defect is found to have come from the female partner, even if this is only inferred, construed or imagined by the man. One may have to be extremely careful in divulging information to a husband or male relative. Not infrequently, a woman may understand little English, and information filtered through the husband may be different from that given originally. In other communities (including much of the author's own South Wales population), men are traditionally peripheral to reproductive decisions, women frequently attending with their own mother, while the husband is left at work, or parking the car.

The traditional pattern of the extended family often runs contrary to the concept of privacy regarded as so important in modern Western society. In such a situation everyone in a family may want to know the result of someone's test, while requests for testing (including decisions on prenatal diagnosis) may be determined by older patriarchs or matriarchs, who may well not have been seen by those giving genetic counselling. Marriages may be arranged in childhood, leading to requests for testing on children that would otherwise have been postponed until adult life.

These are only a few of the complex issues about which anyone giving genetic counselling needs to be aware. However, awareness of cultural difference does not necessarily mean that genetic counselling should always try to fit in with the accepted practices of the relevant society or community. Thus, in eastern Europe, genetic counselling was traditionally directive, and colleagues in these countries frequently assured the author that this was what people expected and wanted. He long suspected that this was largely a reflection of people being faced with authoritarian rules and attitudes in all fields of life, and it has been interesting to see that political changes in these countries have been accompanied by a trend towards a more non-directive approach to genetic counselling.

POPULATION SCREENING FOR GENETIC DISORDERS

The term 'screening' is one that is used widely but often misleadingly in relation to various aspects of medical genetics. It should be confined to those programmes that aim to identify genetic disorders or gene carriers by studying broad groups, either entire populations or large subgroups (e.g. pregnant older women, the newborn, or those with intellectual disability), rather than specific individuals or families. Thus, genetic testing for Huntington's disease, or indeed most genetic testing within a family context, is not a population screening activity.

Screening for genetic disorders may in principle be a clinical activity or involve any form of testing, not just those using DNA-based technologies. For this reason, the term 'genetic screening' needs to be used cautiously and specifically, since DNA-based tests can also be used to screen for non-genetic disorders (e.g. viral infections), while many primary screening tests for genetic disorders do not use genetic technology.

Despite this, screening for genetic disorders does raise important issues over and above the more general ones common to all forms of screening. It is most important that these are not ignored when programmes are being planned and implemented, and there is a real danger of this happening since most of those involved with screening have an epidemiology and public health medicine background and are largely unfamiliar with genetic issues, while most geneticists are equally unfamiliar with epidemiology. Points of fundamental importance include the aim of the screening programme: is it primarily intended to eliminate a disorder or to help individual families and to allow choice? The impact on other family members must be taken into account, while the issues arising from detection of healthy carriers in a programme primarily designed to detect affected homozygotes must also be considered. Thus, if a newborn screening programme for an autosomal recessive disease were to identify every heterozygote, as often happens in screening programmes for sickle cell disease (but not for cystic fibrosis [CF]), the work of informing the parents of the sickle carrier infants and inviting them to be tested could consume much more energy and resources than the identification and management of the much less commonly affected homozygotes.

Most important of all is that, in a screening programme, those tested will mostly have no personal experience of the particular disorder and will not usually have actively requested the test, while the numbers involved may preclude the personal delivery of adequate information, genetic counselling and support.

All of these factors point to major differences between the ethos and practice of screening for genetic disorders and those of genetic counselling. They also help to explain why so many workers in clinical genetics are reluctant to see screening programmes introduced without very careful thought and planning.

Box 34.1 sets out the definition of screening and the key questions drawn up by the UK's National Screening Committee in weighing up whether or not to recommend a proposed screening programme. This list has been reworked from the original World Health Organisation (WHO) criteria for screening of Wilson and Jungner in 1968. Box 9.6 earlier in this volume is a guide to the assessment of screening tests, to clarify terms such as sensitivity, specificity and predictive value.

Box 34.2 summarises the main categories of screening programme that have been introduced or considered in relation to genetic disorders. Although the three main categories of newborn, prenatal and adult screening cannot be separated completely, this provides a reasonable framework for discussing the main issues.

BOX 34.1: Screening

Definition: 'The systematic application of a test or inquiry, to identify individuals at sufficient risk of a specific disorder to warrant further investigation or direct preventive action, amongst persons who have not sought medical attention on account of symptoms of that disorder.'

Key Questions:

The Condition
Is it an important health problem?
Are the epidemiology and natural history understood?
Have all cost-effective primary prevention interventions already been implemented?

The Test
Is there a simple, safe, precise and validated screening test?
Is the distribution of test values in the population known? Is there an agreed cut-off level?
Is it acceptable to the population?
Is there an agreed policy on further diagnostic investigation and the choices available to those who screen positive?

The Treatment
Does early detection lead to an effective treatment or intervention so that better outcomes are achieved?
Are there agreed policies for the offer of appropriate treatment?
Have clinical management and patient outcomes already been optimised?

The Programme
Is there randomised controlled trial (RCT) evidence of improved mortality or morbidity?
Is the complete screening programme acceptable to health professionals and the public?
Do the benefits of participation outweigh the physical and psychological harms?
Is there adequate staffing and are the facilities adequate?
Is there a plan in place for programme management and to monitor it for quality assurance?
Have all other options for managing the condition been considered?

Source: Modified from the UK's National Screening Committee.

BOX 34.2: Population screening for genetic disorders: Current and proposed examples

Newborn Biochemical Screening

Phenylketonuria

Congenital hypothyroidism.

Sickle cell disease

Cystic fibrosis

Duchenne muscular dystrophy (?)

Medium-chain acyl-coenzyme A dehydrogenase (MCAD) deficiency and other metabolic disorders: highly variable (Decisions about screening for specific metabolic disorders depend upon the disease incidence in the local population and the nature of the healthcare system. Screening for a greater range of disorders, sometimes more than 100 disorders, becomes technically possible once the analysis is performed by tandem mass spectrometry.)

Newborn Molecular Genetic Screening

Cystic fibrosis: Entails a secondary, DNA-based step if the serum immunoreactive trypsin (IRT) level is high

High-throughput sequencing (including whole genome sequencing) (!)

Prenatal Population Screening

Down syndrome and other autosomal trisomies (also detecting neural tube defects and other skin lesions): Biochemical testing on the pregnant woman (α-fetoprotein, hormones and other proteins) combined with fetal ultrasound scan. NIPT on cell-free DNA in maternal blood can be used as a secondary screen or (with some caution) as a primary screen; see Chapter 9

Neural tube defects: Fetal ultrasound scan

Presymptomatic (Adult)

Cholesterol: Molecular genetic screening may be offered as a secondary investigation when cholesterol is raised (Screening children has been proposed as a way to identify their affected but presymptomatic parents [?])

Carrier Screening – Adult (screening may be made available in a pregnancy or before conception)

Haemoglobinopathies

Tay-Sachs disease (and other disorders associated with the Ashkenazi Jewish population)

Cystic fibrosis

Wider range of autosomal recessive disorders with testing usually offered on a commercial basis, sometimes by a direct-to-consumer route. It would be important to ensure that the laboratory performing the test has appropriate clinical pathology accreditation and that the test is accompanied by high quality information and pre-test and post-test counselling and support.

Fragile X syndrome (FRAXA) (?): This is offered in Israel, and elsewhere on a commercial basis, but there are good grounds for caution; see Chapter 14

Opportunistic Genomic Screening (?)

This is mentioned here to draw attention to it and to contrast it to 'proper' population screening programmes. This term describes the reporting of additional findings, other than those related to the specific health indication for the genomic investigation that is being performed. These additional findings are often considered in two categories, as 'carrier' information of reproductive significance, and as indicating a risk for late-onset disease that may benefit from strategies to achieve prevention or surveillance (for early detection).

(?) *Indicates situations where the general case for screening has not been proven or where particular attention needs to be paid to the consent process. In the context of newborn screening, for example, this might be a two-tier system of consent.*

(!) *Probably inappropriate except as part of a properly conducted research study.*

NEWBORN SCREENING

Newborn screening in the population is principally established for treatable genetic disorders such as phenylketonuria (PKU), along with less clearly genetic disorders such as congenital hypothyroidism, both of which amply fulfil the traditional criteria of severity if untreated, good response to early (presymptomatic) treatment, simple and satisfactory screening and confirmatory (diagnostic) tests, and a relatively high frequency. A case can similarly be made for the inclusion of screening for sickle cell disease in high-risk populations, in order to provide prompt recognition and treatment of clinical problems. The genetic aspects are not the most important ones in such screening programmes.

More recently, newborn screening has been suggested for genetic disorders that are not fully treatable but where recurrence in sibs could be avoided by early diagnosis in the first child. DMD is a notable example that has raised some controversy. Evaluation of a programme in Wales has led the author to conclude that screening can be recommended but must be subject to two important requirements. First, it must be clearly marked as a very different type of screening from the more traditional, therapeutically oriented screening for PKU or hypothyroidism. To this end, there must be a definite step of parental choice in the screening process, which must be emphasised in a way that is not needed when the screening is for the direct benefit of the individual infant. Second, there must be a robust system in place to provide practical and emotional support for the family.

The question of informed decision, or informed choice, is an important aspect of this. In essence, the parent(s) must be asked what *type of person* they are: 'If it turns out that your child has a serious (life-limiting) and effectively untreatable (incurable) disorder, are you the type of person who would want to know about that at an early stage? Or would you prefer to wait until your child had developed some clear signs of the condition and you had sought medical attention?'

There are other disorders where the reasons for wanting to know – or not to know – that one's child is affected are different but the key distinction between neonatal screening tests that are for the benefit of the child her- or himself and those where the benefit is for someone else (the broader family, society, future patients, research enthusiasts, etc) is clear. Two categories of newborn screening tests can be handled quite simply in discussion and interaction with the parents: those that can be recommended for the sake of the child, where formal parental consent is not of great importance (in some countries, such tests are mandatory), and those where the child is not the primary beneficiary and where thorough discussion and explicit parental consent should be a requirement.

Screening for certain other disorders may combine elements of both settings, as with screening for CF where a case can be made for screening on the grounds of therapy as well as enabling family reproductive choice. In such cases, a decision has to be made as to which category the condition should fall into. In the case of CF, the author would include screening in the therapeutically oriented category alongside PKU, even though the treatments are often not as effective for CF as with PKU, because early diagnosis greatly facilitates the rapid introduction of the full set of treatment approaches.

It is clear that to justify screening for disorders on genetic grounds requires a detailed analysis of the effects of screening on families in addition to the criteria already mentioned.

The methods used in newborn screening for metabolic disorders have shifted over the past two decades from chromatographic approaches to tandem mass spectrometry (TMS). TMS enables the relatively simple detection of many disorders. The process of carefully weighing up conditions, one by one, to see which warrant screening, has been put aside in many places in favour of a single assessment of the technology. The question has become, 'Is TMS superior to chromatography as a laboratory method?', to which the answer is clearly yes. This evasion of the careful assessment of the impact of newborn screening for each disorder has been a temptation. The author's view is that the two categories of metabolic disorder discussed previously should be recognised, with some being tested for in all infants and the others, where the evidence in favour of screening is less compelling, should require careful parental consideration and explicit consent. This would not necessarily require a decision to be made about each disorder separately; the conditions could be grouped into two (or perhaps more) categories as set out earlier.

PRENATAL SCREENING FOR GENETIC DISORDERS

There has been a succession of developments in screening for genetic disorders in pregnancy that have cumulatively had a major impact on the way in which pregnancy is managed and perceived. Whether these are seen as having been a success or not depends largely on what the aims and outcomes of such programmes have been considered to be. If the primary aim is to reduce the birth frequency of a serious disorder, then some have certainly been successful. If the aim is to give maximum information, choice and support to women and their families, then the outcomes have been more questionable. In most cases the relevant issues have still not been adequately examined.

Many prenatal screening programmes have assumed that an affected pregnancy will be, and probably should be, terminated, with one notable exception – Rhesus haemolytic disease detection and immunisation – which stands alone as an example of the successful true (i.e. primary) prevention of a genetic disorder by prenatal screening. Somewhat similar is the single example of the primary prevention of a malformation: folic acid supplements to prevent neural tube defects.

Down syndrome – the most common genetic cause of cognitive impairment – has been the focus of prenatal screening for many years (see Chapters 4 and 9). Initially based on increased maternal age and amniocentesis, and then utilising biochemical testing of maternal serum and sometimes also fetal ultrasound scans for the preliminary screening test, the landscape of prenatal screening has not yet settled. The analysis of cell-free DNA in maternal blood has now become an important approach, either as the primary screening test or as a secondary screen that can greatly reduce the number of invasive tests performed if biochemical and ultrasound methods remain as the first tier of screening.

Prenatal screening for Down syndrome has certainly reduced the birth frequency of Down syndrome in many populations. In some countries, it has stabilised the birth incidence of trisomy 21 (T21) when the distribution of maternal ages has been increasing, so that a higher birth incidence would otherwise have been expected. There have been some concerns about inequity in the availability of screening, but there have also been problems in relation to the quality of information provided about screening, pressure to be tested, proper consent and choice and subsequent support. These latter issues were inadequately considered in the setting up of many programmes. Although now receiving proper evaluation by social scientists, it is difficult to shift long-standing practices that have been routinised within professional practice and the expectations of pregnant women. The primary aims of many programmes have been distorted through an excessive orientation to the 'public health' goal of reducing the birth frequency of Down syndrome in the population instead of giving priority to choice and the benefit of individual women and families.

The same concerns apply to screening for neural tube defects using serum α-fetoprotein (see Chapter 9) and to the more general screening for structural malformations using ultrasound. The lack of prior information and experience concerning a disorder can cause particular difficulties when coming at such a sensitive time.

While antenatal screening programmes have been upheld as beacons of progress, offering important choices to pregnant women, there have been other voices telling a different story that we must also heed. There are women who have felt coerced into compliance with antenatal screening programmes by forceful professionals or who have gone along with a routinised process, only to regret it later once they find it difficult to get off the conveyor belt of increasingly invasive procedures. There are women whose decisions are shaped by their lack of confidence in society's willingness to provide adequate support for them and their children, if their children had a serious disease or disability. Those who choose not to terminate an affected pregnancy – whether the fetus is affected by an inevitably lethal disorder or by a condition that, like Down syndrome, can often be compatible with a happy, healthy life – still sometimes (too often) experience the irritation, judgement or even hostility of their health professionals.

There are also patients with – affected by – some of the conditions that antenatal screening is seeking to detect (and perhaps eliminate), who feel hurt and distressed by the screening programmes that they feel are aimed at (against) them. They are likely already to feel stigmatised, and the decision of 'society' to use antenatal screening to prevent them coming into existence greatly strengthens this experience of imposed worthlessness and exclusion. This experience, voiced eloquently by the disability rights movement, is powerful and has to be weighed in the scale. The impact of screening on these individuals, who must also be of concern to us and may also be our patients, cannot simply be dismissed as irrelevant on the grounds that their view challenges the autonomy of the pregnant woman. This is not the place to resolve these various tensions, if indeed they can be resolved, but it is important at least to note them here.

So far, most prenatal screening approaches have not used modern genetic technology, but this is changing – especially with the use of maternal blood samples (e.g. screening of cell-free DNA from maternal blood to detect fetal autosomal trisomies). Suggestions that CF and fragile X syndrome might be screened for prenatally, whether through testing the mother herself in pregnancy or the fetus through the mother's blood, raise difficult questions. While it may be relatively simple to identify a healthy pregnant woman as 'merely a carrier' of CF, it is harder to be sure that a carrier fetus (with one pathogenic variant identified) is not in fact affected. In relation to fragile X, there are many more carriers of premutation and intermediate repeat sized alleles (nearly 1% in some reports) than there are affected fetuses (1 in 4,000 of either sex). If these women are given such results, it will be difficult to tell them what it means – what it will lead to in the child – and therefore it will be likely to generate great anxiety and little clarity. Furthermore, pregnancy is not the best time to give complex information to carriers of a full fragile X mutation, some of whom will suffer cognitive impairment.

It is fair to say that the entire development of prenatal genetic screening has been unbalanced, based on three powerful forces that have resisted efforts to assess their impact. The process has been technology driven both for its own sake and for the sake of profit, and there has been an underlying eugenic goal of eradicating particular disorders. Those individuals and interests that have driven the process have given inadequate consideration to its potentially toxic effects on individuals caught up in screening and on society as a whole. It is important that this field be radically and critically reassessed from a broader perspective. This is now beginning to happen. Within the United Kingdom, programmes are striving hard to reduce variations between districts and to ensure that the ethos of the programme in operation – as experienced by women – is supportive rather than steering. However, antenatal screening remains very much a 'technology-driven' field where commercial developments outpace the possibility for a measured and incremental development of evidence-based practice.

GENETIC SCREENING IN ADULTS

Population screening in later life for genetic disorders is infrequent at present. Indeed, the potential for identifying one common and serious genetic disorder, familial hypercholesterolaemia, has been largely ignored until recently, and often confused with more general cholesterol screening. It could be argued that the high frequency and treatable nature of familial hypercholesterolaemia make it perhaps the only subgroup of disorders with raised cholesterol levels that everyone would agree is worth detecting. Fortunately, carefully planned programmes, based on both lipid and DNA analysis and following the approach of 'cascade screening' (see later) have been established in several countries. Lipid analysis is needed to focus the DNA-based testing on appropriate individuals and then, when a pathogenic variant has been identified in a family, the DNA-based testing can be used for more reliable cascade testing among relatives.

Detection of the genetic subset of common cancers is an area under considerable discussion in relation to screening, although at present this is largely confined to family-based testing for the high-risk mutations. This is changing, however, with treatment decisions of established malignancies now sometimes being guided by the patient's genetic constitution and sometimes by the genetic constitution of the tumour. The term 'screening' is especially open to confusion in the context of family-based genetic testing, since those at high genetic risk may be offered screening for overt disease (e.g. mammography), while non-genetic screening may be the first-line approach in general population case detection (e.g. cervical cancer screening). At present, it seems unlikely that detection of heritable mutations giving a high cancer risk will be used as a population screening tool, although it has been proposed where one or a few specific pathogenic variants occur at high frequency in a particular population group (e.g. *BRCA* gene variants in Ashkenazi Jewish people). In the unique circumstances of Iceland, with a majority of the (very small) population enrolled in genome-based research, effectively all *BRCA* variants are known, and the problem is how to disseminate the results to those who are at risk but have not asked for their results.

A disorder for which screening has been suggested is haemochromatosis, where recognition of a genotype giving increased susceptibility is now feasible (see Chapter 23). This is a common condition in North-Western Europe as homozygotes for p.Cys282Tyr in the *HFE* gene are frequent, as high as 1% in some areas, although estimates of the penetrance have been so low (cumulatively <2% of homozygotes) that screening has been dismissed as inappropriate and the condition itself may be regarded as an autosomal recessive predisposition rather than a Mendelian disorder. Recent findings from UK Biobank, however, suggest a much higher penetrance in Britons as they age, so the case for screening may need to be reassessed (and the case for eating less meat may be strengthened). This debate will need to be revisited as more evidence emerges. If the case for screening does mount, then the age at which it could be recommended will be an important point to note. In addition, there will need to be agreement as to what (so far) healthy homozygotes should be told and what (if anything) to suggest to heterozygotes.

This example shows how screening for an apparently definite Mendelian disorder can merge into the more general area of susceptibility testing (Chapter 3), where at present even family-based testing is rarely helpful and wider screening is most likely to be positively harmful. It also reminds us how new knowledge can force a reassessment of the evidence and, potentially, a revision of policy.

Screening of particular subgroups, rather than of entire populations, may be appropriate for certain genetic disorders. A case can be made for this in screening those with mental handicap for fragile X syndrome, allowing an explanation to be provided for serious difficulties and allowing a high genetic risk to be recognised that may give options for family members to avoid recurrence of the disorder. Clear information and proper consent, with access to fuller genetic counselling, are essential factors that must be built into any such programmes. This requires adequate resourcing. Such screening of symptomatic, affected groups should be carefully distinguished from more general population and prenatal screening.

The term 'cascade screening' deserves a note here. This refers to the systematic testing of extended families to detect the abnormal genotype or disorder. For some conditions this may allow the detection of more such individuals than would be the case with general population screening, and without some of the problems mentioned previously because family members would often have some direct experience of the condition in their family. Familial hypercholesterolaemia provides an example of its value, and it has also been used in carrier screening for CF (see later).

Finally in this section, there are the direct-to-consumer (DTC) disease susceptibility tests that warrant mention. These screening tests pool the disease associations of multiple single nucleotide polymorphisms (SNPs) to give an estimated lifetime risk of certain diseases, especially the common complex diseases. Such tests are often based on highly significant associations between particular SNPs and the various diseases. However, the effect sizes of these SNP-disease associations are usually very small, which can be described as being both highly significant and essentially trivial, of no clinical utility. While the results may be of value to research, they are useless as clinical investigations. In the limited studies conducted, such test results do not seem to motivate lasting and positive ('medically appropriate') changes in behaviour.

While these DTC risk assessments will often be seen as an unhelpful and exploitative distraction, they may occasionally cause harm. This can arise if someone with an important Mendelian family history (e.g. of cardiac disease or cancer) purchases a DTC susceptibility assessment instead of coming forward for a conventional clinical genetic assessment. If the result they are given is modestly reassuring, as it could easily be, they might be discouraged from a referral to genetics services. Genetics services would be likely to arrange a search for pathogenic variants in the relevant genes. The DTC result would be unlikely to detect those, although this limitation may change once DTC testing comes to be based on exome or whole genome sequencing.

CARRIER SCREENING FOR AUTOSOMAL RECESSIVE DISORDERS

Much of our experience with carrier screening has come from historical work on the haemoglobin disorders, in particular β-thalassaemia, which represents a serious and extremely common problem in many Mediterranean and Asian countries. It is notable that carrier screening only became widely accepted once the option of prenatal diagnosis was available, in particular first-trimester DNA diagnosis. The remarkable degree of acceptance of carrier screening in combination with prenatal diagnosis in widely different countries, many with a traditional society not previously accepting termination of pregnancy, is an indication of how screening programmes can be successful, provided that they are carried out in sympathy with the attitudes of ordinary people. Such programmes must be accompanied by education and full information and must have a tangible result to offer – in this case the possibility of having healthy children without the risk of a progressive and severely disabling disease.

A comparably successful programme has been the introduction of carrier screening for Tay-Sachs disease in people of Ashkenazi Jewish origin. By contrast, sickle cell carrier screening was not successful in early programmes, including in the United States, partly because of the more variable nature of the disorder, and partly because of defects in the necessary educational and information aspects of the programmes.

The identification some 30 years ago of the gene for CF, the most common autosomal recessive disorder in northern Europe, has given the possibility of DNA-based screening for the carrier state. Simple screening tests can be used to identify over 95% of pathogenic variants in Europe and North America. A series of pilot projects were carried out to assess the feasibility and desirability of screening. Aspects studied include the timing and location of carrier screening (in antenatal clinic and primary care settings), the psychological effects on those screened, the attitudes of professionals and families and the costs of testing and counselling.

The results of these pilot programmes have been interesting and were not entirely anticipated. Essentially, they show a high degree of compliance with a thorough and sensitively handled screening programme, but only a low uptake when the initiative is left to individuals or when they are given a time interval in which to make a decision. The launch of 'over-the-counter' or postal DTC testing for CF carrier status, introduced to meet the supposed 'unmet demand' for this, has likewise had only a modest uptake. Thus, the conclusion must be that such carrier testing is a low priority for most people, and there is not a strong case for carrier screening outside families at risk becoming an established part of health services, whether during pregnancy or before conception.

The approach of 'cascade screening', noted earlier, has also been used in CF and some other autosomal recessive disorders. It has the advantage that a much higher proportion of individuals tested will be carriers and that many of them will be aware of the disorder because of its occurrence in the family.

Population screening for a wide range of recessively inherited disorders is now available commercially and has also been introduced in the healthcare system of some countries, notably Finland and Israel, and is in the process of being introduced by political directive in Australia. In both Finland and Israel, a history of population bottlenecks and sometimes also effectively endogamous population sub-groups has resulted in high frequency for a number of serious disease-causing genes. Several countries in the Middle East and North Africa have introduced carrier screening programmes tailored to the specific rare pathogenic variants in their populations. These various approaches will all provide a challenge to ensure satisfactory information and genetic counselling and could cause major problems if such multiple tests are offered as part of a 'laboratory-driven' or commercial venture. The problematic aspects of commercial carrier testing also include the knock-on additional demands placed on the local health services and the use of laboratories without appropriate clinical pathology accreditation.

OPPORTUNISTIC GENOMIC SCREENING

This final category of 'genetic screening' has not been formally launched as a form of population screening, but it has become clear that that is what it is. The essence can be summarised very simply: 'In those having exome- or genome-based DNA sequencing performed for another reason, would it not make sense to include a set of additional genes in the analysis if discovery of a pathogenic variant in one of those genes might lead to helpful medical interventions for the patient and/or their relatives?'

Enthusiasts argue that such additional genome-based investigations, without a particular indication in the patient, would simply entail examining more of their sequence information that has already been generated and would therefore have a low marginal cost. Such searching for additional findings should therefore not be expected to meet the full criteria for screening in the terms of a public health programme. At the same time, this would bring additional direct benefits to the patient and their family members, even when the patient is a child, and their parents are likely to be the first to benefit. Such a scheme would have a helpful educational impact for the public and for (non-genetics) health professionals, and it would help to accumulate experience in the interpretation of variant sequences in important, disease-related genes.

This can be presented as a win-win situation: what is there not to like about it? Well, there are several grounds for caution. First, there will be difficult and time-consuming decisions to be made about which genes to include in the list of those to be searched for additional findings, and which variants in these genes are sufficiently pathogenic to warrant disclosure and reporting. Second, the Inverse Care Law of Julian Tudor Hart predicts that those who will benefit from such opportunistic genomic analysis will usually come from the wealthier, less needy and better provided for section of the population, so that the additional resources committed to this extended analysis and the follow-on medical surveillance will lead to yet more investment of resources in the healthcare of the healthy: it will exacerbate inequity. Further, if the penetrance of the variants found is lower than expected – as may well be the case when their penetrance in this group is compared with their penetrance in the previously reported, high-penetrance families – then the benefits will rapidly diminish and the commitment of funds to long-term continuing medical care, such as repeated cardiac assessments and surveillance for malignancies, will escalate. The opportunity costs of this 'opportunistic screening' will therefore mount and become unsustainable. While this may not cause concern in a market-oriented system of healthcare, as those who cannot pay are invisible to the system, it will be a major problem in countries that strive to deliver equitable health to the whole population.

CONCLUSION

When genetic counselling is dealing with the individual family, it is often capable of being precise and helpful, and of profoundly affecting the decisions of individual couples. This is rarely true at the population level, and here the clinician should be sceptical about whether genetic counselling is having any significant effect, either beneficial or adverse, except in a few specific situations. This is perhaps fortunate, for it means that there is rarely any ethical conflict for either physician or patient between the course that is most beneficial for an individual or a family and that which is beneficial for society as a whole.

Finally, it should be borne in mind that variation is the basis of life and of evolution, for humans as for all other organisms, and that genetic characteristics today considered harmful may not always remain so. The 'thrifty genotype' of the diabetic patient may once have been associated with advantageous factors and may yet be again in a world with shrinking food resources. The evolutionary impact of copy number variants detected by chromosomal microarray, some of which have an adverse but reduced penetrance impact on development or mental health, is likely to reduce fertility. The phenylketonuric genotype, genetically lethal until very recently, is now almost of neutral effect, at least for males. The advent of successful treatment will undoubtedly ameliorate many other genetic diseases. However, while some evolutionary pressures and influences may appear to be waning, other factors will be shaping the direction of the continuing journey of human evolution. All we can know with confidence is that there will be differential reproductive success, so that human evolution will continue although we can only speculate as to how it will modify our successors.

35

Genetics, society and the future

INTRODUCTION

The previous chapter examined some of the ways by which new genetic advances can be delivered more generally to the population, rather than just to those who are already aware of their own need. It also addressed the advances that are being made in genetic (and genomic) screening and some of the associated problems. In this final chapter, the broader issues involving society itself are considered.

These new advances are having powerful effects on our social attitudes, widely disseminated through media publicity and often resulting in concern and controversy. This process also affects how genetics as a whole, including medical genetics, is perceived by the general population, a perception that is often ambivalent, even at times antagonistic, and which will have powerful effects on whether and how people use medical genetics services.

It may be argued that these wider issues are not directly relevant to genetic counselling, but this is not the case. The services we try to offer, at both individual family and population levels, are strongly influenced by the societal background and the attitudes of the community involved. Our approach needs to be adapted to those factors and respond to the interest or concern of society at large or specific sections of the community. One need look no further than such topics as prenatal diagnosis and consanguineous marriage to see how broader social factors have influenced the development of genetics services in different populations. Furthermore, there can be short-lived or sustained surges in demand when public attention is drawn to a specific disease or intervention; this can happen when a sensitive issue is discussed in a popular TV soap or when a high-profile personality uses genetics services, such as the actress Angelina Jolie.

Many of these issues have already been raised in the specific chapters of this book, but it is useful to bring them together here. No attempt is made to cover general ethical and philosophical topics, but rather those that impinge directly on clinical genetic practice, whether carried out by a specialist or by other clinicians in their particular field. It is important to recognise that, as genetic applications become increasingly used by all clinicians in their own particular fields – as the genetic approach to human health is 'mainstreamed' – some non-genetics specialists may have less prior awareness of these ethical and social issues, and the associated practical pitfalls, than do specialists with experience in medical genetics.

GENETIC TESTING ISSUES

Although genetic testing has been available in practice for many years in the form of chromosome and protein analyses, the large-scale development of DNA-based testing and its progressively greater use outside specialist centres have raised important issues that non-genetics specialists may not yet have encountered in practice even if the concepts are familiar. Some of these are raised here and have already stimulated considerable thinking and debate among workers in medical genetics, a healthy sign and one that is now spreading to those involved from more general fields.

What do we mean by genetic testing?

The original author offered the following working definition:

> Genetic testing is the analysis of a specific gene, its product or function, or other DNA and chromosome analysis, to detect or exclude an alteration likely to be associated with a genetic disorder.

Although most genetic testing is DNA based, it is the aim of the test, rather than the technology employed, that is important. Thus, phenotypic or protein-based tests such as electrophysiology in Charcot-Marie-Tooth disease or haemoglobin analysis in sickle cell disease can be regarded in principle as genetic tests when used to detect asymptomatic gene carriers (see Chapters 7 and 8), while DNA-based tests used for diagnosing infectious diseases are clearly not. Despite this lack of absolute distinction, though, it is principally the analysis of specific genes, especially in healthy individuals, that we are concerned with here.

Presymptomatic testing for late-onset disorders

This important topic has been largely covered in Chapter 8, but here the broader societal impact needs consideration. Experience from Huntington's disease and familial cancers has shown the need for the cautious handling of such testing, with proper consent, information and support. The perception of those tested and found to have an abnormal result is that they frequently consider themselves as already 'affected'. This misapprehension is often mirrored by professionals and by society in general and may powerfully affect society's attitude towards those carrying genes for serious late-onset disorders.

As such presymptomatic testing becomes more widespread, a population of asymptomatic gene carriers destined to develop serious genetic disorders has developed, the 'worried well' or 'patients-in-waiting'. The situation is not unlike that for HIV carriers in the past, before AIDS could be managed so effectively, and the potential for stigmatisation and discrimination is comparable, whether this be for employment, insurance or social relationships. One could suggest that the way in which society treats such individuals is an indicator of its maturity and humanity.

Genetic testing of children

The independence of DNA testing from a person's age makes it possible to test for a disorder at any stage of life, regardless of the usual time of onset. To test young children for a late-onset disorder that is not likely to have effects until adult life, and which is untreatable, poses serious problems. This first arose in relation to Huntington's disease when genetics clinics received requests to test children from parents and social workers. Testing was refused on the grounds that it would not benefit the child and would remove any later choice, and subsequently guidelines from professional organisations and disease support groups have supported the view that, unless there is clinical benefit to being tested earlier, predictive genetic testing for late-onset disorders should normally be postponed until the individual can give full consent. Clearly, the situation may vary according to whether treatment exists or whether the condition may also have childhood onset; individual circumstances need careful consideration, but the general principle remains valid.

Different issues arise when adolescents themselves request genetic testing (although the two situations are often confused). Again, current guidelines suggest postponement of testing until an individual becomes an adult, but the topic will need full discussion with the individual, and the maturity of the adolescent will be an important factor. A request for testing can often be a mask for a more general need for information and support, making it all the more important that sensitive discussion precedes any decision on actual testing. In the United Kingdom, decisions on genetic testing and the privacy of results need to be considered in light of the 1985 *Gillick* case, which considers individuals over 16 years old to be competent in relation to contraception and other reproductive issues, and for them and professionals to have the right to withhold information from parents, if necessary. Children of less than 16 years may also be regarded as competent if they are sufficiently mature. How, or even whether, one might become sufficiently mature for such predictive testing before the age of 16 years – or any arbitrary age – has not been determined. Instead, it is assessed using the regular guidance for testing mental capacity in the law of England and Wales: the ability of a person to understand the information given to them, to retain that information (for long enough to make the decision), to weigh the available information and to communicate their decision.

Paediatricians have been giving careful thought to this important topic – not only in relation to genetic testing but more generally to the question of consent to medical treatment – but many other specialists have not yet done so. There has been a convergence of paediatricians' views, at least in the United Kingdom, with those outlined previously, already held by most clinical geneticists.

The rather different context of 'opportunistic genomic screening' is discussed in Chapter 34, but it should be noted that there are particular implications when the sample concerned comes from a child. Whereas predictive genetic testing for a known family disorder can be framed for the developing child by the parents and by the relevant professionals as a decision that is being explicitly left for them to make when older, that situation cannot apply when the family is unaware that their child is at risk of a late-onset inherited disorder. Rather, to exclude children from genomic screening that would be regarded as helpful when applied to adults would be to deny important potential benefits not only to those children but also to their at-risk parents. Testing children in such circumstances would not cut across and undermine a carefully planned process of informing the child and leading them to the possibility of making their own decision at an appropriate time. Instead, it would give them the chance to gain from such medical information both directly and, perhaps, indirectly too, if it proved helpful in preserving the life and health of their parent(s).

Use of research samples

Most research on genetic disorders requires samples from patients, and many workers have a large series of stored DNA samples from both affected and at-risk family members. When the genetic basis of a particular disease is discovered, what should one do – or not do – with these samples?

Using the samples from affected individuals does not pose serious problems, but to test samples from those at risk carries grave consequences, since it is likely that some will show the relevant pathogenic (or, at least, risk-increasing) genotype. The research worker is then in the serious situation of having important information on people without their knowledge, often not knowing whether they would have wished to be tested or what they originally gave consent for. Such samples should not have been used in the first place; if the person requests testing, it is better to take a separate sample specifically for this, after appropriate counselling (i.e. explanation and consideration). Comparable issues can arise when genetic tests are incorporated into a more general research study, identifying individuals with a genetic basis for their disease among a larger group of patients (e.g. in studies of cancer).

As with the other topics in this chapter, there is also the 'opportunistic genomic screening' dimension. Special care must be taken not to make assumptions about what additional investigations would be wanted by research participants, even when the enthusiastic and well-meaning researcher imagines that they would clearly be 'A Good Thing'. If health screening of some form is to be incorporated into research and reported back to the patient/participant, this must be with full information, choice and considered agreement in advance.

Insurance and genetic testing

The past 25 years have seen a long-standing struggle between the insurance industry, unwilling to accept any regulation and insisting that genetic tests on healthy individuals are 'no different from other medical information', and professionals in genetics, supported by a series of independent government reports in several countries, who have pointed out the dangers of individuals being forced to disclose information on genetic tests that they have had for entirely different purposes. Detailed actuarial studies have now confirmed the authors' view that, at least for life insurance, the industry would suffer little from not demanding such results except when very large sums would be at stake. An agreement is in place in the United Kingdom between government and the insurers that such information should only be used by the industry in very restricted circumstances, and legislation restricting use of this information in insurance is now in place in the United States and some European countries. The adverse publicity that this issue generated for the insurance industry is an indication of how society is becoming reluctant to see new advances used to harm, rather than to benefit, its members.

How can we ensure that the expansion in positive and helpful applications of genetic testing to health and healthcare is not constrained by fears of how it will be used to people's disadvantage by insurance companies (and in other ways)? The best approach will be to ensure that there is a system of high-quality healthcare provided either by the state or through a comprehensive (compulsory) health insurance scheme, along with full support for those who cannot afford this. There will then be a strong motivation for the providers of healthcare to bring into practice those advances in genetic medicine that are shown to improve outcomes at a reasonable, proportionate cost. This is to everyone's advantage and is superior to a system in which the effectiveness of marketing strategies can (all too easily) drive the application of gene-based (or other) methods in screening, diagnosis and treatment that are not based on sound evidence assessed through a transparent mechanism.

Without such protection from the adverse effects of genetic disease (and the effects of the risk of genetic disease), there is a danger that genetics services will only be accessible to those in employment and with comfortable incomes. Genetics would then exacerbate social inequalities. This effect would be greater where inequality is already more marked, because more people would be unable to afford adequate health insurance and would therefore be more easily bankrupted by the costs of healthcare and then left without healthcare. Some form of social healthcare or social health insurance is therefore necessary if society is to realise the potential benefit of 'the genetics approach to human health'.

'Direct-to-consumer' genetic testing

The traditional model of investigations, as being tests ordered by a clinician after they have been consulted by the patient with a specific complaint, has served medical genetics well but, as in other fields, is faced by increasing challenges. This is partly because of increasingly consumerist attitudes to medicine, especially in the United States, but also because the internet now provides a means of promoting and delivering such 'direct-to-consumer' (DTC) services without being bound by the regulations and restrictions of specific countries that still restrict 'over-the-counter' genetic testing. The great majority of genetic tests promoted in this way are of minimal or no clinical value, and they are often accompanied by misleading or frankly erroneous information, for purely commercial ends. This is not only a waste of people's money and likely to generate unnecessary anxieties, but it also has serious consequences for the organised and equitable provision of healthcare.

These current and future challenges require critical reflection on where genetics professionals stand in relation to them. This is clearly essential in such a rapidly evolving area. Over-the-counter testing is already widely accepted in such areas as pregnancy testing, cholesterol testing and paternity testing, and in one sense, DTC for genetic tests could be seen as an extension of the outward diffusion of genetic testing from specialist geneticists to more general clinical workers that is now largely established in many parts of medicine. However, it raises many concerns and challenges, and these cannot simply be dismissed. These problems can arise in several ways:

1. Lack of a clear distinction between 'recreational' genetic testing and testing that may have serious health or social consequences, as when 'ancestry' testing unexpectedly provides information about medical risks (e.g. of cancer) or about paternity (when the results are compared with those of other family members).
2. Commercial marketing that achieves uptake by misleading the public, through generating inappropriate fears, exaggerating the benefits from testing or making clearly false claims that actively mislead (beware the blurring between 'marketing' and 'counselling').
3. Providing inadequate information in advance of a test, failing to provide appropriate support for making decisions, or inadequate explanation of the results afterwards.
4. The knock-on imposition of costs on regular health services, such as the National Health Service in the United Kingdom, because the results of testing have either generated inappropriate fears or raised appropriate concerns but without meeting the needs so created. This undermines the equitable provision of care to the population because of the opportunity costs of responding to such concerns.

5. The use of tests, such as non-invasive prenatal testing (NIPT) screening for fetal abnormality, outside their area of acceptable performance. While the performance of NIPT in screening for autosomal trisomies may be acceptable, it may be extended inappropriately to other disorders, such as certain chromosomal microdeletions. Such practices arise when tests are promoted dishonestly – to obtain a competitive advantage – either through a failure to give a clear description of their performance (e.g. not reporting the test's positive predictive value) or as detecting more abnormalities than is warranted (extending the scope of the test to include screening for microdeletions, where its performance may be ill-defined).

Commercial DTC testing began with carrier screening, especially for cystic fibrosis and other autosomal recessive conditions, and then moved into disease susceptibility profiling based on genome-wide (disease) association studies (GWAS). The carrier screening aspects have since diversified, and current carrier screening tests now cover many conditions and are marketed to those in their reproductive years, sometimes through private antenatal clinics. Susceptibility screening has come up against some thorny biological and psychological facts. Biologically, while many disease associations with specific single nucleotide polymorphism variants have been identified, they are mostly very weak (with relative risks usually of less than 1:1.05) although often achieving high levels of statistical significance. It has only proved possible through GWAS to identify a rather modest fraction of the genetic variation that contributes to the heritability of many complex disorders, presumably because of complexities such as gene-gene and gene-environment interactions that are difficult to measure. Psychologically, it seems that those given advice based on these GWAS usually fail to make lasting changes to their lifestyle and their health-related behaviours in light of this advice (which, in any case, has often consisted of 'exercise more' and 'eat more fruits and vegetables, less meat and calories', whatever the pattern of test results).

As exome sequencing and whole genome sequencing have been taken up by private laboratories and healthcare companies, they have become available to the healthy wealthy despite the difficulties of interpretation that are encountered in the bioinformatic analysis of samples from those with a genetic disorder. Interpreting the whole genome sequence of a healthy person may identify some useful information but is even more likely than focussed investigation of a patient (with a problem) to raise questions that it takes further, and inappropriate, medicalisation to resolve. Such tests have been greeted with uncritical enthusiasm for widespread testing by basic (non-clinical) genetics researchers, many of whom should know better, together with corresponding commercial enthusiasm from companies that wish to see a return on their investment. These two, often overlapping, groups have generated a degree of 'hype' that risks bringing more reputable and justified genetic testing into disrepute.

Fortunately, a brake on unhelpful developments is provided in those countries (mainly European at present) fortunate enough to have a universal system of healthcare, by regulatory mechanisms that not only discourage DTC approaches, but which fund only those tests for which there is a satisfactory evidence base of both scientific validity and clinical utility. In such countries, testing for most of the serious genetic disorders covered by this book is already available without charge, as is the proper professional advice that goes with it, which most families regard as helpful rather than as a barrier to genetic testing.

At present, it is difficult to know whether there is indeed any significant demand for, as opposed to promotion of, these DTC services. Data on uptake are normally unavailable, and the main guide to future trends is likely to be the number of genetic counselling referrals prompted by anxiety or confusion resulting from such testing. From experience in South Wales (United Kingdom), it seems that such referrals are still infrequent, suggesting that actual use of DTC tests remains minimal in relation to serious genetic disorders, contrasting with what one might conclude from media publicity. Rather more frequent are referrals resulting from the use of genetic tests by poorly informed clinicians who are not always aware of the complexities and sensitive issues in medical genetics. However, the experience of other geographical areas in the United Kingdom, especially south-east England, may be different as the uptake of private medical care is greater there.

Regulation of genetic testing

Until recently, there have been few regulations, advisory or mandatory, in the field of genetic testing. Fortunately, this has now changed in two respects. First, a number of UK advisory bodies have taken a real interest in the applications of genetic testing within healthcare and have produced reports on many of the major issues, both practical and ethical. These include the Human Genetics Commission (HGC), the Nuffield Council on Bioethics, and the PHG Foundation, whose recommendations are likely to be as influential as the passing of actual laws in such a rapidly changing field as medical genetics. There have also been very helpful reports on comparable topics from the relevant committees of the British Society for Genetic Medicine, the European, American and Australasian Societies of Human Genetics, and the American College of Medical Genetics and Genomics (see Appendix 1). One recurrent question raised in such reports is how the validity and clinical utility of genetic investigations can be built into the processes of licensing for such tests, an important way to restrain inappropriate commercial developments.

Second, there have been developments in the regulation of medical tests and devices, especially within the framework of the European Union, and there have been developments in English law – both statute law and case law – in relation to the capacity to consent, the duty of confidentiality and data protection. These have mostly been helpful although perhaps appearing monolithic and threatening from a distance. We are now adjusting to the requirements of the EU's GDPR (General Data Protection Regulations) and are waiting to see the outcome of a potentially landmark case about the obligation of health professionals to breach patient confidentiality and pass information about one family member to others who may benefit from access to that information. These various developments are likely to have substantial implications for how medical genetics is practised in the future.

One of the few areas of genetic work in the United Kingdom that is legally controlled is that of pre-implantation genetic diagnosis and *in vitro* fertilisation, with oversight by the Human Fertilisation and Embryology Authority.

The United Kingdom used to benefit from a well-established and independent advisory committee, the HGC, mentioned previously. This dealt with broad social and ethical issues in genetics and produced helpful reports on matters such as genetic testing and insurance, genetic privacy, over-the-counter testing, reproductive decision-making, carrier screening, and genetic testing for late-onset disorders. It was a broad-based body with only a minority of expert professionals. It is missed. (I should confess that both the original and the current author of this book served on the HGC and so this opinion may not be thought of as being as independent as the commission certainly was.)

In some parts of the United States, state (not federal) laws have been passed limiting the use of genetic testing, particularly in relation to insurance. However, a much more important federal law, the Genetic Information Nondiscrimination Act, took effect at the end of 2009. This prevents insurance companies making use of certain information in deciding whether or not to provide health insurance (it does not apply to life insurance) or what premiums to charge. The protected types of information concern family health history, the results of genetic tests, the use of genetic counselling and other genetics services, and participation in genetics research. The scope of the law has been restricted somewhat. President Trump acted (in 2017) to enable employers to require their workers to disclose genetic information. This is of concern because in the United States, health insurance coverage is often provided through employers.

AIMS AND OUTCOME MEASURES IN GENETIC COUNSELLING

Any professional activity, especially if it is being supported by public funding, needs to be able to produce clear goals as to what it is trying to achieve, and objective evidence that it is being successful in meeting those goals. In relation to genetic counselling, the whole area of aims and outcome measures is extremely complex, and it is as well to recognise that there are no simple answers. It is somewhat easier to indicate which aims and outcome measures are inappropriate, especially since some of these have already been, and continue to be, used.

The reduction or elimination of genetic disorders is not (at least in the view of the author and most professionals in the field) an aim of genetic counselling, even though it could perhaps, in carefully defined circumstances, be a valid aim of a broader population programme. Correspondingly, outcome measures such as the number of pregnancies terminated or estimated financial savings from a reduced number of births of affected infants are not appropriate measures in any assessment of genetic counselling, or indeed for medical genetics services as a whole.

A key difficulty in determining the outcomes of genetic counselling is that the aim of each consultation is set by the patient and negotiated between the patient and the professional: a global aim is therefore hard to define. Attempts to assess such areas as understanding of information given, reproductive plans and behaviour, patient satisfaction and the measurement of process aspects of the care provided have all been attempted. While they may assess certain aspects of the quality of a service, they do not address outcomes. However, real progress has been made by my colleague Dr Marion McAllister in her development and validation of a 24-item questionnaire that can define the impact of genetics services when used before and after an episode of care: this is the Genetic Counselling Outcome Scale (GCOS24). It focuses particularly on the sense of empowerment of patients and families, given their understanding of their condition and their adjustment to their situation. An abbreviated, six-item form of this scale (Genomics Outcome Scale, GOS) has been developed to assess the impact of addressing genetic aspects of care in non-genetics medical services (i.e. in the context of 'mainstreaming').

PRIVACY AND CONFIDENTIALITY

Genetic counselling raises some extremely difficult issues in this important area, something that is inevitable since the process so often depends on having accurate information on family members and since its implications may extend far beyond those individuals seeking advice.

It should be stressed that, in practice, most difficulties can be resolved provided that time and trouble are taken to ask people's permission, to explain why information is being requested and, in the case of risks to the extended family, to ascertain as far as possible whether they wish for information to be shared.

Given such a careful and sensitive approach, most family members will prove helpful and reasonable, although the process may take considerable time. The temptation to 'cut corners' and assume consent when it has not been specifically given must be strongly resisted. Written permission is increasingly the rule, and is a valuable safeguard if problems arise at a later stage.

In the very few situations where relatives persist in refusing to give access to their records or test results after appropriate approaches have been made, this usually reflects family conflict or sometimes fear and denial of a genetic disorder. It has been suggested that the need of relatives may in some circumstances override the basic principles of confidentiality, but the author's view is that such situations are exceptional and must be based on clear evidence of the harm that would result if the information were not available. Against such abandonment of confidentiality must be set the effects of a general loss of trust if individuals were to feel that their personal genetic data could be divulged in situations other than dire need.

Having said this, it may be perfectly reasonable for a laboratory to make use of information about the details of the genetic test result of one family member in arranging a genetic investigation on another, even without consent, as long as the second individual is not given any personal information about the first that he or she does not already know. Indeed, they will usually have come forward for genetic testing precisely because they already know of the condition affecting their relative. Making use of such technical information within the laboratory would not, in the author's view of the ethics, entail a breach of confidence, although the situation in law may be different and will vary between jurisdictions.

Much more common, in the author's experience, are requests for information from third parties which can and should be firmly denied unless specific permission is given. These include requests from insurers, employers, social services, adoption agencies and various other bodies. There is no case for 'public health interest' disclosure of information as may be present for certain infectious diseases.

At a practical level, difficulty may arise when one is seeing several members of a family separately and is unaware of what information they have shared between themselves. It is best to assume that nothing has been shared and to keep information compartmentalised unless one has clear permission to the contrary. Sometimes it can be preferable for a colleague to see a different branch of a family if it becomes too complicated for one practitioner to keep them separate.

General issues of privacy, confidentiality and consent have become of increasing concern in medicine overall and the consequences of ignoring this have been shown in a series of high-profile cases involving pathology (see Chapter 10). Legislation is increasingly being introduced (e.g. the *Gillick* ruling mentioned previously in relation to testing adolescent minors), but in the practical situations involving genetic counselling one is only rarely in serious difficulty if one follows the broad lines indicated earlier.

REPRODUCTION, EUGENICS AND THE ABUSE OF GENETICS

Everyone working in medicine, whether clinician or scientist, likes to believe that their own field is making a special contribution to human health and well-being. Those of us in medical genetics are no exception, and indeed the advances of recent years have helped families in ways that were unthought of only a generation ago. There is a darker side, though, which needs to be recognised, not ignored. This relates to what is generally known as eugenics, in which the principles of genetics (as understood in the past) were applied to attempting to change the genetic makeup of the population in general, rather than to individual families.

The language and 'science' of eugenics had their origins in nineteenth-century Britain but later became widespread in other European countries and in the United States. Eugenics was closely bound up with the social systems of the time, notably the rigidities of class and the deprivation of much of the population. It was convenient to find a biological explanation in terms of genetic inferiority for these deep-seated problems, with solutions that justified the maintenance of the social status quo. The newly emerging concepts of quantitative and Mendelian inheritance were enthusiastically applied not just to clearly inherited disorders but to a whole series of diseases and characteristics that today would be regarded as heterogeneous and complex in their basis, such as cognitive impairment, mental illness, epilepsy, alcoholism and criminality.

These and other studies, enthusiastic but largely uncritical in nature, provided the scientific justification for a series of coercive measures, including the segregation, institutionalisation and (particularly in the United States) sterilisation of mentally impaired people and other groups. Restrictive legislation on proposed immigrants was another aspect in the United States and Australia. While politicians were responsible for the implementation of these measures, they were enthusiastically promoted and supported by many scientists (notably Charles Davenport, director of the Cold Spring Harbor Laboratory, New York).

The lowest point in the history of eugenics was reached in Nazi Germany, where in 1933 a national eugenics law was one of the first measures introduced, and where compulsory sterilisation of those with mental illness or impairment, along with people suffering from disorders such as Huntington's disease, was followed by the active killing of such individuals, together with those with mental handicap and with congenital malformations. Again, it is tempting to regard this terrible chapter in history as an aberration and to blame the politicians, but this would be wrong. The entire basis for these policies was provided by scientists, including some of the most eminent geneticists of the time, and by clinicians, notably psychiatrists. It should not be forgotten that Josef Mengele was himself a human geneticist.

Eugenics is now a largely discredited field, but it has recently, to the great concern of many people, re-emerged in China, where a frankly eugenic law has been introduced under the guise of 'maternal and child health'. Fortunately, continuing opposition among many professionals seems – perhaps, and for the present – to have resulted in the application of this being quietly abandoned.

If serious abuses of new genetic developments are not to occur again, everyone – especially those working in medical genetics – must be aware of the past and its potential threat to the future. The increase in the power of technology, especially in computing and molecular genetics, makes it especially necessary to ensure that safeguards are introduced as these techniques are applied.

CONCLUSION

The range and depth of the many societal issues arising in genetic counselling, including those outlined, may seem daunting for the professionals involved, and it is easy to feel at times that one's own concepts of 'good practice' are likely to be submerged beneath an avalanche of inappropriate or even harmful developments. The views of both authors – the original author and the present one – are somewhat more optimistic. It is remarkable to see how issues recognised and views held by the relatively small number of practising clinical geneticists and genetic counsellors have gradually permeated not only the medical genetics community, but also the work of clinicians and laboratory colleagues more generally, until they have eventually become acknowledged as standard good practice.

There are three pressing challenges of today for genetic counselling, within western healthcare, which appear to the present author to be as follows: (1) excessive enthusiasm on the part of scientists, (2) institutional constraints on good practice and (3) inequity of access to healthcare that is actually exacerbated by the system of healthcare.

The excessive and uncritical enthusiasm arises in part from a natural wish to see benefit come from one's scientific insights. However, this will sometimes drive the too early implementation of technologies that should be handled with greater initial caution and wariness. Some scientists are so enthusiastic, and so focussed on progress, that they appear willing for the patients of today to suffer (if that is what it takes to climb the learning curve) for the sake of this progress, as if they were promoting a revolution. However, any risks or distress that arise will usually not be experienced by these scientists but by others: their patients or research participants. Some enthusiastic scientists may also have their judgement clouded by their commercial involvement in genome-based corporations. The declaration that a scientist has a commercial conflict of interest in relation to judgements about their science is too often understood by journals, conferences and advisory bodies to neutralise this conflict, when it does not do that at all.

The institutional constraints on good genetic counselling practice arise both in national healthcare systems and in private systems, being driven by the desire to cut costs. This takes the form of a pressure to see more patients in a given time than is compatible with high-quality practice, as staff costs will often exceed most other costs of a genetic counselling service. It will often entail a division of labour that separates tasks and leads to a less personal approach to care. Thus, one practitioner may collect family history information by phone while a second meets the patient or family at an initial clinic appointment and a third sees them at a second, follow-up appointment if that is deemed necessary (i.e. if that can be justified in terms of the institution's policies). Such cost-driven approaches make it much more difficult for strong patient-professional relationships to develop and be sustained. We know these are highly valued by patients and their loss is damaging, although this may not be so important when (for example) genetic tests are being used to address straightforward medical questions. However, when the patient's concerns relate to reproductive decisions, family communication and perhaps the offer of family cascade testing, predictive testing (with no clear medical indication for testing), or a difficult diagnostic process of a child with complex problems, a continuing relationship between counsellor and family is key. Those who have not experienced such a service may not appreciate the difference it makes to the patients involved and their families.

Inequity of access to healthcare – one aspect of the more general 'Inverse Care Law' of Tudor Hart (1971) – is an important fact that applies to the provision of healthcare, even within a state-supported system such as the UK's National Health Service. Unless we build an awareness of this into plans for developing genetics services, there will be numerous opportunities for those with more needs and lower expectations to be further disadvantaged by genomics: it could exacerbate inequity in healthcare and inequalities in health. For example, expecting patients to prompt reassessment in the genetics clinics, 'in a few years, once we understand this better', or to 'contact us again once you hear about advances in treating the disease', will function well for some but not for those in poverty, or those who are exhausted by coping with disease or disability in themselves or in family members, or who have learning difficulties, or who lack internet access or who depend on public transport. We have to develop systems that can function to benefit everyone across the whole of society.

Working in the field of medical genetics and genetic counselling offers remarkable opportunities for being in the forefront of, and helping to shape, new patterns of medical practice. It provides challenges, too, in trying to ensure that one's own practice can set an example to others, and in one's efforts to educate colleagues more generally to adopt comparable standards. Medical genetics in general, and genetic counselling in particular, is now an activity that extends far beyond the boundaries of medical genetics as a specialty, and how families are best helped is increasingly dependent on those whose main background and training lie outside this field. This book has been written – and revised – in the hope that such workers can recognise the facts, problems and issues that arise in relation to genetic disorders, and can use this understanding with a practical wisdom and sensitivity to help the families with whom they are involved.

Glossary

The following list includes only those genetic terms used in this book that may be unfamiliar. A more complete list can be found in King RC, Stansfield WD, Mulligan PK, 2006, *A Dictionary of Genetics*, Oxford University Press, Oxford.

allele: One of several alternative forms of a gene

amniocentesis: The procedure of taking a sample of amniotic fluid from the pregnant uterus

aneuploidy: The occurrence of an additional or missing chromosome to give an unbalanced chromosome complement

anticipation: The occurrence of a genetic disorder at earlier age of onset and/or at greater severity in successive generations

autosomal: Determined by a gene on one of the chromosomes other than the sex chromosomes

Barr body: The sex chromatin body visible beneath the nuclear membrane of a cell from a female, representing the inactive X chromosome

candidate gene: A gene suspected as being the gene mutated in a given disorder

Caenorhabditis elegans: A simple nematode worm, used as a model organism, whose genome has been completely sequenced

cDNA (complementary DNA): A DNA sequence corresponding to the messenger RNA produced by a gene, and lacking the non-coding regions (introns) of the gene

centromere: The portion of the chromosome joining the two chromatids and separating the long and short arms of the chromosome

chimaera: An individual containing cells of more than a single genetic origin

chorion biopsy (chorionic villus sampling): The sampling of tissue from the chorionic membrane of the embryo

chromatid: A single DNA strand of a dividing chromosome (i.e. one double helix), joined to its 'sister chromatid' at the centromere

chromatin: The proteins and other materials composing the structure of the chromosomes in conjunction with the DNA itself

chromosome: A structure within the nucleus (normally numbering 46 in humans), consisting of a long molecule of double-stranded DNA, bearing a linear arrangement of genes, which is associated with nucleoproteins and RNA; it condenses to become visible under the microscope at cell division, and it is able to reproduce its molecular structure with great fidelity through successive cell divisions and in transmission from generation to generation

clone: An identical copy of a DNA sequence, cell or whole organism; 'to clone' also means to isolate and replicate a specific DNA sequence or gene

comparative genomic hybridixation (CGH): A method for detecting increased or decreased copies of a gene sequence, either constitutional or somatic

congenital: Present at birth

consanguinity: Mating between close relatives

consultand: The individual (not always affected) through whom a family with a genetic disorder comes to clinical attention

cytogenetics: The study of chromosomes, their structure, function and abnormalities

deletion: Loss of genetic material (may be applied to a chromosome or a gene)

disomy, uniparental: The transmission of both copies of a chromosome from a single parent, instead of one from each parent

dizygotic twins: Twins originating from two fertilised eggs

DNA: Deoxyribonucleic acid, the molecule whose sequence and replication determine the genetic information present in genes and chromosomes

dominant: A characteristic or disorder expressed in the heterozygote, i.e. requiring only one altered copy to show itself

Drosophila: The fruit fly, a classical experimental organism for genetic studies, whose genome has been completely sequenced

duplication (as applied to a gene or chromosome): Presence of an additional copy of part of a gene or chromosome

dysmorphology: The study of malformation syndromes

empirical risks: Risk estimates based on those actually observed, rather than on general principles

epigenetic: Genetic changes due to processes involving chromatin and methylation, among others, rather than to DNA sequence changes

eugenics: The use of genetic measures to attempt to alter and improve the genetic nature of a whole population

exon: The segments of a gene whose sequence is expressed by formation of messenger RNA and (usually) protein

FISH: Fluorescence *in situ* hybridisation of DNA, allowing microscopic detection of abnormalities

fragile site: A chromosomal site where there is a localised failure of condensation of the chromatin at cell division, giving the appearance of a break in the chromosome (as in fragile X syndrome)

gamete: Egg or sperm

gene: The unit of inheritance, consisting of a DNA sequence coding for a specific protein or component of a protein, arranged in a linear manner on chromosomes

genome: The entire genetic material of a cell or organism

genomics: Study of the genetic material overall

genotype: The genetic constitution of an individual (either overall or referring to a specific gene locus)

germ line: The cell lineages resulting in eggs or sperm

gonadal (germ line) mosaicism: The occurrence of more than one genetic constitution in the precursor cells of eggs or sperm

haploid: Having only a single set of genes (as in sperm or egg)

haplotype: A series of alleles found at linked loci on a single chromosome

hemizygous: The presence of a gene in only a single copy, e.g. X-linked genes in males, but also autosomal genes where one copy is deleted

heritability: The proportion of variance of a characteristic due to genetic rather than environmental factors

heterogeneity (genetic): The occurrence of a single phenotype due to mutation of more than one gene (usually implies more than one genetic locus)

heteroplasmy: Presence of two or more different forms of mitochondrial DNA

heterozygote: An individual with two different alleles at a particular locus

HLA system: The major histocompatibility region, determined by a complex of genetic loci on chromosome 6

homozygote: An individual with identical alleles at a particular locus

imprinting (genomic/genetic): The differential expression of the copy of a gene, or a genetic characteristic or disease, depending on the parent of origin, often related to differences in methylation

in situ **hybridisation:** The technique of applying molecular probes to a chromosome spread or section

interphase: The stage of the nucleus between cell divisions

intron: The DNA sequences in a gene that are not converted into messenger RNA, and which separate the coding regions (exons)

inversion: The turning round of a chromosomal segment with consequent alteration of its fine structure and sometimes its function

isochromosome: An abnormal chromosome composed of two identical arms

karyotype: The chromosome constitution as displayed by a microscopic preparation of dividing chromosomes photographed and arranged in homologous pairs

linkage, genetic: The occurrence of two genetic loci close enough on the same chromosome to interfere with independent assortment at cell division (so that the parental arrangement of genes is not broken up as it usually is)

locus: The specific site of a gene on a chromosome

Lyon hypothesis: The principle of inactivation of one of the two X chromosomes in normal female cells (first proposed by Dr Mary Lyon)

lysosome: An intracellular body containing important enzymes involved in the breakdown of cell components

meiosis: The process of cell division leading to formation of eggs and sperm, with halving of the chromosome number

Mendelian: Following the patterns of inheritance proposed originally by Gregor Mendel

microdeletion: A small or invisible loss of genetic material on a chromosome; often detectable by FISH techniques

mitochondrial inheritance: Exclusively maternal inheritance determined by DNA in the mitochondria, cytoplasmic bodies that also contain key enzymes

mitosis: The process of cell division of somatic cells, in which the daughter cells are normally genetically identical to the parent

monosomy: The occurrence of only a single member of a chromosome pair

monozygotic twins: Twins derived from a single fertilised egg

mosaicism: The occurrence in an individual of more than one genetic constitution, arising after fertilisation (cf. chimaera)

multiplex ligation-dependent probe amplification (MLPA): A method to count the number of copies of different sequences in the genome (e.g. the number of copies of all exons in the dystrophin gene)

mutation/mutant: The change from the normal to an altered form of a particular gene/the individual who has undergone such a change

non-disjunction: Failure of the normal separation of chromosomes at cell division, giving an unbalanced chromosome number (as in trisomy 21)

oncogene: A gene involved in cell proliferation whose abnormal activation or over-expression is important in turning a normal cell into a tumorous cell

p: The short arm of a chromosome

penetrance: The proportion of individuals with a particular genetic constitution who show its effect

pericentric inversion: An inversion of genetic material around the centromere of a chromosome

phenotype: The visible expression of the action of a particular gene; the clinical picture resulting from a genetic disorder

polygenic/multifactorial: Determined by multiple genes and usually also by non-genetic factors

polymerase chain reaction (PCR): The amplification of DNA using a specific technique, which allows analysis of very small quantities of short segments of DNA (up to several thousand base pairs, occasionally longer)

polymorphism: Frequent hereditary variations at a genetic locus

positional cloning: Gene isolation based on the mapping position of that gene rather than on its nature or function

pre-mutation: A clinically insignificant change in a gene that predisposes to a subsequent full mutation

proband: The affected individual through whom a family with a genetic disorder is ascertained (also called propositus)

probe: A labelled DNA sequence that can be used to identify a corresponding sequence by hybridisation

propositus, proposita: Proband (see earlier)

q: The long arm of a chromosome

qPCR: Quantitative PCR, a variant form of PCR which permits accurate quantitation of the number of copies in the genome of the target sequence being amplified

recessive: A characteristic or disorder only expressed when both alleles at a genetic locus are altered

recombination: The separation of alleles that are close together on the same chromosome by crossing over of homologous chromosomes at meiosis

restriction enzyme: A group of bacterial enzymes that cleaves the DNA chain at sequence-specific sites

RFLP: Restriction fragment length polymorphism: inherited variation in DNA detected by the cutting of DNA at different points by a restriction enzyme

ring chromosome: A chromosome in which breakage close to the ends has been followed by rejoining to form a ring

RNA: Ribonucleic acid: the nucleic acid for which DNA forms a template before protein is produced

Robertsonian translocation: The formation of a single abnormal chromosome by the joining of two chromosomes at or close to the centromeres, losing their short (p) arms

somatic: Involving the body cells rather than the germ line

Southern blotting: Transfer of DNA fragments from an electrophoretic gel to a membrane prior to DNA hybridisation

stem cell: A cell capable of reproducing and giving rise to different cell types in its descendants

syndrome: A combination of clinical features forming a recognisable entity

telomere: The terminal region of the chromosome arms

teratogen: An agent that can cause developmental abnormalities in the embryo

translocation: Transfer and exchange of genetic material between different chromosomes, usually not members of the same pair

trinucleotide repeat: A repeated sequence of three bases (e.g. CAG) expanded and unstable in a group of genetic disorders

triploid: Having three rather than two complete sets of chromosomes (usually lethal in humans)

trisomy: The presence of three copies of a specific chromosome

X inactivation: Inactivation (usually at random) of one of the two X chromosomes in a normal female cell (see Lyon hypothesis)

Y chromosome: The small chromosome possessed by males only, whose principal function is involvement in sex determination

zygote: The fertilised egg

Appendix 1: Further Reading and Information

The pace and volume of contemporary medical publishing makes it very difficult to produce a comprehensive list of recommended papers, chapters or even books for a volume such as this, especially if there may not be another edition for several years. Accordingly, I will not even attempt that task.

However, I can point to some information sources that I frequently employ. The GeneReviews element of the National Center for Biotechnology Information (NCBI) website (https://www.ncbi.nlm.nih.gov/books/NBK1116/) is immensely helpful, and the whole medical genetics community must thank the authors of each article, who keep these up to date. A search there, and/or a brief, focussed literature review, will often be very helpful before meeting a patient with a known or likely diagnosis.

Despite the short life of any research paper, there are still some reference sources that are valuable in helping the practitioner think through the differential diagnoses that may be relevant when meeting a patient with an unfamiliar condition. And there are some excellent works focussed on the history or mechanisms of a specific disorder or a category of disease.

What I present is a set of books and papers that I would recommend because I find their approach pleasing: this is a personal list. I present 'Topics' first, then 'Selected web resources', then 'Clinical disorders', then 'Social and ethical aspects' and finally, 'Policy documents'. However, the categories I have used and the selection of books and papers to include in each are entirely personal – even idiosyncratic – and would be difficult to defend objectively. I heartily apologise to those who feel that their valuable contributions should have been included.

A: TOPICS

Clinical genetics

Firth HV, Hurst JA. 2017. *Oxford Desk Reference: Clinical Genetics and Genomics*. Oxford University Press. (This excellent book gives the details where the present volume sets the scene. Indispensable to anyone working in Clinical Genetics.)

Read A, Donnai D. 2015. *The New Clinical Genetics* (3rd ed.). Scion Press.

Common (complex) disorders

Clarke A. 1995. Population screening for genetic susceptibility to disease. *BMJ* 311: 35–38.

Janssens ACJW, Joyner MJ. 2019. Polygenic risk scores that predict common diseases using millions of single nucleotide polymorphisms: Is more, better? *Clin Chem*. Published February 2019 (online ahead of print). doi:10.1373/clinchem.2018.296103
(And see other papers by Cécile Janssens, who has a healthily cautious approach to the application of genome-wide association studies in clinical practice.)

King KA, Rotter JI, Motulsky AG. 2002. *Genetic Basis of Common Diseases* (2nd ed.). Oxford University Press.

McKay TFC. 2004. The genetic architecture of quantitative traits: Lessons from *Drosophila*. *Curr Opin Genet Devel* 14: 253–257.

Vieira C, Pasyukova EG, Zeng Z-B, Hackett JB, Lyman RF, Mackay TFC. 2000. Genotype-environment interaction for quantitative trait loci affecting life span in *Drosophila melanogaster*. *Genetics* 154: 213–227.

Wald NJ, Old R. 2019. The illusion of polygenic disease risk prediction. *Genetics in Medicine*. https://doi.org/10.1038/s41436-018-0418-5

Weatherall DJ. 2000. *The Role of Nature and Nurture in Common Diseases*. Garrod's legacy. The Harveian Oration. Royal College of Physicians.

Wilkie AO. 2006. Polygenetic inheritance and genetic susceptibility screening. Published online in Wiley's *eLS* (*Encyclopedia of Life Sciences*).

Wright A, Hastie N. 2007. *Genes and Common Diseases*. Cambridge University Press.

Consanguinity

Bittles AH. 2013. Consanguineous marriage and congenital anomalies. *Lancet* 382: 1316–1317.

Modell B, Darr A. 2002. Genetic counselling and customary consanguineous marriage. *Nat Rev Genet* 3: 225–229.

Sheridan E, Wright J, Small N. 2013. Risk factors for congenital anomaly in a multiethnic birth cohort: An analysis of the born in Bradford study. *Lancet* 382(9901): 1350–1359.

Counselling

Egan G, Reese RJ. 2018. *The Skilled Helper* (11th ed.). Cengage.

Heron J. 2009. *Helping the Client: A Creative Practical Guide* (5th ed.). Sage.

Cytogenetics

Gardner RJM, Amor DJ. 2018. *Gardner and Sutherland's Chromosome Abnormalities and Genetic Counselling* (5th ed.). Oxford University Press.

McGowan-Jordan J, Simons A, Schmid M. (Eds.). 2016. *ISCN 2016: An International System for Human Cytogenomic Nomenclature*. Karger Medical Scientific.

Mitelman F. *Catalog of Chromosome Aberrations in Cancer*. Now online as Mitelman Database of Chromosome Aberrations in Cancer: http://cgap.nci.nih.gov/chromosomes/Mitelman.

Morris JK, Mutton DE, Alberman E. 2002. Revised estimates of the maternal age specific live birth prevalence of Down's syndrome. *J Med Screen* 9: 2–6.

Schinzel A. 2001. *Catalogue of Unbalanced Chromosome Aberrations in Man*. De Gruyter. (Now largely superseded by access to websites [especially DECIPHER] and online literature searches.)

Slavotinek AM. 2008. Novel microdeletion syndromes detected by chromosome microassays. *Hum Genet* 124: 1–17.

Development

Erickson EP, Wynshaw-Boris A. (Eds.). 2016. *Epstein's Inborn Errors of Development* (3rd ed.). Oxford University Press.

General genetics

Cooper DN, Krawczak M, Polychronakos C, Tyler-Smith C, Kehrer-Sawatzki H. 2013. Where genotype is not predictive of phenotype: Towards an understanding of the molecular basis of reduced penetrance in human inherited disease. *Hum Genet* 132: 1077–1130.

Girirajan S, Rosenfeld JA, Cooper GM. 2010. A recurrent 16p12.1 microdeletion supports a two-hit model for severe developmental delay. *Nat Genet* 42(3): 203–209.

Griffiths AJF, Wessler SR, Carroll SB, Doebley J. 2015. *Introduction to Genetic Analysis* (11th ed.). WH Freeman.

Harper PS, Harley HG, Reardon W, Shaw DJ. 1992. Anticipation in myotonic dystrophy: New light on an old problem. *Am J Hum Genet* 51: 1016.

Herskowitz I. 1987. Functional inactivation of genes by dominant negative mutations. *Nature* 329: 219–222.

Pauli RM, Motulsky AG. 1981. Risk counselling in autosomal disorders with undetermined penetrance, *J Med Genet* 15: 339–345.

Wilkie AOM. 1994. The molecular basis of genetic dominance. *J Med Genet* 31: 89–98.

Genetic counselling

Austin J, Semaka A, Hadjipavlou G. 2014. Conceptualizing genetic counseling as psychotherapy in the era of genomic medicine. *J Genet Couns* 23(6): 903–909.

Elwyn G, Gray J, Clarke A. 2000. Shared decision making and non-directiveness in genetic counselling. *J Med Genet* 37: 135–138.

Evans C. 2006. *Genetic Counselling: A Psychological Approach*. Cambridge University Press.

McCarthy Veach P, Bartels DM, LeRoy BS. 2007. Coming full circle: A reciprocal-engagement model of genetic counseling practice. *J Genet Couns* 16: 713–728.

Resta R. 2006. Defining and redefining the scope and goals of genetic counseling. *Am J Med Genet C* 142C: 269–275.

Resta R, Biesecker BB, Bennett RL, Blum S, Hahn SE, Strecker MN, Williams JL. 2006. A new definition of genetic counseling: National Society of Genetic Counselors' Task Force report. *J Genet Couns* 15(2):77–83.

Skirton H. 2001. The client's perspective of genetic counseling—A grounded theory study. *J Genet Couns* 10(4): 311–329.

Uhlmann WR, Schuette JL, Yashar BM. 2009. *A Guide to Genetic Counseling* (2nd ed.). Wiley-Blackwell.

Weil J. 2000. *Psychosocial Genetic Counseling*. Oxford University Press.

Weil J. 2003. Psychosocial genetic counseling in the post-nondirective era: A point of view. *J Genet Couns* 12(3): 199–211.

Wolff G, Jung C. 1995. Nondirectiveness and genetic counseling. *J Gen Couns* 4: 3–25.

See also chapters in Harper PS, Clarke A. 1997. *Genetics, Society and Clinical Practice*. Bios Scientific Publishers.

History

Harper PS. 1992. Huntington's disease and the abuse of genetics. *Am J Hum Genet* 50: 460–464.

Harper PS. 1996. The naming of syndromes and unethical activities: The case of Hallervordern and Spatz. *Lancet* 348: 1224–1225.

Harper PS. (Ed.). 2004. *Landmarks in Medical Genetics: Classic Papers with Commentaries.* Oxford University Press.

Harper PS. 2006. *First Years of Human Chromosomes: The Beginnings of Human Cytogenetics.* Scion. (This is an historical account, based on interviews with those involved.)

Harper PS. 2008. *A Short History of Medical Genetics.* Oxford University Press.

Harper PS. 2012. *History of medical genetics. Chapter 1.* In: Rimoin DL, Pyeritz RE, Korf BR. (Eds.). Emery & Rimoin's Principles and Practice of Medical Genetics (6th ed.). Churchill Livingstone, pp. 1–39.

Hsu TC. 1979. *Human and Mammalian Cytogenetics: An Historical Perspective.* Springer-Verlag.

Mazumdar PMH. 1992. *Eugenics, Human Genetics and Human Failings.* The Eugenics Society, its Sources and its Critics in Britain. Routledge.

Petermann HI, Harper PS, Doetz S. (Eds.). 2017. *History of Human Genetics: Aspects of Its Development and Global Perspectives.* Springer-Verlag.

Proctor RN. 1988. *Racial Hygiene. Medicine Under the Nazis.* Harvard University Press.

Reed SC. 1955. *Counseling in Medical Genetics.* W.B. Saunders.

Reed SC. 1974. A short history of genetic counseling. *Soc Biol* 21: 332–339.

Human and medical genetics

Bridge PJ. 1997. *The Calculation of Genetic Risks: Worked Examples in DNA Diagnostics* (2nd ed.). Johns Hopkins University Press.

Clarke A, Cooper DN. 2010. GWAS: Heritability missing in action. *Eur J Hum Genet* 18: 859–861.

Emery AEH. 1986. *Methodology in Medical Genetics. An Introduction to Statistical Methods* (2nd ed.). Churchill Livingstone.

Gluckman P, Hanson M. 2005. *The Fetal Matrix. Evolution, Development and Disease.* Cambridge University Press.

Migeon BR. 2007. *Females are Mosaics: X Inactivation and Sex Differences in Disease.* Oxford University Press.

Ørstavik K. 2009. X-chromosome inactivation in clinical practice. *Hum Genet* 126, 363–373.

Ostrer H. 1998. *Non-Mendelian Inheritance in Humans.* Oxford University Press. (This book gives a valuable account of the exceptions to Mendelian inheritance.)

Speicher MR, Antonorakis SE, Motulsky AG. 2010. *Vogel and Motulsky's Human Genetics: Problems and Approaches* (4th ed.). Springer-Verlag.

Stearns SC, Koella JC. 2008. *Evolution in Health and Disease* (2nd ed.). Oxford.

Stewart A, Brice P, Burton H, Pharoah P, Sanderson S, Zimmern R. 2007. *Genetics, Health and Public Policy.* Cambridge University Press.

Vogel F, Motulsky AG. 1997. *Human Genetics: Problems and Approaches* (3rd ed.). Springer-Verlag. (This is still valuable for its in-depth treatment of some topics and has not been completely displaced by the fourth edition, by Speicher et al.)

Young ID. 2007. *Introduction to Risk Calculation in Genetic Counselling* (3rd ed.). Oxford. (A clearly explained and valuable guide to practical situations and to their underlying principles.)

Molecular genetics

Ellard S, Baple EL, Owens M. 2018. *Association of Clinical Genetics Scientists (ACGS) Best Practice Guidelines for Variant Classification 2018*. ACGS.

Kalia SS, Adelman K, Bale SJ on behalf of the ACMG Secondary Findings Maintenance Working Group. 2017. Recommendations for reporting of secondary findings in clinical exome and genome sequencing, 2016 update: A policy statement of the American College of Medical Genetics and Genomics. *Genet Med* 19(2): 249–255.

Richards S, Aziz N, Bale S on behalf of the ACMG Laboratory Quality Assurance Committee. 2015. Standards and guidelines for the interpretation of sequence variants: A joint consensus recommendation of the American College of Medical Genetics and Genomics and the Association for Molecular Pathology. *Genet Med* 17: 405–424.

Strachan T, Read AP. 2019. *Human Molecular Genetics* (5th ed.). CRC Press, Taylor and Francis (Garland Science).

Newborn screening

Parsons EP, Clarke AJ, Hood K, Lycett E, Bradley DM. 2002. Newborn screening for Duchenne muscular dystrophy: A psychosocial study. *Arch Dis Child Fetal Neonatal Ed* 86: F91–F95.

Ross LF, Clarke AJ. 2017. A historical and current review of newborn screening for neuromuscular disorders from around the world: Lessons for the United States. *Pediatr Neurol* 77: 12–22.

Outcomes and outcome measures for genetics services

Berkenstadt M, Shiloh S, Barkai G. 1999. Perceived personal control (PPC): A new concept in measuring outcome of genetic counselling. *Am J Med Genet* 82: 53–59.

Grant PE, Pampaka M, Payne K, Clarke A, McAllister M. 2019. Developing a short-form of the genetic counselling outcome scale: The genomics outcome scale. *Eur J Med Genet*. Published November 26, 2018 (online ahead of print). doi:10.1016/j.ejmg.2018.11.015

Helderman-van den Enden ATJM, van den Bergen JC, Breuning MH, Verschuuren JJGM, Tibben A, Bakker E, Ginjaar HB. 2011. Duchenne/Becker muscular dystrophy in the family: Have potential carriers been tested at a molecular level? *Clin Genet* 79: 236–242.

McAllister M, Davies L, Payne K, Nicholls S, Donnai D, MacLeod R. 2007. The emotional effects of genetic diseases: Implications for clinical genetics. *Am J Med Genet* Part A 143A: 2651–2661.

McAllister M, Wood AM, Dunn G, Shiloh S, Todd C. 2011. The genetic counseling outcome scale: A new patient-reported outcome measure for clinical genetics services. *Clin Genet* 79: 413–424.

Shiloh S, Sagi M. 1989. Effect of framing on the perception of genetic risk recurrence risks. *Am J Med Genet* 33: 130–135.

Skirton H, Parsons EP, Ewings P. 2005. Development of an audit tool for genetic services. *Am J Med Genet* 136A: 122–127.

B: SELECTED WEB RESOURCES

Web addresses are not all given in full, as many sites are more easily accessed through your browser and search engine rather than by entering the full address.

The pre-eminent route to access many resources – especially perhaps for professionals – is provided courtesy of the U.S. government. The global human genetics community is aware of this and is appreciative. There are many other resources based elsewhere and worthy of recognition, such as at the Wellcome Sanger Institute at Hinxton, England, but NCBI is the first port of call for many enquiries:

National Center for Biotechnology Information (NCBI): https://www.ncbi.nlm.nih.gov

This is the gateway to a vast range of powerful databases and other resources, not least PubMed, ClinVar and GeneReviews, and is also a route for accessing Online Mendelian Inheritance in Man (OMIM).

- GeneReviews: https://www.ncbi.nlm.nih.gov/books/NBK1116/
- ClinVar: https://www.ncbi.nlm.nih.gov/clinvar/

Professional societies

American College of Medical Genetics and Genomics	https://www.acmg.net
American Society of Human Genetics	http://www.ashg.org
British Society for Genetic Medicine (BSGM)	https://www.bsgm.org.uk
	This site gives access to the organisations that constitute the BSGM (the Clinical Genetics Society, the Association of Genetic Nurses and Counsellors [AGNC] and the Association for Clinical Genomic Science [ACGS]).
European Board of Medical Genetics	https://www.ebmg.eu
European Society of Human Genetics	https://www.eshg.org
Human Genetics Society of Australasia	https://www.hgsa.org.au
National Society of Genetic Counselors (United States)	https://www.nsgc.org

Clinical, molecular and patient sites

Centers for Disease Control and Prevention (CDC) Genomics	https://www.cdc.gov/genomics/
Clinical Genome Resource	https://www.clinicalgenome.org
Decipher	https://decipher.sanger.ac.uk
Deciphering Developmental Disorders/ Gene2Phenotype (part of the European Bioinformatics Institute [EMBL-EBI])	https://www.ebi.ac.uk/gene2phenotype/about
Ensembl (including the Ensembl Genome Browser)	http://www.ensembl.org
EUROCAT (European Surveillance of Congenital Anomalies)	https://www.eurocat-network.eu

EuroGenTest	http://www.eurogentest.org www.eurogentest.org/index.php?id=226 (Patient leaflets in many languages.)
European Directory of DNA Diagnostic Laboratories	http://www.eddnal.com
ExAc (Exome Aggregation Consortium, hosted at the Broad Institute):	http://exac.broadinstitute.org
Gen-Equip: Genetics Education for Primary Care	https://www.primarycaregenetics.org
Genetic Alliance UK (an umbrella organisation for UK rare disease groups)	https://www.geneticalliance.org.uk
Genetics Home Reference	https://ghr.nlm.nih.gov (for patients)
Genomics Education Programme of Health Education England	https://www.genomicseducation.hee.nhs.uk
Genomics England	https://www.genomicsengland.co.uk
Genomics England PanelApp	https://panelapp.genomicsengland.co.uk
Genomics Partnership Wales (Partneriaeth Genomeg Cymru)	http://www.walesgenepark.cardiff.ac.uk/genomics-partnership-wales/
Genomics Quality Assessment	https://www.genqa.org
Global Alliance for Genomics and Health:	https://www.ga4gh.org
HUGO Gene Nomenclature Committee	https://www.genenames.org
Human Gene Mutation Database	http://www.hgmd.org (A valuable general database of the range and types of mutation found in genetic disorders.)
Human Genome Organisation:	http://www.hugo-international.org
Human Variome Project	http://www.humanvariomeproject.org
Locus-Specific Mutation Databases	These are increasing in number and often also contain helpful general information. They can be accessed through the Human Gene Mutation Database (see earlier). Two valuable examples are the Phenylalanine Hydroxylase Mutation Database (for PKU) and the Cystic Fibrosis Mutation Database.
Mitelman Database of Chromosome Aberrations in Cancer	http://cgap.nci.nih.gov/chromosomes/Mitelman
National Institute for Health and Care Excellence (NICE): guidance on approach to family history of breast cancer	https://www.nice.org.uk/guidance/cg164
National Organization for Rare Disorders (NORD) (U.S.-based)	https://rarediseases.org
OMIM (Online Mendelian Inheritance in Man)	https://www.omim.org
Orphanet: a valuable European resource for all aspects of rare diseases	https://www.orpha.net/consor/cgi-bin/index.php

POSSUM Dysmorphology Database	https://www.possum.net.au
Public Health Genomics Foundation	http://www.phgfoundation.org
Rare Disease UK	https://www.raredisease.org.uk
Scottish Genomes Partnership	https://www.scottishgenomespartnership.org
Transforming Genetic Medicine Initiative	https://www.thetgmi.org
UCSC (University of California at Santa Cruz) Genome Browser	http://genome.ucsc.edu
UNIQUE (Understanding Rare Chromosome and Genetic Disorders)	https://www.rarechromo.org
Winter-Baraitser Dysmorphology Database (also known as the London Dysmorphology Database, and previously accessed through Oxford Medical Databases) is now accessed through Face2Gene	https://www.face2gene.com/lmd-library-london-medical-database-dysmorphology/
World Health Organization	https://www.who.int/genomics/en/
1,000 Genome Project (1KGP)	https://www.internationalgenome.org

C: CLINICAL DISORDERS

General reference

Pyeritz RE, Korf BR, Grody WW. (Eds.). 2018–19. *Emery and Rimoin's Principles and Practice of Medical Genetics* (7th ed.). Academic Press. (This reference work has evolved – and expanded – over many years and now consists of 11 volumes available as hard copy or e-book, with many outstanding chapters on particular groups of diseases.)

Cancer

Campeau PM, Foulkes WD, Tischkowitz MD. 2008. Hereditary breast cancer: New genetic developments, new therapeutic avenues. *Hum Genet* 124: 31–42.

Draper GJ, Heaf MM, Wilson LMK. 1977. Occurrence of childhood cancers among sibs and estimation of familial risks. *J Med Genet* 14: 81–90.

Evans DGR, Eccles DM, Rahman N, Young K, Bulman M, Amir E, Shenton A, Howell A, Lalloo F. 2004. A new scoring system for the chances of identifying a *BRCA1/2* mutation outperforms existing models including BRCAPRO. *J Med Genet* 41(6): 474–480.

Hodgson SV, Foulkes WD, Eng V, Maher ER. 2014. *A Practical Guide to Human Cancer Genetics* (4th ed.). Cambridge University Press.

Pharoah PDP, Antoniou AC, Easton DF, Ponder BAJ. 2010. Polygenes, risk prediction, and targeted prevention of breast cancer. *NEJM* 358(26): 2796–2803.

Vasen H, Watson P, Mecklin J-P, Lynch H. 1999. New clinical criteria for hereditary nonpolyposis colorectal cancer (HNPCC, Lynch syndrome) proposed by the International Collaborative Group on HNPCC. *Gastroenterology* 116(6): 1453–1456.

Cardiac and cardiovascular

Bruneau BG, Burn J, Srivastaca D. 2010. Aetiology of congenital cardiac disease. Chapter 9. In: Anderson HR, Baker EJ, Penny D, Redington AN, Rigby ML, Wernovsky G. (Eds.). *Paediatric Cardiology* (3rd ed.). Churchill Livingstone, pp. 161–171.

Burn J, Goodship J. 2007. Congenital heart disease. In: Rimoin DL, Connor JM, Pyeritz RE, Korf BR. (Eds.). *Emery and Rimoin's Principles and Practice of Medical Genetics* (5th ed.). Churchill Livingstone, pp. 1083–1159.

Kumar D, Elliott P. (Eds.). 2018. *Clinical Cardiovascular Genetics and Genomics: Principles and Clinical Practice.* Oxford University Press.

Nora JJ, Berg K, Nora AH. 1991. *Cardiovascular Diseases: Genetics, Epidemiology and Prevention.* Oxford: Oxford University Press, pp. 49–52.

Pyeritz RE. 2014. Heritable thoracic aortic disorders. *Curr Opin Cardiol* 29: 97–102.

Connective tissue

Beighton P. (Ed.). 1993. *McKusick's Heritable Disorders of Connective Tissue.* Mosby.

Loeys BL, Dietz HC, Braverman AC. 2010. The revised Ghent nosology for the Marfan syndrome. *J Med Genet* 47: 476–485.

Deafness and hearing loss

Toriello HV, Smith SD. (Eds.). 2013. *Hereditary Hearing Loss and Its Syndromes* (3rd ed.). Oxford University Press.

Duchenne muscular dystrophy

As an exemplar of evidence-based practice for rare diseases, this three-part set of guidelines:

Birnkrant DJ, Bushby K, Bann CM; DMD Care Considerations Working Group. 2018. Diagnosis and management of Duchenne muscular dystrophy, part 1: Diagnosis, and neuromuscular, rehabilitation, endocrine, and gastrointestinal and nutritional management. *Lancet Neurol* 17(3): 251–267.

Birnkrant DJ, Bushby K, Bann CM; DMD Care Considerations Working Group. 2018. Diagnosis and management of Duchenne muscular dystrophy, part 2: Respiratory, cardiac, bone health, and orthopaedic management. *Lancet Neurol* 17(4): 347–361.

Birnkrant DJ, Bushby K, Bann CM; DMD Care Considerations Working Group. 2018. Diagnosis and management of Duchenne muscular dystrophy, part 3: Primary care, emergency management, psychosocial care, and transitions of care across the lifespan. *Lancet Neurol* 17(5): 445–455.

Emery AEH, Emery MLH. 2011. *The History of a Genetic Disease: Duchenne Muscular Dystrophy or Meryon's Disease* (2nd ed.). Oxford University Press.

Emery AEH, Muntoni F. 2015. *Duchenne Muscular Dystrophy* (4th ed.). Oxford University Press.

Muntoni F, Torelli S, Ferlini A. 2003. Dystrophin and mutations: One gene, several proteins, multiple phenotypes. *Lancet Neurology* 2: 731–740.

Dysmorphology

Graham JM, Sanchez-Lara PA. 2016. *Smith's Recognizable Patterns of Human Deformation* (4th ed.). Elsevier.

Gripp KW, Slavotinek AM, Hall JG, Allanson JE. 2013. *Handbook of Physical Measurements*. Oxford University Press.

Hennekam RJM, Krantz ID, Allanson JE. 2010. *Gorlin's Syndromes of the Head and Neck* (5th ed.). Oxford University Press. (This is a book on dysmorphology, but it has to be supplemented, of course, by databases, especially the Oxford Medical Dysmorphology Database.)

Jones KL, Jones MC, Casanelles M del C. 2013. *Smith's Recognizable Patterns of Human Malformation* (7th ed.). Elsevier.

Neri G, Boccuto L, Stevenson RE. 2019. *Overgrowth Syndromes; a Clinical Guide*. Oxford University Press.

Reardon W. 2008. *The Bedside Dysmorphologist*. Classic Clinical Signs in Human Malformation Syndromes and Their Diagnostic Significance. Oxford.

Schrander-Stumpel CTRM. 1998. What's in a name? *Am J Med Genet* 79: 228.

Tewfik TL, der Kaloustian VM. 1997. *Congenital Anomalies of the Ear, Nose and Throat*. Oxford University Press.

Fetal alcohol syndrome

British Medical Association. 2016. Alcohol and pregnancy. Preventing and managing fetal alcohol spectrum disorders. June 2007 (updated February 2016).

Cook JL, Green CR, Lilley CM; for the Canada Fetal Alcohol Spectrum Disorder Research Network. 2016. Fetal alcohol spectrum disorder: A guideline for diagnosis across the lifespan. *CMAJ* 188(3): 191–197.

Healthcare Improvement Scotland. 2019. *Children and Young People Exposed Prenatally to Alcohol. A National Clinical Guideline*. NHS Scotland.

Hoyme HE, Kalberg WO, Elliott AJ. 2016. Updated clinical guidelines for diagnosing fetal alcohol spectrum disorders. *Pediatrics* 138(2): e20154256.

Haemochromatosis

Fitzsimons EJ, Cullis JO, Thomas DW, Tsochatzis E, Griffiths WJH on behalf of the British Society for Haematology. 2018. Diagnosis and therapy of genetic haemochromatosis (review and 2017 update). *Br J Haematol* 181: 293–303.

McCune CA, Ravine D, Worwood M. 2003. Screening for hereditary haemochromatosis in families and beyond. *Lancet* 362: 1897–1898.

Pilling LC, Tamosauskaite J, Jones G, Wood AR, Jones L, Kuo C-L, Kuchel GA, Ferrucci L, Melzer D. 2019. Common conditions associated with hereditary haemochromatosis genetic variants: Cohort study in UK Biobank. *BMJ* 364: k5222.

Tamosauskaite J, Atkins JL, Pilling LC, Kuo C-L, Kuchel GA, Ferrucci L, Melzer D. 2019. Hereditary hemochromatosis associations with frailty, sarcopenia and chronic pain: Evidence from 200,975 Older UK Biobank participants. *J Gerontol A Biol Sci Med Sci* 74(3): 337–342.

Metabolic disease

Scriver CR, Beaudet AL, Sly W, Valle D. (Eds.). 2001. *The Metabolic and Molecular Bases of Inherited Disease*. McGraw-Hill. (The definitive source of information on all inborn errors of metabolism and related metabolic disorders, which is now online and continually updated at: https://ommbid.mhmedical.com/ [The Online Metabolic and Molecular Bases of Inherited Disease.])

Whittaker M. 1986. *Cholinesterase*. Karger.

Mitochondrial disorders

Chinnery PF, Hudson G. 2013. Mitochondrial genetics. *Br Med Bull* 106: 135–159.

Mosaicism

Hall JG. 1988. Somatic mosaicism: Observations related to clinical genetics. *Am J Hum Genet* 43: 355–363.

Neurological and neuromuscular (see also Duchenne muscular dystrophy and mitochondrial disorders)

Arzimanoglou A, O'Hare, A, Johnston MV, Ouvrier R. 2018. *Aicardi's Diseases of the Nervous System in Childhood* (4th ed.). *(Clinics in Developmental Medicine)*. MacKeith Press.

Baraitser M. 1997. *The Genetics of Neurological Disorders*. Oxford University Press.

Bates GP, Tabrizi SJ, Jones L. (Eds.). 2014. *Huntington's Disease* (4th ed.). Oxford University Press.

Clarke C, Howard R, Rossor M, Shorvon S. (Eds.). 2016. *Neurology: A Queen Square Textbook* (2nd ed.). Wiley-Blackwell.

Emery AEH. (Ed.). 2001. *The Muscular Dystrophies*. Oxford University Press.

Karpati G, Hilton-Jones D, Bushby K, Griggs RC. (Eds.). 2010. *Disorders of Voluntary Muscle* (8th ed.). Cambridge University Press.

Kay C, Collins JA, Miedzybrodzka Z, Madore SJ, Gordon ES, Gerry N, Davidson M, Slama RA, Hayden MR. 2016. Huntington disease reduced penetrance alleles occur at high frequency in the general population. *Clin Genet* 87: 1–7.

Langbehn DR, Brinkman RR, Falush D, Paulsen JS, Hayden MR on behalf of an International Huntington's Disease Collaborative Group. 2004. A new model for prediction of the age of onset and penetrance for Huntington's disease based on CAG length. *Clin Genet* 65: 267–277.

Straub V, Murphy A, Udd B on behalf of the LGMD workshop study group. 2017. 229th ENMC international workshop: Limb girdle muscular dystrophies – Nomenclature and reformed classification Naarden, the Netherlands, March 17–19. *Neuromusc Dis* 28(8): 702–710.

Upadhyaya M, Cooper DN. (Eds.). 2013. *Neurofibromatosis Type 1: Molecular and Cellular Biology*. Springer Verlag.

Ophthalmology

Traboulsi El. 2012. *Genetic Diseases of the Eye* (2nd ed.). Oxford University Press.

Prenatal genetics

Abramsky L, Chapple J. 2003. *Prenatal Diagnosis: The Human Side* (2nd ed.). Chapman and Hall.
Clarke A. 1997. Prenatal genetic screening: Paradigms and perspectives. In: Harper PS, Clarke A. (Eds.). *Genetics, Society and Clinical Practice*. BIOS, pp. 119–140.
Milunsky A, Milunsky JM. (Eds.). 2016. *Genetic Disorders and the Fetus* (7th ed.). Wiley-Blackwell.
Nuffield Council on Bioethics. 2017. *Non-Invasive Prenatal Diagnosis*. Report of a Working Party. Nuffield Council on Bioethics.
Prenatal Diagnosis (Wiley InterScience), a journal that is a valuable source of recent advances.
Taylor-Phillips S, Freeman K, Geppert J, Agbebiyi A, Uthman O, Madan J, Clarke AJ, Quenby S, Clarke AE. 2016. Accuracy of non-invasive prenatal testing using cell-free DNA for detection of Down, Edwards and Patau syndromes: A systematic review and meta-analysis. *BMJ Open* 6: e010002.
Wilson RD, Gagnon A, Audibert F, Campagnolo C, Carroll J; for the Society of Obstetricians and Gynaecologists of Canada. 2015. Prenatal diagnosis procedures and techniques to obtain a diagnostic fetal specimen or tissue: Maternal and fetal risks and benefits. SOGC Clinical Practice Guideline No. 326, July 2015. *J Obstet Gynaecol Can* 37(7): 656–668.
Wright C. 2009. *Cell-free fetal nucleic acids for non-invasive prenatal diagnosis*. Report of the UK expert working group. Public Health Genetics Foundation.

Radiation

Doll R. 1993. Epidemiological evidence of effects of small doses of ionising radiation with a note on the causation of clusters of childhood leukaemia. *J Radiol Prot* 13: 233–241.
International Atomic Energy Authority. 1991. *International Chernobyl Project: An Overview*. United Nations.
Mole H. 1979. Radiation effects on prenatal development and their radiological significance. *Br J Radiol* 52: 89–101.
Neel JV. 1993. *Physician to the Gene Pool*. Wiley.
Searle A. 1987. Radiation: The genetic risk. *Trends Genet* 3: 152–157.
UNSCEAR report. 1982. *Ionizing Radiation: Sources and Biological Effects. Annex 1: Genetic Effects of Radiation*. United Nations.

Respiratory disorders

Silverman EK. 2004. *Respiratory Genetics*. Hodder.

Skeletal dysplasias

Spranger JW, Brill PW, Hall C, Nishimura G, Superti-Furga A, Unger S. 2018. *Bone Dysplasias: An Atlas of Genetic Disorders of Skeletal Development* (4th ed.). Oxford University Press.

Skin

Irvine A, Hoeger P, Yan A. 2011. *Harper's Textbook of Pediatric Dermatology* (3rd ed.). Wiley-Blackwell.

Sybert VP. 2017. *Genetic Skin Disorders* (3rd ed.). Oxford University Press.

Teratology (including web-based resources)

European Network of Teratology Information Services (ENTIS): https://www.entis-org.eu

Clinical Teratology Web is a project of the TERIS (Teratogen Information System) Program at the University of Washington, Seattle, Washington http://depts.washington.edu/terisdb/terisweb/index.html

Smithells RW, Newman CGH. 1992. Recognition of thalidomide defects. *J Med Genet* 29: 716–723.

UK Teratology Information Service:
http://www.uktis.org
https://www.toxbase.org

Treatments for specific genetic disorders

Clarke AJ, Abdala Sheikh AP. 2018. A perspective on "cure" for Rett syndrome. *Orphanet J Rare Dis* 13: 44.

Gaide O, Schneider P. 2003. Permanent correction of an inherited ectodermal dysplasia with recombinant EDA. *Nat Med* 9: 614–618.

Guy J, Gan J, Selfridge J, Cobb S, Bird A. 2007. Reversal of neurological defects in a mouse model of Rett syndrome. *Science* 315: 1143–1147.

Hammond SM, Hazell G, Shabanpoor F, Saleh AF, Bowerman M, Sleigh JN, Meijboom KE, Zhou H, Muntoni F, Talbot K, Gait MJ, Wood MJA. 2016. Systemic peptide-mediated oligonucleotide therapy improves long-term survival in spinal muscular atrophy. *PNAS* 113(39): 10962–10967.

Schneider H, Faschingbauer F, Schuepbach-Mallepell S. 2018. Prenatal correction of X-linked hypohidrotic ectodermal dysplasia. *N Engl J Med* 378:1604–1610.

Tabrizi SJ, Leavitt BR, Landwehrmeyer GB, Wild EJ, Saft C, Barker RA, Blair NF, Craufurd D, Priller J, Rickards H, Rosser A, Kordasiewicz HB, Czech C, Swayze EE, Norris DA, Baumann T, Gerlach I, Schobel SA, Paz E, Smith AV, Bennett CF, Lane RM. Targeting Huntingtin Expression in Patients with Huntington's Disease. *N Engl J Med* 2019;380:2307–2316.

von Knebel Doeberitz M, Kloor M. 2013. Vaccine against Lynch syndrome cancers. *Fam Cancer* 12(2): 307–312.

Wirth T, Parker N, Ylä-Herttuala S. 2013. History of gene therapy. *Gene* 525(2): 162–169.

D: SOCIAL AND ETHICAL ASPECTS (A PERSONAL SELECTION)

Books

Arribas-Ayllon M, Sarangi S, Clarke A. 2011. *Genetic Testing: Accounts of Autonomy, Responsibility and Blame*. Routledge.

Ashcroft R, Lucassen A, Parker M, Verkerk M, Widdershoven G. (Eds.). 2005. *Case Analysis in Clinical Ethics*. Cambridge.

Bosk C. 1992. *All God's Mistakes. Genetic Counseling in a Pediatric Hospital*. Chicago University Press.

Browner C, Mabel Preloran HM. 2010. *Neurogenetic Diagnoses. The Power of Hope, and the Limits of Today's Medicine*. Routledge.

Clarke A. (Ed.). 1994. *Genetic Counselling: Practice and Principles*. Routledge.

Clarke A. (Ed.). 1998. *The Genetic Testing of Children*. Bios Scientific Publishers.

Clarke A, Parsons EP. (Eds.). 1997. *Culture, Kinship and Genes*. Macmillan.

Duster T. 1990. *Backdoor to Eugenics*. Routledge, Chapman and Hall.

Ebtehaj F, Lindley B, Richards M. (Eds.). 2006. *Kinship Matters*. Cambridge.

Featherstone K, Bharadwaj A, Clarke A, Atkinson P. 2006. *Risky Relations. Family and Kinship in the Era of New Genetics*. Berg Publishers.

Gaff CL, Bylund CL. 2010. *Family Communication about Genetics: Theory and Practice*. Oxford University Press.

Glover J. 2006. *Choosing Children*. Oxford.

Goffman E. 1963. *Stigma*. Penguin Books.

Harper PS, Clarke A. 1997. *Genetics, Society and Clinical Practice*. Bios Scientific Publishers. (Now two decades old but many of the chapters remain pertinent, as with the volume edited by Marteau and Richards.)

Kessler S. (ed. Resta R). 2000. *Psyche and Helix*. Wiley Liss. (A most useful compilation of the papers written by Seymour Kessler about the counselling aspects of genetic counselling.)

Kevles DJ. 1986. *In the Name of Eugenics*. Knopf.

Konrad M. 2005. *Narrating the New Predictive Genetics*. Cambridge.

Latimer J. 2013. *The Gene, the Clinic and the Family: Diagnosing Dysmorphology, Reviving Medical Dominance*. Routledge.

Manson N, O'Neill O. 2007. *Rethinking Informed Consent in Bioethics*. Cambridge University Press.

Marteau T, Richards M. (Eds.). 1996. *The Troubled Helix: Social and Psychological Implications of the New Genetics*. Cambridge University Press.

Müller-Hill B. 1998. *Murderous Science*. Oxford University Press. (are-issue of the English translation of this important and disturbing book, even more relevant now than when first published [and should be compulsory reading for all those involved in medical genetics].)

Palsson G. 2007. *Anthropology and the New Genetics*. Cambridge University Press.

Parens E, Asch A. (Eds.). 2000. *Prenatal Testing and Disability Rights*. Georgetown University Press.

Parker M. 2012. *Ethical Problems and Genetics Practice*. Cambridge University Press.

Rapp R. 2000. *Testing the Woman, Testing the Fetus*. Routledge.

Rehmann-Sutter C, Müller H-J. 2009. *Disclosure Dilemmas: Ethics of Genetic Prognosis after the 'Right to Know/Not to Know' Debate*. Ashgate.

Rothman BK. 1988. *The Tentative Pregnancy*. Pandora.

Rozario S. 2013. *Genetic Disorders and Islamic Identity among British Bangladeshis*. Carolina University Press.

Schwartz Cowan R. 2008. *Heredity and Hope: The Case for Genetic Screening*. Harvard.

Scully JL. 2008. *Disability Bioethics: Moral Bodies, Moral Difference*. Rowman & Littlefield.

Shaw A. 2009. *Negotiating Risk: British Pakistani Experiences of Genetics*. Berghahn Books.

Shakespeare T. 2006. *Disability Rights and Wrongs*. Routledge.

Wilkinson S, Garrard E. 2013. *Eugenics and the Ethics of Selective Reproduction*. Keele University (for The Wellcome Trust).

Papers

Arribas-Ayllon M, Sarangi S, Clarke A. 2009. Professional ambivalence: Accounts of ethical practice in childhood genetic testing. *J Genet Couns* 18: 173–184.

Boardman FK. 2017. Experience as knowledge: Disability, distillation and (reprogenetic) decision-making. *Soc Sci Med* 191: 186–193.

Chokoshvili D, Vears D, Borry P. 2018. Expanded carrier screening for monogenic disorders: Where are we now? *Prenat Diagn* 38: 59–66.

Clarke A. 1991. Is non-directive genetic counselling possible? *Lancet* 338: 998–1001.

Clarke A. 2016. Anticipated stigma and blameless guilt: Mothers' evaluation of life with the sex-linked disorder, hypohidrotic ectodermal dysplasia (XHED). *Soc Sci Med* 158: 141–148.

Clarke A, Sarangi S, Verrier Jones K. 2011. Voicing the lifeworld: Parental accounts of responsibility in genetic consultations for polycystic kidney disease. *Soc Sci Med* 72: 1743–1751.

Clarke A, Thirlaway K. 2011. 'Genomic counseling'? Genetic counseling in the genomic era. *Genome Med* 3: 7.

Clarke A, Wallgren-Pettersson C. 2019. Ethics in genetic counselling. *J Community Genet* 10(1): 3–33.

Clarke AJ. 2013. Stigma, self-esteem and reproduction: Talking with men about life with hypohidrotic ectodermal dysplasia. *Sociology* 47(5): 975–993.

Clarke AJ. 2014. Managing the ethical challenges of next generation sequencing in genomic medicine. *Br Med Bull* 111(1): 17–30.

Dheensa S, Carrieri D, Kelly S, Clarke A, Doheny S, Turnpenny P, Lucassen A. 2017. A 'joint venture' model of recontacting in clinical genomics: Challenges for responsible implementation. *Eur J Med Genet* 60(7): 403–409.

Doheny S, Clarke A, Carrieri D, Dheensa S, Hawkins N, Lucassen A, Turnpenny P, Kelly S. 2018. Dimensions of responsibility in medical genetics: Exploring the complexity of the 'duty to recontact'. *New Genet Soc* 37(3): 187–206.

Downing C. 2005. Negotiating responsibility: Case studies of reproductive decision-making and prenatal genetic testing in families facing HD. *J Gen Couns* 14: 219–234.

Forrest K, Simpson SA, Wilson BJ, van Teijlingen ER, McKee L, Haites N, Matthews E. 2003. To tell or not to tell: Barriers and facilitators in family communication about genetic risk. *Clin Genet* 64: 317–326.

Geelen E, van Hoyweghen I, Doevendans PA, Marcelis CLM, Horstman K. 2011. Constructing 'best interests': Genetic testing of children in families with hypertrophic cardiomyopathy. *Am J Med Genet A* 155A(8): 1930–1938.

Hallowell N, Arden-Jones A, Eeles R, Foster C, Lucassen A, Moynihan C, Watson M. 2006. Guilt, blame and responsibility: Men's understanding of their role in the transmission of *BRCA1/2* mutations within the family. *Sociol Health Illn* 28(7): 969–988.

Hallowell N, Foster C, Eeles R, Ardern-Jones A, Murday V, Watson M. 2003. Balancing autonomy and responsibility: The ethics of generating and disclosing genetic information. *J Med Ethics* 29: 74–79.

Harper PS, Clarke AJ. 1990. Should we test children for 'adult' genetic diseases? *Lancet* 335(8699): 1205–1206.

Hart JT. 1971. The Inverse Care Law. *Lancet* 297: 405–412.

Holt K. 2006. What do we tell the children? Contrasting the disclosure choices of two HD families regarding risk status and predictive genetic testing. *J Gen Couns* 5: 253 onwards.

Liddell K. 2017. Informed Consent in Human Genetic Research. Published online in Wiley's *eLS* (*Encyclopedia of Life Sciences*).

Lippman A. 1991. Prenatal genetic testing. Constructing needs and reinforcing inequities. *Am J Law Med* 17: 15–50. (Reprinted in Clarke [Ed.]. 1994. *Genetic Counselling: Practice and Principles*. Routledge).

Lucassen A, Parker M. 2001. Revealing false paternity: Some ethical considerations, *Lancet* 357: 1033–1035.

Manjoney DM, McKegnay FP. 1978. Individual and family coping with polycystic kidney disease: The harvest of denial. *Int J Psychiatry Med* 9: 19–31.

McDermott R. 1998. Ethics, epidemiology and the thrifty gene: Biological determinism as a health hazard. *Soc Sci Med* 47: 1189–1195.

McDougall R. 2007. Parental virtue: A new way of thinking about the morality of reproductive actions. *Bioethics* 21: 181–189.

Mendes A, Sousa L, Sequeiros J, Clarke A. 2017. Discredited legacy: Stigma and familial amyloid polyneuropathy in Northwestern Portugal. *Soc Sci Med* 182: 73–80.

Parker M, Lucassen A. 2003. Concern for families and individuals in clinical genetics. *J Med Ethics* 29: 70–73.

Pilnick A. 2002. What 'most people' do: Exploring the ethical implications of genetic counselling. *New Genet Soc* 21: 339–350.

Ross LF. 2013. Predictive genetic testing of children and the role of the best interest standard. *J Law, Med Ethics Winter* 2013: 899–906.

Ross LF, Clarke AJ. 2017. A historical and current review of newborn screening for neuromuscular disorders from around the world: Lessons for the United States. *Pediatr Neurol* 77: 12–22.

Sarangi S, Bennert K, Howell L, Clarke A, Harper P, Gray J. 2004. Initiation of reflective frames in counselling for Huntington's disease predictive testing. *J Genet Couns* 13: 135–155.

Sarangi S, Bennert K, Howell L, Clarke A, Harper P, Gray J. 2005. (Mis)alignments in counselling for Huntington's disease predictive testing: Clients' responses to reflective frames. *J Genet Couns* 14: 29–42.

Scully JL, Porz R, Rehman-Sutter C. 2007. 'You don't make genetic test decisions from one day to the next' – Using time to preserve moral space. *Bioethics* 21: 208–217.

Shakespeare T. 1998. Choices and rights: Eugenics, genetics and disability equality. *Disabil Soc* 13: 665–681.

Sobel S, Cowan DB. 2000. Impact of genetic testing for Huntington disease on the family system. *Am J Med Genet* 90: 49–59.

Timmermans S. 2015. Trust in standards: Transitioning clinical exome sequencing from bench to bedside. *Soc Stud Sci* 45: 77–99.

Timmermans S, Buchbinder M. 2010. Patients-in-waiting: Living between sickness and health in the genomics era. *J Health Soc Behav* 51(4): 408–423.

Vos J, Jansen AM, Menko F, van Asperen CJ, Stiggelbout AM, Tibben A. 2011. Family communication matters: The impact of telling relatives about unclassified variants and uninformative DNA-test results. *Genet Med* 13: 333–341.

Wadrup F, Holden S, MacLeod R, Miedzybrodzka Z, Németh AH, Owens S, Pasalodos S, Quarrell O, Clarke AJ on behalf of the UK Huntington's disease predictive testing consortium. 2019. A case-note review of continued pregnancies found to be at a high risk of Huntington's disease: Considerations for clinical practice. *Eur J Human Genet* 27: 1215–1224.

Zola IK. 1993. Self, identity and the naming question: Reflections on the language of disability. *Soc Sci Med* 36: 167–173.

E: POLICY DOCUMENTS (A SELECTION)

American College of Medical Genetics and Genomics

American College of Medical Genetics and Genomics (ACMGG). 2013. Incidental findings in clinical genomics: A clarification. A policy statement of the American College of Medical Genetics and Genomics, Bethesda, MD. *Genet Med* 15(8): 664–666. (And see Kalia et al. 2017, in Section A: Molecular Genetics.)

(With the American Academy of Pediatrics). 2013. Ethical and policy issues in genetic testing and screening of children. *Pediatrics* 131: 620–622 (and see Ross 2013 later).

Edwards JG, Feldman G, Goldberg J, Gregg AR, Norton ME, Rose NC, Schneider A, Stoll K, Wapner R, Watson MS. 2015. Expanded carrier screening in reproductive medicine – Points to consider. A joint statement of the ACMG, ACOG, NSGC, Perinatal Quality Foundation and Society for Maternal-Fetal Medicine. *Obs Gynecol* 125(3): 653–662.

Green RC MD, Berg JS, Grody WW. 2013. ACMG recommendations for reporting of incidental findings in clinical exome and genome sequencing. *Genet Med* 15(7): 565–574.

Kalia SS, Adelman K, Bale SJ. 2017. ACMG Recommendations for reporting of secondary findings in clinical exome and genome sequencing, 2016 update. (As in Section A: Molecular Genetics.)

Richards S, Aziz N, Bale S on behalf of the ACMG Laboratory Quality Assurance Committee. 2015. Standards and guidelines for the interpretation of sequence variants: A joint consensus recommendation of the American College of Medical Genetics and Genomics and the Association for Molecular Pathology. *Genet Med* 17: 405–424.

Ross LF, Saal HM, David KL, Anderson RR; American Academy of Pediatrics; American College of Medical Genetics and Genomics. 2013. Technical Report: Ethical and policy issues in genetic testing and screening of children. *Genet Med* 15(3): 234–245.

American Society of Human Genetics

American Society of Human Genetics, Social Issues Subcommittee on Familial Disclosure. 1998. ASHG Statement. Professional disclosure of familial genetic information. *Am J Hum Genet* 62: 474–483.

Botkin JR, Belmont JW, Berg JS. 2015. American Society of Human Genetics Position Statement. Points to consider: Ethical, legal and psychosocial implications of genetic testing in children and adolescents. *Am J Hum Genet* 97: 6–21.

Bombard Y, Brothers KB, Fitzgerald-Butt S, Garrison NA, Jamal L, James CA, Jarvik GP, McCormick JB, Nelson TN, Ormond KE, ehm HL, Richer J, Souzeau E, Vassy JL, Wagner JK, Levy HP. 2019. The responsibility to recontact research participants after reinterpretation of genetic and genomic research results. *Am J Hum Genet* 104(4): 578–595.

British Society for Genetic Medicine

British Society for Human Genetics (BSHG). 2010. *Genetic testing of children*. Report of a working party of the British Society for Human Genetics.

European Huntington Disease Network

MacLeod R, Tibben A, Frontali M, Evers-Kiebooms G, Jones A, Martinez-Descales A, Roos RA; Editorial Committee and Working Group 'Genetic Testing Counselling' of the European Huntington Disease Network. 2013. Recommendations for the predictive genetic test in Huntington's disease. *Clin Genet* 83: 221–231.

European Society of Human Genetics

Borry P, Evers-Kiebooms G, Cornel MC, Clarke A, Dierickx K, Public and Professional Policy Committee (PPPC) of the European Society of Human Genetics (ESHG). 2009. Genetic testing in asymptomatic minors: Background considerations towards ESHG Recommendations. *Eur J Hum Genet* 17(6): 711–719. (And Recommendations on pages 720–721.)

Dondorp W, de Wert G, Bombard Y on behalf of the European Society of Human Genetics (ESHG) and the American Society of Human Genetics (ASHG). 2015. Non-invasive prenatal testing for aneuploidy and beyond: Challenges of responsible innovation in prenatal screening. *Eur J Hum Genet* 23: 1438–1450.

European Society of Human Genetics (ESHG). 2009. Genetic testing in asymptomatic minors: Recommendations of the European Society of Human Genetics. *Eur J Hum Genet* 17(6): 720–721.

van El CG, Cornel MC, Borry P; ESHG Public and Professional Policy Committee. 2013. Whole-genome sequencing in health care. Recommendations of the European Society of Human Genetics. *Eur J Hum Genet* 21(Suppl 1): S1–S5.

Hastings Center

Johnston J, Lantos JD, Goldenberg A, Chen F, Parens E, Koenig BA; members of the NSIGHT Ethics and Policy Advisory Board. 2018. *'Sequencing Newborns: A Call for Nuanced Use of Genomic Technologies,' The ethics of sequencing newborns: Recommendations and reflections, special report.* Hastings Center Report 48(4): S2+ (20 pages). doi:10.1002/hast.874

Human Genetics Commission (reports)

Inside information. 2002
Making babies. 2006
More genes direct. A report on developments in the availability, marketing and regulation of genetic tests supplied directly to the public. 2007.
A common framework of principles for direct to consumer genetic testing services. 2010.
Increasing options, informing choice: A report on preconception genetic testing and screening. 2011.

Joint Committee on Genomics in Medicine (formerly the Joint Committee on Medical Genetics)

Burton H, Cole T, Farndon P. 2012. *Genomics in medicine: Delivering genomics through clinical practice.* A Report of the Joint Committee on Medical Genetics. PHG Foundation.

Gardiner C, Wellesley D, Kilby MD, Kerr B. 2015. Recommendations for the use of chromosome microarray in pregnancy. *A Report of the Joint Committee on Medical Genetics.*

Lucassen A, Hall A for the Joint Committee on Medical Genetics. 2019. *Consent and confidentiality in genomic medicine: Guidance on use of genetic and genomic information in the clinic* (3rd ed.). Royal College of Physicians and Royal College of Pathologists.

National Academies of Sciences (United States)

Committee on Human Gene Editing: Scientific, Medical, and Ethical Considerations. A Report of the National Academies of Sciences, Engineering and Medicine. 2017. Human genome editing: Science, ethics, and governance. National Academies Press.

National Screening Committee (UK)

Criteria for appraising the viability, effectiveness and appropriateness of a screening programme. Updated 2016 (on website).

Nuffield Council on Bioethics (reports)

Genetic screening: Ethical aspects. 1993.
Mental disorders and genetics. 1998.
Stem cell therapy. 2000.
Patenting DNA. 2002.
Genetics and behaviour. 2002.
Pharmacogenetics. 2003.
Genetic screening (update). 2006.
Medical profiling and online medicine: The ethics of 'personalised healthcare' in a consumer age. 2010.
New techniques for the prevention of mitochondrial DNA disorders. 2012.
Noninvasive prenatal genetic testing: Ethical issues. 2017.
Genome editing and human reproduction. 2018.

Public Health Genomics Foundation

Burton H, Hall A, Kroese M, Raza S. 2018. *Genomics in mainstream clinical pathways.*

Cameron L, Burton H. 2016. A conversation with clinicians: Shaping the implementation of genomics in mainstream medicine.

Kroese M, Elles R, Zimmern R. 2007. The evaluation of clinical validity and clinical utility of genetic tests.

Raza S, Luheshi L, Hall A. 2014. Sharing clinical genomic data for better diagnostics.

UK Parliament

All Party Parliamentary Group on Rare, Genetic and Undiagnosed Conditions. 2016. *Undiagnosed. Genetic conditions and the impact of genome sequencing.*

Morris JK, Mutton DE, Alberman E. 2002. Revised estimates of the maternal age specific live birth prevalence of Down's syndrome. *J Med Screen* 9: 2–6.

World Health Organisation

Wilson, J. M., and Jungner, G. 1968. *Principles and Practice of Screening for Disease.* Public Health Papers 34. Geneva: World Health Organization.

Appendix 2: *Practical Genetic Counselling* – The life story of a book

As I look at the row of different editions and translations of *Practical Genetic Counselling* on the bookshelf in front of me, I am amazed that it has passed through seven editions, and even more so that it is still in active use and will now be renewed in this eighth edition. Of the various books that I have written over the years, this is the one that seems to have been most widely adopted by the medical genetics and genetic counselling community as part of its regular practice, so I feel it is worthwhile, at least for myself, to put down a few facts and memories about the book itself, its beginnings and its development during more than three decades. Whether this will interest anyone else, I do not know, but at any rate it may help to explain why the book is still around and apparently flourishing after so many years.

BACKGROUND AND BEGINNINGS

In late 1971, I returned from the United States (Baltimore, Maryland) to the United Kingdom to start a new medical genetics unit in Cardiff, Wales, whose remit included a genetic counselling service that within a few years had extended over the whole of Wales (population three million). Being single-handed, I found this a challenge, not only logistically but in finding information that I could communicate to the families referred to me, mainly by family doctors and by hospital-based clinicians such as paediatricians and neurologists. When I looked around for published data that might help, especially on recurrence risks for genetic disorders, I found little that would be of much use to me in the context of a specific consultation, though several books on genetic counselling already existed that were valuable for the general principles; these included Sheldon Reed's 1955 *Counseling in Medical Genetics*, as well as the later *Principles of Genetic Counseling* by Murphy and Chase (1975), *Genetic Counselling* by Stevenson et al. (1976), and *Genetic Counseling: A Guide for the Practicing Physician* by Fuhrmann and Vogel (1976).

As I have found repeatedly over the years, the only way to fill this gap was to write something myself, so with some trepidation I set out to write this book. Since by 1980 I had been doing genetic counselling for over 10 years, I also felt that my experience (and my mistakes) might be helpful to others. I was fortunate in having a number of colleagues around the United Kingdom who were generous in their time spent suggesting improvements or correcting mistakes after reading the whole manuscript; these included Ian Young, then a trainee with me, later a professor in Leicester; Alan Emery in Edinburgh, and Cedric Carter in London.

Cedric Carter later told me that he had planned to write a similar book himself after he retired; I felt guilty at first about this, but with hindsight it was good that I did not know his plans at the time, as I might have been dissuaded from writing anything myself. In the event, he sadly died shortly after he retired.

Who did I have in mind as potential readers? Clearly there were people like myself in medical genetics, but we were a small group in those days, certainly not enough to form a market for a book, even worldwide. And in any case, this was planned as a small book that could be carried around, not a large and detailed volume. The book's original preface makes it clear:

> [T]his book is written primarily for practising clinicians, whether in family practice or hospital specialties. It does not attempt to provide the extent or depth of knowledge needed for the medical geneticist running a genetic counselling clinic.

I am sure that the book's compactness has been a major factor in its success.

THE FIRST EDITION, 1980–1981

Any author will know the pleasure of holding the actual published book in one's hand after the many months of planning, preparation, writing and correcting. As I look at my shelf copy of the first edition now, almost 40 years after its birth, it shows signs of its advancing age: a bright orange-red cover (but very faded), scuffed and rather battered, while my separate 'working copy' is almost unreadable from all the changes made by hand for the next edition. I must have been optimistic about its future even then to be thinking ahead, and certainly the reviews were encouraging, while I received numerous corrections and suggestions from friends and colleagues which I tried my best to incorporate.

Looking inside the book, I see the date of publication given as 1981, but this cannot be strictly correct since my wife Elaine has a copy inscribed for her saying 'Christmas 1980' – a rather inadequate Christmas present in light of the neglect of her and the children resulting from writing the book. The children themselves feature in the dedication; only four of them at this point, number five appearing for the second edition.

The publisher can be seen to be John Wright & Sons Ltd, at 42–44 Triangle West, Bristol. This small, mainly medical, regional publisher has, alas, long ago succumbed to takeover by a succession of larger multinational conglomerates, like almost all of its fellow independent publishers. In 1980 publishing was a different world, leisurely and personal, rather old-fashioned and gentlemanly, with the concept of deadlines a purely notional one. I cannot remember why I chose Wright for *Practical Genetic Counselling*, but I should say that they and their successors have served it (and myself) well over the years, having put up with much pestering from me over how they could best publicise the book and tolerating numerous late changes (Table A2.1).

Nowadays, with all aspects of book production computerised, one gets little sense of a book as a physical object until it finally appears, but back in 1980 matters were very different, with successive 'galley proofs' and 'page proofs' forming important landmarks in the book's gestation. I soon found that one had to be eagle-eyed in looking for errors, even up to the last moment, and to check items such as the cover details that might be thought to be entirely the publisher's domain.

Unexpected hazards might arise, too, such as holidays, since the proofs had a deadline which really was of importance. *Practical Genetic Counselling* narrowly avoided one such disaster. The proofs for (I think) the first edition were scheduled to reach me while on holiday with the family in the remote Outer Hebrides, and the postman duly delivered them from the ferry as a battered

Table A2.1 *Practical Genetic Counselling* – Successive editions and publishers

Edition	Year	Publisher
1	1981	John Wright
2	1984	John Wright
3	1988	John Wright
4	1993	Butterworth-Heinemann
5	1998	Butterworth-Heinemann
6	2004	Hodder
7	2010	Hodder-Arnold

and somewhat wave-soaked package, which was fortunately still legible after drying out. The following day my 10-year-old son was insistent that the two of us should camp overnight on a small islet that one could cross to at low tide, and unwisely I took my proofs with me. We had not reckoned with the ferocity of the Scottish midge, however, and soon after the rising tide had made us irrevocably isolated, a cloud of midges descended to devour us. Smoke was the only solution, but firewood on the beach was scanty and damp, while the only paper we had was my son's diary – and my set of proofs. We used successive blank pages of the diary in vain and I began to think that *Practical Genetic Counselling* would soon be consigned to the flames, when the final blank page successfully kindled the fire, banished the midges, and saved the proofs for return to the publishers next day.

THE BOOK ITSELF: STRUCTURE AND EVOLUTION

When I look at the structure of *Practical Genetic Counselling* as it is in the last edition (the seventh) written by myself, the list of contents seems similar to what it was in the original edition. First comes a general section giving outlines of inheritance patterns and how to recognise them, especially Mendelian inheritance and the risks deriving from it; then common non-Mendelian conditions; chromosomes and their disorders; prenatal diagnosis and carrier detection; and finally suggestions on organising a genetic counselling clinic. The topic of syndromes and dysmorphology is in this seventh edition rightly given a full chapter, rather than just a section of one. But the biggest change was the appearance of a chapter on molecular genetics, first seen in the second edition (1984) and greatly expanded and modified thereafter. Actually, 1984 is an early date for this innovation and reflects the involvement of the Cardiff unit in this field from the beginning, the biggest change in the practice of medical genetics in its history until now.

This development also allowed me to shorten other sections, an important aim for me since I have always felt that brevity is one of the main attractions of the book. The increasingly long tables of disorders where prenatal diagnosis and carrier detection might be possible could now largely be eliminated since with molecular techniques these applications were now potentially feasible for all Mendelian disorders. The original edition did have a specific chapter on prenatal diagnosis, but this was mostly limited to amniocentesis for chromosome disorders and neural tube defects. Chorionic villus sampling was still in the future and pre-implantation diagnosis unknown, as was molecular prenatal diagnosis, though the just-discovered application to sickle cell disease gets a brief mention.

The final chapter in this section of the first edition, 'The Genetic Counselling Clinic', now seems very old-fashioned in the way it is written, reflecting my own background as a practising clinician and providing a traditional 'medical model' for the framework of a genetic counselling clinic. Yet in some ways it is starting to look modern again, with its clear statement that:

> The author believes strongly that genetic counselling should preferably be undertaken by people who are medically trained, largely for the reason that it is quite impossible to separate the actual counselling from the associated aspects of clinical diagnosis.

With the 'mainstreaming' of genetics in medicine overall now in vogue, I have begun to realise that I have been around long enough to be in fashion again, since I have never stopped being 'mainstream' myself. However, I have never felt as my mentor Cyril Clarke once did, that a greater involvement of practicing clinicians would avoid the need for specialists in medical genetics.

In 1980 specialist non-medical genetic counsellors hardly existed, at least in Europe, though a number of 'associates' with nursing or social work backgrounds were already playing valuable roles. The past 30 years have seen the evolution and dramatic expansion in both numbers and the scope for such genetic counsellors, and I am proud to have been associated both with their training and day-to-day genetic counselling work. This change has, at least in the United Kingdom, been largely a harmonious and productive one, and genetic counsellors seem to have become one of the main groups worldwide who use *Practical Genetic Counselling*, despite the fact that it is rarely recommended, or even mentioned, in the formal genetic counselling literature. I suspect that this extensive use is because it deals with the day-to-day problems which one meets in genetic counselling, regardless of whether one is medical or non-medical. At any rate I am grateful for this appreciation from genetic counsellors, whatever the reasons, and one of the greatest pleasures of going to meetings around the world is meeting some of these workers face to face and hearing how they have enjoyed the book.

Turning to the central section of the book, dealing with individual organ systems and disorders, the general structure likewise changed little over the years through successive editions, but this conceals some radical advances, such as the emergence of Mendelian subsets of the common cancers, which has had major consequences for genetic counselling. Not only have risk estimates been greatly affected, but cancer genetics has now evolved into a clear sub-specialty, redefining the relationship between medical genetics and oncology, as well as providing particular scope for specialist non-medical genetic counsellors. A somewhat similar development is progressively happening in other areas such as heart disorders, while previously undifferentiated fields such as mental handicap are becoming resolved into individual, often Mendelian entities with a defined molecular basis, where specific genetic counselling is now possible, rather than an approximate empiric risk. In fact, every chapter in this part of the book changed remarkably between the first and the seventh editions in terms of genetic applications to diagnosis, carrier detection, prenatal diagnosis and prediction.

The final section of the book, 'Genetics and Society', in some ways changed the most, and became greatly expanded from the original short chapter. This shows how those practising in the field of medical genetics have led the way in identifying the ethical and social issues arising in genetic counselling, particularly when applied to whole populations in screening programmes, but also for specific families with the widespread use of predictive genetic testing. In the first edition such prediction and screening were almost non-existent, but now are feasible in many situations, and increasingly used by other specialties, giving emphasis to the original aim of the book to be useful for clinicians outside the field of medical genetics. The seventh edition also contained a section on eugenics, reminding the reader how uncomfortably close to this some aspects of medical genetics have been in the past, and could be again in the future unless we are vigilant.

Are there parts of the original book that I regret writing? Actually, very few, though there were plenty of mostly minor errors that I tried to correct along the way. The broad philosophy of the book has been, I feel, sound, and I do not think it would still be in use today if this were otherwise. But certainly, the field has changed over the years, not just in terms of specific advances but also in attitudes. By being in active practice over this time and by close contacts with my younger colleagues, I think the successive editions have marked how the field of genetic counselling overall, not just my own views, has changed over the past decades.

An example of this can be seen in my somewhat casual approach to confidentiality in the early editions, where several figures show pedigrees that are readily identifiable. I hope that I have learned from these and other mistakes, and indeed I have always been convinced that others learn much more from a description of one's problems and failures than of one's successes.

'PRACTICAL GENETIC COUNSELLING' AROUND THE WORLD

When I first wrote the book, I gave little thought to where its readership might be living and working. Having worked myself in both Britain and the United States, I think I was aiming primarily at the English-speaking countries, and certainly they proved receptive, with interest in Canada and Australia also. Initially the book was little publicised in the United States, until Oxford University Press became its distributor there, which immediately increased its U.S. sales to much more than in the rest of the world put together.

Much less expected was the interest in translating the book, resulting in a series of translations in distant countries, as well as into several European languages. More than anything else resulting from the book, this has given me great pleasure, as well as forming the basis for lasting links and friendships. Interestingly there were two early German translations, both in 1988, one for West Germany and one for the East, at the time isolated and only just recovering from the disastrous imposition on genetics of Lysenko's doctrines. Recently historians documenting post-war East Germany's genetics have noted that the publication of the East German translation was a factor that helped in the reintegration and rebuilding of human genetics in the country.

Translation into Russian was certainly not something that I had expected, but a remarkably large edition was produced (the figure 300,000 sticks in my mind). Unfortunately Russia at that time did not recognise copyright, so any hopes for financial benefit were short lived. Who actually read this large number of copies remains a mystery for me, but that some were indeed read became clear when in 2005 I attended the All-Russia Medical Genetics Congress in Ufa, near the Ural Mountains, and was approached by a fellow medical geneticist working in the Russian Far East holding a copy of the Russian translation of the first edition. It had taken him 3 days by train to reach Ufa, and he assured me that he used the book every day in his clinic. When I expressed concern over it now being 25 years out of date, he replied with a phrase citing 'imperishable truths', but both he and I felt happy that I was able to give him the copy of the current (English) edition that I had with me.

At this same Ufa meeting I learned for the first time that the Russian translation had been recommended by Nikolai Bochkov, the first director of the restored Moscow Medical Genetics Institute. After 30 years of genetics being totally banned in Russia, it was good to be part of its renewal.

The Chinese translation (also of the first edition) was also unexpected, but especially welcome as the country had recently announced its controversial and counterproductive 'eugenics law'. Given that it comprises a third of the world's population, it was good to feel that one was making at least some small contribution to help establish a form of genetic counselling that was humanistic rather than authoritarian. Now that China is making huge technological advances, notably in genome sequencing, it has become all the more important that genetic counselling is developed too, so I am pleased to learn that a new translation has recently been made.

In all these countries genetic counselling, where it existed at all, initially seemed likely to follow an authoritarian pattern, not surprisingly, since this was the approach to all aspects of people's lives. I remember in particular one visiting East European medical geneticist who described how she always insisted on seeing members of a couple separately and who, when the genetic risk was high, separately advised each member not to marry the other. I am assured that non-directive genetic counselling is now the norm in all these countries, though whether this applies to the great majority receiving their information from non-geneticist clinicians I very much doubt.

LOOKING TO THE FUTURE

If there is any single reason for the long-lasting popularity of *Practical Genetic Counselling*, I think it is because it has been written by someone actively and personally involved in what they are writing about. I can no longer claim this, so there will be no more editions written by me. Having decided this, my initial inclination was to let the book die peacefully and wait to see what emerged to replace it. But others seemed to feel that there was still life in it, so I was especially happy when my friend and colleague Angus Clarke offered to take on the preparation of a new version. I insisted that he should have a totally free hand in this and should regard it as a new book, keeping only those parts, if any, that seemed truly relevant after such a long time. This year (2019) should see the book appear, and I shall read it with interest then; I have deliberately tried not to follow its progress, but know for certain that it will be valuable, and equally that it will be different from and better than anything which I could have attempted to write now.

This, then, is for me a personal farewell to *Practical Genetic Counselling*, which has been a part of my own life for most of the time since I first entered medical genetics, and which now seems set fair to continue in an independent life without me. It has brought me great pleasure and satisfaction, and likewise seems to have done so for a large number of readers across the world, so I wish the book and those who use it, past, present and future, well.

Peter Harper

Index

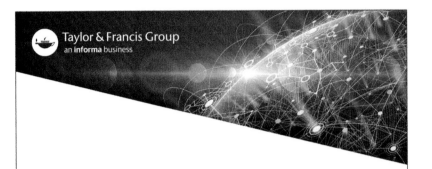